Dietary Behavior and Physical Activity in Children and Adolescents

Dietary Behavior and Physical Activity in Children and Adolescents

Special Issue Editors

Antje Hebestreit
Leonie-Helen Bogl

MDPI • Basel • Beijing • Wuhan • Barcelona • Belgrade

MDPI

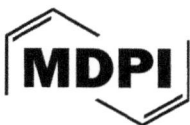

Special Issue Editors

Antje Hebestreit
Leibniz Institute for Prevention
Research and Epidemiology
Germany

Leonie-Helen Bogl
Medical University of Vienna
Austria

Editorial Office
MDPI
St. Alban-Anlage 66
4052 Basel, Switzerland

This is a reprint of articles from the Special Issue published online in the open access journal *Nutrients* (ISSN 2072-6643) from 2018 to 2019 (available at: https://www.mdpi.com/journal/nutrients/special_issues/Dietary_Behavior_Physical_Activity)

For citation purposes, cite each article independently as indicated on the article page online and as indicated below:

LastName, A.A.; LastName, B.B.; LastName, C.C. Article Title. *Journal Name* **Year**, *Article Number*, Page Range.

ISBN 978-3-03921-600-0 (Pbk)
ISBN 978-3-03921-601-7 (PDF)

Cover image courtesy of Adobe Stock Photos user missmimimina.

Contents

About the Special Issue Editors

Antje Hebestreit is head of the Unit Lifestyle-Related Disorders at the Leibniz Institute for Prevention Research and Epidemiology—BIPS, in Bremen, Germany. After her diploma in Nutritional Sciences and Home Economics in 1999, and further training in epidemiology, she conducted the main part of the research for her Ph.D. in the Kilimanjaro Region (2000–2001), Tanzania. After her Ph.D. in 2004, she worked as a Postdoctoral Research Fellow for the Harvard University in Tanzania and as a consultant for the UN World Food Programme.

Over the years, her work has focused on studying the role of dietary intake, dietary behavior, physical activity, and sedentary behaviors, together with their determinants, and their association with non-communicable diseases, as well as primary prevention strategies for childhood obesity.

Leonie-Helen Bogl is currently a Senior Postdoc at the Department of Epidemiology at the Medical University of Vienna, Austria, while maintaining a Visiting Researcher status at the Twin Study group at FIMM in Helsinki (Finland). She completed her doctoral dissertation at the Faculty of Medicine in 2014 on the associations of dietary factors, obesity, and serum lipoprotein profile among young adult twins. She has worked extensively with family and twin data in order to better tease apart the influences of genes and the environment in explaining individual differences in traits, such as obesity and dietary intake.

nutrients

MDPI

Editorial

Dietary Behavior and Physical Activity in Children and Adolescents

Antje Hebestreit [1] and Leonie H. Bogl [2,*]

[1] Leibniz Institute for Prevention Research and Epidemiology—BIPS, D-28359 Bremen, Germany
[2] Department of Epidemiology, Center for Public Health, Medical University of Vienna, Kinderspitalgasse 15, 1. Floor, A-1090 Vienna, Austria
* Correspondence: leonie-helen.bogl@meduniwien.ac.at; Tel.: +43-(0)1-40160-34703

Received: 2 August 2019; Accepted: 7 August 2019; Published: 9 August 2019

Keywords: dietary behavior; physical activity; young populations; surveillance; epidemiology; public health

---

In recent years, diet- and lifestyle-related disorders have become a major health threat in Europe and worldwide. Globally, optimal infant and child feeding practices include exclusive breastfeeding for the first six months of life, age-appropriate and safe complementary feeding, and the prevention of micronutrient deficiencies; they also target a balanced diet during childhood and adolescence to prevent childhood obesity and associated cardiovascular and metabolic sequelae [1]. The promotion of as well as a general increase in physical activity across all ages is one target across numerous settings and communities [2]. Contributions in this monograph include two review articles [3,4] and 19 original contributions from several countries, providing new information to existing research and elucidating important aspects of children's and adolescents' nutrition and lifestyle behavior.

Data included in this Special Issue are from large epidemiological studies including several multi-center [5,6] and multinational studies [3,7] as well as datasets from surveillance initiatives, such as the German Health Interview and Examination Survey for Children and Adolescents (KiGGS) [8,9], the U.S. National Health and Nutrition Examination Survey (NHANES) [10], and the WHO European Childhood Obesity Surveillance Initiative (WHO COSI) [11]. Three of the studies in this Special Issue reported on the co-occurrence of multiple health behaviors in the same children [6,8,11], in particular the clustering of low levels of physical activity levels and/or high screen times with a higher consumption of energy-dense foods [6,8]. These findings encourage future community-based intervention studies to target multiple lifestyle behaviors simultaneously to reduce the burden of lifestyle-related diseases.

The role of parenting and early feeding practices was investigated in four studies within this Special Issue [5,12–14]. Of particular interest, Walton K. et al. videotaped families during dinner and reported associations between food parenting practices and preschooler's risk of poor nutrition. Physical restriction of food from a child was associated with higher nutrition risk whereas positive comments about a child's food was associated with a lower nutrition risk in children [12]. These results suggest that the use of positive encouragement by supporting parents, rather than restriction, may improve preschoolers' nutrition; they further highlight the previously described role of parents as gatekeepers [15].

Ensuring validity of dietary intake data is a prerequisite for any investigation into diet–disease associations. Three U.S. studies [10,16,17] and one Finnish study [18] focused on the validity of self-reported dietary intake data and derived dietary patterns. Validity refers to the extent to which a measurement actually measures what it is intended to measure. There are several types of validity, including criterion-related validity, construct validity, content validity, and face validity [19]. Hibbs-Shipp S.K. et al. [16] derived a diet quality score for the home food environment and carefully evaluated all four validity measures. Face validity was evaluated by expert reviews of representative foods and food amounts, considering whether representative foods can be realistically found in the target population's home. Content validity was assessed by iterative runs and via the removal of each food individually from the score database to determine whether the representative food was loading into the component scores as theorized Criterion validity was assessed by testing the contributions of each food to component and total scores. Finally, construct validity was evaluated by testing five hypothetical home food environments that resulted in a range of scores in the expected directions. Using a validated FFQ, Wolters M. et al. confirmed a positive association between frequent fast food consumption and adverse changes in body composition indicators in two German pediatric cohorts [20].

Two European studies evaluated the prevalence and determinants of dietary supplement use in children and adolescents, an important research question given that dietary supplement use has been implicated in preventable adverse drug events and emergency department visits in children and adolescents [21,22]. Data from the KiGGS Module EsKiMo II study showed that around 16% of adolescents in Germany use dietary supplements [9], and data from Eastern Poland reported that around 30% of children and adolescents use vitamin or mineral supplements [23]. Notably, the time frame for which supplement intake was queried was different in these two studies; in Germany the time frame was the previous four weeks and in Poland the past 12 months. In comparison, 33% of children and adolescents in the United States use dietary supplements [21]. In the two European studies, supplement users were more often female, living in urban areas, from more highly educated families, more likely to be physically active, and less likely to be overweight or obese [9,23].

Growing up in lower socio-economic environments or vulnerable groups such as ethnic minorities may increase susceptibility to unhealthy dietary patterns [24]. The study in this Special Issue from New Caledonia reported that the proportion of adolescents regularly consuming sugar-sweetened beverages was high (90%) and was related to living in rural areas and belonging to a particular ethnic community [25]. Results from the WHO Health Behavior in School-Aged Children survey in Belgium are in line with previous findings which showed that eating culture plays a role in inequalities of eating habits among immigrants when socioeconomic conditions are considered [26]. Mustafa N. et al. [27] further highlighted that the type of foods consumed at breakfast are highly dependent on culture. Malaysian adolescents consume breakfast that is of low nutrient quality, such as cereal-based and often primarily rice dishes, chocolate and confectionary, hot and powered drinks, and noodles. The Malaysian study suggests that breakfast consumption is related to lower cardiovascular risk because of the earlier timing of food intake rather than the types of foods consumed at breakfast. This interesting hypothesis remains to be established in randomized trials.

The diverse articles in this Special Issue highlight the complexity and extent to which nutrition and physical activity behaviors may influence different health aspects of children and adolescents. Few studies in this Special Issue combined genetic data with nutritional data [28], a likely expanding research area in the coming years, with the goal to provide personalized and gene-based dietary recommendations in the future. As seen by the various findings and recommendations, not only is more work in this area required but the translation of this work to practice and policy is imperative if we are to address the challenges impacting the nutrition, physical activity, and health of young populations.

Conflicts of Interest: The authors declare no conflict of interest.

References

1. United Nations Children's Fund (UNICEF). *Improving Child Nutrition: The Achievable Imperative for Global Progress*; UNICEF, Ed.; United Nations Publications: New York, NY, USA, 2013.
2. World Health Organization. *WHO Global Action Plan for the Prevention and Control of Noncommunicable Diseases 2013-2020*; WHO: Geneva, Switzerland, 2013.
3. Katzmarzyk, P.T.; Chaput, J.P.; Fogelholm, M.; Hu, G.; Maher, C.; Maia, J.; Olds, T.; Sarmiento, O.L.; Standage, M.; Tremblay, M.S.; et al. International Study of Childhood Obesity, Lifestyle and the Environment (ISCOLE): Contributions to Understanding the Global Obesity Epidemic. *Nutrients* **2019**, *11*, 848. [CrossRef]

4. Srbely, V.; Janjua, I.; Buchholz, A.C.; Newton, G. Interventions Aimed at Increasing Dairy and/or Calcium Consumption of Preschool-Aged Children: A Systematic Literature Review. *Nutrients* **2019**, *11*, 714. [CrossRef] [PubMed]
5. Sina, E.; Buck, C.; Jilani, H.; Tornaritis, M.; Veidebaum, T.; Russo, P.; Moreno, L.A.; Molnar, D.; Eiben, G.; Marild, S.; et al. Association of Infant Feeding Patterns with Taste Preferences in European Children and Adolescents: A Retrospective Latent Profile Analysis. *Nutrients* **2019**, *11*, 1040. [CrossRef] [PubMed]
6. Miguel-Berges, M.L.; Santaliestra-Pasias, A.M.; Mouratidou, T.; De Miguel-Etayo, P.; Androutsos, O.; De Craemer, M.; Galcheva, S.; Koletzko, B.; Kulaga, Z.; Manios, Y.; et al. Combined Longitudinal Effect of Physical Activity and Screen Time on Food and Beverage Consumption in European Preschool Children: The ToyBox-Study. *Nutrients* **2019**, *11*, 1048. [CrossRef] [PubMed]
7. Jalo, E.; Konttinen, H.; Vepsalainen, H.; Chaput, J.P.; Hu, G.; Maher, C.; Maia, J.; Sarmiento, O.L.; Standage, M.; Tudor-Locke, C.; et al. Emotional Eating, Health Behaviours, and Obesity in Children: A 12-Country Cross-Sectional Study. *Nutrients* **2019**, *11*, 351. [CrossRef]
8. Manz, K.; Mensink, G.B.M.; Finger, J.D.; Haftenberger, M.; Brettschneider, A.K.; Lage Barbosa, C.; Krug, S.; Schienkiewitz, A. Associations between Physical Activity and Food Intake among Children and Adolescents: Results of KiGGS Wave 2. *Nutrients* **2019**, *11*, 1060. [CrossRef]
9. Perlitz, H.; Mensink, G.B.M.; Barbosa, C.L.; Richter, A.; Brettschneider, A.K.; Lehmann, F.; Patelakis, E.; Frank, M.; Heide, K.; Haftenberger, M. Use of vitamin and mineral supplements among 2 adolescents living in Germany—Results from 3 EsKiMo II. *Nutrients* **2019**, *11*, 1208. [CrossRef]
10. Khan, S.; Wirth, M.D.; Ortaglia, A.; Alvarado, C.R.; Shivappa, N.; Hurley, T.G.; Hebert, J.R. Design, Development and Construct Validation of the Children's Dietary Inflammatory Index. *Nutrients* **2018**, *10*, 993. [CrossRef] [PubMed]
11. Bel-Serrat, S.; Ojeda-Rodriguez, A.; Heinen, M.M.; Buoncristiano, M.; Abdrakhmanova, S.; Duleva, V.; Sant'Angelo, V.F.; Fijalkowska, A.; Hejgaard, T.; Huidumac, C.; et al. Clustering of Multiple Energy Balance-Related Behaviors in School Children and its Association with Overweight and Obesity—WHO European Childhood Obesity Surveillance Initiative (COSI 2015(–)2017). *Nutrients* **2019**, *11*, 511. [CrossRef]
12. Walton, K.; Haycraft, E.; Jewell, K.; Breen, A.; Randall Simpson, J.; Haines, J. The family mealtime observation study (FaMOS): Exploring the Role of Family Functioning in the Association between Mothers' and fathers' Food Parenting Practices and Children's Nutrition Risk. *Nutrients* **2019**, *11*, 630. [CrossRef]
13. Groele, B.; Głąbska, D.; Gutkowska, K.; Guzek, D. Mothers' vegetable consumption behaviors and preferences as a factor limiting the possibility of increasing vegetable consumption in children in a national sample of Polish and Romanian respondents. *Nutrients* **2019**, *11*, 1078. [CrossRef] [PubMed]
14. Lovell, A.L.; Milne, T.; Jiang, Y.; Chen, R.X.; Grant, C.C.; Wall, C.R. Evaluation of the Effect of a Growing up Milk Lite vs. Cow's Milk on Diet Quality and Dietary Intakes in Early Childhood: The Growing up Milk Lite (GUMLI) Randomised Controlled Trial. *Nutrients* **2019**, *11*, 203. [CrossRef] [PubMed]
15. Hebestreit, A.; Intemann, T.; Siani, A.; De Henauw, S.; Eiben, G.; Kourides, Y.A.; Kovacs, E.; Moreno, L.A.; Veidebaum, T.; Krogh, V.; et al. Dietary Patterns of European Children and Their Parents in Association with Family Food Environment: Results from the I. Family Study. *Nutrients* **2017**, *9*, 126. [CrossRef] [PubMed]
16. Hibbs-Shipp, S.K.; Boles, R.E.; Johnson, S.L.; McCloskey, M.L.; Hobbs, S.; Bellows, L.L. Development of a Quality Score for the Home Food Environment Using the Home—IDEA2 and the Healthy Eating Index—2010. *Nutrients* **2019**, *11*, 372. [CrossRef] [PubMed]
17. Vosburgh, K.; Smith, S.R.; Oldman, S.; Huedo-Medina, T.; Duffy, V.B. Pediatric-Adapted Liking Survey (PALS): A Brief and 2 Valid Lifestyle Behavior Screener in Pediatric Care. *Nutrients* **2019**, *11*, 1641.
18. Korkalo, L.; Vepsalainen, H.; Ray, C.; Skaffari, E.; Lehto, R.; Hauta-Alus, H.H.; Nissinen, K.; Meinila, J.; Roos, E.; Erkkola, M. Parents' Reports of Preschoolers' Diets: Relative Validity of a Food Frequency Questionnaire and Dietary Patterns. *Nutrients* **2019**, *11*, 159. [CrossRef]
19. Kirkpatrick, S.; Raffoul, A. Measures Registry User Guide: Individual Diet. Washington (DC): National Collaborative on Childhood Obesity Research. Available online: http://www.nccor.org/downloads/NCCOR_MR_User_Guide-Individual_Diet-v6.pdf (accessed on 3 August 2019).
20. Wolters, M.; Joslowski, G.; Plachta-Danielzik, S.; Standl, M.; Muller, M.J.; Ahrens, W.; Buyken, A.E. Dietary Patterns in Primary School are of Prospective Relevance for the Development of Body Composition in Two German Pediatric Populations. *Nutrients* **2018**, *10*, 1442. [CrossRef]

21. Qato, D.M.; Alexander, G.C.; Guadamuz, J.S.; Lindau, S.T. Prevalence of Dietary Supplement Use in US Children and Adolescents, 2003-2014. *JAMA Pediatr.* **2018**, *172*, 780–782. [CrossRef] [PubMed]

22. Geller, A.I.; Shehab, N.; Weidle, N.J.; Lovegrove, M.C.; Wolpert, B.J.; Timbo, B.B.; Mozersky, R.P.; Budnitz, D.S. Emergency Department Visits for Adverse events Related to Dietary Supplements. *N. Engl. J. Med.* **2015**, *373*, 1531–1540. [CrossRef] [PubMed]

23. Sicinska, E.; Pietruszka, B.; Januszko, O.; Kaluza, J. Different Socio-Demographic and Lifestyle Factors Can Determine the Dietary Supplement Use in Children and Adolescents in Central-Eastern Poland. *Nutrients* **2019**, *11*, 658. [CrossRef] [PubMed]

24. Fernandez-Alvira, J.M.; Bornhorst, C.; Bammann, K.; Gwozdz, W.; Krogh, V.; Hebestreit, A.; Barba, G.; Reisch, L.; Eiben, G.; Iglesia, I.; et al. Prospective associations between socio-economic status and dietary patterns in European children: The Identification and Prevention of Dietary and Lifestyle—induced Health Effects in Children and Infants (IDEFICS) Study. *Br. J. Nutr.* **2015**, *113*, 517–525. [CrossRef] [PubMed]

25. Wattelez, G.; Frayon, S.; Cavaloc, Y.; Cherrier, S.; Lerrant, Y.; Galy, O. Sugar-Sweetened Beverage Consumption and Associated Factors in School-Going Adolescents of New Caledonia. *Nutrients* **2019**, *11*, 452. [CrossRef] [PubMed]

26. Rouche, M.; de Clercq, B.; Lebacq, T.; Dierckens, M.; Moreau, N.; Desbouys, L.; Godin, I.; Castetbon, K. Socioeconomic Disparities in Diet Vary According to Migration Status among Adolescents in Belgium. *Nutrients* **2019**, *11*, 812. [CrossRef] [PubMed]

27. Mustafa, N.; Abd Majid, H.; Toumpakari, Z.; Carroll, H.A.; Yazid Jalaludin, M.; Al Sadat, N.; Johnson, L. The Association of Breakfast Frequency and Cardiovascular Disease (CVD) Risk Factors among Adolescents in Malaysia. *Nutrients* **2019**, *11*, 973. [CrossRef]

28. Morell-Azanza, L.; Ojeda-Rodriguez, A.; Giuranna, J.; Azcona-SanJulian, M.C.; Hebebrand, J.; Marti, A.; Hinney, A. Melanocortin-4 Receptor and Lipocalin 2 Gene Variants in Spanish Children with Abdominal Obesity: Effects on BMI-SDS After a Lifestyle Intervention. *Nutrients* **2019**, *11*, 960. [CrossRef]

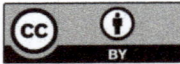

nutrients

MDPI

Article

Association of Infant Feeding Patterns with Taste Preferences in European Children and Adolescents: A Retrospective Latent Profile Analysis

Elida Sina [1,†], Christoph Buck [1,†], Hannah Jilani [1,2], Michael Tornaritis [3], Toomas Veidebaum [4], Paola Russo [5], Luis A. Moreno [6], Denes Molnar [7], Gabriele Eiben [8], Staffan Marild [9], Valeria Pala [10], Wolfgang Ahrens [1,11] and Antje Hebestreit [1,*] (on behalf of the I.Family Consortium)

[1] Leibniz Institute for Prevention Research and Epidemiology—BIPS, Achterstr. 30, 28359 Bremen, Germany; sina@leibniz-bips.de (E.S.); buck@leibniz-bips.de (C.B.); jilani@leibniz-bips.de (H.J.); ahrens@leibniz-bips.de (W.A.)
[2] Institute for Public Health and Nursing Research—IPP, University of Bremen, 28359 Bremen, Germany
[3] Research and Education Institute of Child Health, 2035 Lefcosia, Cyprus; tor.michael@cytanet.com.cy
[4] Department of Chronic Diseases, National Institute for Health Development, 11619 Tallin, Estonia; toomas.veidebaum@tai.ee
[5] Institute of Food Sciences, National Research Council, 83100 Avellino, Italy; prusso@isa.cnr.it
[6] GENUD (Growth, Exercise, Nutrition and Development) Research Group, Instituto Agroalimentario de Aragón (IA2), Instituto de Investigación Sanitaria Aragón (IIS Aragón), Centro de Investigación Biomédica en Red Fisiopatología de la Obesidad y Nutrición (CIBERObn), University of Zaragoza, 50009 Zaragoza, Spain; lmoreno@unizar.es
[7] Department of Pediatrics, Medical School, University of Pécs, 7623 Pécs, Hungary; denes.molnar@aok.pte.hu
[8] Department of Biomedicine and Public Health, School of Health and Education, University of Skövde, 54128 Skövde, Sweden; gabriele.eiben@his.se
[9] Department. of Pediatrics, Institute of Clinical Sciences, Sahlgrenska Academy at University of Gothenburg, 40530 Gothenburg, Sweden; staffan.marild@pediat.gu.se
[10] Department of Preventive and Predictive Medicine, Fondazione IRCCS, Istituto Nazionale dei Tumori, 20133 Milan, Italy; Valeria.Pala@istitutotumori.mi.it
[11] Faculty of Mathematics/Computer Science, University of Bremen, 28359 Bremen, Germany
[*] Correspondence: hebestr@leibniz-bips.de; Tel.: +49-421-218.56849; Fax: +49-421-218.56821
[†] Shared first authorship.

Received: 14 April 2019; Accepted: 6 May 2019; Published: 9 May 2019

Abstract: The aim was to investigate associations between the duration of infant feeding practices (FP) and taste preferences (TP) in European children and adolescents. A total of 5526 children (6–16 years old) of the I.Family study completed a Food and Beverage Preference Questionnaire to measure their preferences for sweet, fatty and bitter tastes. Mothers retrospectively reported the FPs duration in months: exclusive breastfeeding (EBF), exclusive formula milk feeding (EFMF), combined breastfeeding (BF&FMF) and the age at the introduction of complementary foods (CF). Using logistic regression analyses and latent class analysis (latent profiles of FP and CF were identified), we explored associations between profiles and TP, adjusting for various covariates, including the Healthy Diet Adherence Score (HDAS). A total of 48% of children had short durations of EBF (≤4 months) and BF&FMF (≤6 months) and were introduced to CF early (<6 months). No significant relationship was observed between the single FPs and TP, even when considering common profiles of FP. HDAS was inversely associated with sweet and fatty TP, but positively with bitter TP. Contrary to our hypotheses, we did not observe associations between FP and children's TP later in life. Further studies with higher FP variation and longitudinal design are needed to investigate the causal associations between infant FP and taste preferences later in life.

Keywords: breastfeeding; formula milk; taste preference; healthy diet adherence; children; IDEFICS study; I.Family

1. Introduction

Taste preference (TP) is one of the factors that affect the children's food intake and eating habits [1]. Humans can perceive 6 main basic tastes: (1) Sweet taste is caused by sugar and its derivatives such as fructose or lactose, but other substances such as amino acids and alcohol in fruit juices or alcoholic drinks can also activate the sensory cells that respond to sweetness; (2) Sour taste is mostly perceived via acidic solutions such as lemon juice or organic acids and is caused by hydrogen ions; (3) Salty taste is mainly perceived through foods containing table salt. Its chemical basis is the salt crystal, which consists of sodium and chloride. The sensation of saltiness can be caused by other mineral salts such as potassium or magnesium salts [2]; (4) Bitter taste is brought by a variety of components such as 6-*n*-propylthiouracil (PROP), sinigrin and goitrin, found in cruciferous vegetables (e.g., broccoli). There are 25 bitter taste receptors in humans but the most studied is *TAS2R38*. Genetic variations in this receptor cause different responses in taste sensitivity to bitter compounds from one human to another [3]; (5) Umami taste is caused by glutamic acid or aspartic acid and is similar to the taste of meat broth. It is also found in some plants, such as ripe tomatoes or asparagus [4]; (6) Fatty taste, called Oleogustus, has been described as the sixth basic taste. The stimuli devoted to the detection of dietary fat taste are the Non-Esterified Fatty Acids (NEFA). In particular, medium and long-chain fatty acids have a distinct taste sensation compared to other basic tastes (sweet, bitter, sour and salty) [5,6].

Evidence for the influencing role of genetic and environmental factors on the development of TP is well established [7]. Infants prefer the sweet taste and reject the sour and bitter tastes [7], while the preference for salt appears at about 4 months postnatally [8,9]. TP are learned during contact with food and the eating environment. An infant's experience with flavors begins in the mother's womb and during lactation, when flavors from the mother's diet are transmitted to her amniotic fluid, and later to her colostrum and milk. The infant-feeding method parents choose, whether it is breast or formula milk, will later influence their child-feeding practices [10,11] and the development of their children's food preferences and food acceptance patterns [12].

The fundamental role of breastfeeding on different physiological functions and on the infant's early immunity has been recognized through international nutritional policies, such as the World Health Organization guidelines on early life feeding, which recommends the exclusive breastfeeding of infants up to the age of 6 months and at least for the first 4 months of life [13]. Exclusive breastfeeding is crucial for the growth and development of infants [14], has a long term impact in shaping children's eating behaviors, and predicts the Body Mass Index (BMI) during childhood [15] and later in adult life [16]. Previous studies have pointed out the positive influence of breastfeeding duration on food variety and higher intake of fruits and vegetables in preschoolers [17,18], including in 4 European cohorts [19] and in school-aged children [20,21]. Vital compounds in the human milk provide a specific taste, such as lactose for the sweet taste, glutamate for the umami or savory taste, sodium for the salty taste, urea for the bitter taste and long-chain fatty acids for the fatty taste [22,23].

The introduction of formula milk and other complementary foods represents a crucial period for establishing infants' taste preferences and attitudes towards food, as well as for obesity prevention [24]. Children who were fed exclusively with formula milk do not benefit from the rich flavor profile of their mother's milk: their flavor experience is poorer as they don't experience the flavors from the variety of foods in the mother's diet. Various types and brands of formula milk products offer a diversity of flavors: milk-based formulas are described as having low levels of sweetness and 'sour and cereal-type'; soy-based formulas are described as tasting sweeter, more sour and bitter, and having a 'hay/beany' odor, whereas the hydrolysate formulas are extremely unpalatable to adults due to their sourness and bitterness [25]. Formula-fed infants learn to prefer the flavors associated with the formula milk they were fed and this has been found to influence taste preferences later in life [3,25]. Infant formulas might differ in protein, fat and carbohydrate composition and/or structure, and these differences may, in turn, affect growth, health outcomes and taste preferences [26].

Scott et al. demonstrated that breastfeeding duration is directly associated with the food variety at two years of age [18], independent of factors that are known to influence diet quality in children, such as maternal age and education [27,28]. Another study found that having been breastfed was positively associated with a healthier dietary pattern amongst older Australian children [20]. Burnier et al. [29] investigated longitudinal data from the Quebec Longitudinal Study of Child Development and observed that 3 or more months of exclusive breastfeeding appeared to be a predictive factor for the higher consumption of vegetables in preschool age children. Nicklaus and colleagues found that 2–8 year old children who were breastfed for at least three or more months were more likely to eat vegetables compared to those who were breastfed for a shorter time [30]. A number of animal studies [31,32] and experimental studies in humans [33,34] indicated that breastfeeding is associated with a greater acceptability of new food and flavors during the weaning period. Breastfeeding can contribute towards reducing infants' fears to try new foods and facilitate the transition from milk feeding to solid food eating with lower resistance. Consequently, this can lead to an intake of a higher food variety in breastfed children [3,21,35,36].

Although research has shown that breastfeeding influences infants' food acceptance [22,37–39], to our knowledge, no studies have examined whether it shapes taste preferences in later stages of life. This study seeks to fill this gap by examining how breastfeeding practices—in comparison to formula milk feeding—during infancy, affect food TP in later childhood and adolescence, in a population-based cohort of normal, healthy developing children aged 6 to 16 years old, in 7 European countries: Cyprus, Estonia, Germany, Hungary, Italy, Spain and Sweden.

To be exact, we examined the association between infant feeding practices duration (FP): (1) exclusive breastfeeding (EBF), (2) exclusive formula milk feeding (EFMF) and (3) combined strategy (BF&FMF), and taste preferences (TP) evaluated in our study: sweet, fatty and bitter. We further considered a latent class analysis to identify feeding patterns from a combination of feeding practices and food introduction, and their association with taste preferences.

2. Materials and Methods

2.1. Study Sample

I.Family builds on the IDEFICS (Identification and prevention of Dietary and lifestyle-induced health Effects in Children and InfantS) study, whereby it additionally engages the families of the children who were examined during the IDEFICS baseline (T0) and/or follow-up survey (T1) [40,41]. During the IDEFICS study in 2007/2008, 16,229 children aged 2–9 years from Belgium, Cyprus, Estonia, Germany, Hungary, Italy, Spain and Sweden participated in the baseline survey (T0). Two years later (T1), 13,596 children were examined, 11,041 of whom had previously participated in T0 (68%). In 2013/2014, I.Family (T3) collected further data on the lifestyle-related diseases of 7105 (52% of T1) children, who were then between 7 and 17 years old [42]. Data of 5526 children aged 6–16 years old who completed the Food and Beverage Preference Questionnaire (FBP) during I.Family were used. For the purpose of this investigation, Belgian participants were excluded as their data on food and beverage preference were not collected. Further, retrospective information from the Pregnancy and Early Childhood Questionnaire concerning breastfeeding and formula milk feeding practices and their respective durations during infancy and early childhood reported by mothers in both the IDEFICS study and I.Family were linked. Parents provided written informed consent for all examinations. Each child was informed orally about the measurements by field workers and asked for his/her consent immediately before the examination.

2.2. Core Questionnaire

Information on sex, age, country, migration and socio-economic status (SES) of I.Family participants were collected using a self-administered questionnaire. A validated [43,44] and reproducibility tested [45] food frequency questionnaire (FFQ) containing 59 food and beverage items was completed for each participant. The response categories were 'never/less than once a week', '1–3 times a week', '4–6 times a week', '1 time/day', '2 times a day', '3 times a day' and 'I have no idea'. Based on the FFQ data, a Healthy Diet Adherence Score (HDAS) was developed for all 7 countries [46,47], as a proxy-indicator of children's adherence to healthy dietary guidelines including a high consumption of fruits and vegetables, of whole meals, fish consumption of 2–3 times per week and a reduced intake of refined sugars and fat. The HDAS was used for the present analyses as a continuous variable and ranged from 0 to 50. A higher score represented a higher adherence to healthy dietary guidelines. The self-reported educational level of parents was assessed based on the International Standard Classification of Education (ISCED) [48] and used as a proxy indicator for SES. For the present analyses, it was classified into two main categories: "low-medium education", and "high education". Children's migration background was assessed based on whether the parents were born outside the respective country of residence and recorded as the migration status in the categories "both parents", "one parent", "none of the parents".

All questionnaires were developed in English and translated into the respective national languages. They were then back-translated into English to check for translation errors. Children aged 12 years and above self-completed the questionnaire, while parents proxy-reported the relevant questions for children below 12 years of age. The cut-off of 12 years was chosen because children have been shown to be reliable reporters of their food intake at this age [49].

2.3. Food and Beverage Preference Questionnaire

The questionnaire was constructed as part of the I.Family survey to assess the preferences for sweet, fatty, bitter and salty tasting foods and beverages and was administered to children and adolescents. It contained food photographs of 63 items, including single foods (e.g., broccoli, banana, lettuce), mixed foods (e.g., lasagna, donut), condiments (e.g., nougat spread, butter), and drinks (e.g., fruit juice, lemonade). Using a 1–5 point Likert (smiley) scale, children indicated how much they like the taste of the food given in the photograph, with 1 meaning "do not like at all" and 5 meaning "I like it very much". Participants were also given the chance to indicate if they had never tried (don't know) a specific food/drink item (Figure 1). A pre-test was conducted in every center to ensure the availability of all food items across countries. Furthermore, the FBP questionnaire has been shown to provide valid data that are useful for characterizing taste phenotypes in epidemiological studies [50]. For the present analyses, the preferences for sweet and fatty taste were used as proxy-indicators for unhealthy foods [51,52], while bitter taste was used as a proxy-indicator for healthy foods [3]. Our study only focused on taste preferences that are linked to current obesogenic dietary intake in children, characterized by nutrient-dense foods high in fat and sugar and low in fiber [53,54], hence, salty and sour taste were not assessed. Umami taste is under discussion for healthy (e.g., tomatoes) and unhealthy food preferences (e.g., crisps); thus we also did not consider the preference for umami taste. For the sake of clarity, the term "taste preference" will be used instead of preferences for sweet, fatty and bitter tasting foods and beverages, hereafter.

Please indicate how much you like the taste of the following foods and drinks. Please tick the circle below the corresponding smiley for each food or drink. If there are any foods or drinks, you never tried, you don't know or where you don't know how much you like the taste of them, please tick "Never tried/don't know".

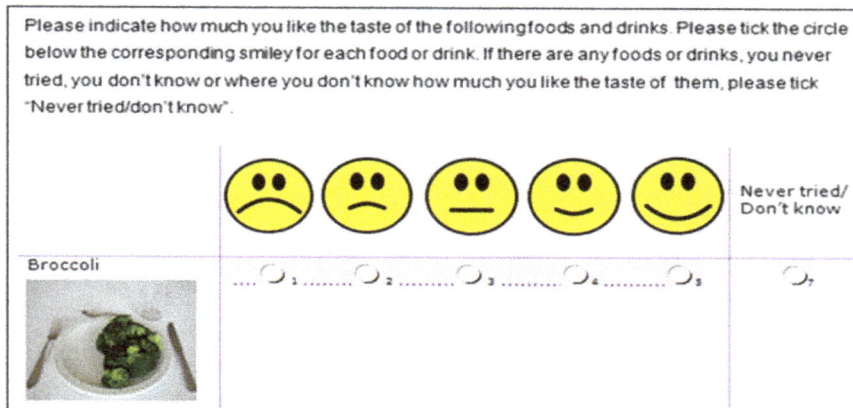

Figure 1. A screenshot of a food item from the Food and Beverage Preference Questionnaire [55].

2.4. Taste Preference Scores

The food and beverages included in our analyses were chosen based on factor analyses conducted by Jilani and colleagues [55] that assigned foods to respective taste modalities. In accordance with the factor analyses, we computed scores for the liking of three specific taste modalities: sweet, fatty and bitter, by calculating the mean liking of the foods and drinks included in each of the 3 categories. To control for differences of age and sex in the liking of each taste, the scores were first calculated separately for boys under 12 years old, girls under 12 years, boys aged 12 years and above and girls aged 12 years and above. The cut off of 12 years was chosen as the median age where children enter the age of puberty and further physiological and anatomical developments occur [56]. The scores were then merged into one unique score for each taste modality, in order to assess the association between taste preference scores and infant FP, independent of the age and sex of subjects. The sum of the ratings for the foods and drinks was then calculated and divided by the total number of foods and drinks that were included in the specific taste modality group. The taste preference scores were then categorized as "high" vs. "low", depending on the children's answers. Based on the median value, those who reported 4 or 5 on the smiley scale were included in the "high" preference category, while children who reported 3 or below on the Likert scale were categorized in the "low" preference category. Due to missing values in the taste preference scores, the sample size varied. For instance, when analyzing the sweet score, the sample size was higher than for the bitter score, because children recognized the sweet tasting foods more than the bitter tasting ones.

2.5. Pregnancy and Early Childhood Questionnaire

During the IDEFICS surveys (2007/2008 and 2009/2010) and the I.Family survey (2013/2014), mothers were asked to retrospectively report on the feeding strategies they had chosen during infancy and the early life stage of their children. The FP included the duration of

1. Exclusive breastfeeding (EBF): calculated as the difference in months between age at start of other forms of feeding (formula or other complementary foods) and the age at the start of EBF (at birth); EBF was then classified in categories "None", "Up to 4 months" and "More than 4 months",

2. Combined breastfeeding (BF&FMF): calculated as the total duration of breastfeeding after birth (breastfeeding combined with any other type of feeding, formula or complementary foods) and classified as "None", "Up to 6 months" and "More than 6 months".

3. Exclusive formula milk feeding (EFMF): calculated as the difference of total duration of formula milk feeding in combination with other types of feeding and the duration of either EBF or BF&FMF. It was then categorized as "None", "Up to 6 months", "More than 6 months".

The categories for the infant feeding variables were chosen to try and accommodate the restricted sample size for smaller categories and to facilitate the interpretability of the results. The cut off of 4 months for EBF was chosen based on the WHO recommendations to breastfeed infants exclusively with breastmilk for at least the first 4 months of life [13]., As the introduction of complementary foods and the duration of FP in many countries varies, the cut off of 6 months was chosen for the BF&FMF and EFMF. This is in accordance with WHO observations and findings of other studies [13,22]. Mothers also provided information on the age at first introduction of any of the five food categories: cereals (or foods containing rye, wheat or barley), vegetables, fruits, meat and cow milk. These categories were then merged into one unique variable—the minimum age at the first introduction of any food category—which was then categorized as "up to 6 months", "later than 6 months" and "missing". This was again based on WHO observations of the introduction of complementary feeding [13]. From here on, we will refer to these categories as complementary food introduction (CF).

2.6. Statistical Analyses

Descriptive analyses of FP during infancy were conducted by calculating the mean, median and range of the duration of EBF, BF&FMF and EFMF. Furthermore, the following study characteristics were described, i.e., N and proportions, based on categories of BF&FMF for categorical covariates included in the analyses, such as age groups, sex, SES, migration status, the age of the first introduction of complementary food categories, preference scores for each taste modality and country. In order to evaluate the association between each of the three different FP (independent variables) and taste preferences (dependent variables), i.e., sweet, fatty and bitter, logistic regression analyses to calculate Odds Ratios (OR) and 95% confidence limits adjusted for covariates (country, age, sex, HDAS, CF introduction, parents' migration status and SES) were conducted. As a combined analysis showed a high multicollinearity of feeding practices and did not yield interpretable results, a latent class analysis (LCA) was conducted in order to identify latent profiles considering categories of FP and age of complementary food introduction [57]. LCA was conducted considering three, four or five latent profiles of seven variables (three FP variables and four separate variables for the introduction of food items). The different LCA were compared by considering the Bayesian Information Criterium (BIC) and a clear distinction of latent profiles in terms of conditional probabilities. The chosen profiles were then used in logistic regression models as independent variables for each of the TP to again calculate Odds Ratios and 95% confidence limits adjusted for the remaining covariates. All statistical analyses were performed using the statistical software SAS, version 9.3 (Statistical Analyses System, SAS Institute Inc., Cary, NC, USA). The latent class analysis was conducted using the PROC LCA Macro (version 1.3.2, University Park: The Methodology Center, Penn State, PA, USA) [58] in SAS 9.3. Level of significance was set to $\alpha = 0.05$.

3. Results

3.1. Study Characteristics

The descriptive analyses of the three main feeding practices, as shown in Table 1, indicated that the median for EBF was 4 months, ranging from not breastfed at all to 36 months of EBF. The BF&FMF had a median of 6 months, varying from 0 to 36 months of total breastfeeding (BF combined with other types of feeding). The EFMF had a maximum of 48 months, with a median of 0 months of formula milk feeding.

Half of the study population was female (Table 2) and the mean age was 11.6 years (SD = 1.9), whereby 53.3 % of the participants were less than 12 years old. Both parents of a small proportion of the children were migrants (5.4%), while 9.8 % had one parent who was a migrant. Half of the children (50.5%) came from highly educated families and 78.1% of them were introduced to complementary foods early (≤6 months). The HDAS ranged from 0 to 44, with a median of 18.

Table 1. The duration of feeding practices during infancy.

Types of Feeding Practices (N = 5526) Duration in Months	Mean/SD	Median	Min/Max
Exclusive Breastfeeding (EBF)	3.3/2.7	4.0	0.0/36.0
Combined Breastfeeding (BF&FMF)	7.2/6.3	6.0	0.0/36.0
Exclusive Formula Milk Feeding (EFMF)	4.1/8.1	0	0.0/48.0

Table 2. The study characteristics of participants according to the duration of combined breastfeeding (BF&FMF).

Variables	Combined Breastfeeding (BF&FMF)						All	
	None		Up to 6 Months		More Than 6 Months			
	N	%	N	%	N	%	N	%
All	798	100.0	2318	100.0	2410	100.0	5526	100.0
Age Groups								
<12 years	404	50.6	1184	51.1	1359	56.4	2947	53.3
≥12 years	394	49.4	1134	48.9	1051	43.6	2579	46.7
Sex								
Boys	410	51.4	1147	49.5	1203	49.9	2760	49.9
Girls	388	48.6	1171	50.5	1207	50.1	2766	50.1
SES								
Low –Medium	511	64.0	1306	56.3	921	38.2	2738	49.5
High	287	36.0	1012	43.7	1489	61.8	2788	50.5
Migrant Status								
Both Parents	69	8.6	107	4.6	122	5.1	298	5.4
One parent	94	11.8	276	11.9	170	7.1	540	9.8
Neitherparent	635	79.6	1935	83.5	2118	87.9	4688	84.8
Complementary Food Introduction								
Missing	76	9.5	153	6.6	86	3.6	315	5.7
≤6 months	592	74.2	1892	81.6	1833	76.1	4317	78.1
>6 months	130	16.3	273	11.8	491	20.4	894	16.2
Sweet Taste Preference								
Low	350	43.9	950	41.0	918	38.1	2218	40.1
High	448	56.1	1368	59.0	1485	61.6	3301	59.7
Missing [1]	0	0	0	0	7	0.3	7	0.1
Fatty Taste Preference								
Low	317	39.7	855	36.9	948	39.3	2120	38.4
High	481	60.3	1463	63.1	1460	60.6	3404	61.6
Missing [1]	0	0	0	0	2	0.1	2	0.0
Bitter Taste Preference								
Low	546	68.4	1583	68.3	1624	67.4	3753	67.9
High	223	27.9	666	28.7	707	29.3	1596	28.9
Missing [1]	29	3.6	69	3.0	79	3.3	177	3.2
Country								
Italy	170	21.3	652	28.1	224	9.3	1046	18.9
Estonia	57	7.1	265	11.4	554	23.0	876	15.9
Cyprus	228	28.6	508	21.9	169	7.0	905	16.4
Sweden	41	5.1	208	9.0	433	18.0	682	12.3
Germany	181	22.7	310	13.4	315	13.1	806	14.6
Hungary	60	7.5	242	10.4	509	21.1	811	14.7
Spain	61	7.6	133	5.7	206	8.5	400	7.2

[1] Missing values were generated when calculating the taste preference scores for each taste group. N is the number of participants in the BF&FMF categories.

Almost 42% of the study population was breastfed for up to 6 months, while 43.6% had a longer duration of more than 6 months and 14.4% were never breastfed. Looking at the proportions of taste preference categories (low vs. high) according to BF&FMF, the children reported high sweet and fatty taste preferences, independent of the duration of BF&FMF during infancy. The contrary was however shown for bitter taste preferences.

3.2. Association between Exclusive Breastfeeding and Taste Preference

The results of the logistic regression analyses showed no associations between EBF and preferences for sweet, fatty and bitter tastes (Table 3). An increase in the HDAS was observed to significantly decrease the chance for high sweet taste preferences (OR = 0.88, 95% CI [0.82; 0.96]) and high-fat taste preferences (OR = 0.88, 95% CI [0.81; 0.95]), while on the other hand significantly increasing the chance for a high bitter taste preference (OR = 1.31, 95% CI [1.20; 1.43]). A late introduction to complementary foods (≤6 months) was found to significantly decrease the odds for a high-fat taste preference (OR = 0.81, 95% CI [0.68; 0.95]). Compared to having parents with a high SES, having parents with a low/medium SES significantly increased the odds for a high-fat taste preference (OR = 1.14, 95% CI [1.009; 1.30]).

Table 3. The association between exclusive breastfeeding (EBF) duration and taste preferences in 6–16 year old children and adolescents who participated in the IDEFICS/I.Family studies.

	Sweet Taste (*N* = 5191)			Fatty Taste (*N* = 5196)			Bitter Taste (*N* = 5029)		
	OR	95% CI		OR	95% CI		OR	95% CI	
EBF									
(ref: None)	1.00			1.00			1.00		
≤4 months	1.12	0.97	1.29	1.04	0.90	1.21	0.98	0.84	1.15
>4 months	1.10	0.95	1.29	1.02	0.87	1.19	0.95	0.80	1.12
Healthy Diet Adherence Score (HDAS) $	0.88	0.82	0.96	0.88	0.81	0.95	1.31	1.20	1.43
Complementary Food Introduction									
(ref. ≤6 months)									
>6 months	0.91	0.77	1.07	0.81	0.68	0.95	1.02	0.86	1.22
Missing	0.88	0.67	1.14	0.82	0.62	1.07	1.02	0.75	1.38
SES									
(ref. high)									
Low- medium	1.11	0.98	1.26	1.14	1.009	1.30	0.88	0.77	1.017

$ OR is calculated for difference in one unit from the mean. (Logistic regression models were adjusted also for age, sex, migrant background and country—OR not reported).

3.3. Association between Combined Breastfeeding and Taste Preference

The logistic regression analyses did not show an association between the duration of BF&FMF and taste preferences (sweet, fatty and bitter) (Table 4). As observed for EBF, significant associations were observed between HDAS and taste preferences, with having a higher HDAS significantly decreasing the odds for high sweet and fatty taste preference but significantly increasing the odds for high bitter taste preference (Table 4). A late introduction of complementary foods significantly decreased the odds for a high-fat taste preference (OR = 0.82, 95% CI [0.70; 0.97]) compared to an introduction of complementary foods before the age of 6 months. Having parents with a low/medium SES again significantly increased the odds for a high-fat taste preference (OR = 1.14, 95% CI [1.004; −1.29]).

Table 4. The association between combined breastfeeding (BF&FMF) duration and taste preference in 6–16 year old children and adolescents who participated in the IDEFICS/I.Family studies.

	Sweet Taste (*N* = 5191)			Fatty Taste (*N* = 5196)			Bitter Taste (*N* = 5029)		
	OR	95% CI		OR	95% CI		OR	95% CI	
BF&FMF									
(ref. None)	1.00			1.00			1.00		
≤6 months	1.11	0.93	1.32	1.15	0.96	1.37	0.98	0.81	1.19
>6 months	1.10	0.92	1.32	1.03	0.85	1.24	1.09	0.89	1.33
HDAS [$]	0.88	0.81	0.96	0.88	0.81	0.95	1.31	1.20	1.43
Complementary Food									
Introduction									
(ref. ≤6 months)									
>6 months	0.91	0.78	1.07	0.82	0.70	0.97	0.99	0.83	1.18
Missing	0.88	0.67	1.15	0.82	0.63	1.08	1.01	0.74	1.37
SES									
(ref. High)									
Low- medium	1.11	0.98	1.26	1.14	1.004	1.29	0.90	0.78	1.03

[$] OR is calculated for difference in one unit from the mean. (Logistic regression models were adjusted also for age, sex, migration status and country—OR not reported.

3.4. Association between Exclusive Formula Feeding and Taste Preference

No significant association was observed between the EFMF duration and preferences for sweet, fatty and bitter taste (Table 5). HDAS was again significantly associated with sweet and fatty taste preferences, (OR = 0.88, 95% CI [0.81; 0.96]) and OR = 0.88, 95% CI [0.81; 0.95]) respectively, as well as with a high bitter taste preference (OR = 1.31, 95% CI [1.20; 1.42]). Furthermore, a late introduction of complementary foods decreased the chance for a high preference of fatty taste (OR = 0.82, 95% CI [0,70; 0.97]) at a later age, compared to an early introduction. Compared to having a high SES background, having a low/medium SES background increased the odds to prefer a high-fat taste (OR = 1.14, 95% CI [1.00; 1.29]).

Table 5. The association between exclusive formula milk feeding (EFMF) duration and taste preference in 6–16 years old children and adolescents who participated in the IDEFICS/I.Family studies.

	Sweet Taste (*N* = 5191)			Fatty Taste (*N* = 5196)			Bitter Taste (*N* = 5029)		
	OR	95% CI		OR	95% CI		OR	95% CI	
EFMF									
(ref. None)									
≤6 months	1.001	0.84	1.18	1.09	0.92	1.29	0.85	0.71	1.02
>6 months	1.009	0.85	1.18	1.008	0.85	1.18	0.95	0.80	1.13
HDAS [$]	0.88	0.82	0.96	0.88	0.81	0.96	1.31	1.20	1.43
Complementary Food									
Introduction									
(ref. ≤6 months)									
>6 months	0.91	0.78	1.07	0.81	0.69	0.95	1.004	0.84	1.19
Missing	0.87	0.67	1.14	0.82	0.62	1.07	1.01	0.75	1.37
SES									
(ref. High)									
Low- medium	1.10	0.97	1.25	1.14	1.004	1.29	0.90	0.78	1.03

[$] OR is calculated for difference in one unit from the mean. (Logistic regression models were adjusted also for age, sex, migration status and country—OR not reported).

3.5. Association between Latent Profiles of Feeding Practices and Taste Preferences

With regard to the four latent profiles, the LCA showed the lowest BIC and a clear interpretable distinction of conditional probabilities for the respective variables. Results of the latent class profiles are presented in Table 6, where names of the profiles were chosen according to the highest conditional probabilities. Almost half of the children and adolescents (48%) had a short duration of EBF (up to

4 months), then were breastfed in combination with formula milk and introduced to complementary foods early (before 6 months). About a quarter (24%) were exclusively breastfed for a long period, were never exclusively fed formula milk and had a late introduction to complementary foods (later than 6 months). A total of 14% were fed formula milk as the main alternative to breastmilk and were as well introduced to complementary foods at a later age. Only 13% were exclusively fed formula milk and were introduced to complementary foods early.

Table 6. The latent class profiles and highest conditional probabilities (ϱ-estimate) of categories within each profile.

Latent Profiles of Feeding Practices			Frequency	%
1. Long period of EBF and mixed breastfeeding, no exclusive use of formula milk, late introduction of complementary foods			1334	24.14
Variable	Category	ϱ-estimate		
Mixed feeding	more than 6 months	0.869		
Exclusive breastfeeding	more than 4 months	0.853		
Exclusive formula milk feeding	None	0.952		
Introduction of vegetables	after month 6	0.674		
Introduction of fruit	after month 6	0.562		
Introduction of meat	after month 6	0.981		
Introduction of cow milk	after month 6	0.988		
2. Predominantly formula milk feeding (mixed and exclusive) and late introduction of complementary foods			774	14.01
Variable	Category	ϱ-estimate		
Mixed feeding	0–6 months	0.702		
Exclusive breastfeeding	0–4 months	0.464		
Exclusive formula milk feeding	more than 6 months	0.619		
Introduction of vegetables	after month 6	0.832		
Introduction of fruit	after month 6	0.657		
Introduction of meat	after month 6	0.997		
Introduction of cow milk	after month 6	0.973		
3. Short duration of EBF and mixed BF without exclusive formula milk use, early introduction of main complementary foods			2700	48.86
Variable	Category	ϱ-estimate		
Mixed feeding	0–6 months	0.541		
Exclusive breastfeeding	0–4 months	0.627		
Exclusive formula milk feeding	None	0.764		
Introduction of vegetables	before month 6	0.964		
Introduction of fruit	before month 6	0.988		
Introduction of meat	before month 6	0.681		
Introduction of cow milk	after month 6	0.824		
4. No breastfeeding, but exclusive formula milk use, early introduction of main complementary foods.			718	12.99
Variable	Category	ϱ-estimate		
Mixed feeding	None	0.841		
Exclusive breastfeeding	None	0.994		
Exclusive formula milk feeding	more than 6 months	0.583		
Introduction of vegetables	before month 6	0.911		
Introduction of fruit	before month 6	0.983		
Introduction of meat	before month 6	0.645		
Introduction of cow milk	after month 6	0.806		

Profile number 4 was considered to reflect the least advisable feeding strategy (no breastfeeding, only formula milk, early introduction) and served as a reference for the logistic regression analyses presented in Table 7. No significant associations of profiles of feeding practices with taste preferences for sweet, fatty and bitter tastes were observed. Again, the HDAS was significantly negatively associated with sweet (OR = 0.88, 95% CI [0.82; 0.96]) and fatty taste preferences (OR = 0.88, 95% CI [0.81; 0.95]) and significantly positively associated with a bitter taste preference (OR = 1.31, 95% CI [1.20; 1.43]).

In addition, children from low/medium SES families were observed to have a higher chance of having a high-fat taste preference (OR = 1.14, 95% CI [1.00; 1.29]).

Table 7. The results of logistic regression models investigating the association between latent profiles of feeding practices (FP) and taste preferences of 6–16 year old children and adolescents who participated in the IDEFICS/I.Family studies.

	Sweet Taste (*N* = 5191)			Fatty Taste (*N* = 5196)			Bitter Taste (*N* = 5029)		
Variables	**OR**	**95% CI**		**OR**	**95% CI**		**OR**	**95% CI**	
Profile of FP									
(ref: profile 4)	1.00			1.00			1.00		
Profile 1	0.99	0.81	1.20	0.97	0.79	1.19	1.09	0.88	1.36
Profile 2	0.90	0.72	1.13	1.13	0.90	1.43	1.05	0.82	1.35
Profile 3	1.09	0.91	1.30	1.11	0.92	1.33	1.06	0.87	1.29
HDAS [$]	0.88	0.82	0.96	0.88	0.81	0.95	1.31	1.20	1.43
SES (ref: high)									
Low/medium	1.11	0.97	1.25	1.14	1.004	1.29	0.89	0.78	1.02

[$] OR is calculated for difference in one unit from the mean. (Logistic regression models were adjusted also for age, sex, migration status and country—OR not reported).

4. Discussion

To our knowledge, this is the first study assessing the association between different infant FPs and children's taste preferences in later stages in life which included retrospective and current data from 7 European countries. Our results indicate that European children were predominantly breastfed exclusively for at least 4 months, which is in line with the WHO guidelines [13]. In addition, almost half of the subjects had a long duration of BF&FMF and only a minority (13%) was exclusively fed FM. The feeding strategy parents used seemed not to play a role in the development of taste preferences later in life, irrespective of whether it was EBF, EFMF or a combination. Using both single logistic regression analyses and LCA methods, in which latent profiles of all FP and introduction of complementary food categories were identified, a higher quality diet (HDAS) was observed to be associated with lower chances for a high sweet and high-fat taste preference and increased chances for high bitter taste preference. This suggests that current food choices can actually mold children's preferences for sweet, fat and bitter tastes, independent of their infant feeding patterns. SES also seemed to play a role, as children who came from a lower SES background were more likely to prefer the fatty taste compared to those from a higher SES background. Our results indicate that a variation in food choice and parental education can affect children's behaviors towards healthy food choices and preferences.

Our findings are supported by the current evidence, which suggests that children have innate preferences for sweet taste as signalers of high energy foods [3,8]. Further, Schwartz et al. reported that infants' sweet acceptance was not related to longer durations of EBF [22]. In a longitudinal study, Desor and colleagues measured the sweet preference in children at the age of 11–15 years and again when they were 19–25 years of age, and found that the preferred levels of sucrose decreased over time [59]. Other studies have suggested that children learn to prefer flavors associated with a high dietary fat content [60,61]. Previous findings from the IDEFICS study indicated that children from low educational backgrounds tended to eat more high energy-dense foods, such as sugar-rich and fat-rich foods, compared to those whose parents had a high education [62]. In contrast, children of parents with a higher education tended to eat more fruits and vegetables, generally eating less unhealthy foods. They were also more likely to eat breakfast on a daily basis, emphasizing the influence of parental education on children's eating habits [47,63–67]. Furthermore, a higher number of fruits and vegetables at 14 months has been shown to increase the preference for these foods and improve the quality of the diet at 3.7 years of age [68]. Our results, which are supported by the current evidence, suggest that taste preferences in children are learned via food experience and are significantly influenced by the food choice and diet literacy of parents. Thus, public health education programs should emphasize the role of food variety in shaping children's preferences for bitter tasting foods in the long term. Particular attention needs to be paid to parents and other caretakers of low to medium socio-economic status families in order to help them reduce their children's preferences for high energy-dense foods.

5. Strengths and Limitations

One of the main strengths of our study is the large sample size of 5526 children and adolescents from 7 European countries, which allowed us to have a detailed picture of FP and its potential association with taste preferences in later stages of life. The standardized protocol and the pre-test conducted in a subsample of children showed that the Food and Beverage Preference Questionnaire is a feasible instrument for assessing preferences of food and beverages in children and adolescents.

Furthermore, having information on covariates such as country of residence, age, sex, HDAS, the timing of the first introduction of complementary feeding, parental education level and migration status allowed us to make adjustments and to control for confounding.

Nevertheless, there are important methodological limits concerning our research. The scale of the taste preference was slightly limited as it was calculated based on measuring the food preference with only 5 points. This limited our ability to clearly distinguish between extreme taste preferences. Further, in the BF&FMF category, information on the proportion of actual formula milk and breastmilk feeding was not provided. Thus, we have to acknowledge this as a limitation as it hampers a critical discussion on the potential effects of a mixed strategy of feeding on taste preference.

Since mothers self-reported the details of their infants' FP (age at starting and termination of infant feeding, the timing of the first introduction of complementary foods) and as adolescents tend to self-report a lower preference for energy-dense (fatty and sweet) foods and beverages [69,70], we cannot entirely exclude social desirability bias. As we used retrospective information on feeding practices, recall bias also potentially affected our data. The reproducibility testing of the early infant parameters showed a weak reproducibility of maternal reports on early infant nutrition, a further potential limitation [71]. Nevertheless, research has shown that mothers recall breastfeeding duration accurately [72,73], while the recall of age at introduction of complementary food is less satisfactory [73]. Moreover, the parents of half of our sample had a high educational status, a fact which might also bias the results with regard to socio-economic status. In addition, we did not have information on other confounding factors such as the role of the maternal diet during breastfeeding and the family diet, factors that have been found to influence taste preference and food intake in children [3,55,74]. Lastly, our research was conducted using only cross-sectional data enriched with retrospective information. We strongly recommend further longitudinal research, e.g., through birth cohorts, that can evaluate the effects of FP during infancy and changes of taste preferences during different stages of life, particularly accounting for the interplay between food choice and socio-economic background.

6. Conclusions

In contrast to our hypotheses, we did not observe an association between infant feeding practices and taste preferences in school children and adolescents, neither regarding the single FPs or as a mixed strategy, nor considering common profiles of FP. Instead, the current diet quality through food choice and educational status of parents consistently showed an association with the current taste preference for sweet, fatty or bitter tastes. Hence, further studies with higher FP variations and using longitudinal data are necessary in order to investigate causal associations between infant feeding practices and taste preferences in later stages of life.

Author Contributions: The authors' responsibilities were as follows: E.S. wrote the paper; E.S., C.B. and A.H. had primary responsibility for the final content; E.S. and C.B. performed the data analysis. H.J., M.T., T.V., P.R., L.A.M., D.M., G.E., S.M., V.P. and W.A. participated in the coordination of the data collection and the project administration. All authors were responsible for critical revisions and final approval of the manuscript. This manuscript represents original work that has not been published previously and is not currently being considered by another journal. If accepted, it will not be published elsewhere, including electronically in the same form, in English or in any other language, without the written consent of the copyright holder.

Funding: This research was funded by the European Community within the Sixth RTD Framework Programme Contract No. 016181 (FOOD) and Seventh RTD Framework Programme Contract No. 266044.

Acknowledgments: This work was done as part of the IDEFICS (http://www.idefics.eu) and I. Family studies (http://www.ifamilystudy.eu/).We thank the IDEFICS and I.Family children and their parents for participating in this extensive examination. We are grateful for the support from school boards, headmasters, and communities.

Conflicts of Interest: The authors declare that they have no conflict of interest.

References

1. Drewnowski, A. Taste preferences and food intake. *Annu. Rev. Nutr.* **1997**, *17*, 237–253. [CrossRef] [PubMed]
2. IQWiG (Institute for Quality and Efficiency in Health Care). *How Does Our Sense of Taste Work?* IQWiG (Institute for Quality and Efficiency in Health Care): Cologne, Germany, 2011.
3. Mennella, J.A. Ontogeny of taste preferences: Basic biology and implications for health. *Am. J. Clin. Nutr.* **2014**, *99*, 704s–711s. [CrossRef]
4. Ikeda, K. New seasonings. *Chem. Senses* **2002**, *27*, 847–849. [CrossRef] [PubMed]
5. Running, C.A.; Craig, B.A.; Mattes, R.D. Oleogustus: The unique taste of fat. *Chem. Senses* **2015**, *40*, 507–516. [CrossRef]
6. Besnard, P.; Passilly-Degrace, P.; Khan, N.A. Taste of fat: A sixth taste modality? *Physiol. Rev.* **2016**, *96*, 151–176. [CrossRef] [PubMed]
7. Birch, L.L. Development of food preferences. *Annu. Rev. Nutr.* **1999**, *19*, 41–62. [CrossRef]
8. Beauchamp, G.K.; Cowart, B.J.; Mennella, J.A.; Marsh, R.R. Infant salt taste: Developmental, methodological, and contextual factors. *Dev. Psychobiol.* **1994**, *27*, 353–365. [CrossRef]
9. Beauchamp, G.K.; Cowart, B.J.; Moran, M. Developmental changes in salt acceptability in human infants. *Dev. Psychobiol.* **1986**, *19*, 17–25. [CrossRef]
10. Fisher, J.O.; Birch, L.L.; Smiciklas-Wright, H.; Picciano, M.F. Breast-feeding through the first year predicts maternal control in feeding and subsequent toddler energy intakes. *J. Am. Diet. Assoc.* **2000**, *100*, 641–646. [CrossRef]
11. Li, R.; Scanlon, K.S.; May, A.; Rose, C.; Birch, L. Bottle-feeding practices during early infancy and eating behaviors at 6 years of age. *Pediatrics* **2014**, *134* (Suppl. 1), S70–S77. [CrossRef]
12. Sullivan, S.A.; Birch, L.L. Infant dietary experience and acceptance of solid foods. *Pediatrics* **1994**, *93*, 271–277.
13. Michaelsen, K.F.; Europe, W.R.O.f.; Europe, W.H.O.R.O.f. *Feeding and Nutrition of Infants and Young Children: Guidelines for the Who European Region, with Emphasis on the Former Soviet Countries*; WHO Regional Office for Europe: Copenhagen, Denmark, 2000.
14. Carling, S.J.; Demment, M.M.; Kjolhede, C.L.; Olson, C.M. Breastfeeding duration and weight gain trajectory in infancy. *Pediatrics* **2015**, *135*, 111–119. [CrossRef] [PubMed]
15. Imai, C.M.; Gunnarsdottir, I.; Thorisdottir, B.; Halldorsson, T.I.; Thorsdottir, I. Associations between infant feeding practice prior to six months and body mass index at six years of age. *Nutrients* **2014**, *6*, 1608–1617. [CrossRef]
16. De Kroon, M.L.; Renders, C.M.; Buskermolen, M.P.; Van Wouwe, J.P.; van Buuren, S.; Hirasing, R.A. The terneuzen birth cohort. Longer exclusive breastfeeding duration is associated with leaner body mass and a healthier diet in young adulthood. *BMC Pediatr.* **2011**, *11*, 33. [CrossRef] [PubMed]
17. Okubo, H.; Miyake, Y.; Sasaki, S.; Tanaka, K.; Hirota, Y. Feeding practices in early life and later intake of fruit and vegetables among Japanese toddlers: The Osaka maternal and child health study. *Public Health Nutr.* **2016**, *19*, 650–657. [CrossRef] [PubMed]
18. Scott, J.; Chih, T.; Oddy, W. Food variety at 2 years of age is related to duration of breastfeeding. *Nutrients* **2012**, *4*, 1464–1474. [CrossRef] [PubMed]
19. De Lauzon-Guillain, B.; Jones, L.; Oliveira, A.; Moschonis, G.; Betoko, A.; Lopes, C.; Moreira, P.; Manios, Y.; Papadopoulos, N.G.; Emmett, P.; et al. The influence of early feeding practices on fruit and vegetable intake among preschool children in 4 European birth cohorts. *Am. J. Clin. Nutr.* **2013**, *98*, 804–812. [CrossRef]
20. Grieger, J.A.; Scott, J.; Cobiac, L. Dietary patterns and breast-feeding in Australian children. *Public Health Nutr.* **2011**, *14*, 1939–1947. [CrossRef]
21. Skinner, J.D.; Carruth, B.R.; Bounds, W.; Ziegler, P.; Reidy, K. Do food-related experiences in the first 2 years of life predict dietary variety in school-aged children? *J. Nutr. Educ. Behav.* **2002**, *34*, 310–315. [CrossRef]

22. Schwartz, C.; Chabanet, C.; Laval, C.; Issanchou, S.; Nicklaus, S. Breast-feeding duration: Influence on taste acceptance over the first year of life. *Br. J. Nutr.* **2013**, *109*, 1154–1161. [CrossRef]
23. Andreas, N.J.; Kampmann, B.; Le-Doare, K.M. Human breast milk: A review on its composition and bioactivity. *Early Hum. Dev.* **2015**, *91*, 629–635. [CrossRef]
24. De Cosmi, V.; Scaglioni, S.; Agostoni, C. Early taste experiences and later food choices. *Nutrients* **2017**, *9*, 107. [CrossRef]
25. Mennella, J.A.; Beauchamp, G.K. Flavor experiences during formula feeding are related to preferences during childhood. *Early Hum. Dev.* **2002**, *68*, 71–82. [CrossRef]
26. Trabulsi, J.C.; Mennella, J.A. Diet, sensitive periods in flavour learning, and growth. *Int. Rev. Psychiatry (Abingdon Engl.)* **2012**, *24*, 219–230. [CrossRef]
27. North, K.; Emmett, P. Multivariate analysis of diet among three-year-old children and associations with socio-demographic characteristics. The Avon longitudinal study of pregnancy and childhood (alspac) study team. *Eur. J. Clin. Nutr.* **2000**, *54*, 73–80. [CrossRef]
28. Robinson, S.; Marriott, L.; Poole, J.; Crozier, S.; Borland, S.; Lawrence, W.; Law, C.; Godfrey, K.; Cooper, C.; Inskip, H. Dietary patterns in infancy: The importance of maternal and family influences on feeding practice. *Br. J. Nutr.* **2007**, *98*, 1029–1037. [CrossRef]
29. Burnier, D.; Dubois, L.; Girard, M. Exclusive breastfeeding duration and later intake of vegetables in preschool children. *Eur. J. Clin. Nutr.* **2011**, *65*, 196–202. [CrossRef] [PubMed]
30. Nicklaus, S. The role of food experiences during early childhood in food pleasure learning. *Appetite* **2016**, *104*, 3–9. [CrossRef]
31. Galef, B.G.; Henderson, P.W. Mother's milk: A determinant of the feeding preferences of weaning rat pups. *J. Comp. Physiol. Psychol.* **1972**, *78*, 213–219. [CrossRef]
32. Galef, B.G.; Sherry, D.F. Mother's milk: A medium for transmission of cues reflecting the flavor of mother's diet. *J. Comp. Physiol. Psychol.* **1973**, *83*, 374–378. [CrossRef]
33. Mennella, J.A.; Forestell, C.A.; Morgan, L.K.; Beauchamp, G.K. Early milk feeding influences taste acceptance and liking during infancy. *Am. J. Clin. Nutr.* **2009**, *90*, 780s–788s. [CrossRef] [PubMed]
34. Mennella, J.A.; Beauchamp, G.K. Mothers' milk enhances the acceptance of cereal during weaning. *Pediatr. Res.* **1997**, *41*, 188–192. [CrossRef]
35. Galloway, A.T.; Lee, Y.; Birch, L.L. Predictors and consequences of food neophobia and pickiness in young girls. *J. Am. Diet. Assoc.* **2003**, *103*, 692–698. [CrossRef]
36. Cooke, L.J.; Wardle, J.; Gibson, E.L.; Sapochnik, M.; Sheiham, A.; Lawson, M. Demographic, familial and trait predictors of fruit and vegetable consumption by pre-school children. *Public Health Nutr.* **2004**, *7*, 295–302. [CrossRef] [PubMed]
37. Mennella, J.A.; Daniels, L.M.; Reiter, A.R. Learning to like vegetables during breastfeeding: A randomized clinical trial of lactating mothers and infants. *Am. J. Clin. Nutr.* **2017**, *106*, 67–76. [CrossRef] [PubMed]
38. Hausner, H.; Nicklaus, S.; Issanchou, S.; Molgaard, C.; Moller, P. Breastfeeding facilitates acceptance of a novel dietary flavour compound. *Clin. Nutr. (Edinb. Scotl.)* **2010**, *29*, 141–148. [CrossRef] [PubMed]
39. Forestell, C.A.; Mennella, J.A. Early determinants of fruit and vegetable acceptance. *Pediatrics* **2007**, *120*, 1247–1254. [CrossRef] [PubMed]
40. Ahrens, W.; Bammann, K.; Siani, A.; Buchecker, K.; De Henauw, S.; Iacoviello, L.; Hebestreit, A.; Krogh, V.; Lissner, L.; Mårild, S.; et al. The idefics cohort: Design, characteristics and participation in the baseline survey. *Int. J. Obes.* **2011**, *35* (Suppl. 1), S3–S15. [CrossRef]
41. Hebestreit, A.; Intemann, T.; Siani, A.; De Henauw, S.; Eiben, G.; Kourides, Y.A.; Kovacs, E.; Moreno, L.A.; Veidebaum, T.; Krogh, V.; et al. Dietary patterns of european children and their parents in association with family food environment: Results from the i.Family study. *Nutrients* **2017**, *9*, 126. [CrossRef]
42. Ahrens, W.; Siani, A.; Adan, R.; De Henauw, S.; Eiben, G.; Gwozdz, W.; Hebestreit, A.; Hunsberger, M.; Kaprio, J.; Krogh, V.; et al. Cohort profile: The transition from childhood to adolescence in European children-how i.Family extends the idefics cohort. *Int. J. Epidemiol.* **2017**, *46*, 1394–1395j. [CrossRef]
43. Bel-Serrat, S.; Mouratidou, T.; Pala, V.; Huybrechts, I.; Börnhorst, C.; Fernández-Alvira, J.; Moreno, L. Relative validity of the children's eating habits questionnaire–food frequency section among young european children: The idefics study. *Public Health Nutr.* **2014**, *17*, 266–276. [CrossRef]

44. Huybrechts, I.; Börnhorst, C.; Pala, V.; Moreno, L.A.; Barba, G.; Lissner, L.; Fraterman, A.; Veidebaum, T.; Hebestreit, A.; Sieri, S.; et al. Evaluation of the children's eating habits questionnaire used in the idefics study by relating urinary calcium and potassium to milk consumption frequencies among european children. *Int. J. Obes.* **2011**, *35* (Suppl. 1), S69–S78. [CrossRef]

45. Lanfer, A.; Hebestreit, A.; Ahrens, W.; Krogh, V.; Sieri, S.; Lissner, L.; Eiben, G.; Siani, A.; Huybrechts, I.; Loit, H.M.; et al. Reproducibility of food consumption frequencies derived from the children's eating habits questionnaire used in the idefics study. *Int. J. Obes.* **2011**, *35* (Suppl. 1), S61–S68. [CrossRef]

46. Arvidsson, L.; Eiben, G.; Hunsberger, M.; De Bourdeaudhuij, I.; Molnar, D.; Jilani, H.; Thumann, B.; Veidebaum, T.; Russo, P.; Tornatitis, M.; et al. Bidirectional associations between psychosocial well-being and adherence to healthy dietary guidelines in european children: Prospective findings from the idefics study. *BMC Public Health* **2017**, *17*, 926. [CrossRef]

47. Jilani, H.S.; Pohlabeln, H.; Buchecker, K.; Gwozdz, W.; De Henauw, S.; Eiben, G.; Molnar, D.; Moreno, L.A.; Pala, V.; Reisch, L.; et al. Association between parental consumer attitudes with their children's sensory taste preferences as well as their food choice. *PLoS ONE* **2018**, *13*, e0200413. [CrossRef]

48. UNESCO. International Standard Classification of Education 2012. Available online: http://uis.Unesco.Org/ sites/default/files/documents/international-standard-classification-of-education-isced-2011-en.Pdf (accessed on 27 October 2016).

49. Livingstone, M.B.; Robson, P.J. Measurement of dietary intake in children. *Proc. Nutr. Soc.* **2000**, *59*, 279–293. [CrossRef] [PubMed]

50. Jilani, H.P.H.; De Henauw, S.; Eiben, G.; Hunsberger, M.; Molnar, D.; Moreno, L.; Pala, V.; Russo, P.; Solea, A.; Veidebaum, T.; et al. Relative validity of a food and beverage preference questionnaire to characterise taste phenotypes in children, adolescents and adult. *Nutrient* **2019**. under revision.

51. Ricketts, C.D. Fat preferences, dietary fat intake and body composition in children. *Eur. J. Clin. Nutr.* **1997**, *51*, 778–781. [CrossRef] [PubMed]

52. Ventura, A.K.; Mennella, J.A. Innate and learned preferences for sweet taste during childhood. *Curr. Opin. Clin. Nutr. Metab. Care* **2011**, *14*, 379–384. [CrossRef]

53. Paes, V.M.; Ong, K.K.; Lakshman, R. Factors influencing obesogenic dietary intake in young children (0–6 years): Systematic review of qualitative evidence. *BMJ Open* **2015**, *5*, e007396. [CrossRef] [PubMed]

54. Johnson, L.; Mander, A.P.; Jones, L.R.; Emmett, P.M.; Jebb, S.A. Energy-dense, low-fiber, high-fat dietary pattern is associated with increased fatness in childhood. *Am. J. Clin. Nutr.* **2008**, *87*, 846–854. [CrossRef]

55. Jilani, H.S.; Intemann, T.; Bogl, L.H.; Eiben, G.; Molnar, D.; Moreno, L.A.; Pala, V.; Russo, P.; Siani, A.; Solea, A.; et al. Familial aggregation and socio-demographic correlates of taste preferences in european children. *BMC Nutr.* **2017**, *3*, 87. [CrossRef]

56. Parent, A.-S.; Teilmann, G.; Juul, A.; Skakkebaek, N.E.; Toppari, J.; Bourguignon, J.-P. The timing of normal puberty and the age limits of sexual precocity: Variations around the world, secular trends, and changes after migration. *Endocr. Rev.* **2003**, *24*, 668–693. [CrossRef] [PubMed]

57. Lanza, S.T.; Flaherty, B.P.; Collins, L.M. Latent class and latent transition analysis. In *Handbook of Psychology*; Weiner, I.B., Ed.; John Wiley & Sons, Inc.: New York, NY, USA, 2003.

58. Lanza, S.T.; Dziak, J.J.; Huang, L.; Xu, S.; Collins, L.M. *PROC LCA & PROC LTA Users' Guide (Version 1.3.2)*; The Methodology Center; Penn State: University Park, PA, USA, 2011.

59. Desor, J.A.; Beauchamp, G.K. Longitudinal changes in sweet preferences in humans. *Physiol. Behav.* **1987**, *39*, 639–641. [CrossRef]

60. Johnson, S.L.; McPhee, L.; Birch, L.L. Conditioned preferences: Young children prefer flavors associated with high dietary fat. *Physiol. Behav.* **1991**, *50*, 1245–1251. [CrossRef]

61. Kern, D.L.; McPhee, L.; Fisher, J.; Johnson, S.; Birch, L.L. The postingestive consequences of fat condition preferences for flavors associated with high dietary fat. *Physiol. Behav.* **1993**, *54*, 71–76. [CrossRef]

62. Fernandez-Alvira, J.M. Parental education and frequency of food consumption in European children: The idefics study. *Public Health Nutr.* **2013**, *16*, 487–498. [CrossRef] [PubMed]

63. Van Ansem, W.J.; Schrijvers, C.T.; Rodenburg, G.; van de Mheen, D. Maternal educational level and children's healthy eating behaviour: Role of the home food environment (cross-sectional results from the inpact study). *Int. J. Behav. Nutr. Phys. Act.* **2014**, *11*, 113. [CrossRef] [PubMed]

64. Cribb, V.L.; Jones, L.R.; Rogers, I.S.; Ness, A.R.; Emmett, P.M. Is maternal education level associated with diet in 10-year-old children? *Public Health Nutr.* **2011**, *14*, 2037–2048. [CrossRef] [PubMed]

65. Sausenthaler, S.; Standl, M.; Buyken, A.; Rzehak, P.; Koletzko, S.; Bauer, C.P.; Schaaf, B.; von Berg, A.; Berdel, D.; Borte, M.; et al. Regional and socio-economic differences in food, nutrient and supplement intake in school-age children in germany: Results from the giniplus and the lisaplus studies. *Public Health Nutr.* **2011**, *14*, 1724–1735. [CrossRef]

66. Sausenthaler, S.; Kompauer, I.; Mielck, A.; Borte, M.; Herbarth, O.; Schaaf, B.; von Berg, A.; Heinrich, J. Impact of parental education and income inequality on children's food intake. *Public Health Nutr.* **2007**, *10*, 24–33. [CrossRef]

67. Lehto, E.; Ray, C.; Te Velde, S.; Petrova, S.; Duleva, V.; Krawinkel, M.; Behrendt, I.; Papadaki, A.; Kristjansdottir, A.; Thorsdottir, I.; et al. Mediation of parental educational level on fruit and vegetable intake among schoolchildren in ten european countries. *Public Health Nutr.* **2015**, *18*, 89–99. [CrossRef]

68. Mallan, K.M.; Fildes, A.; Magarey, A.M.; Daniels, L.A. The relationship between number of fruits, vegetables, and noncore foods tried at age 14 months and food preferences, dietary intake patterns, fussy eating behavior, and weight status at age 3.7 years. *J. Acad. Nutr. Diet.* **2016**, *116*, 630–637. [CrossRef]

69. Perl, M.A.; Mandic, M.L.; Primorac, L.; Klapec, T.; Perl, A. Adolescent acceptance of different foods by obesity status and by sex. *Physiol. Behav.* **1998**, *65*, 241–245. [CrossRef]

70. Tilgner, L.; Wertheim, E.H.; Paxton, S.J. Effect of social desirability on adolescent girls' responses to an eating disorders prevention program. *Int. J. Eat. Disord.* **2004**, *35*, 211–216. [CrossRef]

71. Herrmann, D.; Suling, M.; Reisch, L.; Siani, A.; De Bourdeaudhuij, I.; Maes, L.; Santaliestra-Pasias, A.M.; Veidebaum, T.; Molnar, D.; Pala, V.; et al. Repeatability of maternal report on prenatal, perinatal and early postnatal factors: Findings from the idefics parental questionnaire. *Int. J. Obes. (Lond.)* **2011**, *35* (Suppl. 1), S52–S60. [CrossRef]

72. Natland, S.T.; Andersen, L.F.; Nilsen, T.I.L.; Forsmo, S.; Jacobsen, G.W. Maternal recall of breastfeeding duration twenty years after delivery. *BMC Med. Res. Methodol.* **2012**, *12*, 179. [CrossRef] [PubMed]

73. Li, R.; Scanlon, K.S.; Serdula, M.K. The validity and reliability of maternal recall of breastfeeding practice. *Nutr. Rev.* **2005**, *63*, 103–110. [CrossRef] [PubMed]

74. Birch, L.L. The relationship between children's food preferences and those of their parents. *J. Nutr. Educ.* **1980**, *12*, 14–18. [CrossRef]

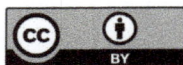

nutrients

MDPI

Article

Associations between Physical Activity and Food Intake among Children and Adolescents: Results of KiGGS Wave 2

Kristin Manz *, Gert B. M. Mensink, Jonas D. Finger, Marjolein Haftenberger, Anna-Kristin Brettschneider, Clarissa Lage Barbosa, Susanne Krug and Anja Schienkiewitz

Department of Epidemiology and Health Monitoring, Robert Koch Institute, 13353 Berlin, Germany; MensinkG@rki.de (G.B.M.M.); FingerJ@rki.de (J.D.F.); HaftenbergerM@rki.de (M.H.); BrettschneiderA@rki.de (A.-K.B.); Lage-BarbosaC@rki.de (C.L.B.); KrugS@rki.de (S.K.); SchienkiewitzA@rki.de (A.S.)
* Correspondence: ManzK@rki.de; Tel.:+49(030)-18754-3567

Received: 12 April 2019; Accepted: 9 May 2019; Published: 11 May 2019

Abstract: A balanced diet and sufficient physical activity are essential for the healthy growth of children and adolescents and for obesity prevention. Data from the second wave of the population-based German Health Interview and Examination Survey for Children and Adolescents (KiGGS Wave 2; 2014–2017) were used to analyse the association between food intake and physical activity among 6- to 17-year-old children and adolescents (n = 9842). Physical exercise (PE) and recommended daily physical activity (RDPA) were assessed with self-administered questionnaires and food intake by a semi-quantitative food frequency questionnaire. Multivariable logistic regression was used to analyse the association between food group intake (dependent variable) and level of PE or RDPA. High levels of physical activity (PE or RDPA) were associated with higher consumption of juice, water, milk, dairy products, fruits, and vegetables among both boys and girls, and among boys with a higher intake of bread, potatoes/pasta/rice, meat, and cereals. Higher PE levels were also less likely to be associated with a high soft drink intake. High levels of RDPA were associated with high intake of energy-dense foods among boys, which was not observed for PE. This study indicates that school-aged children and adolescents with higher levels of physical activity consume more beneficial foods and beverages compared to those with lower physical activity levels.

Keywords: Physical activity; exercise; food intake; diet; children; adolescents; KiGGS

1. Introduction

A balanced diet and sufficient physical activity are essential for a healthy growth and development of children and adolescents and are important determinants of health throughout the life course. Unbalanced dietary patterns (with high amounts of highly processed and energy dense foods) are associated with unfavourable cardiometabolic risk factors (e.g., blood pressure, blood glucose, insulin levels, and lipid profile) among adolescents [1,2]. Higher levels of physical activity are associated with better physical, psychological, and cognitive health of children and adolescents [3], whereas a predominantly sedentary lifestyle is associated with less favourable levels of cardiometabolic risk factors [4]. In addition to genetic predisposition [5], dietary behaviour and physical activity are important determinants of obesity [6,7].

The prevalence of childhood obesity has significantly increased in recent years and is, therefore, a priority for health promotion and prevention policy and action [8]. Current data from KiGGS wave 2 (2014–2017) show that 15% of the 3- to 17-year-old children and adolescents in Germany are overweight; almost 6% are obese [9]. Compared to the KiGGS baseline survey (2003–2006), the prevalence of overweight and obesity has not increased further in the last ten years among children and adolescents, but remains at a high level [9].

There are only a few studies that have comprehensively analysed the relation between the two key components of obesity development, dietary behaviour, and physical activity in children and adolescents. In two studies, one conducted among high school students in the USA and the other among 12-year-old children from France, a higher level of physical activity is associated with a higher intake of fruits and vegetables [10,11]. The international study ISCOLE among 9- to 12-year-old children from 12 countries showed that achieving a higher number of specific physical activity recommendations (for sedentary behaviour, physical activity, and sleep duration) is associated with a more preferable dietary pattern [12]. A review of several studies investigating obesogenic behaviours using cluster analyses indicated that diet, physical activity, and sedentary behaviour cluster in both unhealthy and healthy ways and that cluster patterns differ by sex, age, and socioeconomic status [6].

Most existing studies investigating the relation between physical activity and dietary behaviour cover just a small age-range of childhood and do not indicate how the intake of single food items differ by the level of physical activity. Indicators of the current physical activity levels, as well as consumption of particular food items of children and adolescents have been described for Germany [13,14]. However, the interrelationship between these two behavioural aspects has not yet been analysed.

The aim of this study is to analyse whether children and adolescents aged 6 to 17 years with higher levels of physical activity differ in their food intake compared to those with lower levels of physical activity.

2. Materials and Methods

2.1. Study Design and Study Population

KiGGS (German Health Interview and Examination Survey for Children and Adolescents) is part of the Federal Health Monitoring System of the Robert Koch Institute and consists of regularly conducted representative cross-sectional surveys among children and adolescents aged between 0 and 17 years living in Germany. KiGGS Wave 2 was conducted between 2014 and 2017. The design and methodology of KiGGS Wave 2 have been described in detail elsewhere [15,16]. In brief, the study sample was drawn from the German resident population aged 0 to 17 years using a two-stage cluster sampling approach. Firstly, 167 sample points were randomly selected proportional to the population densities in the federal states and community sizes within the Federal Republic of Germany. Secondly, within each sample point age-stratified samples of individuals were randomly selected from the local population registries. In total, 15,023 children and adolescents (7538 girls; 7,485 boys) participated in the cross-sectional survey of KiGGS Wave 2.

KiGGS Wave 2 was conducted in accordance with the Declaration of Helsinki, and the protocol was approved by the Federal Commissioner for Data Protection and Freedom of Information and by the ethics committee of the Hannover Medical School (Number 2275–2014). A written informed consent was obtained by parents and all participants aged 14 years and above before data collection.

2.2. Data Collection and Aggregation

In KiGGS, parents (or legal guardians) of the 3- to 10-year-olds completed self-administered questionnaires which provided information on their children's health and health behaviour (e.g., food intake and physical activity). Similar questionnaires were filled in by 11- to 17-year-olds themselves.

2.3. Food Intake

KiGGS Wave 2 included a self-administered semi-quantitative food frequency questionnaire (FFQ) to assess the consumption of selected food items [17]. The FFQ starts with a short written introduction about the questionnaire. Participants are instructed how to report the frequency and number of standard portions which were consumed during the last four weeks. An illustration is provided as an example to report two slices of bread that were eaten twice a day during the past four weeks. A further illustration shows how to make corrections in case this is necessary. Finally, a telephone number was provided for further questions about the completion of the questionnaire. The 11- to 17-year-old participants or parents of 3- to 10-year-old participants were asked about the food items they or their children had consumed 'during the last four weeks'. The questionnaire contained 48 food items for younger participants and 53 food items (including alcoholic beverages) for those aged 11 years and above. First, the consumption frequency of each food item was assessed with the question: 'How often did your child/did you eat/drink food/drink X?' and in most cases, examples of the particular food items were given. Answer categories were: 'never', 'once per month', '2–3 times per month', '1–2 times per week', '3–4 times per week', '5–6 times per week', 'daily', '2 times per day', '3 times per day', '4–5 times per day', 'more than five times per day'. Second, portion size information was obtained by questions following the pattern: 'If your child/you eat/drink food/drink X, how much does your child/do you usually eat/drink?' To support portion size estimation, pictures were included as a reference for predefined portion sizes. In each case, five answering categories were given, which varied depending on the food item. These were, for instance, '$\frac{1}{2}$ a glass (or less)', '1 glass', '2 glasses', '3 glasses', and '4 glasses (or more)'. For some food items, a specific aspect of the food consumption was inquired, such as the dilution ratio of juice and water.

For the presented analyses, the information on food consumption frequencies was transformed into the number of occasions of consumption of each food over a four-week period (28 days). The portions were converted into grams or millilitres. For each food item, the estimated amount consumed per day was obtained by multiplying the converted food consumption frequency and the portion amount, and dividing this by 28. The following food groups were used for the analyses, partly constructed by summarising the amounts of multiple food items (in parenthesis): Soft drinks (sugar-sweetened soft drinks; reduced calorie soft drinks), juices (fruit juices; vegetable juices), water, milk, dairy products (cream cheese; cheese; quark, yoghurt or soured milk), fast food (hamburger or doner kebab; grilled sausages; French fries; pizza), fruits (fresh fruits; processed fruits), vegetables (raw vegetables; legumes; cooked vegetables), bread (whole-grain bread or rolls; brown or mixed bread or rolls; white bread or rolls), potatoes, noodles & rice (cooked potatoes; fried potatoes; noodles; rice), meat (poultry; red meat; meat portion in hamburger or doner kebab; grilled sausages; sausage; ham), breakfast cereals (corn flakes; muesli), savoury snacks (potato crisps; salty snacks or crackers), confectionery (cakes, tartes or sweet pastries; biscuits; chocolate; sweets; ice cream; sweet spreads). Based on the consumed amounts of these food groups, participants were ranked into quintiles. Quintiles were calculated separately for boys and girls in the age groups 6–10, 11–13 and 14–17 years in order to account for gender- and age-related differences in energy and nutrient requirements. For each food group, the top two quintiles (40%) were assigned to the category 'high intake'. A table with the threshold values for the category 'high intake' can be found in the Supplemental Table S1.

2.4. Recommended Daily Physical Activity (RDPA) and Physical Exercise (PE)

In KiGGS Wave 2, RDPA and PE information was also obtained using self-administered questionnaires. The indicator RDPA describes the amount of days per week with physical activity (light to vigorous intensity) of at least 60 min. To assess RDPA, participants were asked 'How many days of a normal week are you/is your child physically active for at least 60 min on a single day?' The eight answer categories ranged from 'Seven days' to 'None'. The answers were assigned to the categories 'low' (one hour/day on less than 3 days/week), 'medium' (one hour/day on 3 to 5 days/week) and 'high' (one 1 hour/day on 6 to 7 days/week). The instrument was initially used to verify if participants met the 'at least 60 min daily physical activity' criteria recommended by the World Health Organization [18] and was adapted from Prochaska and colleagues [19] A validation study showed moderate test-retest reliability with a Kappa coefficient of 0.54 and a significant Spearman correlation coefficient of 0.24 for validity when compared with objectively measured physical activity by accelerometers [20]. The indicator PE should include sports activities like running or playing soccer. To obtain information on PE, participants were asked whether they participate in physical exercises, adding that this referred to all kinds of sports regardless if it was within a sports club or not. Physical education at school should not be included. The question could be answered with 'Yes' or 'No'. Participants who answered 'Yes' were consecutively asked how many minutes or hours they usually participate in physical exercises per week. The data on PE was used to assign the persons to categories 'low' (less than one hour of sport/week), 'medium' (1–3 h/week) and 'high' (more than 3 h/week).

2.5. Socioeconomic Status (SES)

In the KiGGS study, an index is used to measure parental socioeconomic status (SES), which is based on information about the parents' education, their occupational status and income [21,22]. A detailed description of the construction of the socioeconomic variables and the SES index can be found elsewhere [22]. Based on the SES index, individuals were categorized into 'low', 'medium' and 'high' SES.

2.6. Body Mass Index (BMI)

In the physical examination component, standardized measurements of body height and weight were obtained [9]. The body mass index (BMI) was calculated from body weight divided by the square of body height. BMI percentiles were modelled as a function of age (BMI-for-age) and transformed to a standard normal distribution (BMI-for-age z-score).

2.7. Data Analysis

Since preschool children have a considerably different physical activity and food consumption pattern from older children, 3- to 5-year-olds were not included in the present analysis. The current analysis was, therefore, restricted to 11,014 participants aged 6 to 17 years (5582 girls and 5432 boys).

Food consumption information was completely set to missing for some cases in the original dataset ($n = 38$). This was done if the frequency answers contained more than 20 missing values or if the calculated total intake was implausibly high (total daily amount of beverages exceeded 15 litres, of solid foods exceeded 10 kg or if there was a combination of the amount of beverages exceeding 4 L and solid foods exceeding 6 kg). In the current analysis, participants with missing information on at least one of the aggregated food intake variables were excluded from the current analysis ($n = 1172$, 10.6%). The sample for multivariable regression analyses among boys comprises 4472 participants for PE and 4557 participants for RDPA, after excluding participants with missing information on PE, RDPA or SES. Among girls, the sample for the multivariable regression comprises 5016 for PE and 5073 participants for RDPA.

Statistical analyses were conducted using Stata SE 15 (StataCorp. 2017. Stata Statistical Software: Release 15. StataCorp LLC, College Station, TX, USA). All analyses were performed with survey design procedures to adjust for the clustered sampling design. A weighting factor was applied to correct deviations within the sample from the German population with regard to age, gender, federal state (as of 31.12.2015), nationality (as of 21.12.2014), and the parents' level of education (Mikrozensus 2013). Multivariable logistic regression was used to analyse if medium and high versus low RDPA and PE were associated with food intake variables. Odds ratios (OR) were reported to describe the odds of having a high intake of a food depending on the variables PE and RDPA. The associations were stepwise adjusted for age (model 1) and parental SES (model 2). In a sensitivity analysis, BMI-for-age z-scores were added to model 2. The criterion for statistical significance was set at $p < 0.05$.

3. Results

Demographic characteristics and physical activity behaviour of the study sample stratified by sex, age, and SES are shown in Table 1. PE was low among 25.7%, medium among 36.7% and high among 37.6% of the participants, while RDPA was low among 25.2%, medium among 47.8% and high among

27.0% of the participants. Boys more often had a high level of PE and RDPA than girls. The proportion of boys and girls with a high PE level was higher among older age groups, whereas the proportion with a high RDPA level was lower among older age groups. The proportion of boys and girls with a high PE level increased with increasing SES, while there were no statistically significant differences in the frequency of high RDPA levels by SES. However, the proportion of participants with low RDPA significantly decreased with increasing SES.

3.1. Binary Associations

A higher PE level was significantly associated with a high intake of water, dairy products, fruits, and vegetables in boys and girls, and a high intake of juice and breakfast cereals in boys (Table 2). A medium or high PE level was less often associated with a high soft drink intake than a low PE level among boys and girls. Furthermore, a low PE level was more often associated with a higher meat intake for girls compared to medium or high PE level, while a low PE level was associated with a high intake of savoury snacks for both genders.

Higher RDPA was significantly associated with a high intake of fruits and vegetables among boys and girls. Furthermore, among boys, higher levels of RDPA were associated with a high intake of water, milk, dairy products, bread, potatoes/pasta/noodles, breakfast cereals, and confectionery (Table 2). Girls with a low RDPA level more often had a high intake of soft drinks, savoury snacks, and confectionery than girls with a medium or high RDPA level.

3.2. Multivariable Analyses

Almost all significant associations in the binary analyses for PE remained significant in the logistic regression analyses after adjustment for age and SES (model 2; Table 3). Exceptions were the associations of PE with water and with meat among girls. Furthermore, the association of PE and a high intake of breakfast cereals and savoury snacks among girls became significant after adjusting for age, but did not remain significant after further adjustment for SES.

For boys, a high compared to a low level of PE was less likely associated with a high soft drink intake (OR 0.7), but was more likely associated with a high intake of juice (OR 1.3), water (OR 1.3), dairy products (OR 1.5), fruits (OR 1.9), vegetables (OR 1.7), and breakfast cereals (OR 1.5) (Table 3). For girls, a high compared to a low level of PE was less likely associated with a high intake of soft drinks (OR 0.7), and more likely associated a high intake of dairy products (OR 1.2), fruits (OR 1.6), and vegetables (OR 1.5).

Many binary associations of RDPA with a certain food group intake remained significant in the multivariable analyses (Table 4). Among boys, the non-significant association observed for a high intake of juice and meat with higher levels of RDPA became significant after adjustment for age and SES. For girls, the significant binary association between RDPA and high soft drink intake did not remain significant after adjusting for age and SES, whereas the associations between RDPA and high intake of juice, water, milk, and dairy products became significant.

For boys, a high compared to a low RDPA was more likely associated with a high intake of juice (OR 1.3), water (OR 1.4), milk (OR 1.7), dairy products (OR 1.4), fruits (OR 2.1), vegetables (OR 1.5) bread (OR 1.5), potatoes/pasta/rice (OR 1.4), meat (OR 1.3), breakfast cereals (OR 1.3), and confectionery (OR 1.6) for boys (Table 4). For girls, a high compared to a low RDPA was more likely associated with a high intake of water (OR 1.3), milk (OR 1.3), dairy products (OR 1.4), fruits (OR 1.9), and vegetables (OR 1.5). A medium compared to a low RDPA was less likely associated with a high intake of savoury snacks (OR 0.8) and confectionery (OR 0.8), and more likely associated with a high intake of juice (OR 1.3) for girls.

The inclusion of BMI-for-age z-scores into model 2 did not alter the relation between PE nor RDPA and food intake (data not shown).

Table 1. Demographic characteristics for categories of physical activity behaviour of the study sample ($N = 9842$).

| | n | Total | | Sex | | | | Age (Years) | | | | | | Socioeconomic Status [a] | | | | | |
		%	95% CI	Boys %	95% CI	Girls %	95% CI	6-10 %	95% CI	11-13 %	95% CI	14-17 %	95% CI	Low %	95% CI	Medium %	95% CI	High %	95% CI
n		100.0	9842	47.2	4646	52.8	5196	32.0	3146	35.2	3464	32.8	3232	12.2	1184	62.3	6065	25.5	2480
Physical exercise [b]																			
Low	2295	25.7	24.4–27.0	22.1	20.4–23.8	29.2	27.4–31.1	23.5	21.1–26.0	23.1	21.1–25.2	29.9	27.7–32.1	44.2	40.4–48.1	24.0	22.6–25.6	12.9	11.3–14.7
Medium	3639	36.7	35.3–38.1	32.5	30.7–34.3	40.7	38.8–42.8	48.3	45.7–50.8	36.4	34.1–38.8	27.3	25.5–29.2	30.4	27.1–34.0	37.6	36.0–39.4	40.0	38.0–42.2
High	3654	37.6	36.2–39.1	45.4	43.2–47.7	30.1	28.3–31.9	28.3	26.3–30.4	40.5	38.0–43.1	42.9	40.8–45.0	25.3	22.5–28.5	38.3	36.5–40.1	47.0	44.5–49.6
Recommended daily physical activity [c]																			
Low	2305	25.2	23.9–26.6	20.3	18.5–22.2	30.1	28.3–31.9	17.1	15.4–18.9	22.8	20.9–24.9	34.2	32.1–36.4	34.1	30.3–38.2	24.1	22.7–25.7	19.7	17.9–21.6
Medium	4786	47.8	46.4–49.2	48.8	46.9–50.6	46.9	44.9–49.0	44.9	42.5–47.3	50.0	47.6–52.5	48.4	46.1–50.6	40.3	36.4–44.2	48.8	47.0–50.5	52.4	50.0–54.8
High	2639	27.0	25.6–28.4	31.0	29.2–32.9	23.0	21.3–24.9	38.0	35.6–40.6	27.1	24.8–29.6	17.4	15.8–19.2	25.6	22.5–29.1	27.1	25.6–28.7	27.9	26.1–29.9

[a] 113 missing; [b] 254 missing; low: < 1 h/week, medium: 1–3 h/week, high: >3 h/week; [c] 112 missing; low: <3 days/week 1 h/day, medium: 3–5 days/week 1 h/day, high: 6–7 days/week 1 h/day; CI—confidence interval.

Table 2. Percentage with high intake of specific foods among 6- to 17-year-old children and adolescents in total and stratified by physical activity variables (binary associations).

High Intake		Total	Physical Exercise [a]				Recommended Daily Physical Activity [b]			
		%	Low %	Medium %	High %	P*	Low %	Medium %	High %	P*
Soft drinks	boys	39.7	48.2	36.3	37.2	<0.001	42.4	37.4	40.5	0.128
	girls	38.0	47.3	33.2	33.9	<0.001	42.0	35.3	36.0	0.008
	total	38.8	47.7	34.6	35.8	<0.001	42.2	36.3	38.6	0.003
Juice	boys	34.5	31.1	33.8	37.3	0.012	31.5	34.9	36.2	0.210
	girls	35.5	32.4	36.0	36.0	0.223	33.2	37.1	35.2	0.231
	total	35.0	31.9	35.0	36.8	0.014	32.5	36.0	35.8	0.092
Water	boys	39.7	36.8	37.0	42.1	0.016	35.9	39.2	42.8	0.045
	girls	33.5	33.7	31.1	36.5	0.042	32.2	32.9	36.7	0.118
	total	36.5	35.0	33.7	39.8	<0.001	33.7	36.1	40.2	<0.001
Milk	boys	25.6	25.5	24.7	27.1	0.496	21.2	25.7	28.3	0.015
	girls	29.9	30.9	27.8	32.1	0.124	30.8	29.6	29.4	0.776
	total	27.8	28.6	26.4	29.1	0.170	27.0	27.6	28.7	0.557
Dairy products	boys	39.0	33.2	38.6	42.5	0.001	33.8	39.7	41.1	0.013
	girls	39.3	36.8	38.6	43.1	0.021	36.0	40.1	41.9	0.057
	total	39.1	35.3	38.6	42.7	<0.001	35.1	39.9	41.5	<0.001
Fast food	boys	40.0	36.6	39.0	41.0	0.220	39.8	40.1	39.2	0.928
	girls	41.4	43.6	40.4	39.8	0.219	41.3	42.0	39.6	0.614
	total	40.7	40.7	39.8	40.5	0.852	40.7	41.0	39.4	0.628
Fruits	boys	36.0	27.4	33.5	41.9	<0.001	24.3	37.7	41.3	<0.001
	girls	37.1	33.5	35.0	43.9	<0.001	30.6	38.5	41.7	<0.001
	total	36.5	30.9	34.4	42.7	<0.001	28.1	38.1	41.5	<0.001
Vegetables	boys	38.4	31.0	35.6	44.1	<0.001	32.1	38.9	41.9	0.001
	girls	40.1	35.3	38.7	47.6	<0.001	34.7	42.0	43.8	<0.001
	total	39.3	33.5	37.4	45.5	<0.001	33.7	40.5	42.7	<0.001
Bread	boys	37.4	39.3	34.7	37.2	0.168	33.5	36.6	40.9	0.016
	girls	38.8	39.7	38.5	37.5	0.689	36.9	37.9	41.5	0.180
	total	38.1	39.5	36.8	37.3	0.295	35.5	37.2	41.1	0.008

Table 2. *Cont.*

High Intake		Total	Physical Exercise [a]				Recommended Daily Physical Activity [b]			
		%	Low %	Medium %	High %	P*	Low %	Medium %	High %	P*
Potatoes/pasta/rice	boys	38.5	36.7	37.2	39.7	0.417	35.6	36.8	42.6	0.013
	girls	39.2	40.5	38.4	38.6	0.596	37.7	40.6	37.5	0.309
	total	38.8	38.9	37.9	39.2	0.663	36.9	38.7	40.4	0.174
Meat	boys	39.8	37.6	38.9	41.1	0.361	37.7	38.6	42.3	0.172
	girls	41.3	45.4	38.9	40.0	0.013	42.2	40.0	42.3	0.438
	total	40.6	42.1	38.9	40.7	0.162	40.4	39.3	42.3	0.159
Breakfast cereals	boys	36.8	31.2	34.0	41.9	<0.001	32.2	38.1	37.7	0.042
	girls	39.3	36.4	39.2	41.6	0.113	37.3	39.3	42.4	0.104
	total	38.0	34.2	37.0	41.8	<0.001	35.3	38.7	39.7	0.020
Savoury snacks	boys	41.0	43.3	39.9	40.1	0.417	40.8	40.9	40.8	0.999
	girls	41.2	44.5	40.0	39.1	0.080	45.0	38.4	41.4	0.011
	total	41.1	44.0	40.0	39.7	0.033	43.3	39.7	41.1	0.098
Confectionery	boys	35.2	31.4	34.2	37.0	0.109	30.7	34.4	39.0	0.009
	girls	40.6	43.9	39.6	40.1	0.143	44.3	37.5	42.8	0.002
	total	37.9	38.6	37.2	38.2	0.719	38.9	35.9	40.6	0.011

[a] n = 9488; boys: n = 4472, girls: n = 5016; low: <1 h/week, medium: 1–3 h/week, high: >3 h/week; [b] n = 9630, boys: n = 4557, girls: n = 5073; low: <3 days/week 1 h/day, medium: 3–5 days/week 1 h/day, high: 6–7 days/week 1 h/day; * P-values of test for differences between groups (chi-square).

Table 3. Results of logistic regression analyses between food intake and physical exercise [a].

High intake of Food Group		Boys (n = 4472) Physical Exercise Level		Girls (n = 5016) Physical Exercise Level	
		Medium	High	Medium	High
		OR (95% CI)	OR (95% CI)	OR (95% CI)	OR (95% CI)
Soft drinks	Model [1]	**0.6 (0.5–0.8)**	**0.6 (0.5–0.8)**	**0.6 (0.5–0.7)**	**0.6 (0.5–0.7)**
	Model [2]	**0.7 (0.6–0.9)**	**0.7 (0.6–0.9)**	**0.7 (0.5–0.8)**	**0.7 (0.6–0.8)**
Juice	Model [1]	1.2 (1.0–1.4)	**1.3 (1.1–1.6)**	1.2 (1.0–1.6)	1.2 (1.0–1.5)
	Model [2]	1.2 (0.9–1.4)	**1.3 (1.0–1.5)**	1.2 (1.0–1.6)	1.2 (1.0–1.5)
Water	Model [1]	1.0 (0.8–1.2)	1.2 (1.0–1.5)	0.9 (0.7–1.1)	1.1 (0.9–1.4)
	Model [2]	1.1 (0.9–1.3)	**1.3 (1.1–1.6)**	0.9 (0.8–1.1)	1.2 (1.0–1.5)
Milk	Model [1]	1.0 (0.8–1.3)	1.0 (0.8–1.4)	1.0 (0.8–1.2)	1.1 (0.9–1.3)
	Model [2]	1.0 (0.8–1.3)	1.0 (0.8–1.4)	1.0 (0.8–1.3)	1.1 (0.9–1.4)
Dairy products	Model [1]	**1.3 (1.0–1.6)**	**1.5 (1.2–1.8)**	1.1 (0.9–1.3)	**1.3 (1.1–1.6)**
	Model [2]	**1.3 (1.0–1.7)**	**1.5 (1.2–1.9)**	1.1 (0.9–1.3)	**1.2 (1.0–1.5)**
Fast food	Model [1]	1.1 (0.9–1.4)	1.2 (1.0–1.5)	0.9 (0.7–1.0)	0.9 (0.7–1.1)
	Model [2]	1.2 (0.9–1.5)	1.2 (1.0–1.5)	1.0 (0.8–1.1)	0.9 (0.8–1.2)
Fruits	Model [1]	1.3 (1.0–1.7)	**2.0 (1.5–2.5)**	1.1 (0.9–1.4)	**1.6 (1.3–1.9)**
	Model [2]	1.2 (1.0–1.6)	**1.9 (1.5–2.4)**	1.1 (0.9–1.4)	**1.6 (1.3–1.9)**
Vegetables	Model [1]	1.2 (1.0–1.6)	**1.7 (1.4–2.2)**	1.2 (1.0–1.4)	**1.7 (1.4–2.0)**
	Model [2]	1.2 (0.9–1.5)	**1.7 (1.3–2.1)**	1.0 (0.8–1.3)	**1.5 (1.2–1.8)**
Bread	Model [1]	0.9 (0.7–1.1)	0.9 (0.7–1.1)	1.0 (0.8–1.2)	0.9 (0.7–1.1)
	Model [2]	0.9 (0.7–1.1)	0.9 (0.8–1.1)	1.0 (0.8–1.2)	0.9 (0.8–1.2)
Potatoes/pasta/rice	Model [1]	1.1 (0.8–1.4)	1.1 (0.9–1.4)	0.9 (0.8–1.1)	0.9 (0.8–1.1)
	Model [2]	1.1 (0.8–1.3)	1.1 (0.9–1.4)	1.0 (0.8–1.1)	0.9 (0.8–1.2)
Meat	Model [1]	1.1 (0.9–1.4)	1.1 (0.9–1.4)	**0.8 (0.7–1.0)**	**0.8 (0.7–1.0)**
	Model [2]	1.1 (0.9–1.5)	1.2 (1.0–1.5)	0.8 (0.7–1.0)	0.9 (0.7–1.1)
Breakfast cereals	Model [1]	1.2 (0.9–1.5)	**1.6 (1.2–2.0)**	1.1 (0.9–1.4)	**1.2 (1.0–1.6)**
	Model [2]	1.1 (0.9–1.4)	**1.5 (1.2–1.8)**	1.1 (0.9–1.3)	1.2 (1.0–1.5)
Savoury snacks	Model [1]	0.9 (0.7–1.1)	0.9 (0.7–1.1)	0.8 (0.7–1.0)	**0.8 (0.6–1.0)**
	Model [2]	1.0 (0.7–1.2)	1.0 (0.8–1.2)	0.9 (0.7–1.1)	0.9 (0.7–1.1)
Confectionery	Model [1]	1.2 (0.9–1.5)	1.2 (1.0–1.6)	0.8 (0.7–1.0)	0.9 (0.7–1.0)
	Model [2]	1.2 (0.9–1.5)	1.3 (1.0–1.6)	0.9 (0.7–1.1)	0.9 (0.7–1.1)

[1] Model adjusted for age; [2] Model adjusted for age and socioeconomic status; [a] low: <1 h/week (reference group), medium: 1–3 h/week, high: >3 h/week; OR—odds ratio; CI—confidence interval; bold: The odds ratio is significantly different from 1 (reference is low PE with $p < 0.05$).

Nutrients **2019**, *11*, 1060

Table 4. Results of logistic regression analyses between food intake and recommended daily physical activity [a].

High intake of Food Group		Boys (n = 4557) Daily Physical Activity Level		Girls (n = 5073) Daily Physical Activity Level	
		Medium	High	Medium	High
		OR (95% CI)	OR (95% CI)	OR (95% CI)	OR (95% CI)
Soft drinks	Model [1]	0.8 (0.7–1.0)	1.0 (0.8–1.2)	**0.8 (0.6–1.0)**	0.8 (0.7–1.1)
	Model [2]	0.9 (0.7–1.1)	1.0 (0.8–1.3)	0.8 (0.7–1.0)	0.9 (0.7–1.1)
Juice	Model [1]	1.2 (0.9–1.5)	**1.3 (1.0–1.6)**	**1.3 (1.0–1.5)**	1.2 (1.0–1.6)
	Model [2]	1.2 (0.9–1.5)	**1.3 (1.0–1.6)**	**1.3 (1.1–1.6)**	**1.3 (1.0–1.6)**
Water	Model [1]	1.2 (0.9–1.4)	**1.4 (1.1–1.8)**	1.0 (0.9–1.2)	**1.3 (1.0–1.6)**
	Model [2]	1.2 (1.0–1.5)	**1.4 (1.1–1.8)**	1.1 (0.9–1.3)	**1.3 (1.0–1.6)**
Milk	Model [1]	**1.3 (1.0–1.7)**	**1.6 (1.2–2.2)**	1.1 (0.9–1.4)	**1.3 (1.0–1.7)**
	Model [2]	**1.3 (1.0–1.7)**	**1.7 (1.3–2.2)**	1.1 (0.9–1.4)	**1.3 (1.0–1.7)**
Dairy products	Model [1]	**1.3 (1.1–1.6)**	**1.4 (1.1–1.8)**	**1.2 (1.0–1.5)**	**1.4 (1.1–1.7)**
	Model [2]	**1.3 (1.1–1.6)**	**1.4 (1.1–1.8)**	**1.2 (1.0–1.5)**	**1.4 (1.1–1.7)**
Fast food	Model [1]	1.0 (0.8–1.3)	1.0 (0.8–1.3)	1.0 (0.9–1.3)	0.9 (0.8–1.2)
	Model [2]	1.0 (0.8–1.3)	1.0 (0.8–1.3)	1.1 (0.9–1.3)	1.0 (0.8–1.2)
Fruits	Model [1]	**1.9 (1.5–2.3)**	**2.1 (1.7–2.7)**	**1.5 (1.3–1.9)**	**1.9 (1.6–2.4)**
	Model [2]	**1.8 (1.5–2.3)**	**2.1 (1.6–2.7)**	**1.5 (1.3–1.8)**	**1.9 (1.6–2.3)**
Vegetables	Model [1]	**1.4 (1.1–1.7)**	**1.6 (1.2–2.0)**	**1.4 (1.2–1.7)**	**1.6 (1.2–2.0)**
	Model [2]	**1.3 (1.1–1.6)**	**1.5 (1.2–2.0)**	**1.3 (1.1–1.6)**	**1.5 (1.2–1.9)**
Bread	Model [1]	1.2 (1.0–1.4)	**1.5 (1.2–1.8)**	1.1 (0.9–1.3)	1.2 (1.0–1.6)
	Model [2]	1.2 (1.0–1.5)	**1.5 (1.2–1.9)**	1.1 (0.9–1.3)	1.3 (1.0–1.6)
Potatoes/pasta/rice	Model [1]	1.1 (0.8–1.3)	**1.4 (1.1–1.8)**	1.2 (1.0–1.4)	1.1 (0.9–1.3)
	Model [2]	1.1 (0.8–1.3)	**1.4 (1.1–1.8)**	1.2 (1.0–1.5)	1.1 (0.9–1.3)
Meat	Model [1]	1.0 (0.8–1.3)	1.3 (1.0–1.6)	1.0 (0.8–1.1)	1.1 (0.9–1.4)
	Model [2]	1.1 (0.9–1.3)	1.3 (1.0–1.6)	1.0 (0.8–1.2)	1.1 (0.9–1.4)
Breakfast cereals	Model [1]	**1.3 (1.1–1.6)**	**1.4 (1.1–1.7)**	1.1 (0.9–1.3)	1.2 (1.0–1.5)
	Model [2]	1.3 (1.0–1.6)	**1.3 (1.1–1.6)**	1.1 (0.9–1.3)	1.2 (1.0–1.5)
Savoury snacks	Model [1]	1.0 (0.8–1.2)	1.0 (0.8–1.3)	**0.8 (0.6–0.9)**	0.9 (0.7–1.1)
	Model [2]	1.1 (0.9–1.3)	1.1 (0.9–1.4)	0.8 (0.7–1.0)	0.9 (0.7–1.1)
Confectionery	Model [1]	1.2 (0.9–1.5)	**1.6 (1.2–2.0)**	**0.8 (0.6–0.9)**	0.9 (0.8–1.1)
	Model [2]	1.2 (0.9–1.5)	**1.6 (1.2–2.0)**	**0.8 (0.6–0.9)**	1.0 (0.8–1.2)

[1] Model adjusted for age; [2] Model adjusted for age and socioeconomic status; [a] low: <3 days/week 1 h/day (reference group), medium: 3–5 days/week 1 h/day, high: 6–7 days/week 1 h/day; OR—odds ratio; CI—confidence interval; bold: The odds ratio is significantly different from 1 (reference is low RDPA with $p < 0.05$).

4. Discussion

Adequate levels of physical activity and a balanced diet are important requirements for an optimal physiological and cognitive development, as well as for the maintenance of good physical conditions and health in general. A good balance between physical activity and diet may also help to prevent or reduce the occurrence of obesity [23]. For a holistic prevention approach, it is important to understand and take into account that these health behaviours may interact with each other. The aim of the current study was, therefore, to analyse differences in intake of various food groups between low, medium and high physical activity behaviour groups among children and adolescents. To our knowledge, this study is the first study to investigate the associations between two different aspects of physical activity behaviour and 14 different food groups based on representative data from children and adolescents living in Germany. These analyses among boys and girls aged 6 to 17 years indicate that higher physical activity levels are more often associated with a high intake of predominantly preferable foods (with some exceptions) and a less frequent high intake of some less beneficial foods. For example, boys and girls with a high RDPA level were twice as likely to consume fruits in high amounts and had 50% higher odds to consume vegetables in high amounts than those with a lower RDPA. Furthermore, the odds ratio of a high soft drink intake was 30% lower in children and adolescents with a high compared to a low PE level.

The more often observed high intake of several food groups among children and adolescents with higher physical activity levels (PE and RDPA), some of which are dairy products, fruits, and vegetables, may partly be explained by a higher energy requirement due to a higher physical activity. A derivation of accurate estimates of the energy intake is not possible due to the relatively short food frequency questionnaire used in KiGGS Wave 2. Nevertheless, a high RDPA level was more often associated with a high intake for many food groups for boys, which may suggest a higher energy intake for this group. Among girls, high intakes of some food groups, i.e., for water, fruits, and vegetables, were associated with higher RDPA levels, although these are not energy-dense foods. Overall, this suggests that differences in energy needs may not explain all observed differences in food intake. The observed association of high intake of water and higher physical activity levels may be related to higher transpiration losses during enhanced physical activity. The authors of a review summarised that the relation between energy expenditure caused by physical activity and energy intake in children and adolescents are still inconclusive due to a lack of data [24]. However, it was observed that nutritional adaptation occurs as a response to physical activity, not only to compensate for the expended energy [24,25]. These adaptations may be changes in food choices as well as in appetite sensation, depending on duration, intensity, and type of physical activity [26,27]. Differences in duration, intensity and type of physical activity between boys and girls might also explain why, in this present analysis, more food groups were associated with physical activity in boys compared to girls. The higher levels of RDPA and PE among boys than girls [13] might have a stronger impact on their food choices. Furthermore, our results confirm that different types of physical activity are differently associated with a high consumption of food items: RDPA was more often associated with a high intake of individual foods compared to PE. Various reasons may lead to engagement in more PE or RDPA. These include body weight loss or maintenance, to gain muscle power, to improve body fitness, or physical skills as well as social aspects [28]. These purposes may differ between genders as well as for RDPA and PE, and could partly explain the observed differences in associations with food intake.

Studies comparing the intake of different food groups and physical activity in children and adolescents are rare. The observed higher fruit and vegetable consumption in children with higher physical activity is in line with studies among school-aged children in the USA and France [10,11]. In a representative sample of adolescents attending grade 9 to 12 in the USA, a higher fruit, vegetable, and soft drink consumption was associated with higher daily physical activity [10]. Regarding the soft drink intake, our study showed contradictory results: a lower soft drink intake was associated with a high PE level. There was no significant association observed between a high soft drink intake and RDPA. A study among 12-year-olds from France showed that the consumption of fruits, vegetables, and fruit juice was positively associated with organised physical activity [11]. In our study, in addition to the observed association with fruit and vegetable intake, fruit juice was also positively associated with PE and RDPA in boys and with RDPA in girls.

Most studies regarding physical activity and food intake in children summarise the assessed food intake into the categories 'healthy dietary pattern' and 'unhealthy dietary pattern'. If we apply these categories to the food groups presented in our study, a high intake of water, fruits, and vegetables would be considered as components of a healthy dietary behaviour, whereas a high intake of soft drinks, fast food, savoury snacks, and confectionery would be unhealthy [29]. From this perspective, the current results suggest that a high PE level is more likely associated with a healthy food pattern, reflected by high intakes of fruit and vegetables and low intakes of soft drinks. High RDPA also seems to be associated with more beneficial intakes of fruits, vegetables, and drinking water. Additionally, high RDPA seems to be associated with higher intakes of energy-dense food groups and less beneficial food groups, like confectionery and meat, among boys. Among girls, higher RDPA was associated with a lower intake of savoury snacks and confectionery. The positive association between PE and a healthy food intake might be explained by a higher overall health consciousness which influences multiple health behaviours [30,31]. For younger children, the motivation of the parents and family to live a healthy lifestyle will be relevant rather than the individual preference [32].

The authors of a review about the clustering of physical activity, sedentary behaviour and diet in children and adolescents concluded that these behaviours show inconsistent clustering patterns, sometimes corresponding with healthy behaviours and sometimes not [6]. Two studies found a consistency in preferable physical activity and dietary behaviour which confirms our results. However, in a cluster analysis conducted with children and adolescents aged 11 to 17 years living in Germany no cluster with high scores in physical activity and healthy diet was observed [33].

Data of the International Study of Childhood Obesity, Lifestyle and the Environment (ISCOLE) were used to examine if meeting recommendations related to physical activity, screen-time and sleep ($\geq$60 min/day moderate-to-vigorous physical activity; $\leq$2 h/day screen time; 9 to 11 h/night sleep duration) were associated with dietary patterns among 9- to 11-year-old children from 12 different countries [12]. Results showed that a healthier diet was observed when more recommendations were met, which confirm partly a positive relation between sufficient physical activity and a healthy diet.

A strength of the study is that it is based on a large nationwide and representative sample of young persons living in Germany. In addition, the information on two different aspects of physical activity, as well as on the intake of many food groups, allows a broad analysis of the association between physical activity and food intake among children and adolescents. Our analyses have some limitations that should be considered. The assessment of physical activity and food intake was based on self-reports which is subject to recall and social desirability bias [34,35]. This may lead to overreporting of healthy behaviours (e.g., physical activity, intake of fruits, and vegetables) and an underreporting of unhealthy behaviours (e.g., intake of soft drinks, snacks, and sweets). The use of objective methods, such as activity monitors, may help to reduce such bias for physical activity. However, bias might still be present, since the measurement of specific physical activities by activity monitors is only possible in combination with a self-reported diary, and the consciousness of activity being measured may also alter actual behaviour [36]. In a free-living population setting, it is hardly possible to objectively measure dietary intake. The food frequency instrument used in this survey is not comprehensive and detailed enough to give a complete and precise overview of food consumption and energy intake. In addition, the specific information on food consumption and physical activity behaviour is gathered from parents for the younger children (up to the age of 11 years) and from those above 11 years themselves, which could have biased the results. Although this is inevitable because young children cannot give reliable information on major parts of the requested items, parents may also not have a complete overview of what their children eat (especially out of home) and how physically active they are. So for the different age groups the level of misreporting could be different. However, we constructed age-specific quintiles for the reported food intakes, so persons are ranked according to reported consumption relative to those within their age group. This may at least reduce in some extent the possible bias introduced by the responder. Furthermore, the association between physical activity and food intake may be confounded by other variables, which we have not considered for adjustment. We adjusted for age and SES because these dimensions could bias the association between physical activity and food intake. In a sensitivity analysis, we additionally adjusted for BMI-for-age z-scores. This, however, had no substantial impact on the regression results (data not shown). Due to the cross-sectional nature of the data, causal inferences cannot be derived. Finally, around 10% of the participants were excluded because of missing values in the analysed items which might have biased the results. These excluded participants were more often boys, younger children, and participants with lower SES.

5. Conclusions

The analysis of the association between RDPA and PE with food intake among school-aged children and adolescents indicates that higher levels of RDPA and PE are associated with more beneficial intakes of particular food items, such as a high fruit and vegetable intake and a lower soft drink intake. RDPA is additionally more often associated with high intakes of some energy-dense foods among boys, but not among girls. Detailed information on activity patterns and food intake can make a considerable contribution to focused primary prevention strategies which promote a healthy lifestyle of children and adolescents.

Supplementary Materials: The following are available online at http://www.mdpi.com/2072-6643/11/5/1060/s1, Table S1: Threshold values for high intake (top two quintiles) of specific foods in millilitre or gram per day.

Author Contributions: K.M. conducted the present analysis and drafted the manuscript. K.M., J.D.F., A.S. and G.B.M.M. conceptualised the present study and statistical analyses. K.M. and J.D.F. conducted the statistical analyses. A.S., A.K.-B., K.M., J.D.F. and G.B.M.M. were involved in the design and conduct of KiGGS Wave 2. G.B.M.M. was responsible for the construction and conversion of the food frequency questionnaire. All authors contributed to the writing, interpretation of findings, reviewed, edited and approved the final manuscript.

Funding: The KiGGS study was funded by the Federal Ministry of Health and the Robert Koch Institute.

Acknowledgments: First: we would like to thank the participants and their parents as well as everyone at the 167 study sites who provided us with space and active support on site. KiGGS Wave 2 could not have been conducted without the dedication of numerous colleagues at the Robert Koch Institute. We would especially like to thank the study teams for their excellent work and their exceptional commitment during the three-year data collection phase.

Conflicts of Interest: The authors declare that they have no competing interests.

References

1. Cunha, C.M.; Costa, P.R.F.; de Oliveira, L.P.M.; Queiroz, V.A.O.; Pitangueira, J.C.D.; Oliveira, A.M. Dietary patterns and cardiometabolic risk factors among adolescents: Systematic review and meta-analysis. *Br. J. Nutr.* **2018**, *119*, 859–879. [CrossRef]
2. Rocha, N.P.; Milagres, L.C.; Longo, G.Z.; Ribeiro, A.Q.; Novaes, J.F. Association between dietary pattern and cardiometabolic risk in children and adolescents: A systematic review. *J. Pediatr.* **2017**, *93*, 214–222. [CrossRef]
3. Poitras, V.J.; Gray, C.E.; Borghese, M.M.; Carson, V.; Chaput, J.P.; Janssen, I.; Katzmarzyk, P.T.; Pate, R.R.; Connor Gorber, S.; Kho, M.E.; et al. Systematic review of the relationships between objectively measured physical activity and health indicators in school-aged children and youth. *Appl. Physiol. Nutr. Metab.* **2016**, *41*, S197–S239. [CrossRef]
4. Carson, V.; Hunter, S.; Kuzik, N.; Gray, C.E.; Poitras, V.J.; Chaput, J.P.; Saunders, T.J.; Katzmarzyk, P.T.; Okely, A.D.; Connor Gorber, S.; et al. Systematic review of sedentary behaviour and health indicators in school-aged children and youth: An update. *Appl. Physiol. Nutr. Metab.* **2016**, *41*, S240–S265. [CrossRef]
5. Hebebrand, J.; Bammann, K.; Hinney, A. Genetic determinants of obesity. Current issues. *Bundesgesundheitsblatt Gesundheitsforschung Gesundheitsschutz* **2010**, *53*, 674–680. [CrossRef] [PubMed]

6. Leech, R.M.; McNaughton, S.A.; Timperio, A. The clustering of diet, physical activity and sedentary behavior in children and adolescents: A review. *Int. J. Behav. Nutr. Phys. Act.* **2014**, *11*, 4. [CrossRef] [PubMed]

7. Fisberg, M.; Maximino, P.; Kain, J.; Kovalskys, I. Obesogenic environment - intervention opportunities. *J. Pediatr.* **2016**, *92*, S30–S39. [CrossRef] [PubMed]

8. Commission on Ending Childhood Obesity. *Report of the Commission on Ending Childhood Obesity*; World Health Organization: Geneva, Switzerland, 2016.

9. Schienkiewitz, A.; Brettschneider, A.K.; Damerow, S.; Schaffrath Rosario, A. Overweight and obesity among children and adolescents in Germany. Results of the cross-sectional KiGGS Wave 2 study and trends. *J. Health Monit.* **2018**, *3*.

10. Lowry, R.; Michael, S.; Demissie, Z.; Kann, L.; Galuska, D.A. Associations of Physical Activity and Sedentary Behaviors with Dietary Behaviors among US High School Students. *J. Obes.* **2015**, *2015*, 876524. [CrossRef]

11. Platat, C.; Perrin, A.E.; Oujaa, M.; Wagner, A.; Haan, M.C.; Schlienger, J.L.; Simon, C. Diet and physical activity profiles in French preadolescents. *Br. J. Nutr.* **2006**, *96*, 501–507.

12. Thivel, D.; Tremblay, M.S.; Katzmarzyk, P.T.; Fogelholm, M.; Hu, G.; Maher, C.; Maia, J.; Olds, T.; Sarmiento, O.L.; Standage, M.; et al. Associations between meeting combinations of 24-hour movement recommendations and dietary patterns of children: A 12-country study. *Prev. Med.* **2019**, *118*, 159–165. [CrossRef]

13. Krug, S.; Finger, J.D.; Lange, C.; Richter, A.; Mensink, G.B. Sports and dietary behaviour among children and adolescents in Germany. Results of the cross-sectional KiGGS Wave 2 study and trends. *J. Health Monit.* **2018**, *3*. [CrossRef]

14. Finger, J.D.; Varnaccia, G.; Borrmann, A.; Lange, C.; Mensink, G.B. Physical activity among children and adolescents in Germany. Results of the cross-sectional KiGGS Wave 2 study and trends. *J. Health Monit.* **2018**, *3*.

15. Mauz, E.; Gößwald, A.; Kamtsiuris, P.; Hoffmann, R.; Lange, M.; von Schenck, U.; Allen, J.; Butschalowsky, H.; Frank, L.; Hölling, H.; et al. Neue Daten für Taten. Die Datenerhebung zur KiGGS Welle 2 ist beendet. *J. Health Monit.* **2017**, *2*.

16. Hoffmann, R.; Lange, M.; Butschalowsky, H.; Houben, R.; Schmich, P.; Allen, J.; Kuhnert, R.; Schaffrath Rosario, A.; Gößwald, A. Querschnitterhebung von KiGGS Welle 2 – Teilnehmendengewinnung, Response und Repräsentativität. *J. Health Monit.* **2018**, *3*.

17. Haftenberger, M.; Heuer, T.; Heidemann, C.; Kube, F.; Krems, C.; Mensink, G.B. Relative validation of a food frequency questionnaire for national health and nutrition monitoring. *Nutr. J.* **2010**, *9*, 36. [CrossRef]

18. World Health Organization. *Global Recommendations on Physical Activity for Health*; World Health Organization: Geneva, Switzerland, 2010.

19. Prochaska, J.J.; Sallis, J.F.; Long, B. A physical activity screening measure for use with adolescents in primary care. *Arch. Pediatr. Adolesc. Med.* **2001**, *155*, 554–559. [CrossRef]

20. Jekauc, D.; Wagner, M.O.; Kahlert, D.; Woll, A. Reliability and validity of MoMo-Physical-Activity-Questionnaire for Adolescents (MoMo-AFB). *Diagnostica* **2013**, *59*, 100–111. [CrossRef]

21. Lampert, T.; Müters, S.; Stolzenberg, H.; Kroll, L.E. Messung des soziöökonomischen Status in der KiGGS-Studie Erste Folgebefragung (KiGGS Welle 1). *Bundesgesundheitsblatt Gesundheitsforschung Gesundheitsschutz* **2014**, *57*, 762–770. [CrossRef]

22. Lampert, T.; Hoebel, J.; Kuntz, B.; Müters, S.; Kroll, L.E. Socioeconomic status and subjective social status measurement in KiGGS Wave 2. *J. Health Monit.* **2018**, *3*.

23. Sahoo, K.; Sahoo, B.; Choudhury, A.K.; Sofi, N.Y.; Kumar, R.; Bhadoria, A.S. Childhood obesity: Causes and consequences. *J. Family Med. Prim. Care* **2015**, *4*, 187–192. [CrossRef]

24. Thivel, D.; Aucouturier, J.; Doucet, E.; Saunders, T.J.; Chaput, J.P. Daily energy balance in children and adolescents. Does energy expenditure predict subsequent energy intake? *Appetite* **2013**, *60*, 58–64. [CrossRef]

25. King, N.A.; Horner, K.; Hills, A.P.; Byrne, N.M.; Wood, R.E.; Bryant, E.; Caudwell, P.; Finlayson, G.; Gibbons, C.; Hopkins, M.; et al. Exercise, appetite and weight management: Understanding the compensatory responses in eating behaviour and how they contribute to variability in exercise-induced weight loss. *Br. J. Sports Med.* **2012**, *46*, 315–322. [CrossRef]

26. Thivel, D.; Blundell, J.E.; Duche, P.; Morio, B. Acute exercise and subsequent nutritional adaptations: What about obese youths? *Sports Med. (Auckland, N.Z.)* **2012**, *42*, 607–613. [CrossRef]

27. Thivel, D.; Chaput, J.P. Are post-exercise appetite sensations and energy intake coupled in children and adolescents? *Sports Med. (Auckland, N.Z.)* **2014**, *44*, 735–741. [CrossRef]
28. Allender, S.; Cowburn, G.; Foster, C. Understanding participation in sport and physical activity among children and adults: A review of qualitative studies. *Health Educ. Res.* **2006**, *21*, 826–835. [CrossRef]
29. Moreno, L.A.; Rodriguez, G. Dietary risk factors for development of childhood obesity. *Curr. Opin. Clin. Nutr. Metab. Care* **2007**, *10*, 336–341. [CrossRef]
30. Birkenhead, K.L.; Slater, G. A Review of Factors Influencing Athletes' Food Choices. *Sports Med. (Auckland, N.Z.)* **2015**, *45*, 1511–1522. [CrossRef]
31. Elder, S.J.; Roberts, S.B. The effects of exercise on food intake and body fatness: A summary of published studies. *Nut. Rev.* **2007**, *65*, 1–19. [CrossRef]
32. Birch, L.L.; Davison, K.K. Family environmental factors influencing the developing behavioral controls of food intake and childhood overweight. *Pediatr. Clin. North Am.* **2001**, *48*, 893–907. [CrossRef]
33. Spengler, S.; Mess, F.; Mewes, N.; Mensink, G.B.; Woll, A. A cluster-analytic approach towards multidimensional health-related behaviors in adolescents: The MoMo-Study. *BMC Public Health* **2012**, *12*, 1128. [CrossRef]
34. Sallis, J.F.; Saelens, B.E. Assessment of physical activity by self-report: Status, limitations, and future directions. *Res. Q. Exerc. Sport* **2000**, *71*, S1–S14. [CrossRef]
35. Macdiarmid, J.; Blundell, J. Assessing dietary intake: Who, what and why of under-reporting. *Nutr. Res. Rev.* **1998**, *11*, 231–253. [CrossRef]
36. Baumann, S.; Gross, S.; Voigt, L.; Ullrich, A.; Weymar, F.; Schwaneberg, T.; Dorr, M.; Meyer, C.; John, U.; Ulbricht, S. Pitfalls in accelerometer-based measurement of physical activity: The presence of reactivity in an adult population. *Scand. J. Med. Sci. Sports* **2018**, *28*, 1056–1063. [CrossRef]

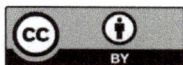

![nutrients logo] *nutrients*

MDPI

Article

Clustering of Multiple Energy Balance-Related Behaviors in School Children and Its Association with Overweight and Obesity—WHO European Childhood Obesity Surveillance Initiative (COSI 2015–2017)

Silvia Bel-Serrat [1,*], Ana Ojeda-Rodríguez [1,2], Mirjam M. Heinen [1], Marta Buoncristiano [3], Shynar Abdrakhmanova [4], Vesselka Duleva [5], Victoria Farrugia Sant'Angelo [6], Anna Fijałkowska [7], Tatjana Hejgaard [8], Constanta Huidumac [9], Jolanda Hyska [10], Enisa Kujundzic [11], Sanja Musić Milanović [12,13], Guljemal Ovezmyradova [14], Napoleón Pérez-Farinós [15], Ausra Petrauskiene [16], Ana Isabel Rito [17], Lela Shengelia [18], Radka Taxová Braunerová [19], Harry Rutter [20], Celine M. Murrin [1], Cecily C. Kelleher [1] and João Breda [3]

[1] National Nutrition Surveillance Centre, School of Public Health, Physiotherapy and Sports Science, University College Dublin, D4 Dublin, Ireland; aojeda.5@alumni.unav.es (A.O.-R.); mirjam.heinen@ucd.ie (M.M.H.); celine.murrin@ucd.ie (C.M.M.); cecily.kelleher@ucd.ie (C.C.K.)
[2] Department of Nutrition, Food Science and Physiology, University of Navarra, 31008 Pamplona, Spain
[3] Division of Noncommunicable Diseases and Promoting Health through the Life-course, WHO European Office for Prevention and Control of Noncommunicable Diseases, 125009 Moscow, Russia; marta.buoncristiano@gmail.com (M.B.); rodriguesdasilvabred@who.int (J.B.)
[4] National Center of Public Health, Ministry of Health of the Republic of Kazakhstan, 010000 Astana, Kazakhstan; shynar_a@mail.ru
[5] National Center of Public Health and Analyses, 1431 Sofia, Bulgaria; v.duleva@ncpha.government.bg
[6] Primary Health Care, 1940 Floriana, Malta; victoria.farrugia-santangelo@gov.mt
[7] Department of Cardiology, Institute of Mother and Child, 01-211 Warsaw, Poland; anna.fijalkowska@imid.med.pl
[8] Danish Health Authority,2300 København, Denmark; thv@sst.dk
[9] National Institute of Public Health, 050463 Bucharest, Romania; constanta.huidumac@insp.gov.ro
[10] Institute of Public Health, 1001 Tirana, Albania; lhyska2002@yahoo.it
[11] Institute of Public Health of Montenegro, 8100 Podgorica, Montenegro; enisa.kujundzic@ijzcg.me
[12] Croatian Institute of Public Health, 10000 Zagreb, Croatia; sanja.music@hzjz.hr
[13] School of Medicine, School of Public Health Andrija Štampar, University of Zagreb, 10000 Zagreb, Croatia
[14] WHO Country Office in Turkmenistan, 744000 Ashgabat, Turkmenistan; ovezmyradovag@who.int
[15] Spanish Agency for Food Safety and Nutrition (AESAN), 28071 Madrid, Spain; estrategianaos@mscbs.es
[16] Department of Preventive Medicine, Lithuanian University of Health Sciences, 44307 Kaunas, Lithuania; Ausra.Petrauskiene@lsmuni.lt
[17] National Institute of Health Doutor Ricardo Jorge, I.P., 1649-016 Lisbon, Portugal; ana.rito@insa.min-saude.pt
[18] National Center for Disease Control and Public Health of Georgia, 0186 Tbilisi, Georgia; lelasheng@gmail.com
[19] Obesity Management Centre, Institute of Endocrinology, 113 94 Prague, Czech Republic; rbraunerova@endo.cz
[20] Department of Social and Policy Sciences, University of Bath, Claverton Down, Bath BA2 7AY, UK; h.r.rutter@bath.ac.uk
*   Correspondence: silvia.belserrat@ucd.ie; Tel.: +353-1-716-3447

Received: 15 January 2019; Accepted: 21 February 2019; Published: 27 February 2019

Abstract: It is unclear how dietary, physical activity and sedentary behaviors co-occur in school-aged children. We investigated the clustering of energy balance-related behaviors and whether the

Nutrients **2019**, *11*, 511

identified clusters were associated with weight status. Participants were 6- to 9-year-old children (n = 63,215, 49.9% girls) from 19 countries participating in the fourth round (2015/2017) of the World Health Organization (WHO) European Childhood Obesity Surveillance Initiative. Energy balance-related behaviors were parentally reported. Weight and height were objectively measured. We performed cluster analysis separately per group of countries (North Europe, East Europe, South Europe/Mediterranean countries and West-Central Asia). Seven clusters were identified in each group. Healthier clusters were common across groups. The pattern of distribution of healthy and unhealthy behaviors within each cluster was group specific. Associations between the clustering of energy balance-related behaviors and weight status varied per group. In South Europe/Mediterranean countries and East Europe, all or most of the cluster solutions were associated with higher risk of overweight/obesity when compared with the cluster 'Physically active and healthy diet'. Few or no associations were observed in North Europe and West-Central Asia, respectively. These findings support the hypothesis that unfavorable weight status is associated with a particular combination of energy balance-related behavior patterns, but only in some groups of countries.

Keywords: cluster analysis; energy balance-related behaviors; physical activity; sedentary behavior; screen time; dietary intake; overweight; obesity; children

---

1. Introduction

Childhood obesity is one of the most serious public health problems of the 21st century [1]. Evidence from a major epidemiological study which evaluated worldwide trends of weight status from 1975 to 2016 revealed that obesity in children has multiplied eightfold in the last 40 years, with a plateauing of body mass index (BMI) in high-income countries [2]. Obesity is a major risk factor of multifactorial etiology. Modifiable factors such as dietary patterns, physical activity and sedentary behaviors play a key role in energy imbalance leading to overweight and obesity in children [3].

Low fruit and vegetable (F&V) intake [4,5], consumption of high energy-dense/nutrient-poor foods [6,7], low physical activity (PA) levels and high sedentary time [8,9] have individually been associated with childhood overweight and obesity in a large number of studies; however, their effects on children's lifestyles are multivariable and interrelated [10]. Previous studies have investigated the clustering of energy balance-related behaviors (EBRB) and its association with childhood obesity to gain some understanding about the potential interplay among different behavior patterns [11–18]. Healthy and unhealthy behaviors seem to co-exist in the same groups of children in complex ways that are not well understood [10]. For instance, it has been shown that isolated unhealthy behaviors may not be related to higher obesity risk when they are compensated with healthy behaviors [15]. However, evidence on the associations between behavior cluster patterns and overweight and obesity remains inconclusive [10]. While some studies have reported higher obesity risk in unhealthy clusters [11,13,14,18], other studies have found no association at all [15,16].

Evaluating the synergetic effect instead of the individual effects of EBRB will help researchers, health professionals and policy makers to understand which behaviors need to be approached simultaneously. This may be helpful to identify and to promote a healthy lifestyle as well as to assist in the development of successful obesity prevention programs. Therefore, this study aimed to identify clusters of EBRB based on dietary patterns, PA and sedentary behaviors, and to investigate their association with obesity, including overweight, in a large sample of children in the World Health Organization (WHO) European region. To date, no studies have addressed these associations in nationally representative samples of primary school children from such a large geographical area including 19 countries spread across Europe and Asia.

2. Materials and Methods

2.1. World Health Organization (WHO) European Childhood Obesity Surveillance Initiative (COSI)

The WHO European Childhood Obesity Surveillance Initiative (COSI) is a collaborative study that was initiated in 2008 by the WHO Regional Office for Europe with 13 member states. Currently, COSI is carried out in 37 European countries that co-operate in relation to survey content, methodology and timing using a common European protocol [19–21]. The study routinely measures overweight and obesity prevalence of primary schoolchildren aged 6 to 9 years old to monitor the progress of the obesity epidemic in this population group, allow between-country comparisons within the WHO European Region and inform action to reverse the trend [22]. The COSI is a unique system that provides a large dataset based on nationally representative samples and standardized weight and height measurements. A total of four rounds have been conducted to date: Round 1 in 2008, Round 2 in 2009/2010, Round 3 in 2012/2013, and Round 4 in 2015/2017.

In addition to the mandatory anthropometric examinations, data on simple indicators of dietary intake, physical activity, screen time use and parental education, amongst others, are collected through an optional family questionnaire [23]. The present study focuses on children from 19 countries (Albania, Bulgaria, Croatia, Czech Republic, Denmark, Georgia, Ireland, Kazakhstan, Latvia, Lithuania, Malta, Montenegro, Poland, Portugal, Romania, Russia (only Moscow), Spain, Tajikistan, and Turkmenistan) who participated in the study in Round 4 (2015/2017) and who had complete information on age, sex, weight, and height and had completed the family questionnaire.

The COSI study is conducted according to the guidelines laid down in the Declaration of Helsinki and all procedures involving human subjects were approved by the local ethics committee at each study site. Parents were fully informed about the study procedures. In some countries, parents had to provide written signed consent to allow their children to participate in the study (opt-in consent approach) whereas other countries adopted the opt-out consent approach. On the measurement day, verbal consent from the child to participate in the study was obtained.

Countries chose the most appropriate professionals to take the anthropometric measurements (e.g., physical education teachers, nationally- or regionally-based health professionals such as nutritionists, physicians, health care nurses, etc.) based on the local arrangements and available budgets. Paper and online versions of the family questionnaire were available for completion to collect information on the child's EBRB and household sociodemographic characteristics. The paper version was either presented to the parent and child during the measurements, sent home with the child, mailed directly to the household, or filled out during parents' meetings in the school. Parents were emailed the link to fill in the online version and completed the questionnaire jointly with their child. More details about the implementation characteristics of COSI rounds can be found elsewhere [23,24].

2.2. Sampling of Children

Main characteristics of study design including the sampling strategy, targeted age range, sample size and participation rates within each country are presented as Supplementary Material in Table S1. Two-stage cluster sampling was applied in most of the countries with the school as primary sampling unit and school classes as the secondary sampling unit to draw nationally representative samples of children. Poland and Bulgaria applied four-stage (region, sub-region, school, class), and three-stage (school, class, 7-year-old children) cluster sampling, respectively, while one-stage cluster sampling was adopted by Croatia (sampling unit = class), Denmark and Latvia (school for both). Primary schools/classes were selected randomly from the list of all primary schools available in each country through the ministry of education or at the national school registry. Bulgaria, Ireland and Lithuania followed a sentinel approach; therefore, the same schools measured in previous rounds were included and classes were randomly selected at each sentinel site. Lithuania followed a sentinel approach combined with the selection of new schools by region and by degree of urbanization. As an exception, the primary sampling unit in Czech Republic was composed of pediatric clinics which were randomly selected from the national list of primary care pediatricians following a cluster sampling design stratified by region and size of residential location. As for other countries, 11 of them stratified their sample: many considered a geographical or administrative division of the national territory (9 countries) and, to a lesser extent, the degree of urbanization of the child's place of residence or school location (4 countries). No specific sampling strategy was used in Malta as all 7-year-old children in the country were included in the study.

COSI targets children aged 6, 7, 8 and 9 years and countries can focus on one or more of these four age groups [21]. Spain targeted children aged 6 to 9 years old, Albania, Croatia, and Poland targeted 8-year-old children, Romania measured children aged 8 and 9 years, Kazakhstan only included those aged 9 years, and the 13 remaining countries targeted 7-year-old children. One class per school was drawn within a grade level when the targeted age group was in the same grade. On the other hand, all grades where children from this age group were present could be sampled if the targeted age group was spread across grades. All children registered in the sampled classes were invited to take part in the study and those who returned a signed parental consent (opt-in consent approach) or did not refuse to take part in the study (opt-out consent approach) and were present on the survey day were examined and received the family questionnaire. Further details about the sampling characteristics have been described elsewhere [23,24].

2.3. Measurements

2.3.1. Anthropometry

Weight and height measurements were carried out by trained fieldworkers following a standardized protocol on anthropometric procedures and data collection drawn up by the WHO [21]. Information on children's age and sex was also collected. Children were asked to wear normal, light, indoor clothing and remove their shoes. Body weight was measured in kilograms, to the nearest 0.1 kg, with portable electronic (digital) scales and was adjusted for the weight of the clothes worn. Children's height was measured in centimeters with stadiometers and the reading taken to the last completed 0.1 cm. Body mass index (BMI) was calculated from the formula: weight (kg) divided by height squared (m^2). The specific equipment used in each country can be found as Supplementary Material (Table S2). The 2007 WHO BMI-for-age (BMI/A) growth charts were used to compute BMI/A z-scores. Children were classified into two weight status categories: underweight/healthy weight and overweight/obese according to the WHO 2007 [25] and the International Obesity Task Force [26,27] and the sex- and age-specific cut-offs.

2.3.2. Energy Balanced-Related Behaviors

The specific questions asked on the EBRB through the family questionnaire are shown as Supplementary Material—Table S3.

Physical Activity

The number of hours per day the child played actively/vigorously (e.g., running, jumping outside or moving and fitness games indoors) in their free time was assessed for both weekdays and weekend days. Numeric answers were assigned to the five answer categories available in the form to convert the variables to a numerical scale: 'never' = 0; '<1 h/day' = 0.5; '1 h/day' = 1; '2 h/day' = 2; '$\geq$3 h/day' = 3. The average hours per day playing actively was computed as [(week days $\times$ 5) + (weekend days $\times$ 2)]/7.

Screen Time

Usual screen time was described in all countries by the time (hours/day) spent watching television (TV) and/or videos or using electronic devices such as computer, tablet, smartphone or other electronic devices (excluding moving or fitness games) either at home or outside home. Responses were provided separately for weekdays and weekend days. In Ireland, Lithuania and Spain, responses included five categories split into weekdays and weekend days. These categories were converted to a numerical scale: 'never' = 0; '<1 h/day' = 0.5; '1 h/day' = 1; '2 h/day' = 2; '≥3 h/day' = 3. Usual screen time (hours/day) was computed as [(week days × 5) + (weekend days × 2)]/7.

Fruit, Vegetable and Sugared Soft Drinks Intake

Fruit, vegetable and sugared soft drinks (SSD) intake during a normal week was obtained through a qualitative food frequency questionnaire. Responses included four frequency categories of consumption: 'never /<once a week', 'some days (1–3 days)', 'most days (4–6 days)', 'every day'. Frequencies were converted into times per week ranging from 0 to 7. Fruit and vegetable responses were grouped into one group.

2.3.3. Parental Education Level

Data was collected separately for the mother and the father using five answer options and regrouped into four categories: 'primary school', 'secondary school/vocational school', 'undergraduate/Bachelor's degree', and 'Master's degree or higher'. One of the parents reported the education level of both parents. The highest level of education attained in the household by either the mother or the father was used for adjustment in multivariable models.

2.4. Statistical Analysis

Following data cleaning, which was performed locally by each country, all country datasets were reviewed in a standard manner for inconsistencies and incompleteness at the WHO Regional Office for Europe before being merged for the intercountry analyses. Children younger than 6 years ($n = 6$) and older than 9 years ($n = 723$) as well as children with biologically implausible BMI/A z-scores below -5 or above $+5$ z-scores ($n = 124$) were excluded from the analyses, as recommended by the WHO [28].

Cluster analyses were performed using the statistical software SPSS version 24.0 (SPSS Inc., IBM Corp., Armonk, NY, USA). Countries were grouped into four groups according to their geographical location and/or cultural similarities as follows: North Europe (Denmark and Ireland), East Europe (Albania, Bulgaria, Czech Republic, Lithuania, Latvia, Montenegro, Poland, Romania and Russia), South Europe/Mediterranean countries (Croatia, Malta, Portugal and Spain) and West-Central Asia (Georgia, Kazakhstan, Tajikistan and Turkmenistan). Clusters were computed specifically for each of the four groups. PA, screen time, F&V and SSD intake were the four EBRB indicators included in the analyses. Variables were standardized prior to data analyses given the variation in means, variances and units among them [29].

Cluster analysis was carried out in two steps applying a combination of hierarchical and non-hierarchical clustering methods [30]. Ward's method based on Euclidean distances [31] was applied in the first step as hierarchical cluster analysis. The high sensitivity of Ward's method to outliers was reduced by removing univariate outliers (z-values > ±3 standard deviation (SD)) and multivariate outliers (those with high values of the Mahalanobis distance) for any of the four variables tested ($n = 383$). In the second step, an iterative on-hierarchical K-means clustering procedure was carried out. Initial cluster centers based on Ward's hierarchical method were used as non-random starting points.

The third step consisted of testing the stability of the cluster solutions. The sample was randomly split into two sub-samples and the clustering procedure was repeated. The agreement between the main sample and two sub-samples was compared with Cohen's kappa (κ). Agreement ranged from 0.985 (North Europe) to 0.932 (South Europe) [32].

Descriptive statistics included mean (SD) values of weight, height, BMI, PA, screen time, and F&V and SSD intake, prevalence estimates for anthropometric indicators, and percentages of sex, parental education level and season of completion of the questionnaire separately per group of countries and per cluster solution.

Mixed-effects regression models with country as the grouping variable were used to investigate the associations between the clusters (independent variables) and anthropometric indicators and the prevalence of overweight/obesity (dependent variables). Univariate and multivariate mixed linear regression models were carried out to examine associations with the continuous dependent variable BMI/A z-score. Univariate and multivariate logistic regression models were conducted between the prevalence of overweight/obesity (dependent variables) and the obtained clusters. Multivariate models were adjusted for sex, age, parental education level and season of completion of the questionnaire. Country was entered as random intercept in all the mixed-effects models. The threshold for statistical significance was set at $p \leq 0.05$. The Stata version 13.0 (StataCorp LP, College Station, TX, USA) was used to perform these analyses.

3. Results

3.1. Sample Characteristics

The final dataset consisted of 63,215 children (49.9% girls) from 19 countries with complete data on age, sex, weight, height and with information on all four EBRB indicators. The main sample characteristics in terms of age, sex, weight, height, BMI, BMI/A, parental education, season of completion of the questionnaire, PA, screen time, F&V intake, and SSD intake are displayed in Table 1 separately for each group of countries. Mean age was around 8 years in all groups except in North Europe where children were younger (mean age = 7.2 years). North Europe had the highest educated sample as nearly 40% of the families were undergraduate or held a Bachelor's degree. The most common highest education level attained in East Europe, South Europe/Mediterranean countries and West-Central Asia was secondary/vocational school with 42.1%, 49.3% and 62.4% of the parents in this category, respectively. The lowest prevalence of overweight/obesity was observed in North Europe (16.6% WHO, 11.3% IOTF) and West-Central Asia (16.4% WHO, 11.5% IOTF) whereas the countries in the South European/Mediterranean group had the highest prevalence (35.3% WHO, 27.5% IOTF).

Table 1. Baseline characteristics of participants in the fourth round of the WHO European Childhood Obesity Surveillance Initiative (COSI), separately by group of countries.

	North Europe		East Europe		South Europe/ Mediterranean Countries		West-Central Asia	
	Mean	SD	Mean	SD	Mean	SD	Mean	SD
Age (years)	7.2	0.4	8.1	0.8	7.9	0.9	8.0	0.9
Weight (kg)	24.9	4.3	28.7	6.7	28.9	7.2	25.5	5.6
Height (cm)	125.1	5.8	130.7	7.4	128.6	8.1	125.4	7.8
BMI (kg/m^2)	15.9	1.8	16.7	2.7	17.3	2.8	16.1	2.4
BMI/A	0.10	1.0	0.29	1.3	0.62	1.3	−0.01	1.16
Physical activity (hours/day)	1.5	0.7	2.0	0.7	1.6	0.8	1.6	0.8
Screen time (hours/day)	1.9	0.9	1.7	1.0	1.4	0.8	1.6	1.1
Fruit and vegetable intake (times/week)	11.0	3.5	8.5	3.8	8.3	3.8	9.2	4.0
Soft drinks (times/week)	0.9	1.1	1.7	2.1	1.3	1.9	2.6	2.6
	n	%	*n*	%	*n*	%	*n*	%
Sex								
Boys	908	51.7	13,975	49.9	10,807	50.1	5966	50.3
Girls	850	48.3	14,018	50.1	10,785	49.9	5906	49.7
Parental education level								
Primary school	11	0.6	1937	7.2	1126	5.4	87	0.8
Secondary and vocational school	517	29.7	11,294	42.1	10,361	49.3	7098	62.4
Undergraduate/Bachelor degree	693	39.9	6223	23.2	7122	33.8	2603	22.9
Master degree or higher	519	29.8	7357	27.5	2419	11.5	1586	13.9
Season questionnaire completion								
Winter	605	34.4	915	3.3	8017	37.1	2681	22.6
Spring	180	10.2	16,596	59.3	7955	36.8	3047	25.7
Summer	252	14.4	1688	6.0	1232	5.7	1	0.01
Autumn	721	41.0	8794	31.4	4388	20.3	6143	51.7
Overweight/obese (WHO 2007)	291	16.6	7644	27.5	7611	35.3	1927	16.4
Overweight/obese (IOTF)	198	11.3	5824	20.9	5929	27.5	1346	11.5

BMI, body mass index; BMI/A, BMI-for-age; IOTF, International Obesity Task Force; WHO, World Health Organization. North Europe: Denmark and Ireland. East Europe: Albania, Bulgaria, Czech Republic, Latvia, Lithuania, Montenegro, Poland, Romania and Russia. South Europe: Malta, Croatia, Portugal and Spain. West-Central Asia: Georgia, Kazakhstan, Tajikistan and Turkmenistan.

PA levels were the highest in East Europe (2.0 h/day) and the lowest in North Europe (1.5 h/day). North Europe had the highest screen time (1.9 h/day) whereas the lowest amount of time spent on this behavior was observed in South Europe/Mediterranean countries (1.4 h/day). The highest and lowest intakes of F&V were observed in North Europe (11.0 times/week) and in South European/Mediterranean countries (8.3 times/week), respectively. West-Central Asia had the highest SSD intake (2.6 times/week) whereas the North European countries had the lowest intake (0.9 times/week).

3.2. Clusters Characteristics

Cluster analyses turned out in a seven-cluster solution as the most adequate, reliable, and stable representation of the clustering of EBRB in the four groups of countries. Figure 1 shows the specific characteristics of each cluster. Cluster labels are based on distinguishing features defined by high or low mean z-scores relative to other clusters. Clusters that were common across groups were given the same cluster number; therefore, a total of 13 distinctive clusters were identified across the four groups.

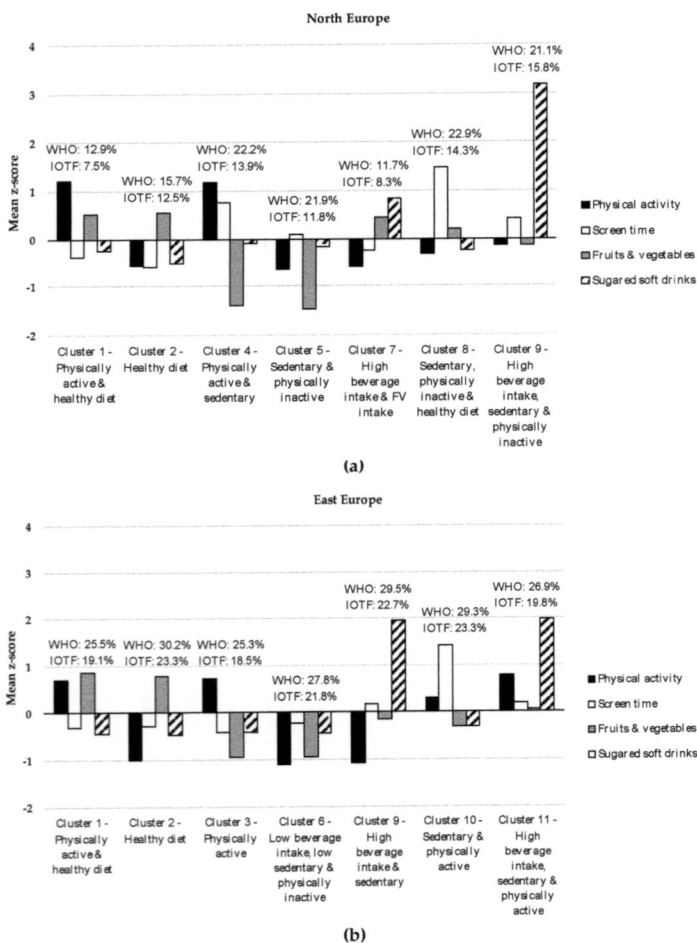

(a)

(b)

Figure 1. *Cont.*

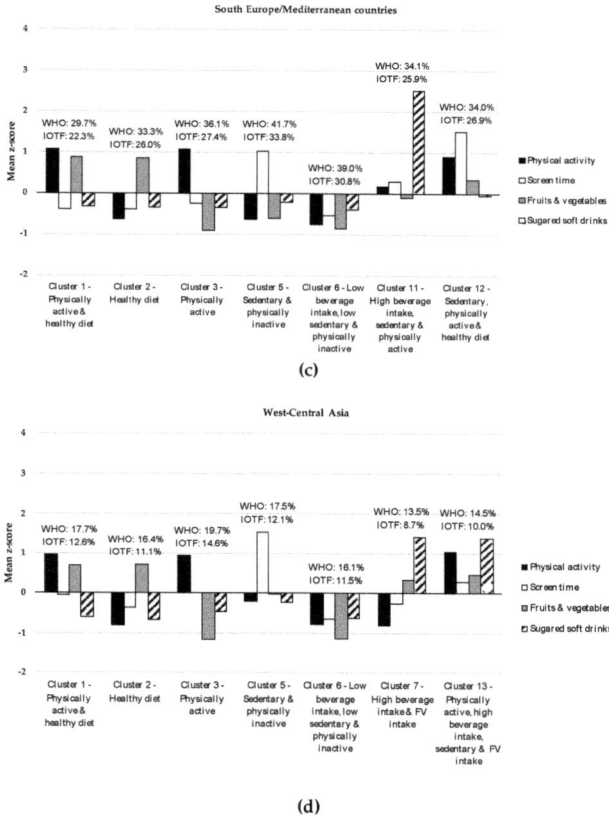

Figure 1. Group-specific cluster solutions (mean z-scores) of the four energy balance-related behaviors (EBRB) patterns among children participating in the fourth round of the World Health Organization European Childhood Obesity Surveillance Initiative: (**a**) Cluster solutions (mean z-scores) of the four EBRB patterns in North Europe; (**b**) Cluster solutions (mean z-scores) of the four EBRB patterns in East Europe; (**c**) Cluster solutions (mean z-scores) of the four EBRB patterns in South Europe/Mediterranean countries; (**d**) Cluster solutions (mean z-scores) of the four EBRB patterns in West-Central Asia. Overweight/obesity prevalence (%) by cluster membership is shown above each cluster. IOTF, International Obesity Task Force; WHO, World Health Organization.

Table 2 shows descriptive data for EBRB indicators and prevalence of overweight/obesity by cluster membership. Cluster 1 (C1, 'Physically active and healthy diet') was characterized by high PA levels and high F&V intake coupled with low screen time use and low intake of SSD. Cluster 2 (C2, 'Healthy diet') comprised children with high F&V intake and low SSD intake. C1 and C2 were observed in all four groups. Cluster 3 (C3, 'Physically active') was observed in East Europe, South Europe/Mediterranean countries and West-Central Asia and was described by high levels of PA. The main features of Cluster 4 (C4, 'Physically active and sedentary'), which only emerged in the North European countries, were high PA levels together with high levels of screen time use. Cluster 5 (C5, 'Sedentary and physically inactive'), with high levels of screen time and low levels of PA, was observed in three groups of countries (North Europe, South Europe/Mediterranean countries and West-Central Asia). Cluster 6 (C6, 'Low beverage intake, low sedentary and physically inactive') was characterized by low levels of all EBRB indicators, that is, low PA levels, low screen time, low F&V intake and low SSD intake. C6 was present in all the groups except in North Europe. Cluster 7 (C7,

'High beverage intake and F&V intake'), described by high intakes of SSD and of F&V, emerged in North Europe and in West-Central Asia.

Cluster 8 (C8, 'Sedentary, physically inactive and healthy diet'), with high levels of screen time, high F&V intake, low PA levels and low SSD intake, was specific to the North European countries. Cluster 9 (C9, 'High beverage intake, sedentary and physically inactive') comprised those in the North European and East European countries with high intake of SSD, high screen time use and low PA levels. Cluster 10 (C10, 'Sedentary and physically active') was only observed in East Europe and was described by high screen time and relatively high PA levels. The main features of Cluster 11 (C11, 'High beverage intake, sedentary and physically active') were high intake of SSD and relatively high screen time and PA levels and emerged in both East Europe and in South Europe/Mediterranean countries. Cluster 12 (C12, 'Sedentary, physically active and healthy diet'), specific to South Europe/Mediterranean countries, was characterized by high screen time use, high PA levels, high intake of F&V and low SSD intake. Cluster 13 (C13, 'Physically active, high beverage intake, sedentary and high F&V intake') was only observed in West-Central Asia and comprised children with high levels of all four EBRB.

In terms of prevalence of overweight/obesity, C9 ('High beverage intake, sedentary and physically inactive') and C8 ('Sedentary, physically inactive and healthy diet') showed, respectively, the highest prevalence with the WHO 2007 definition (22.9%) and with the IOTF definition (15.8%) in the North European countries. The lowest prevalence was observed for C1 ('Physically active and healthy diet', 12.9% WHO, 7.5% IOTF,) and for C7 ('High beverage intake and F&V intake', 11.7% WHO, 8.3% IOTF). C1 also had the lowest overweight/obesity prevalence in East Europe and South Europe/Mediterranean countries regardless of the obesity definition applied. C2 ('Healthy diet'), C9 ('High beverage intake, sedentary and physically inactive') and C10 ('Sedentary and physically active') had very similar high prevalence of overweight/obesity. The highest overweight/obesity prevalence in South Europe/Mediterranean countries was observed for C5 ('Sedentary and physically inactive', 41.7% WHO, 33.8% IOTF). As in the North European countries, C7 ('High beverage intake and F&V intake') in West-Central Asia had the lowest prevalence of overweight/obesity (13.5% WHO, 8.7% IOTF) whereas C3 ('Physically active') had the highest prevalence (19.7% WHO, 14.6% IOFT) regardless of the obesity definition used.

3.3. Associations between Cluster Membership and Anthropometric Indicators

Results from the mixed-effects regression models are shown in Table 3, separately by groups of countries. C1 ('Physically active and healthy diet') was chosen as the reference cluster in all groups as it showed lower overweight/obesity prevalence in most of the groups and it can be considered as the healthiest cluster. After adjusting for confounding factors, all the clusters in South Europe/Mediterranean countries, except C3 ('Physically active') with the IOTF definition, were significantly associated with higher BMI/A and higher odds of overweight/obesity, regardless of the obesity definition applied. In East Europe, a positive significant association was observed between C2 ('Healthy diet') ($\beta = 0.17$, 95% CI = 0.12–0.22), C6 ('Low beverage intake, low sedentary and physically inactive') ($\beta = 0.13$, 95% CI = 0.07–0.18), C9 ('High beverage intake, sedentary and physically inactive') ($\beta = 0.08$, 95% CI = 0.01–0.15) and C10 ('Sedentary and physically active') ($\beta = 0.16$, 95% CI = 0.10–0.22) and BMI/A. Likewise, those children in these clusters (C2, C6, C9 and C10) were at higher risk of overweight/obesity than their peers in C1. In the North European countries, BMI/A was significantly associated with the 'Sedentary, physically inactive and healthy diet' cluster (C8) ($\beta = 0.25$, 95% CI = 0.07–0.42). Children in C8 were also more likely to be overweight/obese (WHO: OR = 1.92, 95% CI = 1.21–3.05; IOTF: OR = 2.15, 95% CI = 1.22–3.77) than those in the 'Physically active and healthy diet' cluster (C1). Moreover, higher odds of being overweight/obese was observed among those in C2 ('Healhty diet') (IOTF: OR = 1.85, 95% CI = 1.15–2.97), C4 ('Physically active and sedentary') (WHO: OR = 1.68, 95% CI = 1.02–2.76), and C5 ('Sedentary and physically inactive') (WHO: OR = 1.63, 95% CI = 1.04–2.54). No significant associations were observed in the West-Central Asian countries between the clusters and BMI/A and the prevalence of overweight/obesity.

Table 2. Descriptive data of energy balance-related behaviors indicators and overweight/obesity prevalence by cluster membership among the participants in the fourth round of the WHO European Childhood Obesity Surveillance Initiative, by groups of countries.

| | n | % | Sex Boys | | Girls | | Physical Activity (Hours/Day) | | Screen Time (Hours/Day) | | Fruit and Vegetables (Times/Week) | | Soft Drinks (Times/Week) | | Overweight/Obesity (WHO 2007) | | Overweight/Obesity (IOTF) | |
			n	%	n	%	Mean	SD	Mean	SD	Mean	SD	Mean	SD	n	%	n	%
North Europe (n = 1758)																		
C1	374	21.3	195	52.1	179	47.9	2.3	0.3	1.6	0.6	12.8	1.7	0.6	0.7	48	12.9	28	7.5
C2	522	29.7	230	44.1	292	55.9	1.1	0.4	1.4	0.5	12.9	1.6	0.3	0.2	82	15.7	65	12.5
C4	158	9.0	86	54.4	72	45.6	2.3	0.4	2.6	0.9	6.0	3.0	0.9	0.8	35	22.2	22	13.9
C5	246	14.0	125	50.8	121	49.2	1.1	0.4	2.0	0.7	5.7	2.5	0.7	0.8	43	21.9	29	11.8
C7	205	11.7	112	54.6	93	45.4	1.1	0.4	1.7	0.6	12.5	1.7	2.0	0.0	24	11.7	17	8.3
C8	196	11.1	125	63.8	71	36.2	1.3	0.6	3.2	0.6	11.7	2.2	0.6	0.7	43	22.9	28	14.3
C9	57	3.2	35	61.4	22	38.6	1.4	0.7	2.3	0.8	10.5	3.1	5.0	0.0	12	21.1	9	15.8
East Europe (n = 27,993)																		
C1	6555	23.4	3174	48.4	3381	51.6	2.5	0.4	1.4	0.7	11.8	1.9	0.8	0.8	1662	25.5	1248	19.1
C2	4798	17.1	2170	45.2	2628	57.8	1.2	0.3	1.4	0.7	11.5	1.9	0.8	0.8	1443	30.2	1113	23.3
C3	4548	16.3	2357	51.8	2191	48.2	2.5	0.4	1.3	0.7	4.9	2.1	0.9	0.8	1146	25.3	837	18.5
C6	4028	14.4	1957	48.6	2071	51.4	1.2	0.4	1.5	0.8	4.9	2.1	0.8	0.8	1117	27.8	876	21.8
C9	1795	6.4	911	50.8	884	49.2	1.2	0.4	1.9	1.0	8.0	3.9	5.9	1.0	527	29.5	406	22.7
C10	3205	11.5	1726	53.9	1479	46.1	2.2	0.6	3.3	0.8	7.4	3.1	1.1	1.0	932	29.3	742	23.3
C11	3064	11.0	1680	54.8	1384	45.2	2.6	0.4	2.0	1.0	8.8	3.8	5.9	1.0	817	26.9	602	19.8
South Europe/Mediterranean countries (n = 21,592)																		
C1	2946	13.6	1556	52.8	1390	47.2	2.4	0.3	1.1	0.5	11.6	1.9	0.7	0.8	874	29.7	657	22.3
C2	5366	24.9	2488	46.4	2878	53.6	1.1	0.4	1.1	0.5	11.5	1.9	0.6	0.8	1789	33.3	1396	26.0
C3	2754	12.8	1501	54.5	1253	45.5	2.4	0.4	1.2	0.6	4.8	2.1	0.6	0.8	993	36.1	754	27.4
C5	2121	9.8	1059	49.9	1032	50.1	1.1	0.4	2.4	0.5	5.9	2.8	0.9	0.9	885	41.7	716	33.8
C6	4244	19.7	2018	47.6	2226	52.4	1.0	0.4	1.0	0.4	5.0	2.1	0.6	0.8	1654	39.0	1306	30.8
C12	1821	8.4	947	52.0	874	48.0	2.3	0.5	2.8	0.6	9.5	3.2	1.2	1.0	621	34.1	472	25.9
C11	2340	10.8	1238	52.9	1102	47.1	1.7	0.8	1.7	0.8	7.8	3.9	6.0	1.0	795	34.0	628	26.9
West-Central Asia (n = 11,872)																		
C1	1787	15.0	875	49.0	912	51.0	2.4	0.4	1.6	0.8	11.9	1.9	1.1	0.8	314	17.7	223	12.6
C2	2086	17.6	993	47.6	1093	52.4	1.0	0.4	1.2	0.7	12.1	1.9	0.9	0.8	339	16.4	230	11.1
C3	1511	12.7	794	52.6	717	47.4	2.4	0.4	1.6	0.9	4.6	2.2	1.4	1.6	296	19.7	220	14.6
C5	1270	10.7	697	54.9	573	45.1	1.5	0.6	3.4	0.8	9.1	3.5	2.0	2.0	220	17.5	152	12.1
C6	1911	16.1	917	48.0	994	52.0	1.0	0.4	0.9	0.7	4.6	2.2	1.0	1.3	303	16.1	217	11.5
C7	1728	14.6	839	48.6	889	51.4	1.0	0.4	1.4	0.9	10.6	3.6	6.3	1.0	230	13.5	149	8.7
C13	1579	13.3	851	53.9	728	46.1	2.5	0.4	2.5	1.0	11.0	3.1	6.2	1.0	225	14.5	155	10.0

Cluster 1 "Physically active and healthy diet"; Cluster 2 "Healthy diet"; Cluster 3 "Physically active"; Cluster 4 "Physically active and sedentary"; Cluster 5 "Sedentary and physically inactive"; Cluster 6 "Low beverage intake, low sedentary and physically inactive"; Cluster 7 "High beverage intake and F&V intake"; Cluster 8 "Sedentary, physically inactive and healthy diet"; Cluster 9 "High beverage intake, sedentary and physically inactive"; Cluster 10 "Sedentary and physically active"; Cluster 11 "High beverage intake, sedentary and physically active"; Cluster 12 "Sedentary, physically active and healthy diet"; Cluster 13 "Physically active, high beverage intake, sedentary and high F&V intake". IOTF, International Obesity Task Force; WHO, World Health Organization. North Europe: Denmark and Ireland. East Europe: Albania, Bulgaria, Czech Republic, Latvia, Lithuania, Montenegro, Poland, Romania and Russia. South Europe: Malta, Croatia, Portugal and Spain. West-Central Asia: Georgia, Kazakhstan, Tajikistan and Turkmenistan.

Table 3. Associations between cluster membership and anthropometric indicators among the participants in the fourth round of the WHO European Childhood Obesity Surveillance Initiative, by groups of countries.

	BMI/A				Overweight/Obesity (WHO 2007)				Overweight/Obesity (IOTF)			
	Crude Model		Adjusted Model [a]		Crude Model		Adjusted Model [a]		Crude Model		Adjusted Model [a]	
	β	95% CI	β	95% CI	OR	95% CI	OR	95% CI	OR	95% CI	OR	95% CI
North Europe (n = 1758)												
C1	ref.		ref.		ref.		ref.		ref.		ref.	
C2	0.07	−0.06–0.21	0.08	−0.05–0.22	1.32	0.89–1.94	1.35	0.91–2.00	1.83	1.15–2.92 *	1.85	1.15–2.97 *
C4	0.12	−0.07–0.31	0.07	−0.12–0.26	1.85	1.14–3.01 *	1.68	1.02–2.76 *	1.92	1.06–3.47 *	1.60	0.86–2.96
C5	0.12	−0.04–0.28	0.11	−0.05–0.27	1.67	1.07–2.60 *	1.63	1.04–2.54 *	1.71	0.99–2.97	1.63	0.94–2.83
C7	0.03	−0.15–0.21	0.04	−0.14–0.21	1.13	0.65–1.95	1.09	0.63–1.87	1.39	0.72–2.69	1.37	0.72–2.63
C8	0.22	0.05–0.40 *	0.25	0.07–0.42 **	1.93	1.22–3.05 **	1.92	1.21–3.05 **	2.08	1.19–3.63 *	2.15	1.22–3.77 **
C9	0.24	−0.05–0.52	0.18	−0.11–0.46	2.18	1.06–4.48 *	1.78	0.85–3.73	2.78	1.22–6.36 *	2.22	0.94–5.26
East Europe (n = 27,993)												
C1	ref.		ref.		ref.		ref.		ref.		ref.	
C2	0.16	0.11–0.21 ***	0.17	0.12–0.22 ***	1.30	1.20–1.42 ***	1.32	1.21–1.44 ***	1.34	1.22–1.47 ***	1.35	1.23–1.49 ***
C3	0.02	−0.04–0.07	0.03	−0.03–0.07	1.01	0.93–1.11	1.03	0.94–1.12	1.00	0.90–1.10	1.01	0.92–1.12
C6	0.12	0.07–0.17 ***	0.13	0.07–0.18 ***	1.17	1.07–1.28 **	1.18	1.08–1.30 ***	1.26	1.14–1.39 ***	1.28	1.15–1.41 ***
C9	0.06	−0.01–0.13	0.08	0.01–0.15 *	1.19	1.06–1.34 **	1.22	1.08–1.38 **	1.23	1.08–1.40 **	1.26	1.11–1.44 **
C10	0.16	0.10–0.21 ***	0.16	0.10–0.22 ***	1.22	1.11–1.34 ***	1.22	1.11–1.35 ***	1.30	1.17–1.45 ***	1.33	1.20–1.49 ***
C11	0.01	−0.05–0.07	0.03	−0.03–0.09	1.03	0.93–1.14	1.05	0.95–1.16	1.00	0.90–1.11	1.04	0.93–1.17
South Europe/Mediterranean countries (n = 21,592)												
C1	ref.		ref.		ref.		ref.		ref.		ref.	
C2	0.08	0.03–0.14 **	0.10	0.04–0.16 **	1.15	1.04–1.26 **	1.14	1.06–1.30 **	1.18	1.06–1.31 **	1.18	1.06–1.32 **
C3	0.11	0.05–0.18 **	0.08	0.01–0.14 *	1.21	1.08–1.35 **	1.17	1.04–1.31 **	1.19	1.05–1.34 **	1.12	0.99–1.27
C5	0.32	0.25–0.39 ***	0.30	0.23–0.37 ***	1.61	1.43–1.81 ***	1.59	1.40–1.79 ***	1.67	1.47–1.90 ***	1.61	1.42–1.84 ***
C6	0.17	0.11–0.23 ***	0.15	0.09–0.21 ***	1.35	1.21–1.49 ***	1.31	1.18–1.46 ***	1.37	1.23–1.54 ***	1.29	1.15–1.45 ***
C11	0.16	0.09–0.23 ***	0.11	0.04–0.18 **	1.29	1.15–1.46 ***	1.21	1.07–1.37 **	1.34	1.18–1.53 ***	1.23	1.08–1.40 **
C12	0.13	0.06–0.21 ***	0.10	0.03–0.18 **	1.26	1.11–1.44 ***	1.22	1.07–1.39 **	1.24	1.08–1.43 **	1.19	1.03–1.37 *
West-Central Asia (n = 11,872)												
C1	ref.		ref.		ref.		ref.		ref.		ref.	
C2	0.04	−0.03–0.12	0.05	−0.02–0.13	0.97	0.81–1.15	0.99	0.73–1.18	0.92	0.76–1.13	0.93	0.76–1.14
C3	−0.01	−0.09–0.07	0.01	−0.08–0.09	0.89	0.75–1.07	0.95	0.79–1.14	0.92	0.75–1.13	0.98	0.79–1.20
C5	0.06	−0.03–0.14	0.06	−0.02–0.15	1.03	0.85–1.25	1.04	0.85–1.26	1.00	0.80–1.25	1.02	0.81–1.28
C6	−0.03	−0.10–0.05	0.01	−0.07–0.08	0.87	0.73–1.04	0.92	0.76–1.10	0.88	0.71–1.08	0.93	0.76–1.15
C7	−0.03	−0.11–0.05	−0.02	−0.10–0.06	0.95	0.78–1.14	0.98	0.81–1.20	0.90	0.72–1.12	0.93	0.74–1.17
C13	0.01	−0.07–0.08	0.02	−0.06–0.10	0.90	0.74–1.08	0.94	0.78–1.14	0.89	0.72–1.11	0.95	0.76–1.19

[a] Adjusted for age, sex, parental education level, season of questionnaire completion. * p < 0.05, ** p < 0.01, *** p < 0.001. Cluster 1 "Physically active and healthy diet"; Cluster 2 "Healthy diet"; Cluster 3 "Physically active"; Cluster 4 "Physically active and sedentary"; Cluster 5 "Sedentary and physically inactive"; Cluster 6 "Low beverage intake, low sedentary and physically inactive"; Cluster 7 "High beverage intake and F&V intake"; Cluster 8 "Sedentary, physically inactive and healthy diet"; Cluster 9 "High beverage intake, sedentary and physically inactive"; Cluster 10 "Sedentary and physically active"; Cluster 11 "High beverage intake, sedentary and physically active"; Cluster 12 "Sedentary, physically active and healthy diet"; Cluster 13 "Physically active, high beverage intake, sedentary and high F&V intake". BMI/A, BMI-for-age; IOTF, International Obesity Task Force; WHO, World Health Organization. North Europe: Denmark and Ireland. East Europe: Albania, Bulgaria, Czech Republic, Latvia, Lithuania, Montenegro, Poland, Romania and Russia. South Europe: Malta, Croatia, Portugal and Spain. West-Central Asia: Georgia, Kazakhstan, Tajikistan and Turkmenistan.

4. Discussion

This study investigated the clustering of F&V and SSD intake patterns, physical activity and sedentary behavior and their cross-sectional associations with anthropometric indicators in a large sample of children in the WHO European region. Our findings showed that (1) some behaviors cluster in the same manner and are common across groups whereas others are specific to the geographical area, and (2) the associations of the clustering of the EBRB and the obesity indicators depend on the group of countries. To the best of our knowledge, this is the first study to examine the clustering of these EBRB and its association with obesity indicators in a large and geographically spread sample of school-aged children.

4.1. Clusters Characteristics

A 7-cluster solution was retained as the best solution within the four groups. While the clustering of some behaviors was common across groups, other behaviors clustered in a unique manner specific to each country grouping. This highlights the complexity of diet, PA and sedentary behavior and their relationships. The current globalization of EBRB [33] could explain the similarity of clusters across groups. On the other hand, group differences in the clustering of these behaviors seem to reflect group-specific EBRB patterns that persist regardless of such globalization, although to a lesser extent as these clusters tended to be less prevalent than the common ones.

4.2. Healthy and Unhealthy Energy Balance-Related Behaviors (EBRB) Clustering

C1 'Physically active and healthy diet' and C2 'Healthy diet', the clusters that represent healthier EBRB, were common across all groups. C3, the 'Physically active' cluster, was common in three groups however (East Europe, South Europe/Mediterranean countries, West-Central Asia). C1, considered as the 'healthy' cluster was characterized by high PA levels and high F&V intake and low levels of screen time and SSD intake. This cluster comprised most of the children in East Europe (23.4%) and was the second most prevalent cluster in North Europe (21.3%). C2 'Healthy diet', with high levels of F&V intake and low SSD intake, was the most prevalent cluster in North Europe (29.7%), South Europe/Mediterranean countries (24.9%) and West-Central Asia (17.6%), and the second that comprised most children in East Europe (17.1%). The healthy clustering of diet and PA in school-aged children has not consistently been observed in the literature. While some studies failed to observe a distinct healthy cluster among children [11,13,34], others reported one cluster in which healthy behaviors co-existed, in line with our results. Sánchez-Oliva et al. [14] identified a 'Healthy Lifestyle' cluster among children aged 8–11 years that was characterized by low levels of screen time and of total sedentary time, high levels of moderate-to-vigorous PA, and average levels of adherence to the Mediterranean diet. Likewise, a 'Healthier lifestyle' cluster with high PA, low sedentary behavior, longer sleep duration and healthier diet was reported in a sample of 9- to 12-year-old Spanish children [16]. In contrast to our findings, this cluster was not the most prevalent in neither of the studies. Another matter is whether children in these healthy clusters met the recommendations for these behaviors. An 'all-round healthy behavior' cluster was observed by Cameron et al. [35] in which children aged 5–12 years met the daily recommendations for moderate-to-vigorous PA, screen time, F&V intake and energy-dense food intake. Our results showed that children in C1 achieved >1 h/day of PA [36], screen time use was below the recommended 2 h/day [37] and SSD consumption was very low (≤once a week). F&V intake was also high; however, due to the nature of the questionnaire, it is very likely that the intake of F&V was underestimated as daily intakes were not available; therefore, it is unknown whether children met the guidelines in this regard.

Consistent with previous literature [14,16–18,34,35], we found clustering of unhealthy behaviors which comprised children with high levels of screen use and high SSD intake. In a review of cross-sectional and longitudinal studies, Pearson and Biddle [38] already reported a positive association between sedentary behaviors and elements of a less healthy diet in children such as energy-dense drinks, snacks and fast food. Nevertheless, this clustering of unhealthy behaviors was the least prevalent in the two groups of countries where it was observed (3.2% North Europe, 6.4% East Europe).

4.3. Co-Occurrence of Healthy and Unhealthy EBRB

As already highlighted by previous studies [11,13,18,34,35], healthy and unhealthy levels of EBRB co-occurred in some regions in all groups, but not in others. Most of these clusters were characterized by high levels of screen time coupled with high levels of PA (C4, C10) and/or high F&V intake (C8, C12). A cluster (C7) combining high F&V intake with high SSD intake was observed in North Europe and West-Central Asia. It is noteworthy that a cluster with high levels of all four behaviors (C13) emerged in West-Central Asia. We found no studies that had already reported such a clustering of EBRB in which individuals had high levels of all healthy and unhealthy behaviors simultaneously. We hypothesized that the co-existence of healthy and unhealthy behaviors in the same cluster could suggest a conscious compensation, by the parents, of the unhealthy behavior by adhering to a healthy one. Parents could engage their children in a particular healthy behavior such as PA performance and/or healthy eating to compensate for engaging in other practices such as high screen time use and/or unhealthier dietary patterns. Although this behavior has only been investigated in adults [39], it may be plausible in our study as data were reported by the parents.

It should be noted that several clusters were characterized by high levels of screen time. In three groups, a sedentary cluster (C5) coupled with low levels of PA emerged comprising children with high screen time use above the recommendations, especially in West-Central Asia (3.4 h/day). Leech et al. [10] already reported in their review a common pattern among several studies in which many clusters were defined by high levels of sedentary behaviors. These findings seem to reflect the current high levels of screen time associated with the use of new technologies and the negative impact that they can already have on the lifestyle of those at still early ages.

4.4. Low EBRB Levels

By contrast, all groups except North Europe had a cluster characterized by low levels of PA, screen time, F&V intake and SSD intake. Likewise, three studies conducted in European children aged 2–9 years [11,13] and 10–12 years [17] found a clustering of low levels on all behaviors. Co-occurrence of low consumption of SSD and low screen time use levels, despite the low PA levels and low F&V intake, could be regarded as positive in terms of health promotion and disease prevention. In fact, the findings in the study from Bel-Serrat et al. [11] suggested that the cardiovascular profile of children with low levels of TV/video/DVD viewing together with low SSD intake was healthier than for those physically active or with high F&V intake. This cluster was considered by the authors as the healthiest cluster solution given that they failed to find a 'healthy' cluster, which could have been associated with an even healthier cardiovascular profile.

Future research should focus on investigating how clusters track over time in this age group. The longitudinal stability of cluster membership was examined among Australian 10–12-year-old children over a 3-year period and was observed to be moderate [12]. While the 'most healthy' clusters showed the lowest stability over time, tracking was highest for the 'high sedentary behavior/low moderate and vigorous PA'. According to the authors, further investigation is still needed to figure out the reason why some clusters tracked better than others [12].

4.5. Associations between Cluster Membership and Anthropometric Indicators

4.5.1. Differences across Groups of Countries

Associations between the clustering of EBRB and anthropometric indicators notably varied per group of countries. All clusters except two were associated with higher BMI/A z-score and higher risk of overweight/obesity regardless of the obesity definition used in South Europe/Mediterranean countries and in East Europe, respectively. Only a small number of associations was observed in North Europe and no associations were observed in West-Central Asia. Although we cannot compare group-specific clusters because they are unique to each area, common clusters were not associated with obesity indicators in the same manner across groups. These differences may represent different stages of evolution of the obesity epidemic in different countries and populations groups, with variable responses in terms of behaviors, norms, and different physical, social, cultural and economic environments. We also hypothesized that countries could be at a different stage of the diffusion of innovation theory from Rogers [40] in terms of obesity prevention strategies and their adoption by the population. Briefly, the diffusion of innovation theory explains how, an idea, behavior or product spreads through a specific population and it is adopted by this population. Adoption, however, does not occur simultaneously within the target population and, there are, indeed, five adopter categories: innovators, early adopters, early majority, late majority and laggards [40]. While in North Europe most of the population may have adopted these strategies in terms of EBRB, in South Europe/Mediterranean countries and in East Europe, the adoption of EBRB strategies is still at earlier stages, which is also reflected by the remarkably higher mean BMI/A and overweight/obesity prevalence observed in these countries.

Nevertheless, it should be kept in mind that the education level in the North European countries was higher than in the other three groups, which could also have an impact on the observed findings as it could imply a healthier cohort of children. In West-Central Asia, however, children could still follow a quite traditional behavior pattern that prevents them from being overweight/obese, even considering that obesity prevention strategies focusing on EBRB in these countries may not be as developed as in Europe given their relatively low overweight/obesity rates as compared with the other countries. Examining the associations between cluster membership and sociodemographic factors in this specific age group deserves more attention and future research. Fernández-Alvira et al. [17] observed that children from seven European countries aged 10–12 years old with lower educated parents were more likely to have unhealthier clustering of EBRB, i.e., low activity/sedentary pattern and sedentary and sugared drinks consumers. Likewise, the 'energy-dense consumers who watch TV' cluster comprised more children with lower educated mothers among Australian 5–6- and 10–12-year-old children [34].

Differences in the observed associations between the clustering of EBRB and overweight/obesity across regions could also be explained by other factors not examined in this study and that have also been shown to play a role in the development of overweight/obesity such as sleep duration, well-being and/or genetic variations, amongst others. Findings from a meta-analysis reported that short sleep duration increased the risk of childhood obesity [41]; however, we did not observe much variation on average sleep time among regions: 11 h/day in the North European countries and 10 h/day in the other three groups of countries. Moreover, obesity has a pronounced genetic component as genetic factors account for between 30–70% of variation in BMI between individuals [42]. The prevalence of obesity also differs between ethnic groups [42]. This could partially explain the low prevalence of overweight/obesity observed in the West-Central Asian countries as opposed to the higher prevalence in the South Europe/Mediterranean countries. On the other hand, the nature of the methodology applied may have a role in explaining the lack of consistent results across regions. A key limitation of self-reported measures is their validity. For that reason, the presence of misclassification bias needs to be considered given that parentally reported measures are subject to possible misreporting of PA, sedentary behaviors and diet.

4.5.2. Synergies among Multiple EBRB and Overweight/Obesity

The synergistic effect of having high levels of PA and high intake of F&V combined with low screen time use and low SSD intake was associated with children being less likely to be overweight/obese. Having only a diet rich in F&V or being physically active did not seem to be associated with children being less overweight/obese as compared with their peers who were engaged in both EBRB simultaneously, even when screen time use and SSD intake were low. The fact that C6 ('Low beverage intake, low sedentary and physically inactive') was also associated with higher odds of overweight/obesity supports this hypothesis. Unlike our findings, Bel-Serrat et al. [11] and Santaliestra-Pasías et al. [13] found that the clustering of low levels of all EBRB was associated with reduced levels of body fat. However, both studies failed to observe a healthy cluster to compare this cluster with. Nevertheless, the evidence on the potential cumulative effect of these behaviors in children is still inconsistent. In the review by Leech et al. [10], five studies found evidence of a possible synergistic effect of multiple EBRB on overweight/obesity whereas seven studies found no association. Differences in the EBRB indicators used, the statistical methods applied to compute the clusters, the culture and/or the specific population studied, amongst others, limit the comparability among studies and could partially explain the lack of agreement.

4.5.3. Measures of EBRB

The low z-scores observed in C6 for all the EBRB could suggest that there might be other underlying factors associated with overweight/obesity that were not captured by either these EBRB measures, i.e., engagement in other eating and/or movement behaviors like light PA, or beyond these EBRB, as mentioned earlier. Therefore, future studies in children may need to target more comprehensive measures of EBRB. In terms of PA, this could include light PA in addition to moderate and vigorous PA, structured and unstructured PA, and PA performance during school time and outside school hours. Assessment of both multiple sedentary behaviors (e.g., screen use (TV, videos, computer, table, smartphone, etc.), reading, socializing) and of domain-specific behaviors (e.g., sitting at school or at home, motorized travel) should be considered [43] in future research. Furthermore, the dietary assessment methodologies applied should provide information not only on the individual foods consumed but on the overall diet to obtain a better understanding of the dietary factors that are related to health outcomes. The combination of several dietary assessment methods, such as food frequency questionnaires and 24-h dietary recalls, is frequently used to fulfill this need. However, the nature of information to be collected and the methodology should be specified by the survey itself. For instance, while accelerometry offers a convenient and accurate measurement of PA, it should be kept in mind that questionnaires are cost-effective, readily accessible to most of the population and have a relatively low participant burden [43]. These aspects are crucial in surveillance where data are collected in an ongoing and systematic basis.

4.5.4. Role of Sedentary Behaviors

Our findings showed that most of the clusters that were associated with an increased risk of overweight/obesity were characterized by high levels of screen time use, regardless of being combined with other healthy/unhealthy behaviors or not. This suggests that high screen time use could mask the potential positive role of PA and of a healthy diet on reducing the obesogenic risk. This 'outweighing' effect of one particular behavior over another has been reported previously [10,18]. In agreement with our results, four studies in the review by Leech et al. [10] found a positive association between overweight and high sedentary behavior. Similarly, Dumuid et al. [18] and Sánchez-Oliva [14] observed that membership of the high sedentary time cluster was associated with higher BMI and higher risk of overweight/obesity and with higher body fat percentage, respectively.

4.5.5. Role of Sedentary Behaviors and Sugared Soft Drinks (SSD) Consumption

It deserves attention the fact that clusters that combined both high levels of screen time use and high consumption of SSD comprised children who were more likely to be overweight/obese. Leech et al. [12] already showed that TV viewing in combination with energy-dense food and drinks consumption predicted overweight and obesity among Australian children. Evidence form cross-sectional, longitudinal, interventional studies carried out in children supports the link between SSD intake and not only unhealthy weight gain, but other adverse health outcomes such as dental caries, high blood pressure, earlier timing of puberty, poor sleep and hyperactivity/inattention [44]. This is a matter of concern given that children in these clusters are simultaneously engaged in two unhealthy behaviors and, therefore, could be at an increased risk of developing health issues linked to these behaviors not only during childhood, but also during adolescence and adulthood.

4.6. Strengths

The main strengths of this study include the application of standardized data collection procedures across countries, the large sample size of more than 60,000 children from diverse geographical areas of Europe and Asia, and the country-based sampling strategies designed to yield nationally representative samples. The inclusion of important obesity-related EBRB, the use of objectively measured height and weight, and the adjustment of regression models for important confounders can also be regarded as study strengths. Furthermore, cluster analysis, a data-driven approach, is able to identify clusters of EBRB patterns, which offers certain superiority as opposed to a priori methods such as indexes [34].

4.7. Limitations

These findings should be interpreted in the context of several limitations. The cross-sectional design of this study does not allow us to make any causal inferences. Differences in sampling methods and target age group(s) across countries should be regarded as a study limitation. Despite the large sample size and the fact that countries selected nationally representative samples, the survey nature of the data and the differences in each country contribution to both the groups sample and population were not considered in the analyses. Therefore, it should be kept in mind when interpreting these findings that they refer to the study sample rather than to any population. Moreover, some degree of selection bias cannot be precluded given the low levels of participation observed in some countries.

Further limitations include the parentally reported EBRB variables which are subject to measurement error, recall bias and socially desirable answers. Therefore, a certain degree of differential misreporting, i.e., over-reporting of healthier behaviors and under-reporting of those regarded as less healthy, cannot be precluded. Also, the parental estimates of their children's behavior patterns may be error-prone, especially when these behaviors took place out of home or in the child's bedroom. School-based PA was not captured by the questionnaire and, therefore, estimates rely only on PA during free time. One of the major challenges in nutritional epidemiology is the measurement error in dietary intake data and, therefore, misreporting cannot be ruled out, especially among parents with overweight/obese children [45]. Furthermore, the nature of the questionnaire could lead to an underestimation of those food items that were consumed several times a day such as F&V intake. Therefore, intakes of F&V in this sample could be higher than those observed in these analyses. The fact that the reliability of the questionnaire has not been examined yet should be regarded as another study limitation. Nevertheless, the COSI food frequency consumption list was designed as an easily applicable monitoring tool to get an overall indication of the children's usual consumption frequencies of a food group, but it did not include portion sizes. Besides, the low cost and ease of administration of the questionnaires makes them the most common tool used in large epidemiological and surveillance studies, despite their methodological limitations.

It should be acknowledged that the grouping of the countries was not perfect and that the use of another grouping system could have resulted in a more accurate grouping. For example, Georgia is not an Asian country as it is located between Western Asia and Eastern Europe. However, the grouping of the countries was limited by the number of countries with available data. Furthermore, the clustering of EBRB and the prevalence of overweight and obesity observed within each group do not represent the current picture of the entire region as many countries were not included in the analyses. Therefore, no attempts should be made to compare data across regions/groups of countries. Nevertheless, it was preferred to group the countries rather than following a country by country approach given the advantages of the former approach in terms of data analysis and reporting and interpretation of the results.

The data-driven and person-centered nature of the cluster analysis approach is also subject to several limitations such as a high degree of subjectivity and lack of generalization of findings to other populations. This implies the need for caution when comparing our results with other studies. Furthermore, there is no agreement on how to best minimize subjectivity when determining the optimal number of clusters [46]. Several clusters were common across groups with similar characteristics;

however, they did not necessarily have the same exact characteristics such as identical levels of a given EBRB indicator. Furthermore, data was collected across all four seasons and, therefore, cluster membership could be different between seasons.

5. Conclusions

Our study identified clustering patterns of diet, PA and screen time in children, and across European and Asian countries. These findings showed the importance of following a healthy lifestyle to prevent overweight/obesity and support the hypothesis that unfavorable weight status is associated with a particular combination of EBRB patterns. However, associations differed by group of countries and cluster characteristics. These discrepancies might suggest that more behaviors beyond these four may need to be targeted. Obesity prevention strategies need to consider the synergistic effect of these behaviors, and future public health initiatives should target a reduction in screen time use and SSD intake coupled with increased levels of PA and F&V intake. Examining the stability or evolution of the clusters over time in this age group and the associations between cluster membership and sociodemographic factors are potential areas of further research.

Supplementary Materials: The following are available online at http://www.mdpi.com/2072-6643/11/3/511/s1, Table S1: Main characteristics of study design within each country participating in the fourth round of the WHO Europe Childhood Obesity Surveillance Initiative (2015/2017); Table S2: Measuring equipment used within each country participating in the fourth round of the WHO Europe Childhood Obesity Surveillance Initiative (2015/2017); Table S3: Questions on energy balance-related behaviors asked through the family survey questionnaire in the fourth round of the WHO Europe Childhood Obesity Surveillance Initiative (2015/2017).

Author Contributions: S.B.-S. conceptualized the manuscript and conducted all analyses; S.B.-S. and A.O.-R drafted the manuscript; C.C.K., M.M.H. and C.M.M. made substantial contributions to the conception, interpretation of the results and drafts of the manuscript; M.M.H., M.B., S.A., V.D., V.F.S.A., A.F., T.H., C.H., J.H., E.K., S.M.M., G.O., N.P.-F., A.P., A.I.R., L.S., R.T.B., H.R., C.M.M., C.C.K. and J.B. contributed with data collection and data cleaning, and critically reviewed the manuscript. All authors contributed to and approved the final manuscript.

Funding: Data collection in the countries was made possible through funding by: Albania: World Health Organization through the Joint Programme on Children, Food Security and Nutrition "Reducing Malnutrition in Children", funded by the Millennium Development Goals Achievement Fund, and the Institute of Public Health; Bulgaria: Ministry of Health, National Center of Public Health and Analyses, World Health Organization Regional Office for Europe; Croatia: Croatian Institute of Public Health and World Health Organization Regional Office for Europe; Czech Republic: grants AZV MZČR 17-31670 A and MZČR—RVO EÚ 00023761; Denmark: Danish Ministry of Health; Georgia: World Health Organization; Ireland: Health Service Executive; Kazakhstan: Ministry of Health of the Republic of Kazakhstan and World Health Organization Country Office; Latvia: n/a; Lithuania: World Health Organization; Malta: Ministry of Health; Montenegro: World Health Organization and Institute of Public Health of Montenegro; Poland: National Health Programme, Ministry of Health; Portugal: Ministry of Health Institutions, the National Institute of Health, Directorate General of Health, Regional Health Directorates and the kind technical support of Centro de Estudos e Investigação em Dinâmicas Sociais e Saúde (CEIDSS); Romania: Ministry of Health; Russia (Moscow): n/a; Spain: Spanish Agency for Food Safety and Nutrition (AESAN); Tajikistan: n/a; Turkmenistan: World Health Organization Country Office in Turkmenistan and Ministry of Health.

Acknowledgments: We gratefully acknowledge all participating children, their parents, and school teachers and principals for kindly volunteering to participate in the study. We also thank the researchers who collected data in each country.

Conflicts of Interest: The authors declare no conflict of interest. The funders had no role in the design of the study; in the collection, analyses, or interpretation of data; in the writing of the manuscript, or in the decision to publish the results.

Disclaimer: The authors alone are responsible for the views expressed in this article and they do not necessarily represent the views, decisions or policies of the institutions they are affiliated with. Dr João Breda, Dr Marta Buoncristiano and Mrs Guljemal Ovezmyradova are staff members of the WHO Regional Office for Europe. The World Health Organization is not liable for any use that may be made of the information contained therein.

References

1. Commision on Ending Childhood Obesity. Facts and Figures on Childhood Obesity. Available online: http://www.who.int/end-childhood-obesity/facts/en/ (accessed on 8 December 2018).

2. Abarca-Gómez, L.; Abdeen, Z.A.; Hamid, Z.A.; Abu-Rmeileh, N.M.; Acosta-Cazares, B.; Acuin, C.; Adams, R.J.; Aekplakorn, W.; Afsana, K.; Aguilar-Salinas, C.A.; et al. Worldwide trends in body-mass index, underweight, overweight, and obesity from 1975 to 2016: A pooled analysis of 2416 population-based measurement studies in 128.9 million children, adolescents, and adults. *Lancet* **2017**, *390*, 2627–2642. [CrossRef]

3. Bischoff, S.C.; Boirie, Y.; Cederholm, T.; Chourdakis, M.; Cuerda, C.; Delzenne, N.M.; Deutz, N.E.; Fouque, D.; Genton, L.; Gil, C.; et al. Towards a multidisciplinary approach to understand and manage obesity and related diseases. *Clin. Nutr.* **2017**, *36*, 917–938. [CrossRef] [PubMed]

4. Bradlee, M.L.; Singer, M.R.; Qureshi, M.M.; Moore, L.L. Food group intake and central obesity among children and adolescents in the Third National Health and Nutrition Examination Survey (NHANES III). *Public Health Nutr.* **2010**, *13*, 797–805. [CrossRef] [PubMed]

5. Mellendick, K.; Shanahan, L.; Wideman, L.; Calkins, S.; Keane, S.; Lovelady, C. Diets Rich in Fruits and Vegetables Are Associated with Lower Cardiovascular Disease Risk in Adolescents. *Nutrients* **2018**, *10*, 136. [CrossRef] [PubMed]

6. DeBoer, M.D.; Scharf, R.J.; Demmer, R.T. Sugar-sweetened beverages and weight gain in 2- to 5-year-old children. *Pediatrics* **2013**, *132*, 413–420. [CrossRef] [PubMed]

7. Malik, V.S.; Pan, A.; Willett, W.C.; Hu, F.B. Sugar-sweetened beverages and weight gain in children and adults: A systematic review and meta-analysis. *Am. J. Clin. Nutr.* **2013**, *98*, 1084–1102. [CrossRef] [PubMed]

8. Wei, X.; Zang, Y.; Jia, X.; He, X.; Zou, S.; Wang, H.; Shen, M.; Zang, J. Age, period and cohort effects and the predictors of physical activity and sedentary behaviour among Chinese children, from 2004 to 2011. *BMC Public Health* **2017**, *17*, 353. [CrossRef] [PubMed]

9. Falbe, J.; Rosner, B.; Willett, W.C.; Sonneville, K.R.; Hu, F.B.; Field, A.E. Adiposity and different types of screen time. *Pediatrics* **2013**, *132*, e1497–e1505. [CrossRef] [PubMed]

10. Leech, R.M.; McNaughton, S.A.; Timperio, A. The clustering of diet, physical activity and sedentary behavior in children and adolescents: A review. *Int. J. Behav. Nutr. Phys. Act.* **2014**, *11*, 4. [CrossRef] [PubMed]

11. Bel-Serrat, S.; Mouratidou, T.; Santaliestra-Pasias, A.M.; Iacoviello, L.; Kourides, Y.A.; Marild, S.; Molnar, D.; Reisch, L.; Siani, A.; Stomfai, S.; et al. Clustering of multiple lifestyle behaviours and its association to cardiovascular risk factors in children: The IDEFICS study. *Eur. J. Clin. Nutr.* **2013**, *67*, 848–854. [CrossRef] [PubMed]

12. Leech, R.M.; McNaughton, S.A.; Timperio, A. Clustering of diet, physical activity and sedentary behaviour among Australian children: Cross-sectional and longitudinal associations with overweight and obesity. *Int. J. Obes.* **2015**, *39*, 1079–1085. [CrossRef] [PubMed]

13. Santaliestra-Pasias, A.M.; Mouratidou, T.; Reisch, L.; Pigeot, I.; Ahrens, W.; Marild, S.; Molnar, D.; Siani, A.; Sieri, S.; Tornatiris, M.; et al. Clustering of lifestyle behaviours and relation to body composition in European children. The IDEFICS study. *Eur. J. Clin. Nutr.* **2015**, *69*, 811–816. [CrossRef] [PubMed]

14. Sanchez-Oliva, D.; Grao-Cruces, A.; Carbonell-Baeza, A.; Cabanas-Sanchez, V.; Veiga, O.L.; Castro-Pinero, J. Lifestyle Clusters in School-Aged Youth and Longitudinal Associations with Fatness: The UP & DOWN Study. *J. Pediatr.* **2018**, *203*, 317–324. [CrossRef] [PubMed]

15. Seghers, J.; Rutten, C. Clustering of multiple lifestyle behaviours and its relationship with weight status and cardiorespiratory fitness in a sample of Flemish 11- to 12-year-olds. *Public Health Nutr.* **2010**, *13*, 1838–1846. [CrossRef] [PubMed]

16. Perez-Rodrigo, C.; Gil, A.; Gonzalez-Gross, M.; Ortega, R.M.; Serra-Majem, L.; Varela-Moreiras, G.; Aranceta-Bartrina, J. Clustering of Dietary Patterns, Lifestyles, and Overweight among Spanish Children and Adolescents in the ANIBES Study. *Nutrients* **2016**, *8*, 11. [CrossRef] [PubMed]

17. Fernandez-Alvira, J.M.; De Bourdeaudhuij, I.; Singh, A.S.; Vik, F.N.; Manios, Y.; Kovacs, E.; Jan, N.; Brug, J.; Moreno, L.A. Clustering of energy balance-related behaviors and parental education in European children: The ENERGY-project. *Int. J. Behav. Nutr. Phys. Act.* **2013**, *10*, 5. [CrossRef] [PubMed]

18. Dumuid, D.; Olds, T.; Lewis, L.K.; Martin-Fernandez, J.A.; Barreira, T.; Broyles, S.; Chaput, J.P.; Fogelholm, M.; Hu, G.; Kuriyan, R.; et al. The adiposity of children is associated with their lifestyle behaviours: A cluster analysis of school-aged children from 12 nations. *Pediatr. Obes.* **2018**, *13*, 111–119. [CrossRef] [PubMed]

19. Wijnhoven, T.; Branca, F.; WHO European Childhood Obesity Surveillance Initiative. *Protocol, Version January 2008*; WHO Regional Office for Europe: Copenhagen, Denmark, 2008.

20. WHO European Childhood Obesity Surveillance Initiative. *Protocol, Version October 2012*; WHO Regional Office for Europe: Copenhagen, Denmark, 2012.

21. WHO European Childhood Obesity Surveillance Initiative. *Protocol, Version October 2016*; World Health Organization Regional Office for Europe: Copenhagen, Denmark, 2016. Available online: http://www.euro. who.int/__data/assets/pdf_file/0018/333900/COSI-protocol-en.pdf?ua=1 (accessed on 8 December 2018).

22. Wijnhoven, T.M.; van Raaij, J.M.; Spinelli, A.; Starc, G.; Hassapidou, M.; Spiroski, I.; Rutter, H.; Martos, E.; Rito, A.I.; Hovengen, R.; et al. WHO European Childhood Obesity Surveillance Initiative: Body mass index and level of overweight among 6–9-year-old children from school year 2007/2008 to school year 2009/2010. *BMC Public Health* **2014**, *14*, 806. [CrossRef] [PubMed]

23. WHO European Childhood Obesity Surveillance Initiative. *Overweight and Obesity among 6-to-9-Year-Old Children. Results of the Third Round of Data Collection 2012–2013*; World Health Organisation: Copenhagen, Denmark, 2018. Available online: http://www.euro.who.int/__data/assets/pdf_file/0010/378865/COSI-3. pdf?ua=1 (accessed on 8 December 2018).

24. Wijnhoven, T.; van Raaij, J.; Breda, J. *WHO European Childhood Obesity Surveillance Initiative: Implementation of Round 1 (2007/2008) and Round 2 (2009/2010)*; WHO Regional Office for Europe: Conpenhagen, Denmark, 2014. Available online: http://www.euro.who.int/__data/assets/pdf_file/0004/258781/COSI-report-round-1-and-2_final-for-web.pdf?ua=1 (accessed on 8 December 2018).

25. de Onis, M.; Onyango, A.W.; Borghi, E.; Siyam, A.; Nishida, C.; Siekmann, J. Development of a WHO growth reference for school-aged children and adolescents. *Bull. World Health Organ.* **2007**, *85*, 660–667. [CrossRef] [PubMed]

26. Cole, T.J.; Bellizzi, M.C.; Flegal, K.M.; Dietz, W.H. Establishing a standard definition for child overweight and obesity worldwide: International survey. *BMJ* **2000**, *320*, 1240–1243. [CrossRef] [PubMed]

27. Cole, T.J.; Flegal, K.M.; Nicholls, D.; Jackson, A.A. Body mass index cut offs to define thinness in children and adolescents: International survey. *BMJ* **2007**, *335*, 194. [CrossRef] [PubMed]

28. World Health Organization (WHO). *AnthroPlus for Personal Computers Manual: Software for Assessing Growth of the World's Children and Adolescents*; World Health Organization: Geneva, Switzerland, 2009. Available online: http://www.who.int/entity/growthref/tools/who_anthroplus_manual.pdf (accessed on 8 December 2018).

29. Milligan, C.W.; Cooper, M.C. Methodology review: Clustering methods. *Appl. Psychol. Meas.* **1987**, *11*, 329–354. [CrossRef]

30. Gore, P.A. Cluster analysis. In *Handbook of Applied Multivariate Statistics and Mathematical Modeling*, 1st ed.; Tinsley, H.E.A., Brown, S.D., Eds.; Academic Press: San Diego, CA, USA, 2000; pp. 297–321.

31. Everitt, B. *Cluster Analysis*; Heinemann Educational Books: London, UK, 1980.

32. Viera, A.J.; Garrett, J.M. Understanding interobserver agreement: The kappa statistic. *Fam. Med.* **2005**, *37*, 360–363. [PubMed]

33. Popkin, B.M.; Adair, L.S.; Ng, S.W. Global nutrition transition and the pandemic of obesity in developing countries. *Nutr. Rev.* **2012**, *70*, 3–21. [CrossRef] [PubMed]

34. Leech, R.M.; McNaughton, S.A.; Timperio, A. Clustering of children's obesity-related behaviours: Associations with sociodemographic indicators. *Eur. J. Clin. Nutr.* **2014**, *68*, 623–628. [CrossRef] [PubMed]

35. Cameron, A.J.; Crawford, D.A.; Salmon, J.; Campbell, K.; McNaughton, S.A.; Mishra, G.D.; Ball, K. Clustering of obesity-related risk behaviors in children and their mothers. *Ann. Epidemiol.* **2011**, *21*, 95–102. [CrossRef] [PubMed]

36. Physical Activity and Young People. Recommended Levels of Physical Activity for Children Aged 5–17 Years. Available online: https://www.who.int/dietphysicalactivity/factsheet_young_people/en/ (accessed on 8 December 2018).

37. Strasburger, V.C.; Hogan, M.J.; Mulligan, D.A.; Ameenuddin, N.; Christakis, D.A.; Cross, C.; Fagbuyi, D.B.; Hill, D.L.; Levine, A.E.; McCarthy, C.; et al. Children, Adolescents, and the Media. *Pediatrics* **2013**, *132*, 958–961. [CrossRef]

38. Pearson, N.; Biddle, S.J. Sedentary behavior and dietary intake in children, adolescents, and adults. A systematic review. *Am. J. Prev. Med.* **2011**, *41*, 178–188. [CrossRef] [PubMed]

39. Vingerhoets, A.M.; Croon, M.; Jeninga, A.; Menges, L. Personality and health habits. *Psychol. Health* **1990**, *4*, 333–342. [CrossRef]

40. Rogers, E.M. *Diffussion of Innovations*; Free Press of Glencoe: New York, NY, USA, 1962.

41. Li, L.; Zhang, S.; Huang, Y.; Chen, K. Sleep duration and obesity in children: A systematic review and meta-analysis of prospective cohort studies. *J. Pediatr. Child Health* **2017**, *53*, 378–385. [CrossRef] [PubMed]

42. Chesi, A.; Grant, S.F.A. The Genetics of Pediatric Obesity. *Trends Endocrinol. Metab.* **2015**, *26*, 711–721. [CrossRef] [PubMed]

43. Atkin, A.J.; Gorely, T.; Clemes, S.A.; Yates, T.; Edwardson, C.; Brage, S.; Salmon, J.; Marshall, S.J.; Biddle, S.J. Methods of measurement in epidemiology: Sedentary behaviour. *Int. J. Epidemiol.* **2012**, *41*, 1460–1471. [CrossRef] [PubMed]

44. Scharf, R.J.; DeBoer, M.D. Sugar-Sweetened Beverages and Children's Health. *Annu. Rev. Public Health* **2016**, *37*, 273–293. [CrossRef] [PubMed]

45. Collins, C.E.; Watson, J.; Burrows, T. Measuring dietary intake in children and adolescents in the context of overweight and obesity. *Int. J. Obes.* **2010**, *34*, 1103–1115. [CrossRef] [PubMed]

46. Everitt, B.S.; Landau, S.; Leese, M.; Stahl, D. *Cluster Analysis*, 5th ed.; John Wiley & Sons Ltd.: West Sussex, UK, 2011.

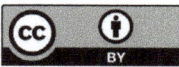

nutrients

MDPI

Article

Emotional Eating, Health Behaviours, and Obesity in Children: A 12-Country Cross-Sectional Study

Elli Jalo [1,*], Hanna Konttinen [1,2], Henna Vepsäläinen [1], Jean-Philippe Chaput [3], Gang Hu [4], Carol Maher [5], José Maia [6], Olga L. Sarmiento [7], Martyn Standage [8], Catrine Tudor-Locke [9], Peter T. Katzmarzyk [4] and Mikael Fogelholm [1]

1   Department of Food and Nutrition, University of Helsinki, 00014 Helsinki, Finland;
    hanna.konttinen@helsinki.fi (H.K.); henna.vepsalainen@helsinki.fi (H.V.);
    mikael.fogelholm@helsinki.fi (M.F.)
2   Sociology, University of Helsinki, 00014 Helsinki, Finland
3   Children's Hospital of Eastern Ontario Research Institute, Ottawa, ON K1H 8L1, Canada;
    jpchaput@cheo.on.ca
4   Pennington Biomedical Research Center, Baton Rouge, LA 70808, USA; gang.hu@pbrc.edu (G.H.);
    peter.katzmarzyk@pbrc.edu (P.T.K.)
5   Alliance for Research In Exercise Nutrition and Activity (ARENA), School of Health Sciences,
    University of South Australia, Adelaide, SA 5001, Australia; carol.maher@unisa.edu.au
6   CIFI2D, Faculdade de Desporto, University of Porto, 4200-450 Porto, Portugal; jmaia@fade.up.pt
7   School of Medicine, Universidad de los Andes, Bogotá 11001000, Colombia; osarmien@uniandes.edu.co
8   Department for Health, University of Bath, Bath BA2 7AY, UK; m.standage@bath.ac.uk
9   Department of Kinesiology, School of Public Health and Health Sciences, University of Massachusetts
    Amherst, MA 01003, USA; ctudorlocke@umass.edu
*   Correspondence: elli.jalo@helsinki.fi; Tel. +358-50-404-6550

Received: 21 December 2018; Accepted: 5 February 2019; Published: 7 February 2019

Abstract: Eating in response to negative emotions (emotional eating, EE) may predispose an individual to obesity. Yet, it is not well known how EE in children is associated with body mass index (BMI) and health behaviours (i.e., diet, physical activity, sleep, and TV-viewing). In the present study, we examined these associations in a cross-sectional sample of 5426 (54% girls) 9–11-year-old children from 12 countries and five continents. EE, food consumption, and TV-viewing were measured using self-administered questionnaires, and physical activity and nocturnal sleep duration were measured with accelerometers. BMI was calculated using measured weights and heights. EE factor scores were computed using confirmatory factor analysis, and dietary patterns were identified using principal components analysis. The associations of EE with health behaviours and BMI z-scores were analyzed using multilevel models including age, gender, and household income as covariates. EE was positively and consistently (across 12 study sites) associated with an unhealthy dietary pattern (β = 0.29, SE = 0.02, p < 0.0001), suggesting that the association is not restricted to Western countries. Positive associations between EE and physical activity and TV viewing were not consistent across sites. Results tended to be similar in boys and girls. EE was unrelated to BMI in this sample, but prospective studies are needed to determine whether higher EE in children predicts the development of undesirable dietary patterns and obesity over time.

Keywords: eating behaviour; psychological eating style; negative emotions; Emotion-Induced Eating Scale; health behaviour; BMI

1. Introduction

Childhood obesity rates are high in both developed and developing countries [1]. It is likely that the most important contributors are the increased availability of energy-dense foods and a reduced need for physical activity—the current obesogenic environment. Many individual characteristics could be relevant for explaining the differential susceptibility to the development of obesity among individuals in the same environment. One example is emotional eating (EE), which refers to a tendency to eat more in response to negative emotions [2,3]. According to the EE theory (also called the psychosomatic theory), individuals with EE use eating to reduce the intensity of negative emotions [2]. This is considered a poor coping strategy, and such difficulties in emotion regulation may be one possible mechanism underlying EE [4]. Foods consumed in response to negative emotions are usually high in sugar and/or fat [3]. These palatable foods provide hedonic pleasure and instant reward, which may distract from the experience of negative emotions [3]. Because an expected normal physiological reaction to negative emotions is a suppressed appetite [3,5], EE may interfere with physiological regulation. It may therefore represent a risk factor for becoming overweight and obese. Several studies have indeed suggested this might be the case in adults, since EE has been found to correlate positively with body mass index (BMI) [6–9] and to predict weight gain [10,11].

However, in children, empirical evidence regarding the association between EE and obesity is far from conclusive. Cross-sectional studies conducted with children (mean age between 7 and 13 years) have reported a positive association [12–18], no association [19,20], or even an inverse association [21–23] between EE and BMI/being overweight. It is possible that some of these inconsistencies are related to the use of different approaches to measure EE in previous work. Even though it has been shown that there is a good agreement between self-reported and parent-reported EE [13], the majority of the studies reporting positive associations with BMI/being overweight have employed parent-reported EE [12,14–18]. In contrast, self-reported EE has been employed in studies reporting an inverse association with BMI/being overweight [21–23]. Regardless, broader measures of emotion dysregulation have also been associated with obesity in children. For example, emotion-driven impulsiveness was associated with increased BMI z-scores in a large sample of 12–18-year-old children [24]. In longitudinal studies, parent-reported EE at the age of 5 to 6 years predicted higher BMI in 7–8-year-old children [25], but parent-reported EE at the age of 6 years was not associated with changes in BMI standard deviation scores in children aged 6 to 8 years [26].

Health behaviours, such as adhering to a healthy diet and getting adequate physical activity and sleep, are potentially important in prevention of childhood obesity [27–29]. As in adults, EE has been associated with a higher consumption of salty and sweet energy-dense foods and soft drinks in 12–15-year-old children [30] and a higher consumption of sweets and soft drinks in 12-year-old girls [31]. In contrast, in children aged between 5 and 12 years, no association between EE and the consumption of snacks [20,32], sweet foods [32], or fatty foods [32] has been reported. Even though these contradictory findings may be due to methodological issues (e.g., crude measure for snacking, and parent- vs. self-reported food consumption data), it is currently unclear whether EE is associated with diet in children under the age of 12 years. The clustering of health behaviours in children [33,34] raises the question of whether EE is also related to physical activity, sedentary behaviour (such as TV viewing), and/or sleep duration. Given that these behaviours do not occur in isolation, it is important to study them simultaneously.

The aim of this study was to examine the associations between self-reported EE, health behaviours (i.e., dietary patterns, physical activity, sleep duration, and TV viewing), and BMI in 9–11-year-old children. Because of inconsistent evidence and the limited number of previous studies, the analyses were exploratory, and we did not have specific hypotheses regarding the directions of these associations. Previous studies on EE in children have been mainly conducted in Western countries (in Europe and North America). In this work, we used a large sample from 12 countries and five continents, which gave us a unique opportunity to examine whether EE is consistently linked to behaviours that predispose individuals to obesity across countries representing diversity in terms of development, culture, socioeconomic status, and ethnic backgrounds.

2. Materials and Methods

2.1. Study Setting and Participants

The present study is a secondary analysis of the International Study of Childhood Obesity, Lifestyle and the Environment (ISCOLE), which aimed to determine the relationships between lifestyle behaviours and obesity in children. The details of the ISCOLE protocol have been reported previously [35]. The cross-sectional sample consisted of 9–11-year-old children from study sites located in urban and semi-urban areas in 12 different countries from all parts of the world (Australia, Brazil, Canada, China, Colombia, Finland, India, Kenya, Portugal, South Africa, the United Kingdom, and the United States). Rural areas were excluded due to logistical concerns. Each study site identified one or more school districts with a sufficient population to provide a sample of 500 children. The primary sampling unit within sites was schools, and the secondary sampling unit was classes within the schools. Schools were stratified by socio-economic status before sampling in order to maximize variability within sites see [35]. The Institutional Review Board at the Pennington Biomedical Research Center (coordinating center) approved the overarching ISCOLE protocol, and the Institutional/Ethical Review Boards at each participating institution approved the local protocols. Parents or legal guardians provided written informed consent, and children provided their written assent before participation, as required by local ethics boards. Data were collected from September 2011 through December 2013.

In total, 7372 children participated in ISCOLE [36], of which 5426 (74%) were included in the present analytical sample. Children who were missing data on one or several of the following variables were excluded: emotional eating (0.7% were excluded due to lacking data on this variable), dietary patterns (2.3%), accelerometry (moderate to vigorous physical activity (MVPA) and/or sleep, 16.5%), TV viewing (0.6%), BMI (0.4%), and household income (11.1%).

2.2. Emotional Eating

EE was measured via the Emotion-Induced Eating Scale (EIES), which was developed using a sample of over 2000 girls aged 9 to 10 years from the United States by Striegel-Moore et al. [21]. Children completed the EIES as part of a six-page questionnaire. The original EIES consists of seven items pertaining to emotionally-induced eating, as follows: eating in response to feeling sad, worried, mad, bored, or happy (e.g., "I eat more when I'm sad"), eating when not hungry, and using food as a reward. Responses were recorded on a 3-point scale (1 = never or almost never, 2 = sometimes, 3 = usually or always). See Supplementary Materials, Figure S1 for item level frequencies of the original EIES. However, taking a closer look at the wordings of the original EIES items reveals that two items out of the seven do not describe eating in response to emotions ("I eat between meals even if I'm not hungry" and "When I do something well I give myself a food treat"), and one item describes eating in response to a positive affective state ("I eat more when I'm happy"). EE is traditionally defined as "eating induced by negative emotions" [2], and it is also suggested that the desire to eat in response to negative emotions vs. positive emotions are two different constructs [5]. We wanted to adhere to this definition, and therefore used only the four items describing eating in response to negative emotions (sad, mad, worried, and bored) to assess EE in this study.

A confirmatory factor analysis (CFA) using a weighted least squares estimation with robust standard errors and a mean and variance adjusted test statistic (Lavaan package version 0.5.-23.1097 in the R system of statistical computing) was applied to test whether the four items describing eating in response to negative emotions loaded onto a one-factor latent construct. The items were used as ordinal variables in the analysis. The CFA was first conducted for the pooled data and then repeated for each study site and both genders separately. When evaluating the model fit, Comparative Fit Index (CFI) and Tucker–Lewis Index (TLI) values $\geq$0.95, a Root Mean Square Error of the Approximation (RMSEA) value $\leq$0.06, and a Standardized Root Square Mean Residuals (SRMR) value $\leq$0.08 were considered to indicate a good fit between the model and data [37]. Based on these criteria, the model showed an excellent fit for the pooled data (χ^2(df) = 2.660(2), p for χ^2 = 0.264, CFI = 1.000, TLI = 1.000,

RMSEA = 0.007 and SRMR = 0.006, Table 1). The Cronbach's alpha value for the four EE items was 0.60. For comparison, we tested also the original 7-item scale. CFA indicated a poorer fit compared to 4-item model (χ^2(df) = 364.68(14), p for χ^2 < 0.001, CFI = 0.96, TLI = 0.94, RMSEA = 0.06, and SRMR = 0.04). Furthermore, the Cronbach's alpha value for the 7-item scale (0.65) was not substantially higher than the respective value for the 4-item scale, especially because alpha always increases when more items are added [38]. These results further supported our initial decision to include only the four items measuring eating in response to negative emotions.

In the gender-stratified analysis, standardized factor loadings were highly comparable between boys and girls (Table 1). The test of the measurement invariance also indicated strong invariance, since CFI values changed less than 0.01 [39] when loadings (ΔCFI = 0.001, p for $\Delta\chi^2$ = 0.416), thresholds (ΔCFI < 0.001, p for $\Delta\chi^2$ = 0.874), and residual variances (ΔCFI = 0.001, p for $\Delta\chi^2$ = 0.182) were forced equal across the genders in a stepwise manner. There were some differences in factor loadings between the study sites in the site-stratified analysis, especially regarding the item about eating in response to boredom (factor loadings ranged from 0.31 to 0.87 between the sites). The test of the measurement invariance also indicated that loadings were not equal across the study sites (ΔCFI = 0.03, p for $\Delta\chi^2$ < 0.001). Yet, since partial metric invariance (equality of factor structure and factor loadings) was achieved after releasing an equality constraint only for one factor loading (the "bored" item, ΔCFI=0.008, p for $\Delta\chi^2$ = 0.064), we decided to use the EE factor scores from the pooled data in the present analyses. However, we also repeated all analyses by using the site-specific EE factor scores and found that the results remained highly similar (data not shown). EE factor scores were computed using the Empirical Bayes approach.

Table 1. Confirmatory factor analysis [a] for Emotion-Induced Eating Scale (EIES) negative emotion items.

	n	χ^2 (df)	p-Value	CFI	TLI	RMSEA	SRMR	Standardized Factor Loadings for EIES Items [b]			
								Sad	Worried	Mad	Bored
All	7319	2.66 (2)	0.264	1.00	1.00	0.01	0.01	0.79	0.69	0.62	0.46
Gender											
Boys	3393	0.32 (2)	0.854	1.00	1.00	<0.01	<0.01	0.79	0.70	0.61	0.44
Girls	3926	6.53 (2)	0.038	1.00	0.99	0.02	0.013	0.78	0.69	0.63	0.49
Country (city/cities)											
Australia (Adelaide)	526	0.89 (2)	0.642	1.00	1.01	<0.01	0.01	0.82	0.69	0.65	0.52
Brazil (Sao Paulo)	569	0.26 (2)	0.878	1.00	1.01	<0.01	0.01	0.75	0.70	0.43	0.85
Canada (Ottawa)	566	0.14 (2)	0.932	1.00	1.02	<0.01	0.01	0.94	0.66	0.66	0.41
China (Tianjin)	549	3.27 (2)	0.195	1.00	0.99	0.03	0.03	0.75	0.61	0.83	0.37
Colombia (Bogota)	919	4.20 (2)	0.123	0.99	0.96	0.04	0.03	0.61	0.55	0.53	0.36
Finland (Helsinki, Espoo, Vantaa)	535	1.29 (2)	0.524	1.00	1.01	<0.01	0.02	0.72	0.79	0.58	0.59
India (Bangalore)	620	0.79 (2)	0.675	1.00	1.03	<0.01	0.02	0.62	0.60	0.48	0.44
Kenya (Nairobi)	559	5.11 (2)	0.078	0.99	0.95	0.05	0.03	0.85	0.58	0.47	0.31
Portugal (Porto)	777	3.42 (2)	0.181	1.00	1.00	0.03	0.02	0.74	0.81	0.79	0.87
South Africa (Cape Town)	541	7.31 (2)	0.026	0.98	0.95	0.07	0.04	0.81	0.62	0.62	0.38
United Kingdom (Bath and Somerset)	525	1.08 (2)	0.583	1.00	1.01	<0.01	0.01	0.85	0.69	0.63	0.52
Unites States of America (Baton Rouge)	633	2.02 (2)	0.365	1.00	1.00	<0.01	0.02	0.84	0.76	0.76	0.60

(a) The weighted least squares estimation with robust standard errors and a mean and variance adjusted test statics was used, and items were used as ordinal variables. The model fit was evaluated with several types of fit indices including Chi-Square statistics, the Comparative Fit Index (CFI), the Tucker–Lewis Index (TLI), the Root Mean Square Error of Approximation (RMSEA), and the Standardized Root Mean Square Residual (SRMR). As suggested by Hu and Bentler [37], CFI and TLI values $\geq$0.95, RMSEA values $\leq$0.06, and SRMR values $\leq$0.08 were considered to indicate a good fit for the data. Results are presented for pooled data and separately for each gender and country (city/cities). (b) Sad = "I eat more when I'm sad", worried = "I eat more, when I'm worried", mad = "I eat when I'm mad", bored = "I eat more, when I'm bored".

2.3. Dietary patterns

Dietary patterns were defined using data from a self-administered food frequency questionnaire (FFQ), in which children reported their usual consumption frequency of 23 different food groups, according to seven response categories ranging from "never" to "more than once a day". The FFQ was validated within ISCOLE against 3-day pre-coded food diaries [40]. The identification of the two dietary patterns has been reported in detail elsewhere [41]. In short, principal components analysis

(PCA) with an orthogonal Varimax transformation was carried out using weekly portions of the FFQ food groups as input variables. From the 23 FFQ food groups, fruit juices were excluded from PCA due to low validity of reporting [40]. Two components were identified and named: (1) an unhealthy diet pattern, with high loadings for fast foods, ice cream, fried food, French fries, potato chips, cakes and sugar-sweetened sodas, and (2) a healthy diet pattern, with high loadings for dark-green vegetables, orange vegetables, vegetables in general, and fruits and berries. The naming was based on previous knowledge of associations between health and food items that loaded highly on the two dietary patterns. In total, the two dietary patterns explained 36% of the total variance in reported food consumption. The unhealthy diet pattern was stronger with an eigenvalue of 4.8 (22% of variance explained), and the healthy diet pattern was slightly weaker with an eigenvalue of 3.1 (14% of variance explained). The PCA was also repeated for each site separately, and the resulting site-specific diet patterns were very similar to the patterns that emerged with the pooled data. In the present paper, we used the pattern scores from the pooled data in accordance with the EE factor scores.

2.4. Physical Activity and Sleep

The average daily time spent in MVPA and average nocturnal sleep duration were assessed using the Actigraph GT3X+ accelerometer (Pensacola, FL, USA). The device was worn at the waist on an elastic belt for 24 hours per day (removing only for water-related activities, such as swimming or taking a shower) for at least seven days. The minimal amount of data considered adequate to calculate the average daily MVPA was at least four days with 10 or more hours of daily awake wear time, including at least one weekend day. MVPA was defined as $\geq$574 counts per 15 s [42]. Nocturnal sleep duration was estimated using an algorithm for 24-h accelerometers that was previously validated for the ISCOLE [43]. This algorithm captures the total nocturnal sleep time from sleep onset to the end of sleep and distinguishes it from daytime sleep episodes, and its accuracy was shown to be acceptable when compared to sleep logs [43]. Only nights with valid sleep (total sleep time $\geq$160 min) were used to calculate the mean nocturnal sleep duration of the week and adequate data for calculating the average value was considered at least 3 valid nights, including one weekend night (Friday or Saturday).

2.5. TV Viewing

TV viewing time was determined with a self-administered questionnaire, which was adapted from the U.S. Youth Risk Behaviour Surveillance system [44]. Children were asked how many hours they typically watched TV for weekdays and weekend days separately. The response categories (respective scores) were "I did not watch TV" (0), less than 1 h (0.5), 1 h (1), 2 h (2), 3 h (3), 4 h (4), and 5 or more h (5). The total score was calculated by weighing the responses for weekdays by 5/7 and weekend days by 2/7. The TV viewing questions were shown to have adequate reliability ($r = 0.55$–0.68) and validity ($r = 0.47$) in a sample of 11–15-year-old U.S. children [45].

2.6. BMI

Anthropometric measurements were conducted during the school day by trained study assistants. Height was measured without shoes using a Seca 213 portable stadiometer (Hamburg, Germany) and weight was measured when participants were barefoot, in light indoor clothing, and without any pocket items, using a portable Tanita SC-240 Body Composition Analyzer (Arlington Heights, IL). Two measurements were obtained, and the average was used for analysis. If the first two measurements were more than 0.5 cm or 0.5 kg apart for height and weight, respectively, a third measurement was done, and the closest two measurements were averaged for analysis. BMI was calculated dividing the weight by the height squared (kg/m^2). Age- and gender-specific reference data from the World Health Organization were used to compute the BMI z-scores [46].

2.7. Covariates

Age, gender, and household income were used as covariates. Parents reported the annual household income using eight to ten predefined categories designed for each study site. Country-specific income categories were merged into four levels. It was not possible to achieve exact quartiles, but the aim of the merging was to ensure the distribution of income was as balanced as possible.

2.8. Statistical analyses

The descriptive results were calculated using IBM SPSS Statistics 24 (IBM SPSS, Chicago, IL, USA). An independent samples t-test and a χ^2 test were used to compare the analytical sample with excluded children. Since the sample was clustered at three levels (students nested within schools nested within study sites), the associations between the EE factor scores and dependent variables were assessed using multilevel linear regression models (PROC MIXED of SAS statistical package version 9.4; SAS Institute Inc., Cary; NC, USA). Study sites and schools nested within study sites were both considered to have random effects. The denominator degrees of freedom for statistical tests pertaining to fixed effects were calculated using the Kenward and Roger approximation [47]. The first adjusted models included age, gender, and household income as covariates. In addition to that, second fully adjusted models included other health behaviours and BMI z-scores. Since a few earlier studies found a gender difference in the association between EE and BMI [22,23], we tested the interaction between the EE factor scores and gender in the fully adjusted models. Multilevel linear regression models were repeated for each site separately, and in these analyses, schools were considered as having random effects. Due to the skewness of the EE factor score variable, it was also studied as a categorical variable with five categories. This variable was formed with two steps: first, children who answered "never" for all four EE items were categorized into one group, and second, remaining children were categorized into quarters based on the EE factor scores.

3. Results

3.1. Descriptive Results

The analytical sample of the present study comprised 5426 children (74% of the overall study sample). Children who were excluded because of missing data showed more tendency towards EE than the included children (mean (SD) score 0.09 (0.58) vs. 0.03 (0.56), $p < 0.001$). In addition, as compared with the analytical sample, they had higher scores for the unhealthy diet pattern (0.22 (1.18) vs. −0.07 (0.93), $p < 0.001$), watched more TV (TV viewing score 1.8 (1.3) vs. 1.7 (1.2), $p = 0.001$), and had higher BMI z scores (0.61 (1.28) vs. 0.44 (1.25), $p < 0.001$). Also, more boys were excluded from the analytical sample than girls (28% vs. 25%, $p = 0.002$). Parents of the excluded children belonged more frequently to the lowest income group compared with those in the analytical sample (30% vs. 25%, $p < 0.001$). There were no differences in the scores for the healthy diet pattern, the amount of MVPA, sleep duration, or age between the excluded and included children.

Out of the analytical sample, 32% of the children answered "never or almost never" to all four EE items, and 25% answered "never or almost never" to three items and "sometimes" to one item. Only 18 (0.3%) children answered "usually or always" to all four EE items. Descriptive results stratified by gender and study site including the EE factor scores are presented in Table 2. There were no significant differences in the EE factor scores between boys and girls (data not shown), except in the United Kingdom, where girls showed a higher tendency towards EE compared with boys (mean (SD) score 0.10 (0.55) in girls vs. −0.04 (0.50) in boys, t-test = −2.37, $p = 0.018$).

Nutrients **2019**, 11, 351

Table 2. Descriptive results of the analytical sample by gender and country (city/cities).

	Number of Participants (% Girls)	Emotional Eating Score [a]	Unhealthy Diet Score [b]	Healthy Diet Score [b]	Mean (SD)			BMI z-Score	Age (years)	Household Classified Lowest Income [e], n (%)	Household Classified Highest Income [e], n (%)
					MVPA (min/day) [c]	Sleep (min/day) [c]	TV Viewing [d]				
All	5426 (55)	0.03 (0.56)	−0.07 (0.93)	0.00 (0.99)	60 (25)	528 (53)	1.7 (1.2)	0.43 (1.25)	10.4 (0.6)	1376 (25)	1466 (27)
Gender											
Boys	2461 (0)	0.03 (0.56)	0.00 (0.98)	−0.06 (1.00)	70 (26)	524 (52)	1.8 (1.2)	0.53 (1.30)	10.4 (0.6)	596 (24)	696 (28)
Girls	2965 (100)	0.03 (0.56)	−0.14 (0.89)	0.04 (0.99)	52 (21)	532 (53)	1.6 (1.2)	0.36 (1.21)	10.4 (0.6)	780 (26)	770 (26)
Country (city/cities)											
Australia (Adelaide)	407 (54)	0.05 (0.54)	−0.30 (0.73)	0.24 (0.94)	65 (23)	565 (43)	1.7 (1.1)	0.57 (1.13)	10.7 (0.4)	88 (22)	94 (23)
Brazil (Sao Paulo)	378 (50)	0.24 (0.61)	0.09 (0.90)	−0.45 (1.05)	60 (27)	512 (49)	2.2 (1.4)	0.92 (1.43)	10.5 (0.5)	144 (38)	52 (14)
Canada (Ottawa)	481 (59)	−0.10 (0.51)	−0.50 (0.57)	0.49 (0.98)	59 (20)	544 (51)	1.4 (1.2)	0.42 (1.21)	10.5 (0.4)	88 (18)	186 (39)
China (Tianjin)	430 (48)	−0.09 (0.47)	−0.24 (0.96)	0.05 (0.90)	45 (16)	527 (39)	1.2 (1.1)	0.73 (1.54)	9.9 (0.5)	86 (20)	135 (31)
Colombia (Bogota)	810 (51)	−0.02 (0.52)	−0.08 (0.55)	−0.45 (0.74)	68 (25)	525 (49)	2.1 (1.1)	0.20 (1.05)	10.5 (0.6)	279 (34)	185 (23)
Finland (Helsinki, Espoo, Vantaa)	426 (55)	−0.08 (0.52)	−0.57 (0.43)	−0.15 (0.85)	70 (27)	508 (56)	1.4 (0.9)	0.27 (1.04)	10.5 (0.4)	81 (19)	174 (41)
India (Bangalore)	500 (55)	0.06 (0.51)	−0.10 (0.83)	−0.09 (0.89)	48 (21)	516 (44)	1.2 (0.9)	0.22 (1.36)	10.4 (0.5)	121 (24)	188 (38)
Kenya (Nairobi)	434 (54)	0.19 (0.57)	0.11 (1.01)	0.28 (0.99)	73 (32)	515 (52)	1.6 (1.3)	−0.06 (1.20)	10.2 (0.7)	101 (23)	126 (29)
Portugal (Porto)	490 (57)	−0.09 (0.56)	−0.36 (0.63)	0.25 (1.04)	56 (22)	497 (51)	1.5 (1.0)	0.83 (1.13)	10.4 (0.3)	96 (20)	105 (21)
South Africa (Cape Town)	267 (60)	0.35 (0.67)	1.08 (1.25)	0.26 (1.08)	62 (25)	552 (43)	2.0 (1.3)	0.20 (1.27)	10.2 (0.7)	133 (45)	37 (13)
United Kingdom (Bath and Somerset)	355 (57)	0.04 (0.53)	−0.17 (0.73)	0.03 (0.91)	64 (23)	569 (43)	1.7 (1.0)	0.40 (1.08)	10.9 (0.4)	95 (27)	81 (23)
Unites States of America (Baton Rouge)	418 (60)	0.00 (0.59)	0.59 (1.36)	−0.14 (1.14)	50 (19)	533 (55)	2.0 (1.4)	0.71 (1.27)	9.9 (0.6)	64 (15)	103 (25)

(a) Confirmatory factor analysis with weighted least squares estimation with robust standard errors and a mean and variance adjusted test statistic was conducted. Factor scores were computed using the Empirical Bayes approach, and the range of scores was −0.55 to 1.93. (b) Component scores identified with principal components analysis with an orthogonal varimax rotation. (c) The average amount of moderate to vigorous physical activity (MVPA) during the day and the average amount of night-time sleep, measured with accelerometers. (d) TV viewing score obtained from a questionnaire: minimum 0 points, maximum 5 points. (e) Annual household income was reported by parents using site-specific categories, which were merged into four levels.

62

3.2. Associations between Emotional Eating, Health Behaviours and BMI

The results from the multilevel linear regression models using the EE score as an independent variable are presented in Table 3. In the unadjusted models, EE was positively associated with the unhealthy diet pattern, MVPA, and TV viewing, and inversely associated with the BMI z-score. No associations were observed between the EE and the healthy diet pattern or sleep duration. The associations with the unhealthy diet pattern, MVPA, and TV viewing remained significant after adjusting for covariates (age, gender, and income), other health behaviours, and BMI z-scores. There was an interaction between the EE score and gender only in association with MVPA ($p = 0.02$). The association between EE and MVPA was positive for both genders, but it was stronger in boys ($\beta = 3.31$, SE = 0.86, $p = 0.0001$) than in girls ($\beta = 1.28$, SE = 0.60, $p = 0.035$, Table 4).

The adjusted multilevel linear regression models were repeated for each site separately (Table 4). The positive association observed between the EE score and the unhealthy diet pattern was consistent across the study sites, but the significant positive association between EE and MVPA was observed only in Colombia and South Africa, and the significant positive association between EE and TV viewing was observed only in Canada and China.

When EE was included in the adjusted multilevel linear regression models as a categorical variable to account for the skewness of the original continuous variable, the results remained highly similar (Table 5). Compared to children with no EE, children in all EE quarters had higher unhealthy diet pattern scores, and this association followed a linear pattern according to the EE score quarters. A linear positive association was also found between the categorical EE variable and MVPA, and there was a significant, but not very strong, interaction with gender ($p = 0.04$). The association was significant for both genders, but it was stronger for boys. The categorical EE variable was also associated with TV viewing, but the association was not linear. Similar to the continuous EE score, the categorical EE variable was not associated with the healthy diet pattern, sleep duration, or BMI z-score.

Table 3. The associations [a] between emotional eating factor scores (as the independent variable) and outcome variables [b]. *n* = 5426.

	Unhealthy Diet Pattern		Healthy Diet Pattern		MVPA		Sleep		TV Viewing		BMI z-Score	
	Beta (SE)	p-Value	Beta (SE)	p-Value	Beta (SE)	p-Value	Beta (SE)	p-Value	Beta (SE)	p-Value	Beta (SE)	p-Value
Unadjusted [c]	0.33 (0.02)	<0.0001	−0.03 (0.02)	0.739	2.95 (0.55)	<0.0001	−0.04 (1.20)	0.977	0.16 (0.03)	<0.0001	−0.09 (0.03)	0.004
1. Adjusted model [d]	0.32 (0.02)	<0.0001	−0.03 (0.02)	0.291	2.65 (0.51)	<0.0001	0.01 (1.19)	0.993	0.15 (0.03)	<0.0001	−0.09 (0.03)	0.004
2. Adjusted model [e]	0.29 (0.02)	<0.0001	−0.04 (0.02)	0.138	2.01 (0.51)	<0.0001	0.65 (1.22)	0.594	0.07 (0.03)	0.010	−0.06 (0.03)	0.055

(a) Analyzed with a multilevel (site, schools nested within sites) linear regression. (b) The unhealthy and healthy diet pattern scores identified using principal components analysis, daily moderate to vigorous physical activity (min, MVPA), nightly sleep duration (min), TV viewing scores, and BMI z-scores. (c) Only using the emotional eating factor score as an independent variable. (d) Adjusted by age, gender, and household income. (e) Adjusted by age, gender, household income, and other outcome variables.

Table 4. The association between emotional eating [a] and outcome variables [b] in gender-stratified [c] and site-stratified [d] analyses.

	N	Unhealthy Diet Pattern		Healthy Diet Pattern		MVPA		Sleep		TV Viewing		BMI z-Score	
		Beta (SE)	p-Value	Beta (SE)	p-Value	Beta (SE)	p-Value	Beta (SE)	p-Value	Beta (SE)	p-Value	Beta (SE)	p-Value
Gender													
Boys	2461	0.29 (0.03)	<0.0001	−0.03 (0.04)	0.346	3.31 (0.86)	0.0001	−0.91 (1.80)	0.613	0.08 (0.04)	0.068	−0.11 (0.05)	0.014
Girls	2965	0.30 (0.03)	<0.0001	−0.03 (0.03)	0.392	1.28 (0.60)	0.035	1.60 (1.67)	0.337	0.05 (0.04)	0.157	−0.03 (0.04)	0.493
Study sites													
Australia (Adelaide)	407	0.35 (0.06)	<0.0001	−0.01 (0.09)	0.911	0.00 (1.95)	0.998	−2.43 (4.01)	0.544	0.09 (0.10)	0.390	0.17 (0.11)	0.117
Brazil (Sao Paulo)	378	0.19 (0.08)	0.014	−0.06 (0.09)	0.546	3.60 (1.92)	0.062	3.95 (4.04)	0.329	0.05 (0.12)	0.674	0.07 (0.12)	0.562
Canada (Ottawa)	481	0.18 (0.05)	0.0001	−0.01 (0.09)	0.903	1.06 (1.63)	0.515	−0.69 (4.08)	0.867	0.27 (0.10)	0.008	−0.09 (0.11)	0.392
China (Tianjin)	378	0.43 (0.10)	<0.0001	−0.04 (0.10)	0.710	−0.75 (1.57)	0.634	0.66 (4.17)	0.874	0.34 (0.10)	0.001	−0.19 (0.16)	0.227
Colombia (Bogota)	810	0.20 (0.04)	<0.0001	0.10 (0.05)	0.045	3.33 (1.51)	0.028	2.97 (3.44)	0.389	0.10 (0.08)	0.186	−0.16 (0.07)	0.021
Finland (Helsinki; Espoo, Vantaa)	426	0.18 (0.04)	<0.0001	0.02 (0.08)	0.809	1.09 (2.25)	0.630	−2.47 (5.15)	0.632	−0.04 (0.09)	0.624	−0.21 (0.10)	0.032
India (Bangalore)	500	0.21 (0.07)	0.004	−0.10 (0.08)	0.197	−0.10 (1.50)	0.945	1.24 (3.98)	0.756	−0.04 (0.08)	0.583	−0.14 (0.12)	0.246
Kenya (Nairobi)	434	0.30 (0.08)	0.0003	−0.09 (0.09)	0.283	2.80 (1.89)	0.139	1.08 (4.71)	0.819	0.01 (0.11)	0.933	0.12 (0.10)	0.243
Portugal (Porto)	490	0.27 (0.05)	<0.0001	0.05 (0.09)	0.587	2.86 (1.56)	0.068	−0.51 (4.37)	0.907	0.13 (0.08)	0.110	−0.11 (0.10)	0.287
South Africa (Cape Town)	267	0.62 (0.11)	<0.0001	−0.21 (0.11)	0.052	5.12 (2.23)	0.022	2.41 (4.46)	0.589	0.09 (0.13)	0.475	0.06 (0.13)	0.633
United Kingdom (Bath and Somerset)	355	0.23 (0.07)	0.0007	0.01 (0.09)	0.913	−1.98 (1.97)	0.317	−4.68 (4.27)	0.273	−0.04 (0.10)	0.684	0.01 (0.11)	0.920
Unites States of America (Baton Rouge)	418	0.47 (0.09)	<0.0001	−0.03 (0.10)	0.788	0.53 (1.44)	0.715	1.78 (4.52)	0.695	−0.03 (0.11)	0.791	−0.06 (0.11)	0.600

(a) Emotional eating factor scores as the independent variable. (b) The unhealthy and healthy diet pattern scores identified using principal components analysis, daily moderate to vigorous physical activity (min, MVPA), nightly sleep duration (min), TV viewing scores, and BMI z-scores. (c) Analyzed with a multilevel (site, schools nested within sites) linear regression, adjusted with age, household income, and other outcome variables. (d) Analyzed with a multilevel (schools) linear regression, adjusted by age, gender, household income, and other outcome variables.

Table 5. The associations [a] between categorized emotional eating factor scores [b] and outcome variables [c].

	n (%)	Unhealthy Diet Pattern		Healthy Diet Pattern		MVPA		Sleep		TV Viewing		BMI z-Score	
		Beta (SE)	p-Value	Beta (SE)	p-Value	Beta (SE)	p-Value	Beta (SE)	p-Value	Beta (SE)	p-Value	Beta (SE)	p-Value
All	1759 (32)		<0.0001		0.190		0.0008		0.105		0.002		0.248
No emotional eating		ref.		ref.		ref.		ref.		ref.		ref.	
1. quarter	943 (17)	0.11 (0.03)	0.0006	−0.05 (0.04)	0.201	−0.15 (0.82)	0.853	4.42 (1.95)	0.023	0.11 (0.05)	0.014	−0.09 (0.05)	0.065
2. quarter	771 (14)	0.14 (0.03)	<0.0001	−0.08 (0.04)	0.044	0.51 (0.86)	0.551	−1.20 (2.05)	0.557	0.08 (0.05)	0.105	−0.01 (0.05)	0.889
3. quarter	1017 (19)	0.27 (0.03)	<0.0001	−0.06 (0.04)	0.145	1.27 (0.79)	0.109	2.28 (1.89)	0.230	0.18 (0.04)	<0.0001	−0.06 (0.05)	0.239
4. quarter	936 (17)	0.43 (0.03)	<0.0001	−0.08 (0.04)	0.050	3.36 (0.84)	<0.0001	1.74 (2.01)	0.387	0.09 (0.05)	0.047	−0.09 (0.05)	0.093
Boys	789 (32)		<0.0001		0.573		0.001		0.833		0.097		0.052
No emotional eating		ref.		ref.		ref.		ref.		ref.		ref.	
1. quarter	432 (18)	0.10 (0.05)	0.060	−0.03 (0.06)	0.656	−0.96 (1.37)	0.486	−0.09 (2.87)	0.974	0.06 (0.07)	0.371	−0.17 (0.07)	0.021
2. quarter	356 (15)	0.15 (0.05)	0.007	−0.08 (0.06)	0.190	1.45 (1.45)	0.316	−2.40 (3.03)	0.427	0.05 (0.07)	0.512	−0.10 (0.08)	0.215
3. quarter	452 (18)	0.29 (0.05)	<0.0001	−0.08 (0.06)	0.182	2.28 (1.35)	0.093	0.74 (2.83)	0.795	0.19 (0.07)	0.006	−0.17 (0.07)	0.020
4. quarter	432 (18)	0.41 (0.05)	<0.0001	−0.07 (0.06)	0.261	5.09 (1.42)	0.0003	−2.14 (2.96)	0.470	0.09 (0.07)	0.224	−0.18 (0.08)	0.020
Girls	970 (33)		<0.0001		0.615		0.046		0.025		0.038		0.737
No emotional eating		ref.		ref.		ref.		ref.		ref.		ref.	
1. quarter	511 (17)	0.12 (0.04)	0.004	−0.06 (0.05)	0.265	−0.08 (0.96)	0.932	8.01 (2.67)	0.003	0.14 (0.06)	0.017	−0.02 (0.07)	0.727
2. quarter	415 (14)	0.15 (0.04)	0.001	−0.06 (0.06)	0.256	−0.34 (1.01)	0.736	−0.46 (2.81)	0.870	0.09 (0.06)	0.149	0.07 (0.07)	0.321
3. quarter	565 (19)	0.25 (0.04)	<0.0001	−0.03 (0.05)	0.610	−0.08 (0.93)	0.932	3.48 (2.58)	0.177	0.16 (0.06)	0.005	0.02 (0.06)	0.727
4. quarter	504 (17)	0.45 (0.04)	<0.0001	−0.07 (0.05)	0.193	2.62 (1.00)	0.009	4.24 (2.77)	0.126	0.07 (0.06)	0.240	−0.03 (0.07)	0.700

(a) Analyzed with multilevel (site, schools nested within sites) linear regression. All models adjusted with age, household income, other outcome variables, and model for all participants adjusted also for gender. (b) The emotional eating factor scores were categorized by first setting the participants with no emotional eating as reference group and then dividing rest of the participants to quarters based on emotional eating factor scores. The emotional eating score in "No emotional eating" -group was −0.552 and minimum and maximum values of emotional eating factor score was −0.26 and −0.06 in 1st quarter, −0.05 and 0.20 and in 2nd quarter, 0.21 and 0.65 in 3rd quarter, and 0.66 and 1.93 in 4th quarter. (c) The unhealthy and the healthy diet pattern scores identified using principal components analysis, daily moderate to vigorous physical activity (min, MVPA), nightly sleep duration (min), TV viewing (min), and BMI z-scores.

4. Discussion

In this large, international sample of 9–11-year-old children, we found a positive association between EE and an unhealthy diet pattern. The novel finding of this study was that this positive association appeared to be consistent across the 12 study sites representing very different cultural and environmental settings. This is an important contribution to the current literature which has been almost completely focused on Western countries. We also found that EE was positively associated with both MVPA and TV viewing, yet these patterns were not consistent across all study sites. There were no associations between EE and healthy diet pattern, nocturnal sleep duration, or BMI z-score.

Our findings regarding the positive association between EE and the unhealthy diet pattern and the lack of association between EE and the healthy diet pattern support the earlier findings mainly in adults [3] that EE is especially associated with increased consumption of sweet and high-fat foods, which are generally considered to be highly palatable. Previous studies in 12–15-year-old children have also indicated that EE is associated with higher consumption of energy-dense foods and soft drinks, but it is not associated with the consumption of fruits and vegetables [30,31]. It must be noted that in addition to the palatability and nutrient composition of foods, food choice in response to emotional state might also reflect the availability and accessibility of foods. Many foods included in the unhealthy diet pattern (i.e., fast foods, ice cream, fried food, French fries, potato chips, cakes, and sugar-sweetened sodas) are ready to eat and are easily obtainable, even for 9–11-year-olds. However, one cause of EE may be poor emotion regulation in general [4], and it has been shown that adolescents (mean age 13.6 years) who are having difficulties with adequately regulating their negative emotions consume snacks, especially energy-dense snacks, more frequently [48]. Yet, because our study, as well as most of the earlier research regarding the association between emotional eating and diet, was cross-sectional, we cannot rule out the possibility of a reverse relationship. That might be the case if an unhealthier diet is associated with a decreased mood, or impaired hunger control, making it easier to eat in emotional states.

Interestingly, in 5–12-year-old children, an age group closer to the present sample age range, no association between self-reported EE and food consumption has been reported previously [20,32]. One explanation for these contradictory findings may be differences in how diet was measured. Van Strien and Oosterveld [20] asked one simple question about the weekly frequency of consumption of sweet and/or savoury snacks with four answer options (never/sometimes/often/everyday), which might not have allowed enough variance to detect a possible association. In the study by Michels et al. [32], food consumption was reported by the parents, and it is possible that foods eaten in response to emotions are eaten without the knowledge of the parents. It has also been suggested that in children aged 6 to 18 years, self-reporting of dietary intake is more valid than parental reports [49,50].

As mentioned above, the positive association between EE and the unhealthy diet pattern appeared to be similar in all 12 countries. All beta estimates were positive, but there were some differences in the sizes of the estimates. The significance of these differences was not tested, because comparing each country against all of the remaining countries was outside of the scope of this study. Yet, similar findings across different countries suggest that the association between EE and the unhealthy diet pattern is not restricted to Western countries and their cultural and food environments. A normal physiological reaction to negative emotions is expected to be a suppressed appetite [5]. So, rather than being an innate characteristic, EE is most likely learned [51], and, for example, the home environment [52] and parenting [53] may affect this process. Our results suggest that the association between EE and unhealthy food consumption in children is independent, or at least not fully dependent, on the culture and culturally learned behavioural patterns.

We found a small but significant positive association between EE and the amount of both daily MVPA and TV viewing. However, in contrast to the association with the unhealthy diet pattern, these associations were not consistent between all study sites. The significant positive associations between EE and these outcomes were observed only in two out of 12 sites (Colombia and South Africa for of MVPA and Canada and China for TV viewing). These findings need further clarification and replication in other study samples, because unassessed local factors may influence the observed relationships. For example, children undertake MVPA under a variety of contexts, and given that accelerometry was used to measure MVPA, we have detailed information on the level and pattern of MVPA but not the cultural, social or environmental context under which MVPA was performed.

We hypothesized that EE might be related to MVPA and TV-viewing, because unhealthy behaviours tend to cluster in children [33,34]. The observed positive association between EE and MVPA was in contrast to that hypothesis. To our knowledge, only one study has previously examined the association between EE and physical activity in children, with no association between EE and weekly frequency of doing sports reported [20]. However, in that study, the amount of physical activity was measured with one simple question, whereas in the present study, MVPA was measured objectively using accelerometers. A few earlier studies support our finding regarding a positive association between EE and TV viewing. Ouwens et al. [54] reported a small but significant positive correlation between EE and TV viewing, and in another study, a significant positive correlation was found, but only in girls [20].

As the present study was cross-sectional, future studies are needed to determine the causal relationship and possible mechanisms for the association between EE and both MVPA and TV viewing. One might only speculate that children with high EE could compensate for this behaviour with a higher amount of MVPA. On the other hand, it may be that children with high MVPA eat more overall as well as during emotional situations. There is also a possibility that children with high MVPA have more hobbies, including those involving physical activity in competing environments, which might lead to more stress and subsequently EE. TV viewing is associated with higher intakes of sweet and salty snacks and carbonated beverages [55], and Ouwens et al. [54] found that the association between TV viewing and snacking was stronger in children with high EE. Distraction caused by the television can lead to diminished awareness of hunger and satiety, and eating in front of television can be considered "mindless eating", which has been shown to be closely related to EE in children [56]. It is also possible that there is a third unmeasured variable explaining the association. For example, children with high negative affectivity could watch more TV as well as display more EE.

We did not find an association between EE and BMI z-scores in the fully adjusted model. In line with our findings, other studies have also reported no difference in self-reported [20] and parent-reported [19] EE between normal weight and overweight 7 to 15-year-old children. However, several studies have also found a positive association [12–18]. In children, EE has been measured using self-reported or parent-reported questionnaires, and it has been shown that there is good concordance between these two approaches [13]. However, it seems that the majority of the studies reporting positive associations with BMI/being overweight have used parent-reported EE [12,14–18], and some studies using self-reported EE have even found an inverse association with BMI/being overweight [21–23]. It remains an interesting question for future studies as to whether inconsistent findings could be partially explained by the different reporting methods for EE.

We found a weak but significant negative association between self-reported EE and BMI z-scores in the unadjusted model, but after adjusting for other health behaviours (including MVPA), it was no longer significant. This result is probably due to including MVPA in the model, since EE was positively associated with MVPA in our sample, and MVPA was the strongest significant predictor of a lower BMI [36]. In earlier studies that reported a negative association [21–23], physical activity was not taken into account. Altogether, our results strengthen the existing literature that, in children, EE does not seem to be as clearly associated with obesity as in adults.

It is interesting and somewhat controversial that EE was associated with the unhealthy diet pattern but not with BMI. However, in the ISCOLE sample, the unhealthy diet pattern was not associated with BMI [36]. It should be noted that the diet pattern scores describe dietary quality instead of energy intake per se, which may be more closely related to BMI. Nevertheless, it has been shown that food choices determined by dietary patterns track into adulthood [57]. It might be that EE already leads to the unhealthy diet pattern during childhood, but its consequences, such as excess weight gain, are visible only later in life. To our knowledge, there are no prospective studies examining these associations from childhood to adolescence or adulthood, but in one previous study, parent-reported EE of 5 to 6-year-old children predicted a higher BMI in 7 to 8-year-old children [25]. In adults, EE has also been shown to predict weight gain [10,11].

We did not find any interactions between EE and gender in association with dietary patterns, TV viewing, sleep duration, or BMI z-scores. Yet, the positive association between EE and MVPA was significantly stronger in boys. Further studies are needed to clarify and explain this observed interaction. In our study, there was no difference in reported EE between boys and girls, which is consistent with some previous findings [12,23], but not all, since Snoek et al. [22] found that 11–16-year-old girls reported more EE than boys. In site-specific analyses, we found that in the United Kingdom, higher amounts of EE were reported among girls than boys. The difference between mean EE scores was small (0.10 (0.55) in girls vs. −0.04 (0.50) in boys), and it is possible that the significant difference emerged by chance due to multiple testing (type I error).

A potential limitation of the present study was that EE was self-reported. However, Braet et al. [13] compared children's self-reported EE vs. parent-reported EE and found that the agreement between reporting was good enough to conclude that it is possible to rely on either of the informants, especially for children aged 10 years and older. We measured EE using the EIES, which was developed in a similar age group as our sample. Even though the internal consistency was less than optimal for the four EIES items (Cronbach's alpha value 0.6), the excellent fit of the one-factor CFA model and high factor loadings supported the unidimensionality of the scale. In addition, the percentage of children reporting no EE in our study was 32%. Similar percentages have been reported previously, regardless of the questionnaire or the reporter. In one study using the child-version of the Dutch Eating Behaviour Questionnaire to measure self-reported EE, 45% of the children reported that they never expressed EE [54], and in the other study, approximately 35% of the parents reported that their child never displays EE using the Children's Eating Behavior Questionnaire [18]. As well as EE, diet was also self-reported. It has been suggested that in children aged 6 to 18 years, self-reporting of dietary intake is more valid than parental reporting [49,50]. Furthermore, in that age group, a relatively short (20–60 items) FFQ without requirement for portion size estimation, as used in the present study, has been suggested to be a valid method for measuring self-reported diet [49].

A further limitation was that the excluded children reported more EE, had higher scores on the unhealthy dietary pattern, watched more TV, and had higher BMI z-scores. This finding fits well with the hypothesis that unhealthy behaviours tend to cluster [33,34]. It is possible that this selection effect has attenuated the observed associations, and it may affect the generalizability of the results, although the observed differences between two groups were quite small, albeit statistically significant. Furthermore, it should also be mentioned that children's opportunities to eat in response to negative emotions depend on how often they experience these emotions. Unfortunately, no measures of emotions, mood, or stress were included in the present study, because it was a secondary analysis of existing ISCOLE, and the questionnaire was originally designed to address the main research questions. Finally, the cross-sectional nature of the data does not allow any conclusions about the causality of the observed associations or their direction to be formed. However, a particular strength and novel aspect of this study is that the same EE questionnaire and outcome measures were used in a large and truly international study sample. We were also able to study multiple health behaviours simultaneously, and MVPA, sleep duration, and BMI were measured objectively.

5. Conclusions

In conclusion, we found a significant positive association between EE and an unhealthy diet pattern, which was consistent across the 12 different study sites. As previous studies have been almost completely focused on Western countries, this extends the present knowledge by suggesting that the association between EE and unhealthy diet pattern is not restricted to Western countries and their cultural and food environments. It is possible that EE can already lead to an unhealthy diet pattern during childhood, but its consequences, such as excess weight gain, are visible only later in life.

The associations between EE and other health behaviours were either inconsistent between sites or not significant. We observed no association between EE and BMI z-scores. Prospective studies in different cultural contexts are needed to determine whether higher EE in children leads to an undesirable diet and subsequent obesity over time.

Supplementary Materials: The following is available online at http://www.mdpi.com/2072-6643/11/2/351/s1, Figure S1: Item level frequencies of the original Emotion-Induced Eating Scale.

Author Contributions: Conceptualization, E.J., H.K., H.V. and M.F.; Formal analysis, E.J. and H.K.; Investigation, E.J., J.-P.C., G.H., C.M., J.M., O.L.S., M.S., C.T.-L., P.T.K. and M.F.; Methodology, E.J., H.K., H.V., J.-P.C., G.H., J.M., O.L.S., C.T.-L., P.T.K. and M.F.; Project administration, P.T.K. and M.F.; Visualization, E.J.; Writing—original draft, E.J.; Writing—review & editing, H.K., H.V., J.-P.C., G.H., C.M., J.M., O.L.S., M.S., C.T.-L., P.T.K. and M.F.

Funding: ISCOLE was funded by The Coca-Cola Company. With the exception of requiring that the study be global in nature, the study sponsor had no role in study design, data collection and analysis, decision to publish, or preparation of manuscripts. E.J. has received personal grants from Jenny and Antti Wihuri Foundation and Emil Aaltonen Foundation. Preparation of this manuscript has also been funded by the Academy of Finland (grants 314135 and 309157 to H.K.).

Acknowledgments: We wish to thank the ISCOLE External Advisory Board, ISCOLE participants and their families, and the ISCOLE Research Group.

Conflicts of Interest: The authors declare no conflict of interest. With the exception of requiring that the study be global in nature, the funder had no role in the design of the study; in the collection, analyses, or interpretation of data; in the writing of the manuscript, or in the decision to publish the results.

References

1. Ng, M.; Fleming, T.; Robinson, M.; Thomson, B.; Graetz, N.; Margono, C.; Mullany, E.C.; Biryukov, S.; Abbafati, C.; Abera, S.F.; et al. Global, regional, and national prevalence of overweight and obesity in children and adults during 1980–2013: a systematic analysis for the Global Burden of Disease Study 2013. *Lancet (London, England)* **2014**, *384*, 766–781. [CrossRef]

2. Kaplan, H.I.; Kaplan, H.S. The psychosomatic concept of obesity. *J. Nerv. Ment. Dis.* **1957**, *125*, 181–201. [CrossRef] [PubMed]

3. Macht, M. How emotions affect eating: A five-way model. *Appetite* **2008**, *50*, 1–11. [CrossRef] [PubMed]

4. van Strien, T. Causes of Emotional Eating and Matched Treatment of Obesity. *Curr. Diab. Rep.* **2018**, *18*, 35. [CrossRef] [PubMed]

5. van Strien, T.; Donker, M.H.; Ouwens, M.A. Is desire to eat in response to positive emotions an 'obese' eating style: Is Kummerspeck for some people a misnomer? *Appetite* **2016**, *100*, 225–235. [CrossRef] [PubMed]

6. Keskitalo, K.; Tuorila, H.; Spector, T.D.; Cherkas, L.F.; Knaapila, A.; Kaprio, J.; Silventoinen, K.; Perola, M. The Three-Factor Eating Questionnaire, body mass index, and responses to sweet and salty fatty foods: a twin study of genetic and environmental associations. *Am. J. Clin. Nutr.* **2008**, *88*, 263–271. [CrossRef] [PubMed]

7. van Strien, T.; Herman, C.P.; Verheijden, M.W. Eating style, overeating, and overweight in a representative Dutch sample. Does external eating play a role? *Appetite* **2009**, *52*, 380–387. [CrossRef]

8. Konttinen, H.; Silventoinen, K.; Sarlio-Lähteenkorva, S.; Männistö, S.; Haukkala, A. Emotional eating and physical activity self-efficacy as pathways in the association between depressive symptoms and adiposity indicators. *Am. J. Clin. Nutr.* **2010**, *92*, 1031–1039. [CrossRef]

9. Péneau, S.; Ménard, E.; Méjean, C.; Bellisle, F.; Hercberg, S. Sex and dieting modify the association between emotional eating and weight status. *Am. J. Clin. Nutr.* **2013**, *97*, 1307–1313. [CrossRef]

10. Koenders, P.G.; van Strien, T. Emotional eating, rather than lifestyle behavior, drives weight gain in a prospective study in 1562 employees. *J. Occup. Environ. Med.* **2011**, *53*, 1287–1293. [CrossRef]

11. van Strien, T.; Konttinen, H.; Homberg, J.R.; Engels, R.C.M.E.; Winkens, L.H.H. Emotional eating as a mediator between depression and weight gain. *Appetite* **2016**, *100*, 216–224. [CrossRef] [PubMed]

12. Braet, C.; Van Strien, T. Assessment of emotional, externally induced and restrained eating behaviour in nine to twelve-year-old obese and non-obese children. *Behav. Res. Ther.* **1997**, *35*, 863–873. [CrossRef]

13. Braet, C.; Soetens, B.; Moens, E.; Mels, S.; Goossens, L.; Van Vlierberghe, L. Are two informants better than one? Parent–child agreement on the eating styles of children who are overweight. *Eur. Eat. Disord. Rev.* **2007**, *15*, 410–417. [CrossRef] [PubMed]

14. Viana, V.; Sinde, S.; Saxton, J.C. Children's Eating Behaviour Questionnaire: associations with BMI in Portuguese children. *Br. J. Nutr.* **2008**, *100*, 445–450. [CrossRef] [PubMed]

15. Webber, L.; Hill, C.; Saxton, J.; Van Jaarsveld, C.H.M.; Wardle, J. Eating behaviour and weight in children. *Int. J. Obes.* **2009**, *33*, 21–28. [CrossRef] [PubMed]

16. dos Passos, D.R.; Gigante, D.P.; Maciel, F.V.; Matijasevich, A. Children's eating behaviour: comparison between normal and overweight children from a school in Pelotas, Rio Grande do Sul, Brazil. *Rev. Paul. Pediatr.* **2015**, *33*, 42–49. [PubMed]

17. Sánchez, U.; Weisstaub, G.; Santos, J.L.; Corvalán, C.; Uauy, R. GOCS cohort: children's eating behavior scores and BMI. *Eur. J. Clin. Nutr.* **2016**, *70*, 925–928. [CrossRef]

18. Steinsbekk, S.; Barker, E.D.; Llewellyn, C.; Fildes, A.; Wichstrøm, L. Emotional Feeding and Emotional Eating: Reciprocal Processes and the Influence of Negative Affectivity. *Child Dev.* **2017**. [CrossRef] [PubMed]

19. Caccialanza, R.; Nicholls, D.; Cena, H.; Maccarini, L.; Rezzani, C.; Antonioli, L.; Dieli, S.; Roggi, C. Validation of the Dutch Eating Behaviour Questionnaire parent version (DEBQ-P) in the Italian population: A screening tool to detect differences in eating behaviour among obese, overweight and normal-weight preadolescents. *Eur. J. Clin. Nutr.* **2004**, *58*, 1217–1222. [CrossRef] [PubMed]

20. van Strien, T.; Oosterveld, P. The children's DEBQ for assessment of restrained, emotional, and external eating in 7- to 12-year-old children. *Int. J. Eat. Disord.* **2008**, *41*, 72–81. [CrossRef] [PubMed]

21. Striegel-Moore, R.; Morrison, J.A.; Schreiber, G.; Schumann, B.C.; Crawford, P.B.; Obarzanek, E. Emotion-induced eating and sucrose intake in children: the NHLBI Growth and Health Study. *Int. J. Eat. Disord.* **1999**, *25*, 389–398. [CrossRef]

22. Snoek, H.M.; van Strien, T.; Janssens, J.M.A.M.; Engels, R.C.M.E. Emotional, external, restrained eating and overweight in Dutch adolescents. *Scand. J. Psychol.* **2007**, *48*, 23–32. [CrossRef] [PubMed]

23. Braet, C.; Claus, L.; Goossens, L.; Moens, E.; Van Vlierberghe, L.; Soetens, B. Differences in eating style between overweight and normal-weight youngsters. *J. Health Psychol.* **2008**, *13*, 733–743. [CrossRef] [PubMed]

24. Coumans, J.M.J.; Danner, U.N.; Ahrens, W.; Hebestreit, A.; Intemann, T.; Kourides, Y.A.; Lissner, L.; Michels, N.; Moreno, L.A.; Russo, P.; et al. The association of emotion-driven impulsiveness, cognitive inflexibility and decision-making with weight status in European adolescents. *Int. J. Obes.* **2018**, *42*, 655–661. [CrossRef] [PubMed]

25. Parkinson, K.N.; Drewett, R.F.; Le Couteur, A.S.; Adamson, A.J. Do maternal ratings of appetite in infants predict later Child Eating Behaviour Questionnaire scores and body mass index? *Appetite* **2010**, *54*, 186–190. [CrossRef] [PubMed]

26. Steinsbekk, S.; Wichstrøm, L. Predictors of Change in BMI from the Age of 4 to 8. *J. Pediatr. Psychol.* **2015**, *40*, 1056–1064. [CrossRef] [PubMed]

27. Pate, R.R.; O'Neill, J.R.; Liese, A.D.; Janz, K.F.; Granberg, E.M.; Colabianchi, N.; Harsha, D.W.; Condrasky, M.M.; O'Neil, P.M.; Lau, E.Y.; Taverno Ross, S.E. Factors associated with development of excessive fatness in children and adolescents: a review of prospective studies. *Obes. Rev.* **2013**, *14*, 645–658. [CrossRef]

28. Huang, J.; Qi, S. Childhood obesity and food intake. *World J. Pediatr.* **2015**, *11*, 101–107. [CrossRef]

29. Felső, R.; Lohner, S.; Hollódy, K.; Erhardt, É; Molnár, D. Relationship between sleep duration and childhood obesity: Systematic review including the potential underlying mechanisms. *Nutr. Metab. Cardiovasc. Dis.* **2017**, *27*, 751–761.

30. Nguyen-Michel, S.; Unger, J.B.; Spruijt-Metz, D. Dietary correlates of emotional eating in adolescence. *Appetite* **2007**, *49*, 494–499. [CrossRef]

31. Elfhag, K.; Tholin, S.; Rasmussen, F. Consumption of fruit, vegetables, sweets and soft drinks are associated with psychological dimensions of eating behaviour in parents and their 12-year-old children. *Public Health Nutr.* **2008**, *11*, 914–923. [CrossRef] [PubMed]

32. Michels, N.; Sioen, I.; Braet, C.; Eiben, G.; Hebestreit, A.; Huybrechts, I.; Vanaelst, B.; Vyncke, K.; De Henauw, S. Stress, emotional eating behaviour and dietary patterns in children. *Appetite* **2012**, *59*, 762–769. [CrossRef] [PubMed]

33. Fernández-Alvira, J.M.; De Bourdeaudhuij, I.; Singh, A.S.; Vik, F.N.; Manios, Y.; Kovacs, E.; Jan, N.; Brug, J.; Moreno, L.A. Clustering of energy balance-related behaviors and parental education in European children: the ENERGY-project. *Int. J. Behav. Nutr. Phys. Act.* **2013**, *10*, 5. [CrossRef]

34. Leech, R.M.; McNaughton, S.A.; Timperio, A. The clustering of diet, physical activity and sedentary behavior in children and adolescents: A review. *Int. J. Behav. Nutr. Phys. Act.* **2014**, *11*, 4. [CrossRef] [PubMed]

35. Katzmarzyk, P.T.; Barreira, T.V.; Broyles, S.T.; Champagne, C.M.; Chaput, J.; Fogelholm, M.; Hu, G.; Johnson, W.D.; Kuriyan, R.; Kurpad, A.; et al. The International Study of Childhood Obesity, Lifestyle and the Environment (ISCOLE): design and methods. *BMC Public Health* **2013**, *13*, 900.

36. Katzmarzyk, P.T.; Barreira, T.V.; Broyles, S.T.; Champagne, C.M.; Chaput, J.; Fogelholm, M.; Hu, G.; Johnson, W.D.; Kuriyan, R.; Kurpad, A.; et al. Relationship between lifestyle behaviors and obesity in children ages 9–11: Results from a 12-country study. *Obesity (Silver Spring)* **2015**, *23*, 1696–1702. [CrossRef] [PubMed]

37. Hu, L.; Bentler, P.M. Cutoff criteria for fit indexes in covariance structure analysis: Conventional criteria versus new alternatives. *Struct. Equ. Model. Multidiscip. J.* **1999**, *6*, 1–55. [CrossRef]

38. Tavakol, M.; Dennick, R. Making sense of Cronbach's alpha. *Int. J. Med. Educ.* **2011**, *2*, 53–55. [CrossRef]

39. Cheung, G.W.; Rensvold, R.B. Evaluating Goodness-of-Fit Indexes for Testing Measurement Invariance. *Struct. Equ. Model. Multidiscip. J.* **2002**, *9*, 233–255. [CrossRef]

40. Saloheimo, T.; González, S.A.; Erkkola, M.; Milauskas, D.M.; Meisel, J.D.; Champagne, C.M.; Tudor-Locke, C.; Sarmiento, O.; Katzmarzyk, P.T.; Fogelholm, M. The reliability and validity of a short food frequency questionnaire among 9–11-year olds: A multinational study on three middle-income and high-income countries. *Int. J. Obes. Suppl.* **2015**, *5*, S22–S28. [CrossRef]

41. Mikkilä, V.; Vepsäläinen, H.; Saloheimo, T.; Gonzalez, S.A.; Meisel, J.D.; Hu, G.; Champagne, C.M.; Church, T.S.; Katzmarzyk, P.T.; Kuriyan, R.; et al. An international comparison of dietary patterns in 9–11-year-old children. *Int. J. Obes. Suppl.* **2015**, *5*, S17–S21.

42. Evenson, K.R.; Catellier, D.J.; Gill, K.; Ondrak, K.S.; McMurray, R.G. Calibration of two objective measures of physical activity for children. *J. Sports Sci.* **2008**, *26*, 1557–1565. [CrossRef] [PubMed]

43. Barreira, T.V.; Schuna, J.M.; Mire, E.F.; Katzmarzyk, P.T.; Chaput, J.; Leduc, G.; Tudor-Locke, C. Identifying children's nocturnal sleep using 24-h waist accelerometry. *Med. Sci. Sports Exerc.* **2015**, *47*, 937–943. [CrossRef]

44. US Centers for Disease Control and Prevention: Youth Risk Behavior Surveillance System (YRBSS). 2012. Available online: https://www.cdc.gov/healthyyouth/data/yrbs/index.htm (accessed on 21 June 2017).

45. Schmitz, K.H.; Harnack, L.; Fulton, J.E.; Jacobs, D.R.; Gao, S.; Lytle, L.A.; Coevering, P.V. Reliability and Validity of a Brief Questionnaire to Assess Television Viewing and Computer Use by Middle School Children. *J. Sch. Health* **2004**, *74*, 370–377. [CrossRef] [PubMed]

46. de Onis, M.; Onyango, A.W.; Borghi, E.; Siyam, A.; Nishida, C.; Siekmann, J. Development of a WHO growth reference for school-aged children and adolescents. *Bull. World Health Organ.* **2007**, *85*, 660–667. [CrossRef] [PubMed]

47. Kenward, M.G.; Roger, J.H. Small sample inference for fixed effects from restricted maximum likelihood. *Biometrics* **1997**, *53*, 983–997. [CrossRef] [PubMed]

48. Coumans, J.M.J.; Danner, U.N.; Intemann, T.; De Decker, A.; Hadjigeorgiou, C.; Hunsberger, M.; Moreno, L.A.; Russo, P.; Stomfai, S.; Veidebaum, T.; et al. Emotion-driven impulsiveness and snack food consumption of European adolescents: Results from the I.Family study. *Appetite* **2018**, *123*, 152–159. [CrossRef]

49. Kolodziejczyk, J.K.; Merchant, G.; Norman, G.J. Reliability and Validity of Child/Adolescent Food Frequency Questionnaires That Assess Foods and/or Food Groups. *J. Pediatr. Gastroenterol. Nutr.* **2012**, *55*, 4. [CrossRef]

50. Burrows, T.L.; Truby, H.; Morgan, P.J.; Callister, R.; Davies, P.S.W.; Collins, C.E. A comparison and validation of child versus parent reporting of children's energy intake using food frequency questionnaires versus food records: Who's an accurate reporter? *Clin. Nutr.* **2013**, *32*, 613–618. [CrossRef]

51. Herle, M.; Fildes, A.; Steinsbekk, S.; Rijsdijk, F.; Llewellyn, C.H. Emotional over- and under-eating in early childhood are learned not inherited. *Sci. Rep.* **2017**, *7*, 9092. [CrossRef]

52. Herle, M.; Fildes, A.; Rijsdijk, F.; Steinsbekk, S.; Llewellyn, C. The Home Environment Shapes Emotional Eating. *Child Dev.* **2017**. [CrossRef]

53. Bjørklund, O.; Wichstrøm, L.; Llewellyn, C.H.; Steinsbekk, S. Emotional Over-and Undereating in Children: A Longitudinal Analysis of Child and Contextual Predictors. *Child Dev.* **2018**. [CrossRef] [PubMed]

54. Ouwens, M.A.; Cebolla, A.; van Strien, T. Eating style, television viewing and snacking in pre-adolescent children. *Nutr. Hosp.* **2012**, *27*, 1072–1078. [PubMed]

55. Coon, K.A.; Tucker, K.L. Television and children's consumption patterns. A review of the literature. *Minerva Pediatr.* **2002**, *54*, 423–436. [PubMed]

56. Hart, S.R.; Pierson, S.; Goto, K.; Giampaoli, J. Development and initial validation evidence for a mindful eating questionnaire for children. *Appetite* **2018**, *129*, 178–185. [CrossRef] [PubMed]

57. Mikkilä, V.; Räsänen, L.; Raitakari, O.T.; Pietinen, P.; Viikari, J. Consistent dietary patterns identified from childhood to adulthood: The cardiovascular risk in Young Finns Study. *Br. J. Nutr.* **2005**, *93*, 923–931. [CrossRef] [PubMed]

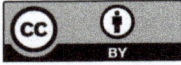

![nutrients logo] *nutrients*

Article

Combined Longitudinal Effect of Physical Activity and Screen Time on Food and Beverage Consumption in European Preschool Children: The ToyBox-Study

María L. Miguel-Berges [1,2,*], Alba M. Santaliestra-Pasias [1,2,3,4], Theodora Mouratidou [1], Pilar De Miguel-Etayo [1,2,4], Odysseas Androutsos [5], Marieke De Craemer [6], Sonya Galcheva [7], Berthold Koletzko [8], Zbigniew Kulaga [9], Yannis Manios [5] and Luis A. Moreno [1,2,3,4] on behalf of the ToyBox-study group

[1] Growth, Exercise, Nutrition and Development (GENUD) Research Group, University of Zaragoza, C/Pedro Cerbuna 12, 50009 Zaragoza, Spain; albasant@unizar.es (A.M.S.-P.); theodoramouratidou@icloud.com (T.M.); pilardm@unizar.es (P.D.M.-E.); lmoreno@unizar.es (L.A.M.)
[2] Instituto Agroalimentario de Aragón (IA2), 50009 Zaragoza, Spain
[3] School of Health Science (EUCS), University of Zaragoza, C/Domingo Miral s/n, 50009 Saragossa, Spain
[4] Centro de Investigación Biomédica en Red de Fisiopatología de la Obesidad y Nutrición (CIBERObn), 50009 Zaragoza, Spain
[5] Department of Nutrition and Dietetics, School of Health Science and Education, Harokopio University, 17671 Athens, Greece; oandrou@hua.gr (O.A.); manios.toybox@hua.gr (Y.M.)
[6] Department of Movement and Sports Sciences, Ghent University, Watersportlaan 2, 9000 Ghent, Belgium; marieke.decraemer@ugent.be
[7] Department of paediatrics. Medical University Varna, 55 Marin Drinov Str., 9002 Varna, Bulgaria; sonya_galcheva@mail.bg
[8] Dr von Hauner Children's Hospital, University of Munich Medical Centre, 80337 Munich, Germany; berthold.koletzko@med.uni-muenchen.de
[9] The Children's Memorial Health Institute, 04-730 Warsaw, Poland; z.kulaga@ipczd.pl
* Correspondence: mlmiguel@unizar.es; Tel.: +0034-638234634

Received: 9 April 2019; Accepted: 8 May 2019; Published: 10 May 2019

Abstract: Lifestyle behavioral habits such as excess screen time (ST), a lack of physical activity (PA), and high energy-dense food consumption are associated with an increased risk of children being overweight or obese. This study aimed to (1) track longitudinal adherence to PA and ST recommendations at baseline (T0) and follow-up (T1) and (2) assess the association between changes in adherence to PA and ST recommendations and food and beverage consumption at follow-up. The present study included 2321 preschool children (3.5 to 6) participating in the multicenter ToyBox-study. A lineal mixed effects model was used to examine the association between different types of food and beverages and their relationship with changes in adherence to PA and ST recommendations. Approximately half of the children (50.4%) did not meet the PA and ST recommendations at both baseline and follow-up. However, only 0.6% of the sample met both PA and ST recommendations. Preschool children who met both recommendations consumed fewer fizzy drinks, juices, sweets, desserts, and salty snacks and consumed more water, fruits and vegetables, and dairy products than did those not meeting both recommendations. In conclusion, the proportion of European preschool children adhering to both PA and ST recommendations was very low and was associated with a low consumption of energy-dense foods.

Keywords: screen time; physical activity; preschool children; food and beverage consumption

1. Introduction

Being overweight or obese during childhood and adolescence is a major public health challenge [1]. Excess weight gain during childhood is associated with long-term health risks and adult diseases such as cardiovascular disease, type 2 diabetes, and hypertension [2]. Behaviors such as excessive screen time (ST), a lack of physical activity (PA), and high consumption of energy-dense foods have been shown to be independently associated with increased risks of being overweight or obese in children, adolescents, and adults [3]. Individually and combined, high sugar-sweetened beverage and low fruit and vegetable consumption are associated with an increased obesity risk [4,5], while behaviors such as PA appear to be protective [6,7]. Hence, it is crucial that interventions during childhood target lifestyle behaviors such as diet, physical activity, and sedentary behavior, which are established in early years and track into adulthood [8].

PA guidelines for preschool children recommend that preschool children should spend at least 180 min per day doing PA [9]. Limited evidence suggests that a total daily physical activity volume of 10,000–14,000 steps per day is associated with 60–100 min of moderate vigorous PA in preschool children [10]. De Craemer et al. [11] proposed using 11,500 steps per day as an attainable and realistic cut-off for PA recommendations, helping to promote PA among preschool children. Regarding ST, established guidelines for preschool children (one- to five-year-olds) state that they should limit TV viewing and use of other electronic media such as computers, DVDs, and other electronic games to less than one hour per day [9].

ST has been shown to be associated with increased energy-dense food and beverage consumption and decreased fruit and vegetable (F & V) consumption in preschool children [12]. In European children participating in the IDEFICS study, low time spent on moderate to vigorous physical activity (MVPA) was associated with a low consumption of vegetables and yogurt and high fast food consumption [13]. A low socioeconomic status was also associated with consumption of high energy-dense foods, increased ST, and low levels of PA [14,15].

To the authors' knowledge, there are no studies that have investigated the individual and combined effects of PA and ST on food consumption in preschool children. For this reason, the current study aimed to (1) track longitudinal adherence to PA and ST recommendations at baseline (T0) and follow-up (T1) and (2) assess the association between changes in the adherence to PA and ST recommendations and food and beverage consumption at follow-up (T1).

2. Methods

2.1. Study Design

The ToyBox-study (www.toybox-study.eu) was were a cluster-randomized clinical trial aiming to prevent obesity in preschool children. It was conducted in six European countries, namely Belgium, Bulgaria, Germany, Greece, Poland, and Spain. The detailed protocol is described elsewhere [16,17]. In total, 309 kindergarteners and 7056 children aged 3.5–6 years were recruited at baseline (T0), and 5529 children continued at follow-up (T1) [18]. The ToyBox intervention aimed to promote preschool children's water consumption, healthy snacking, and PA and limit/interrupt their sedentary time by improving the children's physical and social environment both in kindergarten and at home. In this study, 2321 (33% of the baseline sample) preschool children were included with complete information from a parental questionnaire and also pedometer information at baseline (T0) and follow-up (T1). Data collection was carried out in May–June 2012 (T0) and May–June 2013 (T1). The ToyBox-study adhered to the Declaration of Helsinki and the conventions of the Council of Europe on human rights and biomedicine. In all countries, ethical approval was obtained from their respective ethical committees and local authorities.

2.2. Socioeconomic Variables

Maternal education level (years of education) was recorded in five categories: less than 7 years, 7–12 years, 13–14 years, 15–16 years, and more than 16 years of education. For the purposes of the analysis, this was then recategorized into three categories: less than 7 years to 12 years, between 13 and 16 years, and more than 16 years of education. The selection of this indicator was based on its identification as the best proxy indicator of socioeconomic status [19].

2.3. Anthropometric Measures

Body weight was measured in underwear and without shoes using an electronic scale (Type SECA 861 or SECA 813) to the nearest 0.1 kg, and body height was measured with a telescopic height instrument (Type SECA 225 or SECA 214) to the nearest 0.1 cm. Body mass index (BMI) was calculated as weight (kg) divided by squared height (m^2). BMI z-scores (zBMI) were computed to classify children as being of a normal weight, being overweight, or being obese, for which the Cole et al. criteria were considered [20]. The intra- and interobserver reliability for weight and height was excellent (greater than 99% and 98%) in all participating countries [21].

2.4. Diet Assessment

Food and beverage consumption was assessed via a parentally reported semiquantitative food frequency questionnaire (FFQ) [22]. Low to moderate relative validity was observed, which varied by food and beverage group [23]. Estimated correlations ranged from 0.52 to 0.79. Food and beverage consumption was expressed as the number of portions per week. In the FFQ, 37 items were included, and in the current analysis they were merged into 21 groups according to their nutritional content (the main nutrient being proteins, carbohydrates, or fats). Of those 21, 10 were chosen and entered into the current analysis because they were considered to be associated with obesity development [24]: (1) water; (2) fizzy drinks (soft drinks and light drinks); (3) fresh fruit juices and packed juices; (4) dried, canned, and fresh fruits; (5) dairy products (milk, yogurt, and cheese); (6) sweets (chocolate and chocolate spreads, cakes, biscuits, and pastries); (7) desserts (smoothies, milk-based desserts, and sugar desserts); (8) meat and processed meat; (9) salty snacks; and (10) pasta and rice.

2.5. Physical Activity

In all of the countries except Belgium, PA was assessed by means of pedometers (Omron Walking Style Pro pedometers (HJ-720IT-E2)) assessing the number of steps per day. In Belgium, steps were measured using ActiGraph (Pensacola, FL, USA) accelerometers. Step counts from the accelerometers and pedometers were comparable. Evidence of their validity in preschool children indicated high correlations (daily, $r = 0.89$). In addition, evidence has suggested that the Omron Walking Style Pro pedometer is a valid and accurate measure to assess preschoolers' steps per hour [25]. The devices were worn on the right hip (secured by an elastic waistband) for six consecutive days, including two weekend days [22]. The steps were further categorized into two categories, including ≥11,500 steps per day (if children followed the PA recommendations) and <11,500 steps per day (if children did not follow the PA recommendations). The selected step count cut-off was based on Reilly et al. [26] and De Craemer et al. [11].

2.6. Screen Time

Data on children's screen time was collected via a standardized proxy-administered parental questionnaire (i.e., the Primary Caregivers' Questionnaire). Screen time was used as a proxy indicator of sedentary behavior. The behaviors assessed included watching TV and DVDs and playing computer/video games. Parents/caregivers reported frequency for both weekdays and weekend days. The frequency categories included "never", "less than 30 min/day", "30 min to 1 h/day", "1–2 h/day", "3–4 h/day", "5–6 h/day", "7–8 h/day", "8 h/day", and "more than 8 h/day". Average hours per day of TV/video viewing and personal computer use (separately for weekdays and weekend days) were summed up to obtain the screen time. To obtain the daily screen time, the average minutes per day, both for week- and weekend days, were summed up and divided by 7 days. The answers were further aggregated into two categories, including ≤1 h per day (if children followed the recommendations) and >1 h per day (if children did not follow the recommendations). These categories were based on the Australian and Canadian sedentary behavior recommendations, which state that preschool children should limit their screen time to a maximum of 1 h per day [9,27,28].

2.7. Statistical Analysis

Statistical analyses were performed using Statistical Package for the Social Sciences (version 21.0; SPSS, Inc., Chicago, IL, USA). Analysis was done for the whole sample, as there were no differences by sex in all of the included variables as tested using a *t*-test for continuous variables and a chi-squared test for categorical variables. In order to evaluate possible changes in the adherence to both behaviors (ST and PA) between T0 and T1, seven groups were established, reflecting differential combinations of meeting or not meeting the ST and/or PA recommendations. Figure 1 shows the seven groups derived from possible combinations of ST and/or PA recommendations. Two of them included children who got worse in their behaviors from T0 to T1 (meeting both recommendations at T0 and meeting one of the recommendations at T1; meeting one of the recommendations at T0 and not meeting any recommendations at T1). Two groups included children who improved in their behaviors from T0 to T1 (not meeting any recommendations at T0 and meeting one of the recommendations at T1; meeting one of the recommendations at T0 and meeting both recommendations at T1). The last three groups included children who maintained their behaviors from T0 to T1 (meeting both recommendations at T0 and T1; meeting one of the recommendations at T0 and T1; and not meeting any recommendations at T0 and T1). After establishing the potential combinations of ST and PA recommendations, a lineal mixed effects model with random effects for country and food consumption at T1 as predictor variables and z-BMI, maternal education, and intervention versus control region at T1 as covariates were analyzed. Marginal means and standard deviations (SE) were used to show differences in food and beverage consumption by PA and ST recommendation combinations. All statistical tests and corresponding *p*-values lower than 0.05 were considered statistically significant.

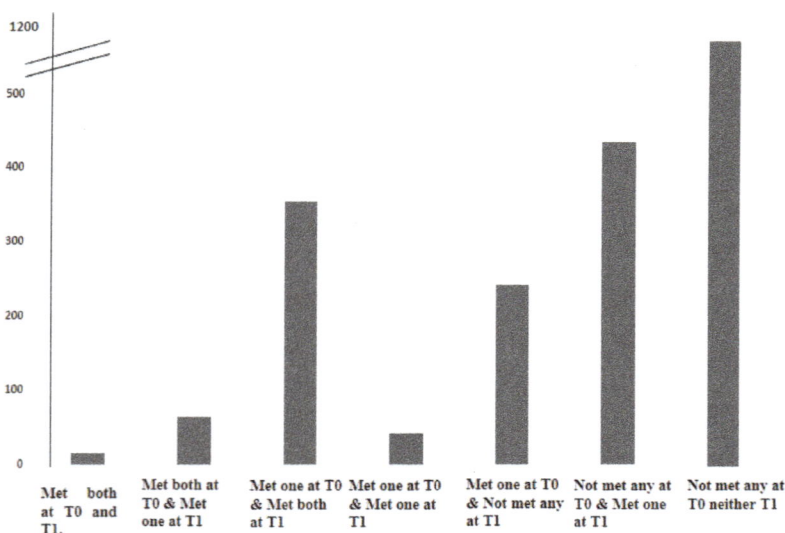

Figure 1. Proportion of European preschool children in each group. Groups are according to whether they met physical activity (PA) and/or screen time (ST) recommendations.

3. Results

Table 1 presents descriptive information on age, gender, BMI categories, z-BMI scores, maternal education, and country for the total sample, both at the T0 and T1 periods. According to BMI, 2.8% of the sample at T0 was obese and 10.6% was overweight, while 3.2% of the sample at T1 was obese and 10.3% was overweight.

Table 1. Descriptive characteristics of European preschool children participating in the ToyBox-study.

		T0	T1	*P*-Figvalue
		Mean (SE)	Mean (SE)	
Age (years)		4.74 (0.4)	5.72 (0.4)	<0.001
Sex	Boys	1209 (52.1)	1210 (52.1)	0.152
	Girls	1111 (47.9)	1111 (47.9)	
BMI status *	Normal weight	1988 (85.7)	1980 (85.3)	
	Overweight	245 (10.6)	240 (10.3)	<0.001
	Obese	64 (2.8)	75 (3.2)	
zBMI		0.20 (1.0)	0.27 (1.0)	<0.001
		n (%)		
Maternal education	<7–12	337 (14.5)		
(years)	13–16	947 (40.8)		0.104
	>16	965 (41.6)		
Center	Belgium	522 (22.5)		
	Bulgaria	74 (3.2)		
	Germany	284 (12.2)		0.645
	Greece	317 (13.7)		
	Poland	688 (29.6)		
	Spain	435 (18.7)		

Abbreviations: BMI, body mass index; zBMI, body mass index z-score; T0, baseline period; T1, follow-up period; * BMI according to Cole's cut-off [20].

Table 2 presents the proportion of the sample adhering to PA and ST recommendations for preschool children at both time points. Only 12.4% of children at T0 and 8.8% at T1 met the PA recommendation. In terms of ST, 30.2% of children at T0 and 27.7% at T1 met the recommendations.

Table 2. Number (%) of European preschool children participating in the ToyBox study that met or did not meet the physical activity and screen time recommendations at baseline (T0) and follow-up (T1) (*n* = 2321).

		T0 *n* (%)	T1 *n* (%)
Physical activity	<11,500 steps/day	2033 (87.6)	2117 (91.2)
recommendations *	≥11,500 steps/day	288 (12.4)	204 (8.8)
Screen time	≤1 h/day	701 (30.2)	644 (27.7)
recommendations **	>1 h/day	1620 (69.8)	1670 (72.3)

* Recommendations according to Reilly et al. [26] and De Craemer et al. [11] ** Recommendations on healthy eating and physical activity guidelines for early childhood settings in Australia [9,27,28].

Derived from the general linear model, Figure 2 presents the marginal means and SDs of eight food and beverage groups (F & V, dairy products, desserts, sweets, water, salty snacks, juices, and fizzy drinks), according to several grouping combinations for meeting or not meeting PA and ST recommendations at baseline (T0) and follow-up (T1). In general, preschool children who met both recommendations (PA and ST) consumed less dessert (Figure 2c), sweets (Figure 2d), salty snacks (Figure 2f), juices (Figure 2g), and fizzy drinks (Figure 2h) and more F & V (Figure 2a), dairy products (Figure 2b), and water (Figure 2e). In contrast, preschool children who failed to meet the recommendations over time had a higher consumption of desserts (Figure 2c), sweets (Figure 2d), juices (Figure 2g), and fizzy drinks (Figure 2h), and lower consumption of F & V (Figure 2a) and water (Figure 2e).

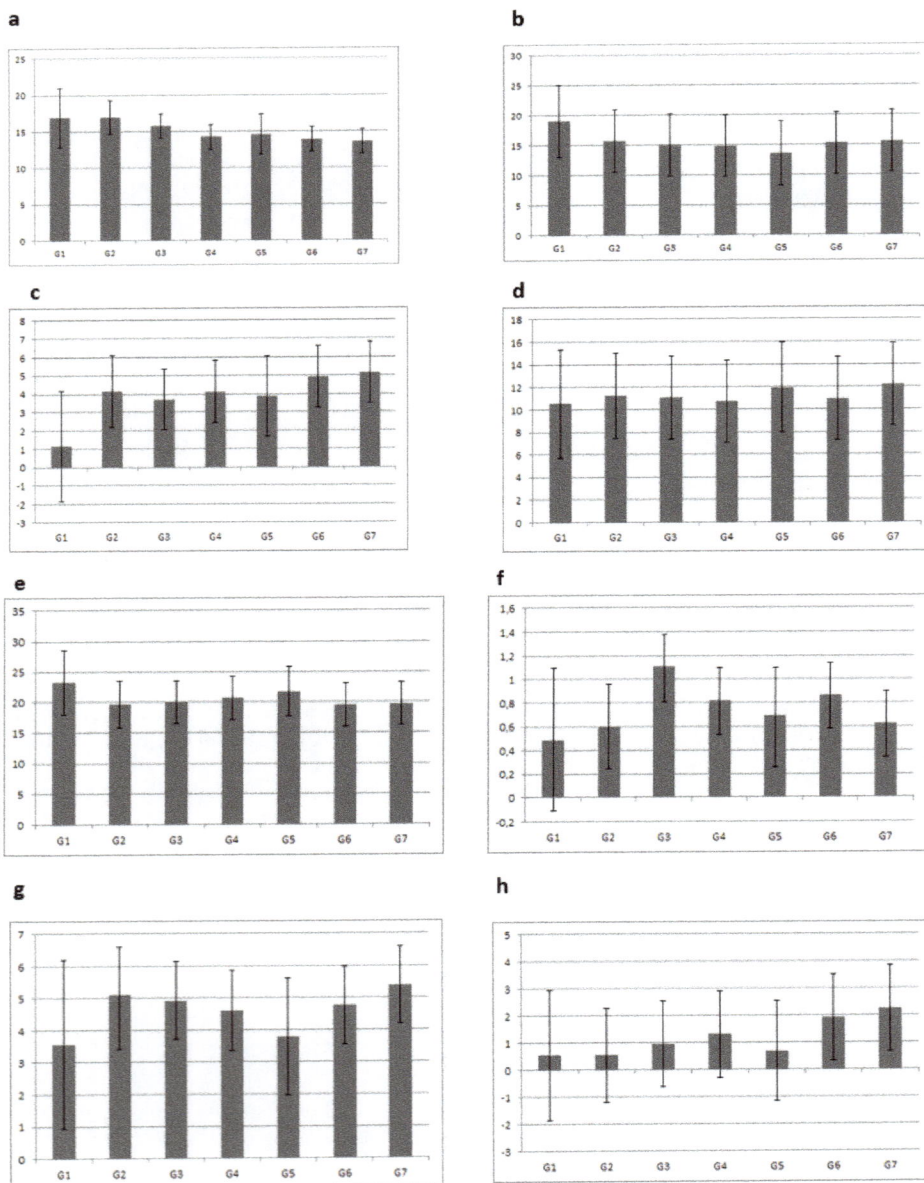

Figure 2. Marginal means and SD of food and beverage consumption (number of portions per week) according to PA and ST recommendations. G1: met both recommendations at T0 and met both recommendations at T1; G2: met both recommendations at T0 and met one of the recommendations at T1; G3: met one of the recommendations at T0 and met both recommendations at T1; G4: met one of the

recommendations at T0 and met one of the recommendations at T1; G5: met one of the recommendations at T0 and did not meet any recommendations at T1; G6: did not meet any recommendations at T0 and met one of the recommendations at T1; G7: did not meet any recommendations at T0 and did not meet any recommendations at T1. Adjusted for maternal education, body mass index z-score at T1, sex, and center. Abbreviations: PA, physical activity; ST, screen time; SD, standard deviation; T0, baseline period; T1, follow-up period; F & V, fruits and vegetables; dairy products (milk, yogurt and cheese); desserts (smoothies, milk-based desserts and sugar desserts); sweets (chocolate and chocolate spreads, cakes, biscuits and pastries); juices (fresh fruit juices and packed juices); fizzy drinks (soft drinks and light drinks). (**a**) F & V, (**b**) dairy products, (**c**) dessert, (**d**) sweets, (**e**) water, (**f**) salty snacks, (**g**) juices, (**h**) fizzy drinks.

Table 3 presents the associations between several grouping combinations of meeting or not meeting the PA and ST recommendations at T0 and at follow-up T1 and food and beverage consumption at follow up (T1). Seven possible combinations were identified. Approximately half of the sample (50.4%) did not meet either the PA or the ST recommendations in either period. With the opposite, only 0.6% of the sample met both PA and ST recommendations at both T0 and T1. Those who did not meet either recommendation at either time point (T0 and T1) were used as the reference group for analysis. Those children who met both recommendations at T0 and T1 consumed significantly fewer milk-based desserts and salty snacks in comparison to those who did not meet either recommendation at either time point. Those who met both recommendations at T0 and only one at T1 had a significantly lower consumption of fizzy drinks and salty snacks and higher consumption of F & V in comparison to the reference group. In addition, those children who met one of the recommendations at T0 and T1 had a significantly lower consumption of fizzy drinks, sweets, desserts, and salty snacks, and higher consumption of F & V. Those children who did not adhere to the recommendations at T0 and met one of them at T1 had a lower consumption of fizzy drinks, juices, sweets, desserts, and salty snacks in comparison to the reference group. At the same time, those children who met one of the recommendations at T0 and both at T1 had a lower consumption of fizzy drinks, juices, and salty snacks in comparison to not meeting either recommendation at either time point. Lastly, a significantly low consumption of juices, sweets, and salty snacks was observed in those children who met one of the recommendations at T0 and did not meet any recommendations at T1 in comparison to those who did not meet the PA and ST recommendations over time.

Table 3. Results of the lineal mixed effects model between food consumption and adherence to physical activity and screen time recommendations at baseline (T0) and follow-up (T1) periods (*n* = 2321).

PA and ST Recommendations at T0	PA and ST Recommendations at T1	n %	Water β (95% CI)	Fizzy Drinks β (95% CI)	Juices β (95% CI)	F & V β (95% CI)	Dairy Products β (95% CI)	Sweets β (95% CI)	Desserts β (95% CI)	Meat and Processed Meat β (95% CI)	Salty Snacks β (95% CI)	Pasta and Rice β (95% CI)
Met both recommendations	Met both recommendations	15 (0.6)	3.41 (-1.22; 8.04)	-1.65 (-3.71; 0.41)	-1.84 (-4.32; 0.65)	3.32 (-0.62; 7.25)	3.43 (-0.77; 7.63)	-1.69 (-5.43; 2.04)	-4.03 (-6.75; -1.29)*	-2.38 (-5.06; 0.29)	-0.60 (-1.18; -0.02)*	0.49 (-0.51; 1.49)
	Met one of the recommendations	64 (2.8)	0.25 (-2.16; 2.67)	-1.75 (-2.80; -0.69)*	-0.38 (-1.67; 0.90)	3.42 (1.41; 5.44)*	0.078 (-2.07; 2.23)	-0.93 (-2.84; 0.98)	-1.04 (-2.44; 0.35)	-0.33 (-1.66; 0.99)	-0.51 (-0.80; -0.20)*	-0.26 (-0.77; 0.25)
Met one of the recommendations	Met both recommendations	354 (15.3)	1.76 (-1.09; 4.62)	-1.47	-1.60 (-3.18; -0.02)*	0.99 (-1.50; 3.49)	-2.07 (-4.73; 0.59)	-0.32 (-2.69; 2.05)	-1.32 (-3.05; 0.40)	-0.10 (-1.77; 1.56)	-0.41 (-0.78; -0.04)*	-0.09 (-0.73; 0.55)
	Met one of the recommendations	41 (1.8)	0.58 (-0.49; 1.66)	-1.34 (-1.82; -0.86)*	-0.47 (-1.05; 011)	2.29 (1.36; 3.20)*	-0.58 (-1.56; 0.40)	-1.15 (-2.03; -0.27)*	-1.45 (-2.08; -0.81)*	-0.56 (-1.17; 0.05)	-0.49 (-0.62; -0.35)*	0.01 (-0.22; 0.25)
Met one of the recommendations	Did not meet any recommendations	241 (10.4)	0.07 (-1.06; 1.21)	-0.34 (-0.85; 0.16)	-0.63 (-1.24; -0.01)*	0.38 (-0.58; 1.34)	-0.34 (-1.37; 0.69)	-1.24 (-2.15; -0.31)*	-0.24 (-0.90; 0.43)	-0.28 (-0.92; 0.35)	-0.24 (-0.38; -0.09)*	-0.21 (-0.46; 0.03)
Did not meet any recommendations	Met one of the recommendations	436 (18.8)	1.05 (-0.30; 2.41)	-0.97 (-1.55; -0.38)*	-0.78 (-1.49; -0.07)*	0.67 (-0.45; 1.79)	-0.74 (-1.92; 0.45)	-1.46 (-2.52; -0.40)*	-1.05 (-1.82; -0.27)*	-0.57 (-1.31; 0.17)	-0.29 (-0.46; -0.12)*	0.03 (-0.26; 0.31)
Did not meet any recommendations	Did not meet any recommendations	1170 (50.4)	REF	REF	REF	REF	REF	REF	REF	REF	REF	REF

Adjusted for maternal education, body mass index z-score at T1, sex, and center. Abbreviations: PA, physical activity; ST, screen time; REF, reference group not meeting any recommendations at either T0 or T1; CI, confidence interval; fizzy drinks (soft drinks and light drinks); juices (fresh fruit juices and packed juices); F & V, fruits and vegetables; dairy products (milk, yogurt, and cheese); sweets (chocolate and chocolate spreads, cakes, biscuits, and pastries); desserts (smoothies, milk-based desserts, and sugar desserts). * *P* < 0.001.

4. Discussion

In this study, associations between lifestyle behaviors, i.e., PA and ST and food and beverage consumption in preschool children, were investigated. The novelty of this report included examining adherence to both PA and ST recommendations across two time points and its relationship with food and beverage consumption in a large sample of European preschool children. The main finding of our study suggests that meeting both PA and ST recommendations at T0 and T1 was associated with a high consumption of foods considered healthy (F & V and water) and a lower consumption of energy-dense products (fizzy drinks, sweets, desserts, and salty snacks). In addition, we also observed a low proportion of children adhering to both recommendations during the follow-up.

The high proportion of children who failed to meet individual PA and ST recommendations at both periods agreed with results from other longitudinal studies, which observed similar trends. To our knowledge, there is no study reporting the proportion of preschool children meeting both PA and ST recommendations at the same time. Studies focusing on PA have reported that the percentage compliance with MVPA recommendations for European children is generally low [29]. The Health Behavior in School-Aged Children (HBSC) Study found that only 26% of its sample spent at least 1 h per day in MVPA [30]. Regarding ST, the HBSC study reported that 39% of the children complied with screen time recommendations [31]. In European children, approximately one-third of the children failed to meet current screen time recommendations [32]. An Australian study with a follow-up of three years reported that less than 20% of the sample met the ST recommendations and that screen time increased over the three-year follow-up. In addition, in an Australian study, participants were less likely to meet ST recommended guidelines as they got older [33].

In our sample, we found low levels of PA and high levels of ST in preschool children. The preschool age is an important period, as lifestyle behaviors such as PA and ST are established. However, different studies have observed that PA decreases during early childhood and adolescence [34,35] and even more so during the transition period from adolescence to adulthood [35,36]. Regarding ST, studies have observed an increase in ST during early childhood and also during the transition from primary to secondary school [37]. Both low PA and high ST have been associated with unfavorable body composition indicators such as BMI and waist circumference [38–40], both being determinants of obesity development in adulthood [33]. It has been suggested that ST, particularly TV, has an important role in the etiology of obesity due to its relationship with other unhealthy behaviors and its displacement of PA [41]. However, there is little evidence about the relationship between PA and ST on the one hand and food and beverage consumption on the other hand.

Previously, several cross-sectional studies analyzed the effects of PA or ST (alone) on food and beverage consumption. In European children (2–10 years old), boys and girls spending less time doing MVPA were more likely to consume fast food and less likely to consume vegetables and yogurt than those spending more time doing MVPA [13]. Similar associations were observed in European adolescents [42]: Those adolescents with the lowest PA levels consumed fewer fruits and dairy products compared to active adolescents. In a previous publication of the ToyBox study, those exceeding baseline ST recommendations had a higher consumption of energy-dense foods (sugar-based desserts, salty snacks, pastries, cakes, and biscuits) and beverages (fizzy drinks, sweet milk, and juices) than those complying with ST recommendations [12]. Another study reported that high TV viewing was related to less healthy food options (consumption of sweets and soft drinks) in children from different countries [43]. A study carried out in Brazil [44] in children less than two years old observed a positive association between time spent watching TV and the consumption of soft drinks. Santaliestra-Pasias et al. [45] reported that increased TV viewing and computer and internet use were associated with higher odds of sugar-sweetened beverage consumption and lower odds of fruit consumption in European adolescents. In an Australian adolescent sample, TV viewing was positively associated with energy-dense snack consumption and with higher availability of energy-dense snack foods at home [46].

There is consistent evidence to show that consumption of energy-dense foods is positively associated with low PA and high ST levels. However, research assessing the relationship between combinations of both PA and ST and food and beverage consumption is very scarce. Although high levels of both PA and ST have been observed in children [5], no studies have observed the combined effects of adherence to PA and ST recommendations on food and beverage consumption in preschool children.

This study had limitations. First, the generalizability of the findings is limited to the specific age group studied in the current study. The method used to assess PA was a pedometer, aside from Belgium. However, pedometers are not the gold standard in measuring preschool child PA, and therefore our results should be interpreted with caution. Nevertheless, the use of a pedometer provided objective information on PA, specifically in this age group. Information on food and beverage consumption and ST were collected via parental self-reported questionnaires, which are prone to over- or underreporting. However, the questionnaires used were developed/adapted and validated for the purposes of the study [22].

The main strengths of our study included the use of a large and culturally and socioeconomically diverse sample of preschool children from six different countries across Europe and its longitudinal design. Information through questionnaires was assessed via standardized and harmonized procedures [22].

5. Conclusions

This study examined the relationship between adherence to PA and ST recommendations and food and beverage consumption. In this sample of preschool children, we found that low PA levels and high ST were associated with an unhealthy food and beverage consumption profile. Preschool children and their parents should try to increase family time spent at activities promoting physical activity and to minimize the time they spend on screen time or being sedentary. In addition, public health interventions should focus on activities aimed at increasing movement in preschool children. Enabling healthier food and physical activity environments, together with the promotion of positive parental role modeling, should be prioritized to achieve higher rates of adherence to PA and ST recommendations.

Author Contributions: Y.M. and O.A. designed research; formal analysis, M.L.M.-B.; investigation M.L.M.-B., writing—original draft preparation, M.L.M.-B.; writing—review and editing, M.L.M.-B.; visualization, A.M.S.-P., T.M. and P.D.M.-E.; supervision, L.A.M.; funding acquisition, Y.M. All authors revised the manuscript for important intellectual content, read and approved the final manuscript.

Funding: The ToyBox-study was funded by the Seventh Framework Programme (CORDIS FP7) of the European Commission under grant agreement number 245200. The content of this article reflects only the authors' views, and the European Community is not liable for any use that may be made of the information contained herein.

Conflicts of Interest: The authors declare no conflict of interest.

References

1. *Obesity: Preventing and Managing the Global Epidemic: Report of a WHO Consultation*; World Health Organization: Geneva, Switzerland, 1999.

2. Dietz, W.H. Health consequences of obesity in youth: Childhood predictors of adult disease. *PEDIATRICS* **1998**, *101*, 518–525.

3. Van Stralen, M.M.; Velde, S.J.T.; Van Nassau, F.; Brug, J.; Grammatikaki, E.; Maes, L.; De Bourdeaudhuij, I.; Verbestel, V.; Galcheva, S.; Iotova, V.; et al. Weight status of European preschool children and associations with family demographics and energy balance-related behaviours: A pooled analysis of six European studies. *Obes. Rev.* **2012**, *13*, 29–41. [CrossRef] [PubMed]

4. Paes, V.M.; Hesketh, K.; O'Malley, C.; Moore, H.; Summerbell, C.; Griffin, S.; Van Sluijs, E.M.F.; Ong, K.K.; Lakshman, R. Determinants of sugar-sweetened beverage consumption in young children: A systematic review. *Obes. Rev.* **2015**, *16*, 903–913. [CrossRef] [PubMed]

5. Santaliestra-Pasías, A.M.; Mouratidou, T.; Reisch, L.; Pigeot, I.; Ahrens, W.; Mårild, S.; Molnár, D.; Siani, A.; Sieri, S.; Tornatiris, M.; et al. Clustering of lifestyle behaviours and relation to body composition in European children. The IDEFICS study. *Eur. J. Clin. Nutr.* **2015**, *69*, 811–816. [CrossRef] [PubMed]

6. Kimm, S.Y.; Glynn, N.W.; Obarzanek, E.; Kriska, A.M.; Daniels, S.R.; Barton, B.A.; Liu, K. Relation between the changes in physical activity and body-mass index during adolescence: A multicentre longitudinal study. *Lancet* **2005**, *366*, 301–307. [CrossRef]

7. Miguel-Berges, M.L.; Reilly, J.J.; Moreno Aznar, L.A.; Jimenez-Pavon, D. Associations Between Pedometer-Determined Physical Activity and Adiposity in Children and Adolescents: Systematic Review. *Clin. J. Sport Med.* **2017**, *28*, 64–75. [CrossRef] [PubMed]

8. Brug, J.; Van Stralen, M.M.; Velde, S.J.T.; Chinapaw, M.J.M.; De Bourdeaudhuij, I.; Lien, N.; Bere, E.; Maskini, V.; Singh, A.S.; Maes, L.; et al. Differences in Weight Status and Energy-Balance Related Behaviors among Schoolchildren across Europe: The ENERGY-Project. *PLoS ONE* **2012**, *7*, e34742. [CrossRef]

9. Australian Department of Health and Aging. *Get Up and Grow: Healthy Eating and Physical Activity for Early Childhood.* Available online: https://www.health.gov.au/internet/main/publishing.nsf/Content/2CDB3A000FE57A4ECA257BF0001916EC/$File/HEPA%20-%20B5%20Book%20-%20Staff%20and%20Carer%20Book_LR.pdf (accessed on 9 May 2019).

10. Tudor-Locke, C.; Craig, C.L.; Beets, M.W.; Belton, S.; Cardon, G.M.; Duncan, S.; Hatano, Y.; Lubans, D.R.; Olds, T.S.; Raustorp, A.; et al. How many steps/day are enough? for children and adolescents. *Int. J. Behav. Nutr. Phys. Act.* **2011**, *8*, 78. [CrossRef]

11. De Craemer, M.; De Decker, E.; De Bourdeaudhuij, I.; Verloigne, M.; Manios, Y.; Cardon, G. The translation of preschoolers' physical activity guidelines into a daily step count target. *J. Sports Sci.* **2014**, *33*, 1051–1057. [CrossRef]

12. Miguel-Berges, M.L.; on behalf of the ToyBox-study Group; Santaliestra-Pasias, A.M.; Mouratidou, T.; Androutsos, O.; De Craemer, M.; Pinket, A.-S.; Birnbaum, J.; Koletzko, B.; Iotova, V.; et al. Associations between food and beverage consumption and different types of sedentary behaviours in European preschoolers: The ToyBox-study. *Eur. J. Nutr.* **2016**, *56*, 1939–1951. [CrossRef]

13. Santaliestra-Pasías, A.M.; Dios, J.E.L.; Sprengeler, O.; Hebestreit, A.; De Henauw, S.; Eiben, G.; Felső, R.; Lauria, F.; Tornaritis, M.; Veidebaum, T.; et al. Food and beverage intakes according to physical activity levels in European children: The IDEFICS (Identification and prevention of Dietary and lifestyle induced health EFfects In Children and infantS) study. *Public Health Nutr.* **2018**, *21*, 1717–1725. [CrossRef] [PubMed]

14. Fernández-Alvira, J.M.; Mouratidou, T.; Bammann, K.; Hebestreit, A.; Barba, G.; Sieri, S.; Reisch, L.; Eiben, G.; Hadjigeorgiou, C.; Kovacs, E.; et al. Parental education and frequency of food consumption in European children: The IDEFICS study. *Public Health Nutr.* **2017**, *16*, 487–498. [CrossRef] [PubMed]

15. Miguel-Berges, M.L.; Zachari, K.; Santaliestra-Pasias, A.M.; Mouratidou, T.; Androutsos, O.; Iotova, V.; Galcheva, S.; De Craemer, M.; Cardon, G.; Koletzko, B.; et al. Clustering of energy balance-related behaviours and parental education in European preschool children: The ToyBox study. *Br. J. Nutr.* **2017**, *118*, 1089–1096. [CrossRef] [PubMed]

16. Androutsos, O.; Apostolidou, E.; Iotova, V.; Socha, P.; Birnbaum, J.; Moreno, L.; De Bourdeaudhuij, I.; Koletzko, B.; Manios, Y. Process evaluation design and tools used in a kindergarten-based, family-involved intervention to prevent obesity in early childhood. The ToyBox-study. *Obes. Rev.* **2014**, *15*, 74–80. [CrossRef] [PubMed]

17. Manios, Y. The 'ToyBox-study' obesity prevention programme in early childhood: An introduction. *Obes. Rev.* **2012**, *13*, 1–2. [CrossRef] [PubMed]

18. Manios, Y.; Androutsos, O.; Katsarou, C.; Iotova, V.; Socha, P.; Geyer, C.; Moreno, L.; Koletzko, B.; De Bourdeaudhuij, I. Designing and implementing a kindergarten-based, family-involved intervention to prevent obesity in early childhood: The ToyBox-study. *Obes. Rev.* **2014**, *15*, 5–13. [CrossRef] [PubMed]

19. Nixon, C.A.; Moore, H.J.; Douthwaite, W.; Gibson, E.L.; Vögele, C.; Kreichauf, S.; Wildgruber, A.; Manios, Y.; Summerbell, C. Identifying effective behavioural models and behaviour change strategies underpinning preschool- and school-based obesity prevention interventions aimed at 4–6-year-olds: A systematic review. *Obes. Rev.* **2012**, *13*, 106–117. [CrossRef]

20. Cole, T.J.; Bellizzi, M.C.; Flegal, K.M.; Dietz, W.H. Establishing a standard definition for child overweight and obesity worldwide: International survey. *BMJ* **2000**, *320*, 1240. [CrossRef]

21. De Miguel-Etayo, P.; Mesana, M.I.; Cardon, G.; De Bourdeaudhuij, I.; Góźdź, M.; Socha, P.; Lateva, M.; Iotova, V.; Koletzko, B.V.; Duvinage, K.; et al. Reliability of anthropometric measurements in European preschool children: The ToyBox-study. *Obes. Rev.* **2014**, *15*, 67–73. [CrossRef]

22. Mouratidou, T.; Miguel, M.L.; Androutsos, O.; Manios, Y.; De Bourdeaudhuij, I.; Cardon, G.; Kulaga, Z.; Socha, P.; Galcheva, S.; Iotova, V.; et al. Tools, harmonization and standardization procedures of the impact and outcome evaluation indices obtained during a kindergarten-based, family-involved intervention to prevent obesity in early childhood: The ToyBox-study. *Obes. Rev.* **2014**, *15*, 53–60. [CrossRef]

23. Mouratidou, T.; Graffe, M.I.M.; Huybrechts, I.; De Decker, E.; De Craemer, M.; Androutsos, O.; Manios, Y.; Galcheva, S.; Lateva, M.; Gurzkowska, B.; et al. Reproducibility and relative validity of a semiquantitative food frequency questionnaire in European preschoolers: The ToyBox study. *Nutrition* **2019**, *65*, 60–67. [CrossRef] [PubMed]

24. Commission of the European Communities. Green Paper: Promoting Healthy Diets and Physical Activity: A European Dimension for the Prevention of Overweight, Obesity, and Chronic Disease. 2005. Available online: https://publications.europa.eu/en/publication-detail/-/publication/fb6264c8-c756-47c4-944d-6d10bc9fce10/language-en (accessed on 9 May 2019).

25. De Craemer, M.; De Decker, E.; Santos-Lozano, A.; Verloigne, M.; De Bourdeaudhuij, I.; Deforche, B.; Cardon, G. Validity of the Omron pedometer and the actigraph step count function in preschoolers. *J. Sci. Med. Sport* **2015**, *18*, 289–293. [CrossRef] [PubMed]

26. Reilly, J.J.; Coyle, J.; Kelly, L.; Burke, G.; Grant, S.; Paton, J.Y. An Objective Method for Measurement of Sedentary Behavior in 3- to 4-Year Olds. *Obes. Res.* **2003**, *11*, 1155–1158. [CrossRef] [PubMed]

27. Leblanc, A.G.; Choquette, L.; Dillman, C.; Duggan, M.; Gordon, M.J.; Hicks, A.; Kho, M.E.; Latimer-Cheung, A.E.; Murumets, K.; Okely, A.D.; et al. Canadian Sedentary Behaviour Guidelines for the Early Years (aged 0–4 years). *Appl. Physiol. Nutr. Metab.* **2012**, *37*, 370–380. [CrossRef] [PubMed]

28. *Guidelines on Physical Activity, Sedentary Behaviour and Sleep for Children under 5 Years of Age*; World Health Organization: Geneva, Switzerland, 2019.

29. Konstabel, K.; on behalf of the IDEFICS consortium; Veidebaum, T.; Verbestel, V.; Moreno, L.A.; Bammann, K.; Tornaritis, M.; Eiben, G.; Molnár, D.; Siani, A.; et al. Objectively measured physical activity in European children: The IDEFICS study. *Int. J. Obes.* **2014**, *38*, S135–S143. [CrossRef] [PubMed]

30. Inequalities in Young People's Health: Health Behaviour in School-Aged Children (HBSC) Study. International Report from the 2005/2006 Survey. Available online: http://www.euro.who.int/__data/assets/pdf_file/0005/53852/E91416.pdf (accessed on 9 May 2019).

31. Sigmundová, D.; Sigmund, E.; Bucksch, J.; Baďura, P.; Kalman, M.; Hamřík, Z. Trends in Screen Time Behaviours in Czech Schoolchildren between 2002 and 2014: HBSC Study. *Cent. Eur. J. Public Health* **2017**, *25*, S15–S20. [CrossRef]

32. Santaliestra-Pasias, A.M.; Mouratidou, T.; Verbestel, V.; Bammann, K.; Molnar, D.; Sieri, S.; Siani, A.; Veidebaum, T.; Marild, S.; Lissner, L.; et al. Physical activity and sedentary behaviour in European children: The IDEFICS study. *Public Health Nutr.* **2014**, *17*, 2295–2306. [CrossRef]

33. Hesketh, K.; Wake, M.; Graham, M.; Waters, E. Stability of television viewing and electronic game/computer use in a prospective cohort study of Australian children: Relationship with body mass index. *Int. J. Behav. Nutr. Phys. Act.* **2007**, *4*, 60. [CrossRef]

34. Dumith, S.C.; Gigante, D.P.; Domingues, M.R.; Kohl, H.W., 3rd. Physical activity change during adolescence: A systematic review and a pooled analysis. *Int. J. Epidemiol.* **2011**, *40*, 685–698. [CrossRef] [PubMed]

35. Jones, R.A.; Hinkley, T.; Okely, A.D.; Salmon, J. Tracking Physical Activity and Sedentary Behavior in Childhood: A Systematic Review. *Am. J. Prev. Med.* **2013**, *44*, 651–658. [CrossRef]

36. Telama, R. Tracking of Physical Activity from Childhood to Adulthood: A Review. *Obes. Facts* **2009**, *2*, 187–195. [CrossRef] [PubMed]

37. Pearson, N.; Haycraft, E.; Johnston, J.P.; Atkin, A.J. Sedentary behaviour across the primary-secondary school transition: A systematic review. *Prev. Med.* **2017**, *94*, 40–47. [CrossRef]

38. Tremblay, M.S.; Leblanc, A.G.; Kho, M.E.; Saunders, T.J.; Larouche, R.; Colley, R.C.; Goldfield, G.; Gorber, S.C. Systematic review of sedentary behaviour and health indicators in school-aged children and youth. *Int. J. Behav. Nutr. Phys. Act.* **2011**, *8*, 98. [CrossRef] [PubMed]

39. Biddle, S.J.; Petrolini, I.; Pearson, N. Interventions designed to reduce sedentary behaviours in young people: A review of reviews. *Br. J. Sports Med.* **2014**, *48*, 182–186. [CrossRef]

40. Strong, W.B.; Malina, R.M.; Blimkie, C.J.; Daniels, S.R.; Dishman, R.K.; Gutin, B.; Hergenroeder, A.C.; Must, A.; Nixon, P.A.; Pivarnik, J.M.; et al. Evidence Based Physical Activity for School-age Youth. *J. Pediatr.* **2005**, *146*, 732–737. [CrossRef] [PubMed]

41. Birch, L.L.; Davison, K.K. Childhood overweight: A contextual model and recommendations for future research. *Obes. Rev.* **2001**, *2*, 159–171.

42. Ottevaere, C.; Huybrechts, I.; Béghin, L.; Cuenca-Garcia, M.; De Bourdeaudhuij, I.; Gottrand, F.; Hagströmer, M.; Kafatos, A.; Le Donne, C.; Moreno, L.A.; et al. Relationship between self-reported dietary intake and physical activity levels among adolescents: The HELENA study. *Int. J. Behav. Nutr. Phys. Act.* **2011**, *8*, 8. [CrossRef]

43. Vereecken, C.A.; Todd, J.; Roberts, C.; Mulvihill, C.; Maes, L. Television viewing behaviour and associations with food habits in different countries. *Publish Health Nutr.* **2006**, *9*, 244–250. [CrossRef]

44. Jaime, P.C.; Prado, R.R.D.; Malta, D.C. Family influence on the consumption of sugary drinks by children under two years old. *Rev. Saude Publica* **2017**, *51*, 13. [CrossRef]

45. Santaliestra-Pasías, A.M.; Mouratidou, T.; Verbestel, V.; Huybrechts, I.; Gottrand, F.; Donne, C.L.; Cuenca-García, M.; Díaz, L.E.; Kafatos, A.; Manios, Y.; et al. Food Consumption and Screen-Based Sedentary Behaviors in European Adolescents: The HELENA Study. *Arch. Pediatr. Adolesc. Med.* **2012**, *166*, 1010–1020. [CrossRef] [PubMed]

46. Pearson, N.; Biddle, S.J.; Williams, L.; Worsley, A.; Crawford, D.; Ball, K. Adolescent television viewing and unhealthy snack food consumption: The mediating role of home availability of unhealthy snack foods. *Public Health Nutr.* **2014**, *17*, 317–323. [CrossRef] [PubMed]

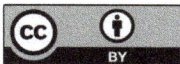

![nutrients logo]

MDPI

Article

The Family Mealtime Observation Study (FaMOS): Exploring the Role of Family Functioning in the Association between Mothers' and Fathers' Food Parenting Practices and Children's Nutrition Risk

Kathryn Walton [1,*], Emma Haycraft [2], Kira Jewell [3], Andrea Breen [3], Janis Randall Simpson [3] and Jess Haines [3]

1   Department of Translational Medicine, The Hospital for Sick Children, Toronto, ON M5G 0A4, Canada
2   School of Sport, Exercise and Health Sciences, Loughborough University, Loughborough, Leicestershire LE11 3TU, UK; e.haycraft@lboro.ac.uk
3   Department of Family Relations & Applied Nutrition, University of Guelph, Guelph, ON N1G 2W1, Canada; kjewell@uoguelph.ca (K.J.); abreen@uoguelph.ca (A.B.); rjanis@uoguelph.ca (J.R.S.); jhaines@uoguelph.ca (J.H.)
*   Correspondence: kathryn.walton@sickkids.ca

Received: 4 March 2019; Accepted: 11 March 2019; Published: 15 March 2019

Abstract: This cross-sectional study explores associations between mothers' and fathers' food parenting practices and children's nutrition risk, while examining whether family functioning modifies or confounds the association. Home observations assessed parents' food parenting practices during dinnertime ($n = 73$ families with preschoolers). Children's nutrition risk was calculated using NutriSTEP®. Linear regression models examined associations between food parenting practices and NutriSTEP® scores. An interaction term (family functioning × food parenting practice) explored effect modification; models were adjusted for family functioning to explore confounding. Among mothers, more frequent physical food restriction was associated with higher nutrition risk in their children ($\beta = 0.40$ NutriSTEP® points, 95% Confidence Interval (CI) = 2.30, 7.58) and among both mothers and fathers, positive comments about the target child's food were associated with lower nutrition risk (mothers: $\beta = -0.31$ NutriSTEP® points, 95% CI = -0.54, -0.08; fathers: $\beta = -0.27$ NutriSTEP® points, 95% CI = -0.75, -0.01) in models adjusted for parent education and child Body Mass Index (BMI) z-score. Family functioning did not modify these associations and they remained significant after adjustment for family functioning. Helping parents to use positive encouragement rather than restriction may help to reduce their children's nutrition risk.

Keywords: family meals; food parenting practices; preschoolers; nutrition risk; direct observation

---

1. Introduction

Nutrition plays a critical role in the growth, development, school readiness, subsequent academic achievement, and overall health status of young children [1]. Eating preferences and patterns are established early in life [2] and longitudinal research shows that food preferences and choices during the preschool years are strongly associated with dietary patterns and food choices later in life [3]. This stability of eating habits from early childhood to adulthood [4,5] suggests that young children's eating habits have important implications not only for children's current health, but also their risk of future chronic disease [6–8]. Despite the evidence that the preschool age is a key time for establishing healthy dietary patterns, few Canadian preschoolers are meeting dietary recommendations [9,10]. It is estimated that 11–30% have moderate risk for poor nutritional intake and 10–17% have high risk, as assessed by the Nutrition Screening Tool for Every Preschooler (NutriSTEP®), a validated measure used to assess eating habits and identify nutrition problems in preschool-aged children [11–13]. Nutrition risk can range from under- to overnutrition and, among preschoolers, is defined as the presence of characteristics that can lead to nutritional deficiencies including poor growth, under or over consumption of certain food groups, and difficulties chewing or swallowing [11].

Parents are the primary influence in young children's lives and there is evidence to suggest that parents' food parenting practices influence children's dietary intake [2,14–16] and their resulting risk of inadequate nutrition, i.e., their nutrition risk [13]. However, existing research exploring the influence of food parenting practices has produced equivocal results. For example, although early research demonstrated that restricting access to less healthful foods was associated with higher subsequent intakes of these foods [17], results from more recent studies suggest that parental restriction may be associated with healthier dietary intakes among young children [18].

Recent scientific reviews [19,20] have identified that these inconsistent findings may be due to the methodological limitations of existing research, including a reliance on parental report to assess food parenting. The validity of such reports is limited due to potential error through inaccurate recall or bias due to social desirability. Recent research has found inverse associations between parental report and observed feeding practices [21], as well as no associations at all [22–24]. Therefore, direct observation is needed to more accurately explore associations between food parenting practices and children's nutrition risk.

In addition to a reliance on parental-report measures, the current literature does not account for the feeding context, including the home environment, in which feeding interactions transpire and the presence of mothers and fathers during mealtimes. Family systems theory posits that individual or family behaviors must be understood within the global family context or system [25]. General family factors, such as family functioning, may moderate the associations of food parenting practices on children's nutrition risk because they influence how the feeding practices are experienced by the child [26]. Family functioning is defined by how family members manage daily routines, communicate and connect emotionally with one another [26]. There is some evidence that family functioning is associated with frequency of fast food consumption among adolescent females [27]; however, the mechanisms by which family functioning influences dietary intake remain largely unknown, especially among young children.

Although mothers have traditionally held the primary role in feeding children, fathers also play an important and increasingly more prominent role during feeding interactions [28]. Unfortunately, fathers have been underrepresented in existing feeding research [28,29]. Mothers and fathers have been found to differ in the food parenting practices they use [13,30], highlighting the need to explore the potentially differential relationship between their food parenting and their children's nutrition risk. Furthermore, the existing body of literature has been based on studies conducted outside of Canada where feeding and parenting norms may differ. To date, only two studies exploring food parenting practices among preschoolers have been conducted in Canada [13,31]; both used parental report of food parenting practices.

The overall aim of this study is to address the limitations of existing research through a cross-sectional study to examine the associations between mothers' and fathers' food parenting practices, assessed via direct observation in the home, and children's nutrition risk among a sample of Canadian families with preschool-aged children. We hypothesized that: (1) the children of parents who engage in controlling and pressuring food parenting would have higher NutriSTEP® nutrition risk scores and therefore poorer nutritional status than those whose parents do not use these food parenting practices; and (2) children whose parents use positive encouragement during meals would have lower NutriSTEP® nutrition risk scores than those whose parents do not use these food parenting practices. The second aim of this study was to examine whether family functioning modifies or confounds the association of food parenting practices and children's nutrition risk. We hypothesized that family functioning would moderate the association between controlling food parenting practices and children's nutrition risk. Compared to children from families with high family functioning, the positive associations between controlling food parenting practices and nutrition risk would be stronger among children from families with low family functioning.

2. Methods

2.1. Participants and Procedure

We recruited families to participate in the Family Mealtime Observation Study (FaMOS) through a variety of methods including Facebook, posters in daycare centers, visits to library story times and word of mouth. Families were eligible to participate if: (1) they had a child between the ages of 18 months and 5 years; (2) it was typical for the family to eat meals together; and (3) parent(s) were able to speak and respond to surveys in English. In families with more than one child within our target age range, the child with the closest birthday to the date of the first home visit was chosen to be the target child; in the case of twins, a coin was flipped to randomly choose the target child.

Once families were confirmed as eligible to participate, a research assistant (RA) visited each family in their home at a time that was convenient for the family. During this visit, parent(s) provided consent on behalf of themselves and their child(ren) to participate. All children in the family provided assent to be video-recorded and the target child provided additional assent to have their height and weight measured. Where possible, in two-parent homes, both parents were asked to be home during this initial visit. The parent(s) decided on which three mealtimes over the following days would be recorded. All observations collected were of the evening meal. The evening meal was chosen as it was identified by parents as the typical "family meal" and, in two-parent homes, the time when both parents usually ate with the target child. Families were reminded that we wanted to see "typical" family mealtime experiences and that there was no reason to do anything special on the nights they recorded their meal. In cases where English was the family's second language, families were reminded to speak English during the recorded mealtimes. Each family was provided with a video camera and tripod to record their meals and the RA assisted the parent(s) with the initial video camera set-up and placement to ensure that all family members were in-view of the recording and that their faces could be seen. The RA measured parents' and target children's heights using a calibrated stadiometer and weights using a calibrated electronic scale. Following the home visit, we emailed parents a link to a 15-min online questionnaire, which asked them to report on their food parenting practices and aspects of their home environment, and to complete a nutrition risk questionnaire for the target child. In two parent families, each parent was sent an individual link to the questionnaire to complete.

On the evenings that a family was scheduled to record, an RA called or texted the family 15 min prior to the scheduled start of their mealtime to remind them to turn on the camera. Families were asked to record their entire meal. Study staff was not present during mealtime recordings. One hour after the family meal, an RA called or texted the family to confirm that they were indeed able to record, and to note any atypical events that may have occurred during the meal (i.e., target child had an atypical temper tantrum during the meal, camera ran out of battery, etc.). If the family was unable to record, another date was chosen for recording.

Following the recording of the three meals, an RA visited the family home again to pick up the camera. During this second home visit, the RA confirmed that three observations were recorded on the camera and that the parent questionnaires had been completed. Families were provided a $50 grocery gift card for participating. This study was approved by the University of Guelph Research Ethics Board (REB#14OC033).

2.2. Measures

Observed food parenting practices: we used the Family Mealtime Coding System (FMCS) [23,32] to measure mothers' and fathers' feeding practices. The FMCS was created to reflect the Child Feeding Questionnaire [33] and seven of its subscales were used in the current study: pressure for target child to eat ("eat three more bites"), physical prompts for target child to eat (spoon feeding child or putting food on the utensil for child to pick up), verbal restriction of target child's food consumption ("you can't have any more"), physical restriction of target child's food consumption (moving a specific food away from child), food rewards to encourage target child to eat ("if you eat your peas, you can have ice cream"), non-food rewards to encourage target child to eat ("if you finish your meal, you can watch TV"), and positive comments about food (either comments about food in general, the parent's own food, or the target child's food, explored separately) [23]. All instances of each food parenting behavior were logged and frequencies of occurrence for each behavior were calculated for the mealtime observation. The FMCS has been found to be a reliable measure of food parenting practices among preschool aged children (inter-rater reliability >86.5%) [23,32].

Target Child's Nutrition Risk: we measured the target child's nutrition risk using the Nutrition Screening Tool for Every Preschooler (NutriSTEP®) [11]. NutriSTEP® was developed by registered dietitians and is a 17-item questionnaire used to assess eating habits and identify nutrition problems in preschool aged children (3–5 years) across five subscales: eating behaviours, dietary intake, parental concerns about food and activity, screen time duration, and the use of supplements [11]. The primary parent (parent who completed the questionnaire first) completed the NutriSTEP® questionnaire for the target child. NutriSTEP® has been validated against registered dietitians' assessment of children's nutritional status (based on medical and nutritional history, three-day food records and anthropometric measurements) among a large sample of ethnically and geographically diverse families in Canada [11]. Scores on NutriSTEP® and registered dietitians' ratings were correlated ($r = 0.48$, $p = 0.01$) and the questionnaire was found to be reliable when completed by parents on two separate occasions, 2–4 weeks apart (kappa >0.75) [11]. Individual questions are answered using a tailored Likert scale, which are then coded into a numerical score through the use of the designated NutriSTEP® coding system. These scores are then summed to generate a nutrition risk score for the target child (ranging from 0 to 68), with higher scores representing greater nutrition risk. For descriptive purposes, scores were tabulated to determine three levels of risk of poor nutrition based on the standardized NutriSTEP® cut-offs: low (scores $\leq$20), medium (scores 21–25), and high (scores >25) [11]. A medium score identifies a level of risk that can be managed by public health services and a high score indicates risk requiring further assessment by a registered dietitian. For regression analyses, NutriSTEP® scores were explored as a continuous variable.

2.3. Covariates and Moderating Variables

Parental Educational Attainment: as an indicator of socio-economic status, mothers and fathers reported their educational attainment individually on an eight-point Likert Scale ranging from eighth grade or less to Postgraduate Training or Degree. Responses were dichotomized to graduated college/university and less than a college/university education.

Child Body Mass Index (BMI): trained research assistants measured children's heights and weights during home visit 1, as described above. Based on the World Health Organization (WHO) growth charts, we calculated BMI z-scores using WHO Anthro Software (version 3.2.2, WHO, Geneva, Switzerland) to assess child weight adjusted for age and gender.

Family Functioning: we measured family functioning using the "general functioning" subscale of the McMaster Family Assessment Device (FAD) [34]. Because family functioning is a family-level variable, we used the primary parent's report of family functioning. The scale consists of statements about families to which participants indicated the degree to which they agreed on a four-point scale (strongly disagree to strongly agree) and includes items that measure the overall health/pathology of the family relating to six dimensions of family functioning: (a) problem solving; (b) communication; (c) roles; (d) affective responsiveness; (e) affective involvement; and (f) behavioral control. The FAD has been validated against experienced family therapists' clinical ratings and found to correspond with clinicians' ratings of healthy and unhealthy families; 'general functioning' subscale (t (39) = 2.49, $p < 0.05$) [35]. Test-retest reliability has also been reported for the 'general functioning' subscale when completed by participants one week later ($r = 0.71$) [35]. We averaged responses to each of the

12 items comprising the 'general functioning' subscale to create an overall score; higher scores indicate lower levels of family functioning [34]. In our sample, the Cronbach's alpha for this subscale was 0.86, indicating strong internal consistency. For descriptive purposes, a cut-off of 2.17 was used to distinguish high and low functioning families (<2.17 = high functioning, ≥2.17 = low functioning) [35]. For regression analyses, family functioning was explored as a continuous variable.

2.4. Data Analysis

Videos of the mealtime observations were coded using Noldus Observer XT 12.5 (Noldus Information Technology, Wageningen, The Netherlands). To reduce camera reactivity, only mealtimes two and three were coded; video one was used as a warm-up for families [23]. Videos were coded by two independent coders who received a standardized training (4 h in length) outlining use of the Observer XT software and the behaviors to code using the FMCS [23,32]. Prior to coding videos for the current study, coders were provided with five sample videos and were required to demonstrate reliability (kappa >0.8) in comparison to pre-determined codes. During analysis, coders met bi-weekly to discuss coding challenges and to code a video together to ensure adherence to the coding scheme. Detailed notes from these meetings were kept to document decisions. Both coders also conducted regular reviews of their own coding to ensure intra-rater reliability during the coding of the full sample. A random sample of 20% of the videos were coded by both coders to ensure reliability [36]. We calculated intra-rater and inter-rater reliability using Observer XT's reliability function. Our inter-rater reliability (kappa = 0.8) and intra-rater reliability (kappa = 0.82) were both excellent [37].

Analyses were run separately for mothers and fathers, as previous research has suggested differences in mothers' and fathers' food parenting practices [28]. For both the mothers and fathers, there were no statistically significant differences in food parenting practices used in videos 2 and 3; thus, scores for parenting practices were averaged across the two observations. We calculated descriptive and frequency statistics for each food parenting practice to understand the practices used during mealtimes, as well as Mann-Whitney U-tests of difference between mothers' and fathers' food parenting practices. We ran linear regression models to examine the association between food parenting practices and children's NutriSTEP® risk scores. To examine whether family functioning modifies the association between food parenting practices and NutriSTEP® risk scores, we ran linear regression models including an interaction term, created using centered variables (family functioning × food parenting practice). There was no evidence of modification by family functioning ($p > 0.05$ for the interaction terms; results not shown); thus, we then included family functioning in the model as a covariate to examine whether family functioning confounds the association between food parenting practices and NutriSTEP® risk scores. Based on previous research, all models were adjusted for parent educational attainment and child BMI z-score [38,39]. Additionally, we explored whether associations between food parenting practices and child nutrition risk score differed by child gender; results from stratified models showed no difference by child gender (results not shown). Statistical analyses were conducted using SPSS version 25 for Mac (PASW, IBM, New York, NY, USA).

3. Results

3.1. Participant and Family-Level Characteristics

Of the families who expressed interest in our study by completing our eligibility screener ($n = 112$), two were ineligible because they did not have a child within our target age range, three lived too far away for RAs to conduct home visits, one indicated that they did not speak English during mealtimes and 29 of the families did not follow-up to schedule a home visit. We scheduled and completed home visits with 77 families. We were unable to obtain video data from four families; one family found that the camera was too distracting for the target child, and three families spoke languages other than English during their meal recordings.

Thus, our final sample for analysis consisted of 73 families (137 parents; 74 mothers, 63 fathers). Most of the parents (n = 73) identified as the "primary parent" (by completing the questionnaire first) were mothers. The majority of parents in this study were married or living with a partner (94.5%; Table 1), 85.3% of parents reported having graduated from College or University or more (i.e., post-graduate degree), and 86.1% of families reported a total household income of $\geq$$50,000/year. Moreover, the majority of parents identified as "white" (84.6%). Most of the families in this study participated in family dinners seven days a week (83.6%) and 90.4% were considered to have high family functioning (scores <2.17).

Table 1. Parent and family-level characteristics of participants in the Family Mealtime Observation Study (FaMOS) (n = 73 Families; 137 Parents).

Parental Characteristics (n = 137)	
	n (%)
Relation to Child	
Mother [i]	74 (54.0)
Father	63 (46.0)
Parental Age in years, mean (SD)	36.1 (9.5)
Parental Educational Attainment	
High School Education or Less	5 (3.7)
Some College or University	15 (11.0)
College Graduate	18 (13.2)
University Graduate	50 (36.8)
Post Graduate Training or Degree	48 (35.3)
Parent Race/Ethnicity	
White	115 (84.6)
Chinese	5 (3.7)
Latin American	6 (4.4)
Other (South Asian, Southeast Asian, West Indian, Black, Aboriginal/Indigenous)	10 (7.3)
Parent Birth Country	
Outside of Canada	18 (14.9)
Parental Weight Status (BMI, kg/m^2) [ii], mean (SD)	**26.9 (6.5)**
Underweight (BMI <18.5)	1 (0.7)
Normal Weight (BMI 18.5–24.9)	56 (43.8)
Overweight/Obese (BMI $\geq$25)	71 (55.5)
Family-Level Characteristics (n = 73)	
	n (%)
Family Structure	
Married or living with a partner	69 (94.5)
Total Household Income	
<$49,999/year	10 (13.9)
$50,000–$99,999/year	25 (34.7)
$\geq$$100,000/year	37 (51.4)
Family Functioning, mean SD	**1.62 (0.39)**
High (<2.17)	66 (90.4)
Low ($\geq$2.17)	7 (9.6)
Family Dinners (days/week)	
Every day (7 days/week)	61 (83.6)
Most days (4–6 days/week)	9 (12.3)
Rarely (<3 days/week)	3 (4.1)

[i] One same-sex couple. [ii] Parent weight missing for pregnant mothers (n = 9). SD standard deviation; BMI: Body Mass Index.

The average age of the target child was 3.3 $\pm$ 1.1 years and 56.2% were female (Table 2). The majority of children (65.3%) were considered to have a healthy weight status and low nutrition risk (89.0%).

Table 2. Characteristics of children participating in the Family Mealtime Observation Study (FaMOS) (*n* = 73).

	n (%)
Child Age mean (SD) 3.3 years (1.1)	
Child Gender	
Female	41 (56.2)
Child Race/Ethnicity	
White	57 (78.1)
Other (including Latin American, Southeast Asian, Chinese, Black and West Indian)	16 (21.9)
Child Weight Status (BMI *z*-score) [i] **mean (SD) 0.9 (1.9)**	
Healthy Weight	47 (65.3)
At risk of Overweight	19 (26.4)
Overweight/Obese	6 (8.3)
NutriSTEP® Score mean (SD) 13.3 (5.2)	
Low risk (≤20)	65 (89.0)
Medium risk (21–25)	6 (8.2)
High risk (>25)	2 (2.7)

[i] Child weight missing for one child who declined measurement. SD: standard deviation; BMI: Body Mass Index.

3.2. Exploration of Mealtime Videos and Food Parenting Practices

The average meal length was 24.5 min. Our results suggest that, overall, mothers were more engaged in food parenting than fathers (Table 3). Mothers used significantly more controlling feeding practices (described as mean frequency of occurrence, times/meal); specifically, more verbal restriction (mothers: 1.31 times/meal ± 1.59; fathers: 0.63 times/meal ± 0.88; $p < 0.05$), food rewards (mothers: 0.75 times/meal ± 1.79; fathers: 0.49 ± 1.13, $p < 0.05$), and non-food rewards (mothers: 0.31 times/meal ± 0.57; fathers: 0.14 times/meal ± 0.36, $p < 0.05$) than fathers. Additionally, mothers used more positive encouragement, specifically towards the target child's food during meals, than fathers (mothers: 7.12 times/meal ± 5.31; fathers: 4.26 times/meal ± 3.45, $p < 0.05$).

Table 3. Descriptive and frequency statistics for mothers' and fathers' observed food parenting practices [a] with target child and Mann-Whitney *U*-tests of difference between mothers' and fathers' observed food parenting.

	Mothers (*n* = 74)			Fathers (*n* = 63)			Mann-Whitney *U*-Test *z*-Scores
	Mean (SD)	Minimum	Maximum	Mean (SD)	Minimum	Maximum	
Verbal Pressure to eat	4.37 (5.22)	0	37.5	3.03 (3.06)	0	11.5	−1.7
Physical Pressure to eat	2.31 (4.22)	0	21	1.63 (2.80)	0	13	−0.67
Verbal Restriction	**1.31 (1.59)**	0	9.5	**0.63 (0.88)**	0	4	**−3.13**
Physical Restriction	0.21 (0.43)	0	2	0.12 (0.35)	0	2	−1.29
Use of Food as Reward	**0.75 (1.79)**	0	14.5	**0.49 (1.13)**	0	6.5	**−2.00**
Use of Non-Food Rewards	**0.31 (0.57)**	0	2.5	**0.14 (0.36)**	0	2	**−2.02**
Positive comments about food in general	3.91 (3.29)	0	14	3.11 (2.96)	0	16	−1.42
Positive comments about own food	1.83 (1.47)	0	7.5	1.78 (1.54)	0	5.5	−0.42
Positive comments about target child's food	**7.12 (5.31)**	0	25	**4.26 (3.45)**	0	14.5	**−3.52**

[a] Measured by the Family Mealtime Coding System. Significant differences at $p < 0.05$ level are bolded. SD standard deviation.

3.3. Exploration of Food Parenting Practices and Target Child's NutriSTEP® Risk Scores

3.3.1. Mothers

Among mothers, more frequent physical restriction of food was associated with higher NutriSTEP® nutrition risk scores in their children (β = 0.40 NutriSTEP® points, 95% CI = 2.30, 7.58) and more frequent positive comments about the target children's food were associated with lower nutrition risk (β = −0.31 NutriSTEP® points, 95% CI = −0.54, −0.08) in models adjusted for parent educational attainment and child BMI z-score (Model 1; Table 4). These associations remained significant after adjustment for family functioning (Model 2; Table 4). No other significant associations between mothers' food parenting practices and the target child's nutrition risk scores were found.

Table 4. Linear Regression models examining associations of Observed Food Parenting Practices with NutriSTEP® Scores.

Observed Food Parenting Practice	Mothers (*n* = 74)		Fathers (*n* = 63)	
	Model 1	Model 2	Model 1	Model 2
	Effect Estimate (95% CI)		Effect Estimate (95% CI)	
Verbal Pressure to eat	−0.01 (−0.25, 0.22)	−0.01 (−0.24, 0.23)	0.03 (−0.37, 0.46)	0.04 (−0.36, 0.50)
Physical Pressure to eat	−0.05 (−0.36, 0.23)	−0.05 (−0.35, 0.24)	0.20 (−0.09, 0.80)	0.21 (−0.10, 0.80)
Verbal Restriction	0.28 (−0.68, 0.88)	0.30 (−0.68, 0.89)	0.13 (−0.73, 2.17)	0.15 (−0.67, 2.29)
Physical Restriction	**0.40 (2.30, 7.58)**	**0.41 (2.39, 7.72)**	0.03 (−3.00, 3.99)	0.06 (−2.88, 4.52)
Use of Food as Reward	−0.14 (−1.10, 0.26)	−0.14 (−1.10, 0.27)	−0.08 (−1.44, 0.79)	−0.08 (−1.45, 0.80)
Use of Non-Food Rewards	−0.16 (−3.59, 0.69)	−0.16 (−3.65, 0.67)	0.01 (−3.43, 3.64)	0.02 (−3.36, 3.79)
Positive comments about food in general	−0.16 (−0.63, 0.11)	−0.16 (−0.63, 0.11)	0.15 (−0.18, 0.67)	0.18 (−0.15, 0.73)
Positive comments about own food	−0.15 (−1.40, 0.29)	−0.15 (−1.40, 0.31)	−0.13 (−1.19, 0.42)	−0.14 (−1.24, 0.40)
Positive comments about target child's food	**−0.31 (−0.54, −0.08)**	**−0.31 (−0.54, −0.08)**	**−0.27 (−0.75, −0.01)**	−0.27 (−0.76, 0.00)

Dependent Variable: NutriSTEP® Risk Score, continuous Model 1. Adjusted for parent educational attainment, dichotomous and child BMI-z score, continuous Model 2. Adjusted for model 1 covariates and family functioning, continuous Estimates where the 95% Confidence Interval (CI) does not include 0.0 are bolded.

3.3.2. Fathers

Among fathers, more frequent positive comments about the target children's food were associated with lower nutrition risk (β = −0.27 NutriSTEP® points, 95% CI = −0.75, −0.01) in models adjusted for parent educational attainment and child BMI z-score (Mode 1; Table 4). The association remained similar, but not significant (CIs just overlapping 0) after adjustment for family functioning (Model 2; Table 4). Similar to our results with mothers, adjustment for family functioning did not otherwise change our results, and no other significant associations between fathers' food parenting practices and the target child's nutrition risk scores were found (Model 2; Table 4).

4. Discussion

In this sample of Canadian parents of preschool aged children, we observed that mothers' use of physical restriction was associated with higher nutrition risk for their child and both mothers' and fathers' use of positive comments towards the target child's food was associated with lower nutrition risk. Family functioning did not modify or confound these associations. To our knowledge, this is the first study to explore the associations of observed food parenting practices with preschool children's nutrition risk while considering the potential influence of family functioning on these associations.

Our finding that maternal use of physical restriction of food was associated with greater risk of nutritional inadequacy supports our hypothesis that controlling food parenting practices would be associated with increased nutrition risk. This finding is consistent with previous longitudinal research that suggests restriction undermines a child's ability to recognize their own hunger and satiety cues [40] and increases eating in the absence of hunger [14], thereby increasing the child's risk for overeating and potential for increased nutrition risk. Similar to previous observational studies, we observed fairly low levels of parental restriction [22,23,30,41,42]. It has been suggested that overt restriction (i.e., taking food away from a child or telling them to stop eating a certain food) may occur more often during less structured eating occasions such as snack time and that covert restriction may occur more during structured mealtimes (i.e., not bringing certain foods into the home or offering them at mealtimes) [43]. Future research should explore the association of restriction and children's dietary intake and eating behaviors throughout the day using a longitudinal study design to help tease out the directionality of the association. It is possible that the mothers in this sample were concerned about their child's nutritional intake and thus used more physical restriction during mealtimes.

Our finding that mothers' and fathers' positive comments about the target child's food were associated with lower nutrition risk among children also supports our initial hypotheses. Research by Holley and colleagues [44] found parental modeling and positive comments to be helpful in increasing children's consumption of disliked vegetables. Positive encouragement, without pressure, has also been related to lower reported levels of fussy eating and greater reports of food enjoyment in preschoolers [45]. Taken together, these results suggest that positive parental comments may be an effective method of both increasing intake of healthful foods and decreasing nutrition risk scores among preschool aged children. Future research should test the ability of interventions to teach parents to use positive encouragement rather than controlling feeding practices to improve dietary intake and reduce nutrition risk among preschoolers.

It has been argued that family dysfunction may diminish the impact of positive role modeling and intensify adverse impacts of controlling feeding practices during mealtimes [46]. However, our results suggest family functioning does not modify or confound the association between parents' food parenting practices and preschoolers' nutrition risk. Contrary to our hypotheses, the associations between controlling food parenting practices and greater nutrition risk were not stronger among children from families with low family functioning. Similarly, effect estimates did not change when family functioning was added to the analytic models. When it comes to reducing children's nutrition risk, our findings suggest that food parenting practices are an important avenue of intervention, regardless of level of family functioning. However, future research should seek to replicate our findings in populations with diverse levels of family functioning; it is possible that the limited variability of family functioning in our sample may have contributed to the null effects of family functioning on the associations explored.

Mothers', but not fathers', use of physical restriction was associated with children's nutrition risk. However, this finding is contrary to previous research using mother and father reports of food parenting. Among a sample of Canadian parents, Watterworth et al. [13] found that fathers, but not mothers, reported 'restriction for health' was associated with higher nutrition risk among children. Comparisons between the two studies are difficult due to Watterworth and colleagues' [13] use of parental report of food parenting practices, as previous research has found little association between observed and reported food parenting practices [21–24]. Mealtime observations only capture overt restriction and parents may use covert restriction, which would not be observed during mealtime videos, but can be captured in food parenting questionnaires. Future research should explore the use of mixed observational and parent-report methods in an attempt to more accurately capture both overt and covert restriction as well as the meaning behind the restriction (e.g., for health or weight control) [47].

We found that mothers used significantly more verbal restriction and food and non-food rewards than fathers during meals. Overall, we found that positive comments about the target child's food (e.g., "your broccoli looks delicious") was the most commonly used food parenting practice among both mothers and fathers, followed by verbal pressure to get the child to eat (e.g., "eat three more bites") for mothers and positive comments about food in general (e.g., "milk helps us grow strong bones and teeth") for fathers, which is similar to previous observational research [30]. Our findings suggest that mothers and fathers differ in the food parenting practices they use. While observational studies including fathers have been limited [28], the research exploring differences in mothers' and fathers' observed food parenting practices has produced conflicting results [23,30]. One U.K.- based study that used the FMCS [23] reported no significant differences in the frequency of mothers' and fathers' food parenting practices. However, similar to our findings, an American study by Orrell-Valente and colleagues [30] found that, overall, mothers used significantly more food parenting practices than fathers and they also tended to use praise more frequently. Interestingly, the study that showed no difference between mothers' and fathers food parenting [23] was conducted in the U.K., suggesting that food parenting practices could be regionally and culturally defined. These inconsistent results highlight the importance of exploring both mothers' and fathers' food parenting practices to further understand how parents may influence each other's food parenting practices and how this interaction between mothers and fathers may impact children's dietary intake. Harris et al., have pioneered work in this area and found that, compared to discordant mother-father pairs, Australian mother-father pairs who concordantly report low levels of pressure to eat had children with lower levels of pickiness [48]. Additional research is needed to understand the impact of concordance/discordance between mothers' and fathers' food parenting practices in Canada.

Our study had a number of key strengths. First, the inclusion of fathers in this study is fairly unique within studies exploring food parenting practices [13,28], or children's health in general [29]. This allowed for a more accurate analysis of the context in which preschoolers from primarily two-parent families are fed. Second, the use of direct observation allowed us to more accurately explore associations between food parenting practices and children's nutrition risk. Furthermore, these observations were conducted in the home, without the presence of an RA, to allow for typical mealtime interactions to occur. Many studies exploring food parenting practices have either been conducted in lab settings or in the home in the presence of an RA where interactions are more likely to be atypical. Third, the use of a validated nutrition risk screening tool also adds to the strength of our study, ensuring an accurate measure of nutrition risk. Finally, this study is the first to observe food parenting practices in a Canadian context, which allows us to better understand the mealtime environments in which Canadian preschoolers are fed.

Despite the many strengths, there are limitations that should be noted when interpreting our results. This study was cross-sectional, and thus, the bi-directional nature of parent-child feeding interactions could not be determined. For example, it is possible that more controlling feeding practices are used with picky eaters; parents may use these practices in an attempt to improve their child's nutritional intake. Prospective research is needed to understand the temporal order of the association between food parenting practices and children's dietary intake as well as the bi-directional nature of these feeding interactions. While families recorded three mealtimes, we only observed food parenting practices during the evening meal. It is possible that food parenting practices differ during less structured eating occasions such as snack time. The level of nutrition risk reported in this study was much lower than previous studies exploring NutriSTEP® risk scores in Canada. Results may differ among families with children who have higher nutrition risk. Similarly, the families in this study also had high levels of family functioning. Results may also differ among families with lower functioning. While we found a significant association between mothers' use of physical restriction and mothers' and fathers' positive comments about the target child's food with NutriSTEP® risk scores, it should be noted that the effect sizes of the associations were relatively small. We have NutriSTEP® data from just one parent (primarily mothers) which may impact our findings and explain the few associations between fathers' food parenting practices and NutriSTEP® scores. Parents may perceive their child's nutrition risk differently; future research should seek to understand differences in how mothers' and fathers' report their child's nutrition risk. We calculated 36 tests (Table 4) and did not account for multiple comparisons. However, of these tests, five were statistically significant at the $p < 0.05$ level, which is larger than the one test we would expect by chance. Finally, the families in this study were highly educated and the majority identified as "white"; our results may not be generalizable to more diverse populations.

5. Conclusions

Mothers' observed use of physical restriction was associated with increased nutrition risk and mothers' and fathers' use of positive comments about the target child's food was associated with lower nutrition risk among preschool aged children. Family functioning did not moderate or confound the associations between parental food parenting practices and children's nutrition risk. Results suggest that supporting parents to use more positive encouragement rather than restriction may help to reduce preschoolers' nutrition risk. Future research should test interventions aimed at changing food parenting practices among families with preschoolers at medium-high nutrition risk. While we found few associations between fathers' food parenting practices and preschoolers' nutrition risk, we found differences among the types and frequency of food parenting practices employed by mothers and fathers. This underscores the importance of including fathers in food parenting research. As this was the first Canadian study to observe food parenting practices, future research is needed among more diverse populations, including those with more socio-economic diversity, higher levels of nutrition risk, and lower levels of family functioning, to further elucidate the association between food parenting practices and children's nutrition risk in Canada.

Availability of Data and Material: The datasets used and/or analyzed during the current study are available from the corresponding author on reasonable request.

Author Contributions: K.W., J.H., and E.H. developed study methods and sought funding. K.W. led the study, data analysis and manuscript preparation. E.H. was part of K.W.'s dissertation committee, developed the mealtime coding scheme, supported video coding and manuscript preparation. K.J. conducted study visits, coded videos and supported study analysis. A.B. was part of K.W.'s dissertation committee, assisted with study methods and manuscript preparation. J.R.S. supported manuscript preparation and assisted with interpretation of results. J.H. was K.W.'s PhD advisor and supported the study, analyses, manuscript preparation and interpretation of results.

Funding: Funding for the Family Mealtime Observation Study (FaMOS) was provided by the Canadian Foundation for Dietetic Research (CFDR).

Acknowledgments: The authors would like to thank the families that participated in FaMOS, who generously welcomed us into their homes to allow us to learn from their mealtimes.

Conflicts of Interest: The authors declare no conflict of interest.

Abbreviations

FaMOS	Family Mealtime Observation Study
FMCS	Family Mealtime Coding Scheme
BMI	Body Mass Index
NutriSTEP®	Nutrition Screening Tool for Every Preschooler
WHO	World Health Organization
FAD	Family Assessment Device

References

1. Nicklas, T.A.; Hayes, D.; Association, A.D. Position of the American Dietetic Association: Nutrition guidance for healthy children ages 2 to 11 years. *J. Am. Diet. Assoc.* **2008**, *108*, 1038–1044. [PubMed]
2. Savage, J.S.; Fisher, J.O.; Birch, L.L. Parental influence on eating behavior: Conception to adolescence. *J. Law Med. Ethics* **2007**, *35*, 22–34. [CrossRef] [PubMed]
3. Birch, L.L.; Fisher, J.O. Development of eating behaviors among children and adolescents. *Pediatrics* **1998**, *101*, 539–549. [PubMed]
4. Birch, L.L. Development of food preferences. *Annu. Rev. Nutr.* **1999**, *19*, 41–62. [CrossRef] [PubMed]
5. Skinner, J.D.; Carruth, B.R.; Wendy, B.; Ziegler, P.J. Children's food preferences: A longitudinal analysis. *J. Am. Diet. Assoc.* **2002**, *102*, 1638–1647. [CrossRef]

6. Freedman, D.S.; Khan, L.K.; Dietz, W.H.; Srinivasan, S.R.; Berenson, G.S. Relationship of childhood obesity to coronary heart disease risk factors in adulthood: The Bogalusa Heart Study. *Pediatrics* **2001**, *108*, 712–718. [CrossRef]

7. Rylatt, L.; Cartwright, T. Parental feeding behaviour and motivations regarding pre-school age children: A thematic synthesis of qualitative studies. *Appetite* **2016**, *99*, 285–297. [CrossRef]

8. Eyre, H.; Kahn, R.; Robertson, R.M.; Clark, N.G.; Doyle, C.; Hong, Y.; Gansler, T.; Glynn, T.; Smith, R.A.; Taubert, K.; et al. Preventing cancer, cardiovascular disease, and diabetes: A common agenda for the American Cancer Society, the American Diabetes Association, and the American Heart Association. *Stroke* **2004**, *35*, 1999–2010. [CrossRef] [PubMed]

9. Jessri, M.; Nishi, S.K.; L'Abbe, M.R. Assessing the nutritional quality of diets of Canadian children and adolescents using the 2014 Health Canada Surveillance Tool Tier System. *BMC Public Health* **2016**, *16*, 381. [CrossRef] [PubMed]

10. Garriguet, D. *Findings from the Canadian Community Health Survey: Overview of Canadians' Eating Habits*; Canada, S., Ed.; Statistics Canada: Ottawa, ON, Canada, 2004.

11. Randall Simpson, J.A.; Keller, H.H.; Rysdale, L.A.; Beyers, J.E. Nutrition Screening Tool for Every Preschooler (NutriSTEP): Validation and test-retest reliability of a parent-administered questionnaire assessing nutrition risk of preschoolers. *Eur. J. Clin. Nutr.* **2008**, *62*, 770–780. [CrossRef]

12. Watson-Jarvis, K.; McNeil, D.; Fenton, T.R.; Campbell, K. Implementing the Nutrition Screening Tool for Every Preschooler (NutriSTEP®) in community health centres. *Can. J. Diet. Pract. Res.* **2011**, *72*, 96–98. [CrossRef] [PubMed]

13. Watterworth, J.C.; Hutchinson, J.M.; Buchholz, A.C.; Darlington, G.; Randall Simpson, J.A.; Ma, D.W.L.; Haines, J.; Study, G.F.H. Food parenting practices and their association with child nutrition risk status: Comparing mothers and fathers. *Appl. Physiol. Nutr. Metab.* **2017**, *42*, 667–671. [CrossRef] [PubMed]

14. Birch, L.L.; Fisher, J.O.; Davison, K.K. Learning to overeat: Maternal use of restrictive feeding practices promotes girls' eating in the absence of hunger. *Am. J. Clin. Nutr.* **2003**, *78*, 215–220. [CrossRef] [PubMed]

15. Faith, M.S.; Berkowitz, R.I.; Stallings, V.A.; Kerns, J.; Storey, M.; Stunkard, A.J. Parental feeding attitudes and styles and child body mass index: Prospective analysis of a gene-environment interaction. *Pediatrics* **2004**, *114*, e429–e436. [CrossRef] [PubMed]

16. Blissett, J.; Meyer, C.; Haycraft, E. Maternal and paternal controlling feeding practices with male and female children. *Appetite* **2006**, *47*, 212–219. [CrossRef] [PubMed]

17. Johannsen, D.L.; Johannsen, N.M.; Specker, B.L. Influence of parents' eating behaviors and child feeding practices on children's weight status. *Obesity (Silver Spring)* **2006**, *14*, 431–439. [CrossRef]

18. Campbell, K.; Andrianopoulos, N.; Hesketh, K.; Ball, K.; Crawford, D.; Brennan, L.; Corsini, N.; Timperio, A. Parental use of restrictive feeding practices and child BMI z-score. A 3-year prospective cohort study. *Appetite* **2010**, *55*, 84–88. [CrossRef]

19. Ventura, A.K.; Birch, L.L. Does parenting affect children's eating and weight status? *Int. J. Behav. Nutr. Phys. Act.* **2008**, *5*, 15. [CrossRef]

20. Skouteris, H.; McCabe, M.; Ricciardelli, A.; Milgrom, J.; Baur, L.; Aksan, N.; Dell'Aquila, D. Parent-child interactions and obesity prevention: A systematic review of the literature. *Early Child Dev. Care* **2012**, *182*, 153–174. [CrossRef]

21. Bergmeier, H.; Skouteris, H.; Haycraft, E.; Haines, J.; Hooley, M. Reported and observed controlling feeding practices predict child eating behavior after 12 months. *J. Nutr.* **2015**, *145*, 1311–1316. [CrossRef]

22. Farrow, C.; Blissett, J.; Haycraft, E. Does child weight influence how mothers report their feeding practices? *Int. J. Pediatr. Obes.* **2011**, *6*, 306–313. [CrossRef] [PubMed]

23. Haycraft, E.L.; Blissett, J.M. Maternal and paternal controlling feeding practices: Reliability and relationships with BMI. *Obesity (Silver Spring)* **2008**, *16*, 1552–1558. [CrossRef] [PubMed]

24. Bergmeier, H.; Skouteris, H.; Hetherington, M. Systematic research review of observational approaches used to evaluate mother-child mealtime interactions during preschool years. *Am. J. Clin. Nutr.* **2015**, *101*, 7–15. [CrossRef] [PubMed]

25. Broderick, C. *Understanding Family Process: Basics of Family Systems Theory*; Sage: Thousand Oaks, CA, USA, 1993.

26. Rhee, K. Childhood overweight and the relationship between parent behaviours, parenting style and family functioning. *Ann. AAPSS* **2008**, *615*, 12–37. [CrossRef]

27. Haines, J.; Rifas-Shiman, S.L.; Horton, N.J.; Kleinman, K.; Bauer, K.W.; Davison, K.K.; Walton, K.; Austin, S.B.; Field, A.E.; Gillman, M.W. Family functioning and quality of parent-adolescent relationship: Cross-sectional associations with adolescent weight-related behaviors and weight status. *Int. J. Behav. Nutr. Phys. Act.* **2016**, *13*, 68. [CrossRef]

28. Khandpur, N.; Blaine, R.E.; Fisher, J.O.; Davison, K.K. Fathers' child feeding practices: A review of the evidence. *Appetite* **2014**, *78*, 110–121. [CrossRef]

29. Davison, K.K.; Kitos, N.; Aftosmes-Tobio, A.; Ash, T.; Agaronov, A.; Sepulveda, M.; Haines, J. The forgotten parent: Fathers' representation in family interventions to prevent childhood obesity. *Prev. Med.* **2018**, *111*, 170–176. [CrossRef]

30. Orrell-Valente, J.K.; Hill, L.G.; Brechwald, W.A.; Dodge, K.A.; Pettit, G.S.; Bates, J.E. "Just three more bites": An observational analysis of parents' socialization of children's eating at mealtime. *Appetite* **2007**, *48*, 37–45. [CrossRef]

31. Shea, C.; Dwyer, J.J.; Heeney, E.S.; Goy, R.; Simpson, J.R. The effect of parental feeding behaviours and participation of children in organized sports/activities on child body mass index. *Can. J. Diet. Pract. Res.* **2010**, *71*, e87–e93. [CrossRef]

32. Haycraft, E. Child Feeding Practices in Fathers and Mothers of Young Children. Ph.D. Thesis, University of Birmingham, Birmingham, UK, 2007.

33. Birch, L.L.; Fisher, J.O.; Grimm-Thomas, K.; Markey, C.N.; Sawyer, R.; Johnson, S.L. Confirmatory factor analysis of the Child Feeding Questionnaire: A measure of parental attitudes, beliefs and practices about child feeding and obesity proneness. *Appetite* **2001**, *36*, 201–210. [CrossRef]

34. Epstein, N.; Baldwin, L.; Bishop, D. The McMaster Family Assessment Device. *J. Marital Fam. Ther.* **1983**, *9*, 171–180. [CrossRef]

35. Miller, I.; Epstein, N.; Bishop, D.; Keitner, G. The McMaster Family Assessment Device: Reliability and validity. *J. Marital Fam. Ther.* **1985**, *11*, 345–356. [CrossRef]

36. Pesch, M.H.; Lumeng, J.C. Methodological considerations for observational coding of eating and feeding behaviors in children and their families. *Int. J. Behav. Nutr. Phys. Act.* **2017**, *14*, 170. [CrossRef] [PubMed]

37. Hallgren, K.A. Computing Inter-Rater Reliability for Observational Data: An Overview and Tutorial. *Tutor. Quant. Methods Psychol.* **2012**, *8*, 23–34. [CrossRef] [PubMed]

38. Shloim, N.; Edelson, L.R.; Martin, N.; Hetherington, M.M. Parenting styles, feeding styles, feeding practices and weight status in 4-12 year-old children: A systematic review of the literature. *Front. Psychol.* **2015**, *6*, 1–20. [CrossRef]

39. Vereecken, C.A.; Keukelier, E.; Maes, L. Influence of mother's educational level on food parenting practices and food habits of young children. *Appetite* **2004**, *43*, 93–103. [CrossRef]

40. Hughes, S.O.; Frazier-Wood, A.C. Satiety and the Self-Regulation of Food Take in Children: A Potential Role for Gene-Environment Interplay. *Curr. Obes. Rep.* **2016**, *5*, 81–87. [CrossRef]

41. Hughes, S.O.; Power, T.G.; Papaioannou, M.A.; Cross, M.B.; Nicklas, T.A.; Hall, S.K.; Shewchuk, R.M. Emotional climate, feeding practices, and feeding styles: An observational analysis of the dinner meal in Head Start families. *Int. J. Behav. Nutr. Phys. Act.* **2011**, *8*, 60. [CrossRef]

42. Farrow, C.V.; Haycraft, E.; Blissett, J.M. Observing Maternal Restriction of Food with 3–5-Year-Old Children: Relationships with Temperament and Later Body Mass Index (BMI). *Int. J. Environ. Res. Public Health* **2018**, *15*. [CrossRef]

43. Fisher, J.O.; Birch, L.L. Restricting access to palatable foods affects children's behavioral response, food selection, and intake. *Am. J. Clin. Nutr.* **1999**, *69*, 1264–1272. [CrossRef]

44. Holley, C.E.; Haycraft, E.; Farrow, C. 'Why don't you try it again?' A comparison of parent led, home based interventions aimed at increasing children's consumption of a disliked vegetable. *Appetite* **2015**, *87*, 215–222. [CrossRef] [PubMed]

45. Powell, F.; Farrow, C.; Meyer, C.; Haycraft, E. The Stability and Continuity of Maternally Reported and Observed Child Eating Behaviours and Feeding Practices across Early Childhood. *Int. J. Environ. Res. Public Health* **2018**, *15*, 1017. [CrossRef] [PubMed]

46. Berge, J.M.; Wall, M.; Larson, N.; Loth, K.A.; Neumark-Sztainer, D. Family functioning: Associations with weight status, eating behaviors, and physical activity in adolescents. *J. Adolesc. Health* **2013**, *52*, 351–357. [CrossRef] [PubMed]

47. Horton, N.J.; Fitzmaurice, G.M. Regression analysis of multiple source and multiple informant data from complex survey samples. *Stat. Med.* **2004**, *23*, 2911–2933. [CrossRef]

48. Harris, H.A.; Jansen, E.; Mallan, K.M.; Daniels, L.; Thorpe, K. Do Dads Make a Difference? Family Feeding Dynamics and Child Fussy Eating. *J. Dev. Behav. Pediatr.* **2018**, *39*, 415–423. [CrossRef] [PubMed]

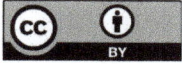

nutrients

MDPI

Article

Mothers' Vegetable Consumption Behaviors and Preferences as Factors Limiting the Possibility of Increasing Vegetable Consumption in Children in a National Sample of Polish and Romanian Respondents

Barbara Groele [1], Dominika Głąbska [1,*], Krystyna Gutkowska [2] and Dominika Guzek [2]

[1] Department of Dietetics, Faculty of Human Nutrition and Consumer Sciences, Warsaw University of Life Sciences (SGGW-WULS), 159C Nowoursynowska Street, 02-787 Warsaw, Poland; barbara_groele@sggw.pl
[2] Department of Organization and Consumption Economics, Faculty of Human Nutrition and Consumer Sciences, Warsaw University of Life Sciences (SGGW-WULS), 159C Nowoursynowska Street, 02-787 Warsaw, Poland; krystyna_gutkowska@sggw.pl (K.G.); dominika_guzek@sggw.pl (D.G.)
* Correspondence: dominika_glabska@sggw.pl; Tel.: +48-22-593-71-26

Received: 11 March 2019; Accepted: 10 May 2019; Published: 15 May 2019

Abstract: Increasing the insufficient intake of vegetables in children may be difficult, due to the influence of parents and at-home accessibility. The aim of this study was to analyze the association between self-reported vegetable consumption behaviors and preferences of mothers and the behaviors and preferences of their children, as declared by them. The nationally representative Polish (n = 1200) and Romanian (n = 1157) samples of mothers of children aged 3–10 were obtained using the random quota sampling method, and interviewed for their and their children's general frequency of consumption and preferences of vegetables in years 2012–2014. A 24 h dietary recall of vegetable consumption was conducted for mothers and their children. Associations were observed for general number of servings consumed per day by mother–child pairs ($p < 0.0001$; $R = 0.6522$, $R = 0.6573$ for Polish and Romanian samples, respectively) and number of types indicated as preferred ($p < 0.0001$; $R = 0.5418$, $R = 0.5433$). The share of children consuming specific vegetables was 33.1–75.3% and 42.6–75.7% while their mothers also consumed, but 0.1–43.2% and 1.2–22.9% while their mothers did not. The share of children preferring specific vegetables was 16.7–74.1% and 15.2–100% when their mother shared the preference, but 1.3–46.9% and 0–38.3% when their mother did not. The mothers' vegetable consumption behaviors and preferences may be a factor limiting the possibility of increasing vegetable consumption in their children.

Keywords: children; mothers; vegetable intake; consumption behaviors; choice; preferences

1. Introduction

The World Health Organization (WHO) advocates regular consumption of vegetables and fruits as an important element of a child's diet, not only in order to prevent non-communicable diet-related diseases, but also to create beneficial dietary patterns that are commonly predictive of their adolescence and adulthood patterns [1]. It is especially stated that vegetable intake patterns and preferences remain stable during childhood and adolescence [2].

Insufficient intake of vegetables and fruits is common worldwide, and the WHO has flagged it as being among the top ten determinants of global mortality [3]. At the same time, in the systematic review and meta-analysis of Touyz et al. [4], it was indicated that children more often meet the nutritional recommendations for fruits than for vegetables, so it is especially important to conduct interventions targeted at vegetables in order to increase their intake.

The '5-a-day' campaign has been carried out in a number of countries in order to increase the vegetable and fruit intake of children and adults, however, both the quantity and the variety consumed are still not adequate [5]. Also, the Cochrane systematic review by Hodder et al. [6] indicated that some interventions may increase the intake of vegetables and fruits by children. However, the observed evidence was stated to be low-quality and the observed increase was stated to be minor, so future research is required [6]. Based on the analysis of consumption trends in 33 countries, it has been observed that the intake of vegetables and fruits is increasing in many countries [7]. However, the trend is not stable, as the Health Survey for England indicated an important decrease in the frequency of meeting the '5-a-day' recommendation for children, from 20% to 17% between 2011 and 2013, even though an increase had been noted earlier [8].

Increasing the intake of vegetables in children may be hindered by a number of barriers associated with both internal and external factors [9,10] associated with sensory attributes, perception, preferences, knowledge, price, convenience, availability and accessibility, and parental, peer, and media influence. One of the most important barriers is low accessibility, which may result from seasonality [11], place of residence [12], and relatively high prices compared to other food products [13]. The other group of barriers results from preferences associated with the sensory attributes of vegetables [14], parental food consumption patterns [15], and food neophobia [16].

In general, a child is dependent on a diet that is prepared at home, being an element of the family environment and under general parental influence, until other influencing factors, such as peers and media, become more prominent [17]. As a result, the diets of children and parents are similar, as was observed in the systematic review and meta-analysis of Yee et al. [18], who concluded that a number of consumption behaviors of parents and their children were correlated.

For a number of the indicated barriers, the influence of parents and at-home accessibility may be crucial to reducing the children's intake of vegetables. Such reduction of intake may be observed in spite of the fact that, in general, parents know that intake of vegetables is important for their children and believe that it will influence their health and vitality [19]. It has already been observed that in order to increase the intake of fruits by children, it is necessary to influence the fruit consumption preferences and behaviors of their mothers [20], but this has not been analyzed for vegetables so far. Taking this into account, the aim of the present study was to analyze the association between self-reported vegetable consumption behaviors and preferences of mothers and the vegetable consumption behaviors and preferences of their children, as reported by them in national samples of Polish and Romanian respondents.

2. Materials and Methods

2.1. Ethical Statement

The study was conducted on a national sample of Polish and Romanian respondents according to the guidelines laid down in the Declaration of Helsinki, and all procedures involving human subjects were approved by the Ethics Committee of the Faculty of Human Nutrition and Consumer Sciences of the Warsaw University of Life Sciences. All participants provided informed consent.

2.2. Studied Sample

The study was conducted on Polish and Romanian subjects, who were recruited using the same procedure and inclusion/exclusion criteria as previously described [20]. The study itself was conducted in Poland and Romania according to the same methodology, with identical questions being asked in the respondent's native language. The data gathering was financed by the National Polish Promotion Fund for Fruits and Vegetables Consumption and Polish Association of Juices Producers within funds of the 5xVFJ (5 Portions of Vegetables, Fruit or Juice) national campaign, as an element of policy development in order to obtain the aim of increasing vegetables and fruits consumption in children.

One thousand and two hundred Polish and 1200 Romanian mothers of children aged 3–10 were planned to be recruited as respondents. The random quota sampling procedure was applied and informed consent was obtained from each respondent. Due to some missing data in the questionnaires obtained in the Romanian sample, 43 recruited respondents (3.6%), who were included in interviewing but did not complete it, were excluded. Finally, 1200 representative Polish respondents and 1157 Romanian respondents were included in years 2012–2014.

Recruitment was done in cooperation with a professional international agency that assesses public opinion and perception, and the agency was responsible for carrying out the random quota sampling. The planned quotas were determined for age, education, and residence (region and size of the city) in order to obtain representative Polish and Romanian samples of mothers of children aged 3–10.

The applied inclusion criteria were as follows: women, mother of child/children aged 3–10, inhabitant of Poland/Romania, aged 25–45. The applied exclusion criteria were as follows: lack of informed consent to participate, any missing data in the questionnaire.

2.3. Methods

The Computer-Assisted Telephone Interviewing (CATI) was done in cooperation with a professional international agency that assesses public opinion and perception, and the agency was hired as a partner responsible for data gathering, as in the previously described study [20]. Women aged 25–45 were randomly recruited while using the national database—they were invited to participate in the study during a telephone call and, if agreeing, they were verified for inclusion/exclusion criteria, as well as quota sampling being applied. The participation was compensated by a low value digital gift voucher code, according to commonly applied standards [21].

The assessment of vegetable consumption behaviors and preferences was conducted using questions that were asked about the mother's own behaviors and preferences (self-reported) and, in separate questions, about the behaviors and preferences of her child (as reported by the mother). A mother who declared she had more than one child aged 3–10 was asked to choose one of them arbitrarily and, afterwards, to inform about vegetable consumption behaviors and preferences of only this child during the whole interview.

In spite of the fact that while parents report the intake of their children, there may be important bias associated with proxy-reporting, there is also a bias associated with self-reporting by children, as it is indicated that they are able to self-report their intake from the age of 8 [22]. As a result, it would not be effective to assess the intake self-reported by children, as in the present study, the nutritional habits of children aged 3–10 were to be assessed. In general, for younger children mothers commonly report their intake [23]. In order to not apply various methodology (proxy-reporting for younger children and self-reporting for older ones), it was decided to assess the behaviors and preferences of children as reported by mothers in all cases, as for mothers.

In addition to the questions that were planned to be analyzed, respondents were also asked additional 'dummy questions'. They were associated with consumed vegetables, but not directly with behaviors and preferences of mothers and their children, as they were related to issues such as the place where vegetables are consumed, applied techniques of preparation of vegetables, known campaigns that promote vegetables consumption, and advantages and disadvantages of increased vegetable consumption. They were applied between main questions, in order to avoid interruptions of answers by the previous questions and answers. Respondents were also informed about the typical serving size (80 g, as defined by Food and Agriculture Organization of the United Nations (FAO) and WHO [24]) that was defined using a few examples of typical household measures for fresh and processed vegetables.

The vegetable consumption behaviors and preferences of mothers were assessed as follows:

- The general frequency of consumption of vegetables—based on the answer to the open-ended question about the number of servings of raw and processed vegetables consumed by them per day (self-reported);

- The previous day's frequency of consumption of vegetables—based on the 24 h dietary recall of the mothers' vegetable intake (self-reported);
- Preferred vegetables—based on the answer to the open-ended question to list the vegetables most preferred by them (self-reported);
- Consumed vegetables—based on the 24 h dietary recall of the mothers' vegetable intake (self-reported).

The vegetable consumption behaviors and preferences of children were assessed as follows:

- The general frequency of consumption of vegetables—based on the answer to the open-ended question about the number of servings of raw and processed vegetables consumed per day by their children (reported by the mothers);
- The previous day's frequency of consumption of vegetables—based on the 24 h dietary recall of the vegetable intake of the children (reported by the mothers);
- Preferred vegetables—based on the answer to the open-ended question to list the vegetables most preferred by their children (reported by the mothers);
- Consumed vegetables—based on the 24 h dietary recall of vegetable intake by children (reported by the mothers).

During the interview, the respondents were instructed to exclude potatoes and dry pulses from the declared number of servings of consumed vegetables. In the case of the 24 h dietary recall of vegetable intake and the list of most preferred vegetables, potatoes, dry pulses, and corn were excluded during analysis if they had been included.

2.4. Statistical Analysis

The normality of the distribution was verified using the Kolmogorov–Smirnov test and, afterwards, an analysis of correlation was carried out using Spearman's rank correlation coefficient due to the non-parametric distribution. The shares of the groups were compared using the chi^2 test and afterwards the obtained results were controlled for the false discovery results (FDR) using the Benjamini–Hochberg procedure.

$P \leq 0.05$ was considered significant. Statistical analysis was conducted using the following software packages: Statgraphics Plus for Windows 5.1 (Statgraphics Technologies Inc., The Plains, VA, USA), Statistica software version 8.0 (StatSoft Inc., Tulsa, OK, USA), and the Benjamini–Hochberg procedure spreadsheet by McDonalds [25].

3. Results

3.1. Analysis of the Association between the Quantity of Vegetables Consumed and Preferred by Mothers and Their Children

An analysis of the correlation between the daily frequency of vegetable consumption of the mothers and their children in nationally representative samples of Polish and Romanian mother–child pairs is presented in Table 1.

Table 1. Analysis of the correlation between the daily frequency of vegetables consumption of mothers and of their children in nationally representative samples of Polish ($n = 1200$) and Romanian ($n = 1157$) mother–child pairs.

Analyzed Correlation		*p*-Value [a]	R
Polish mother–child pairs ($n = 1200$)	general daily frequency	<0.0001	0.6522
	previous day frequency	<0.0001	0.4172
Romanian mother–child pairs ($n = 1157$)	general daily frequency	<0.0001	0.6573
	previous day frequency	<0.0001	0.3897

[a] Spearman's rank correlation coefficient.

The median for the open-ended question about general number of servings of vegetables consumed by mothers in both Polish and Romanian samples was two servings a day, and it ranged from not consuming at all to five servings a day. Similarly, for their children it was also two servings a day, and it ranged from not consuming at all (for the Polish sample) or consuming less than once a week (for the Romanian sample) to five servings a day. For both the Polish and Romanian samples, a significant correlation was observed between the number of servings consumed in general by the mothers and their children ($p < 0.0001$; $R = 0.6522$ for the Polish sample, $R = 0.6573$ for the Romanian sample).

In order to verify the association, the number of servings of vegetables consumed the previous day was analyzed, based on a 24 h dietary recall of vegetable consumption. The median for the number of servings of vegetables consumed the previous day for both mothers and their children in both Polish and Romanian samples was four servings a day, and it varied from not consuming at all to five servings a day. For both Polish and Romanian samples, a significant correlation was observed between the number of servings consumed the previous day by the mothers and their children ($p < 0.0001$; $R = 0.4172$ for the Polish sample, $R = 0.3897$ for the Romanian sample).

An analysis of the correlation between the number of types of vegetables indicated as consumed and preferred by mothers and their children in nationally representative samples of Polish and Romanian mother–child pairs is presented in Table 2.

Table 2. Analysis of the correlation between the number of types of vegetables indicated as consumed and preferred by mothers and by their children in nationally representative samples of Polish ($n = 1200$) and Romanian ($n = 1157$) mother–child pairs.

Analyzed Correlation		*p*-Value [a]	*R*
Polish mother–child pairs ($n = 1200$)	number of vegetables indicated as consumed	<0.0001	0.5418
	number of vegetables indicated as preferred	<0.0001	0.2872
Romanian mother–child pairs ($n = 1157$)	number of vegetables indicated as consumed	<0.0001	0.5433
	number of vegetables indicated as preferred	<0.0001	0.3878

[a] Spearman's rank correlation coefficient.

The median for the general number of types of vegetables indicated as consumed by the mothers in both Polish and Romanian samples was two, and it varied from a lack of types consumed to nine types. Similarly, for the children it was also two types, and it varied from a lack of types consumed to seven types (for the Polish sample) or nine types (for the Romanian sample). For both the Polish and Romanian samples, a significant correlation was observed between the number of types of vegetables indicated as consumed by mothers and their children ($p < 0.0001$; $R = 0.5418$ for the Polish sample, $R = 0.5433$ for the Romanian sample).

The median for the general number of types of vegetables indicated as preferred for both mothers and children in the Polish sample was three, and it ranged from a lack of types preferred to 19 types (for mothers) or 17 types (for children). The median for the general number of types of vegetables indicated as preferred for both mothers and children in the Romanian sample was two, and it ranged from a lack of types preferred to 17 types (for mothers) or 15 types (for children). For both the Polish and Romanian samples, a significant correlation was observed between the number of types of vegetables indicated as preferred by mothers and children ($p < 0.0001$; $R = 0.2772$ for the Polish sample, R = 0.3878 for the Romanian sample).

3.2. Analysis of the Association between the Variety of Vegetables Consumed and Preferred by Mothers and Their Children

An analysis of the association between the vegetable consumption behaviors self-reported by mothers and reported by them for their children in a nationally representative sample of Polish mother–child pairs is presented in Table 3. For all the vegetables that were declared by the mothers as consumed, there was a statistically significant association ($p < 0.0001$ for chi^2 test; $p < 0.0001$ after controlling for the FDR using a Benjamini–Hochberg procedure)—types consumed by the mothers were also consumed by their children, as compared to types not consumed by the mothers. For the specific types consumed by the mothers, the consumption by the children ranged from 33.1% (for peppers) to 75.3% (for carrots), while for types not consumed by the mothers, the consumption by the children ranged from 0.1% (for eggplant) to 43.2% (for tomatoes).

Table 3. Analysis of the association between the vegetable consumption behaviors self-reported by the mothers and reported by them for their children in a nationally representative sample of Polish mother–child pairs ($n = 1200$).

Vegetable [a]	Mothers Consuming the Specified Vegetable [b]		Mothers not Consuming the Specified Vegetable [b]		*p*-Value [c]
	Reporting their Children as also Consuming	Reporting their Children as not Consuming	Reporting their Children as Consuming	Reporting their Children as also not Consuming	
Carrot ($n = 592; n = 608$)	446 (75.3%)	146 (24.7%)	141 (23.2%)	467 (76.8%)	<0.0001
Tomato ($n = 393; n = 807$)	231 (58.8%)	162 (41.2%)	349 (43.2%)	458 (56.8%)	<0.0001
Cucumber ($n = 325; n = 875$)	196 (60.3%)	129 (39.7%)	330 (37.7%)	545 (62.3%)	<0.0001
Cabbage ($n = 167; n = 1033$)	90 (53.9%)	77 (46.1%)	64 (6.2%)	969 (93.8%)	<0.0001
Pepper ($n = 133; n = 1067$)	44 (33.1%)	89 (66.9%)	32 (3.0%)	1035 (97.0%)	<0.0001
Lettuce ($n = 120; n = 1080$)	48 (40.0%)	72 (60.0%)	48 (4.4%)	1032 (95.6%)	<0.0001
Celery ($n = 103; n = 1097$)	40 (38.8%)	63 (61.2%)	25 (2.3%)	1072 (97.7%)	<0.0001
Beetroot ($n = 103; n = 1097$)	73 (70.9%)	30 (29.1%)	52 (4.7%)	1045 (95.3%)	<0.0001
Onion ($n = 97; n = 1103$)	47 (48.5%)	50 (51.5%)	34 (3.1%)	1069 (96.9%)	<0.0001
Broccoli ($n = 88; n = 1112$)	38 (43.2%)	50 (56.8%)	16 (1.4%)	1096 (98.6%)	<0.0001
Cauliflower ($n = 66; n = 1134$)	34 (51.5%)	32 (48.5%)	32 (2.8%)	1102 (97.2%)	<0.0001
Chinese cabbage ($n = 45; n = 1155$)	20 (44.4%)	25 (55.6%)	15 (1.3%)	1140 (98.7%)	<0.0001
Green peas ($n = 38; n = 1162$)	18 (47.4%)	20 (52.6%)	19 (1.6%)	1143 (98.4%)	<0.0001
Beans ($n = 27; n = 1173$)	11 (40.7%)	16 (59.3%)	12 (1%)	1161 (99%)	<0.0001
Zucchini ($n = 23; n = 1177$)	13 (56.5%)	10 (43.5%)	2 (0.2%)	1175 (99.8%)	<0.0001
Eggplant ($n = 5; n = 1195$)	3 (60.0%)	2 (40.0%)	1 (0.1%)	1194 (99.9%)	<0.0001

[a] the number of mothers consuming the specific vegetable, followed by the number of mothers non-consuming the specific vegetable; [b] assessed based on the previous day's vegetable consumption behaviors; [c] chi^2 test.

An analysis of the association between the vegetable consumption behaviors self-reported by the mothers and reported by them for their children in a nationally representative sample of Romanian mother–child pairs is presented in Table 4. There was a statistically significant association ($p < 0.0001$ for chi^2 test; $p < 0.0001$ after controlling for the FDR using a Benjamini–Hochberg procedure) for all vegetables that were declared by the mothers as consumed—types consumed by the mothers were also consumed by their children, as compared to types not consumed by the mothers. For the types consumed by the mothers, the consumption by the children ranged from 42.6% (for eggplant) to 75.7% (for carrots), while for types not consumed by the mothers, the consumption by the children ranged from 1.2% (for broccoli) to 22.9% (for carrots).

Table 4. Analysis of the association between the vegetable consumption behaviors self-reported by the mothers and reported by them for their children, in a nationally representative sample of Romanian mother–child pairs ($n = 1157$).

Vegetable [a]	Mothers Consuming the Specified Vegetable [b]		Mothers not Consuming the Specified Vegetable [b]		p-Value [c]
	Reporting their Children as also Consuming	Reporting their Children as not Consuming	Reporting their Children as Consuming	Reporting their Children as also not Consuming	
Carrot ($n = 568$; $n = 589$)	430 (75.7%)	138 (24.3%)	135 (22.9%)	454 (77.1%)	<0.0001
Pepper ($n = 429$; $n = 728$)	254 (59.2%)	175 (40.8%)	102 (14.0%)	626 (86.0%)	<0.0001
Tomato ($n = 406$; $n = 751$)	243 (59.9%)	163 (40.1%)	93 (12.4%)	658 (87.6%)	<0.0001
Onion ($n = 324$; $n = 833$)	177 (54.6%)	147 (45.4%)	73 (8.8%)	760 (91.2%)	<0.0001
Cucumber ($n = 200$; $n = 957$)	116 (58.0%)	84 (42.0%)	81 (8.5%)	876 (91.5%)	<0.0001
Celery ($n = 191$; $n = 966$)	104 (54.5%)	87 (45.5%)	60 (6.2%)	906 (93.8%)	<0.0001
Cabbage ($n = 103$; $n = 1054$)	56 (54.4%)	47 (45.6%)	44 (4.2%)	1010 (95.8%)	<0.0001
Beans ($n = 91$; $n = 1066$)	44 (48.4%)	47 (51.6%)	26 (2.4%)	1040 (97.6%)	<0.0001
Green peas ($n = 63$; $n = 1094$)	42 (66.7%)	21 (33.3%)	27 (2.5%)	1067 (97.5%)	<0.0001
Eggplant ($n = 61$; $n = 1096$)	26 (42.6%)	35 (57.4%)	17 (1.6%)	1079 (98.4%)	<0.0001
Zucchini ($n = 49$; $n = 1108$)	23 (46.9%)	26 (53.1%)	27 (2.4%)	1081 (97.6%)	<0.0001
Lettuce ($n = 51$; $n = 1106$)	18 (35.3%)	33 (64.7%)	20 (1.8%)	1086 (98.2%)	<0.0001
Cauliflower ($n = 35$; $n = 1122$)	16 (45.7%)	19 (54.3%)	16 (1.4%)	1106 (98.6%)	<0.0001
Broccoli ($n = 27$; $n = 1130$)	17 (63.0%)	10 (37.0%)	13 (1.2%)	1117 (98.8%)	<0.0001
Beetroot ($n = 22$; $n = 1135$)	15 (68.2%)	7 (31.8%)	17 (1.5%)	1118 (98.5%)	<0.0001

[a] the number of mothers consuming the specific vegetable followed by the number of mothers non-consuming the specific vegetable; [b] assessed based on the previous day's vegetable consumption behaviors; [c] chi^2 test.

An analysis of the association between the vegetable preferences self-reported by the mothers and reported by them for their children in a nationally representative sample of Polish mother-child pairs is presented in Table 5. There was a statistically significant association ($p < 0.002$ for chi^2 test; $p < 0.002$ after controlling for the FDR using a Benjamini-Hochberg procedure) for all vegetables that were declared by the mothers as preferred—types preferred by the mothers were also preferred by their children, as compared to types not preferred by the mothers. For specific types preferred by the mothers, children's preferences varied from 16.7% (for eggplant) to 74.1% (for carrots), while for types not preferred by the mothers, children's preferences ranged from 1.3% (for eggplant) to 46.9% (for carrots).

Table 5. Analysis of the association between the vegetable preferences self-reported by the mothers and reported by them for their children in a national representative sample of Polish mother–child pairs ($n = 1200$).

Vegetable [a]	Mothers Indicating the Specified Vegetable as the Most Preferred		Mothers not Indicating the Specified Vegetable as the Most Preferred		*p*-Value [b]
	Reporting their Children as also Preferring	Reporting their Children as not Preferring	Reporting their Children as Preferring	Reporting their Children as also not Preferring	
Carrot ($n = 665; n = 535$)	493 (74.1%)	172 (25.9%)	251 (46.9%)	284 (53.1%)	<0.0001
Tomato ($n = 576; n = 624$)	342 (59.4%)	234 (40.6%)	222 (35.6%)	402 (64.4%)	<0.0001
Cucumber ($n = 433; n = 767$)	313 (72.3%)	120 (27.7%)	345 (45.0%)	422 (55.0%)	<0.0001
Broccoli ($n = 279; n = 921$)	97 (34.8%)	182 (65.2%)	112 (12.2%)	809 (87.8%)	<0.0001
Cauliflower ($n = 269; n = 931$)	123 (45.7%)	146 (54.3%)	192 (20.6%)	739 (79.4%)	<0.0001
Beetroot ($n = 205; n = 995$)	88 (42.9%)	117 (57.1%)	236 (23.7%)	759 (76.3%)	<0.0001
Cabbage ($n = 191; n = 1009$)	71 (37.2%)	120 (62.8%)	154 (15.3%)	855 (84.7%)	<0.0001
Lettuce ($n = 181; n = 1010$)	58 (32.0%)	123 (68%)	166 (16.3%)	853 (83.7%)	<0.0001
Pepper ($n = 153; n = 1047$)	56 (36.6%)	97 (63.4%)	143 (13.7%)	904 (86.3%)	<0.0001
Beans ($n = 92; n = 1108$)	41 (44.6%)	51 (55.4%)	133 (12.0%)	975 (88.0%)	<0.0001
Chinese cabbage ($n = 77; n = 1123$)	21 (27.3%)	56 (72.7%)	147 (13.1%)	976 (86.9%)	0.0010
Celery ($n = 77; n = 1123$)	15 (19.5%)	62 (80.5%)	48 (4.3%)	1075 (95.7%)	<0.0001
Onion ($n = 71; n = 1129$)	14 (19.7%)	57 (80.3%)	79 (7.0%)	1050 (93.0%)	0.0003
Zucchini ($n = 62; n = 1138$)	12 (19.4%)	50 (80.6%)	86 (7.6%)	1052 (92.4%)	0.0022
Green peas ($n = 48; n = 1152$)	21 (43.8%)	27 (56.3%)	146 (12.7%)	1006 (87.3%)	<0.0001
Eggplant ($n = 24; n = 1176$)	4 (16.7%)	20 (83.3%)	15 (1.3%)	1161 (98.7%)	<0.0001

[a] the number of mothers preferring the specific vegetable followed by the number of mothers non-preferring the specific vegetable; [b] chi^2 test.

An analysis of the association between vegetable preferences self-reported by the mothers and reported by them for their children in a nationally representative sample of Romanian mother–child pairs is presented in Table 6. There was a statistically significant association ($p < 0.0001$ for chi^2 test; $p < 0.0001$ after controlling for the FDR using a Benjamini–Hochberg procedure) for all vegetables that were declared by the mothers as preferred—types preferred by the mothers were also preferred by their children as compared to types not preferred by the mothers. For specific types preferred by the mothers, children's preferences varied from 15.2% (for cauliflower) to 100.0% (for Chinese cabbage), while for types not preferred by the mothers, children's preferences ranged from 0.0% (for Chinese cabbage) to 38.3% (for carrot).

Table 6. Analysis of the association between the vegetable preferences self-reported by the mothers and reported by them for their children in a nationally representative sample of Romanian mother–child pairs (n = 1157).

Vegetable [a]	Mothers Indicating the Specified Vegetable as the Most Preferred		Mothers not Indicating the Specified Vegetable as the Most Preferred		p-Value [b]
	Reporting their Children as also Preferring	Reporting their Children as not Preferring	Reporting their Children as Preferring	Reporting their Children as also not Preferring	
Tomato (n = 571; n = 586)	289 (50.6%)	282 (49.4%)	108 (18.4%)	478 (81.6%)	<0.0001
Carrot (n = 447; n = 710)	328 (73.4%)	119 (26.6%)	272 (38.3%)	438 (61.7%)	<0.0001
Pepper (n = 378; n = 779)	136 (36.0%)	242 (64.0%)	111 (14.2%)	668 (85.8%)	<0.0001
Cucumber (n = 341; n = 816)	191 (56.0%)	150 (44.0%)	184 (22.5%)	632 (77.5%)	<0.0001
Cabbage (n = 157; n = 1000)	60 (38.2%)	97 (61.8%)	81 (8.1%)	919 (91.9%)	<0.0001
Eggplant (n = 140; n = 1017)	32 (22.9%)	108 (77.1%)	34 (3.3%)	983 (96.7%)	<0.0001
Onion (n = 130; n = 1027)	30 (23.1%)	100 (76.9%)	43 (4.2%)	984 (95.8%)	<0.0001
Cauliflower (n = 105; n = 1052)	16 (15.2%)	89 (84.8%)	29 (2.8%)	1023 (97.2%)	<0.0001
Beans (n = 91; n = 1066)	24 (26.4%)	67 (73.6%)	32 (3%)	1034 (97%)	<0.0001
Lettuce (n = 87; n = 1070)	17 (19.5%)	70 (80.5%)	25 (2.3%)	1045 (97.7%)	<0.0001
Celery (n = 87; n = 1070)	14 (16.1%)	73 (83.9%)	14 (1.3%)	1056 (98.7%)	<0.0001
Green peas (n = 69; n = 1088)	24 (34.8%)	45 (65.2%)	33 (3%)	1055 (97%)	<0.0001
Zucchini (n = 64; n = 1093)	20 (31.3%)	44 (68.8%)	23 (2.1%)	1070 (97.9%)	<0.0001
Broccoli (n = 63; n = 1094)	20 (31.7%)	43 (68.3%)	14 (1.3%)	1080 (98.7%)	<0.0001
Beetroot (n = 35; n = 1122)	7 (20.0%)	28 (80.0%)	16 (1.4%)	1106 (98.6%)	<0.0001
Chinese cabbage (n = 1; n = 1156)	1 (100.0%)	0 (0.0%)	0 (0.0%)	1156 (100.0%)	<0.0001

[a] the number of mothers preferring the specific vegetable followed by the number of mothers non-preferring the specific vegetable; [b] chi^2 test.

4. Discussion

The strong associations between vegetable consumption preferences and behaviors of mothers and their children were observed both for Polish and Romanian samples. Moreover, they were observed both for assessed quantity and variety of vegetables consumed. This corresponds with the previously observed associations for fruit consumption preferences and behaviors [20], in spite of the fact that for children, fruit and vegetable preferences and exposure commonly differ [26]. As indicated by Korinek et al. [26], this is associated with children's preference for the sweet taste and pleasant texture of fruits, and because of this, parents offer them fruits rather than vegetables, resulting in not only a higher amount, but also a wider variety of consumed fruits as compared to vegetables.

It is stated that repeated exposure may change the preferences, but this is more effective for fruits than vegetables [27]. Moreover, other stimuli are also more effective in increasing the intake of fruits than vegetables [28]. As a result, when comparing vegetables and fruits it may be said that, for children, fruits are not only more preferred over vegetables and a higher amount and variety is consumed, but they are also more frequently offered by parents and their intake is also easier to adopt. So, in order to assess the intake of vegetables, two domains must be analyzed—not only the consumption behaviors, but also consumption preferences, as they may be crucial for correcting nutritional behaviors.

Despite the fact that changing the preferences of vegetables may be more difficult than for fruits, it is still possible, as was proven in a number of intervention studies [29–32]. All the indicated above studies [29–32] allow us to conclude that, for children, it is possible to increase not only vegetable consumption but also preferences for the disliked ones when the exposure is applied at home. This is also confirmed by Cooke's [33] review, which showed that both laboratory studies and interventions conducted so far for assessing the efficacy of exposure confirmed that opportunities to taste unfamiliar food products results in increased consumption and preferences. However, no national-scale studies have been conducted so far, in Poland or Romania, to analyze the association between vegetable consumption behaviors and preferences of mothers and of their children. Such observations would give broader perspective, not only to make a conclusion based on small studies of various stimuli to increase vegetable intake, but also to observe associations in real conditions.

The results of our own study indicate a significant barrier for increasing vegetable exposure at home, as the vegetable consumption behaviors of mothers determine the consumption behaviors of their children. A similar association was observed for vegetable preferences. It may be concluded that, in spite of a number of studies having proven the possibility of increasing the consumption of vegetables, our own study indicates that if mother does not like a vegetable and does not consume it, the exposure of her child to this vegetable does not exist, and this, consequently, results in lack of preference in her child.

Johnson et al. [34] classified the determinants of the size of the serving consumed by a child into child-centered (including individual preferences and general consumption behaviors of the child as well as the previous meals) and mother-centered (including their opinions about the nutritional value of products and the need to avoid wastage of money and time). Such mother-centered determinants are associated not only with child's feeding and cooking for family members but also with her individual diet, and are observed by the child during the process of learning preferences at home [35]. However, for feeding a child there are additional factors, such as maternal feeding self-efficacy, that influence the kind and amount of products offered to the child and the child's final eating behaviors [36].

The association between eating behaviors of mothers and their children that was observed in the conducted study is confirmed by the results of another Polish study, as a similar strong association between eating behaviors of mothers and their adolescent daughters was observed [37], and it also contributed to similar excessive body mass risk [38] and similarities in other health-related consequences [39]. This may be important, as an excessive body mass of children was commonly observed in a recent study of Polish adolescents [40]. However, a mother may also transfer her dislikes to her child and create their preferences similar to her own [41]. This may be associated with the fact that children mimic their parents in a number of behaviors, including nutritional ones [42].

Parents commonly declare that food product preferences of their children are influenced by the marketing of food, and some of them state that they make choices of food products available at home based on those preferences [43]. However, the availability of unhealthy food products at home is associated with the children's choice of such products and the consumption of such products [44], and so if a child prefers unhealthy food products and the mother provides it, the child will consume it. At the same time, a number of parents believe that they provide such products to overcome the negative food product preferences of their children and promote a healthy diet [45]. But the question is, are they really are able to do it if their own preferences set in. A systematic review by Pearson et al. [46] indicated that vegetable and fruit consumption of children is associated not only with at home accessibility, family rules, and parental encouragement, but also with parental intake, and so parents may promote a healthy diet not by just providing it to their children but only if they also have such a diet.

The choice of food products and purchase decisions are influenced by a number of factors, including those related to health [47], nutritional knowledge [48], and the place where the product is purchased [49], but convenience and preferences may be the crucial ones [50]. This was confirmed by the results of a study by Horning et al. [51], where it was observed that the common reasons for choosing pre-packed processed meals instead of non-processed ones are preferences and time. So, even if parents declare that they want to promote healthy food decisions by their children through their own choices, other factors may interfere.

In general, when a child asks the parent for a specific vegetable or fruit, they tend to comply with this request [52]. But for children aged 2–5 years, it was observed that food product choices based on their desire may decrease their preference for healthy food products, including vegetables, as they would rather ask about products other than vegetables [53]. As a result, parents cannot wait for their child to ask for a specific product but should provide at home accessibility. Moreover, in order to provide effective exposure, parents should not only purchase vegetables but also include them in their own diet, in order to influence their child through the role-modeling mechanism, in addition to healthy products being provided in schools and childcare institutions.

In spite of the fact that the presented study was conducted in the nationally representative samples of Polish and Romanian respondents, some limitations must be indicated. The main limitations are associated with the proxy-reporting, due to the fact that the consumption preferences and behaviors of children were declared by their mothers. Moreover, there were the different participation rates in the Polish and Romanian samples, with some missing data in the Romanian sample. It must also be indicated that the mother was able to arbitrarily choose which of her children to discuss, with no randomization. Moreover, the 24 h dietary recall of vegetable consumption turned out to be a tool that over reported the intake, so results of general declared intake rather than the previous day's intake should be taken into account. All the indicated issues may result in some bias and must be taken into account in the further studies.

5. Conclusions

In Polish and Romanian representative samples of mother–child pairs, it was observed that vegetable consumption preferences and behaviors of mothers and their children were associated, both for the quantity and variety of consumed vegetables. A mother's lack of preference for specific vegetables may cause a lack of at-home accessibility (namely, lack of exposure for their children) and a resultant lack of preference of their children. In order to increase the vegetable intake in a child's diet, effective exposure should be provided, not only by purchasing the products and by at home accessibility (exposure), but also by including them in the diet of parents (role-modeling).

Author Contributions: B.G. and D.G. (Dominika Głąbska) made study conception and design; B.G. performed the research; B.G., D.G. (Dominika Głąbska) and D.G. (Dominika Guzek) analyzed the data; B.G., D.G. (Dominika Głąbska) and D.G. (Dominika Guzek) interpreted the data; B.G., D.G. (Dominika Głąbska), K.G. and D.G. (Dominika Guzek) wrote the paper. All authors read and approved the final manuscript.

Funding: The data gathering was financed by the National Polish Promotion Fund for Fruits and Vegetables Consumption and Polish Association of Juices Producers within funds of the 5xVFJ (5 Portions of Vegetables, Fruit or Juice) national Polish campaign (Project of Agricultural Market Agency, no. PP/004/004/PP-1767/W/2011 financed within the Common Agricultural Policy (CAP), action: Support of promotion and information actions for agricultural products).

Acknowledgments: Nothing to declare.

Conflicts of Interest: The authors declare no conflict of interest. The funders had no role in the design of the study; in the collection, analyses, or interpretation of data; in the writing of the manuscript, or in the decision to publish the results.

References

1. World Health Organization (WHO). *Increasing Fruit and Vegetable Consumption to Reduce the Risk of Noncommunicable Diseases*; WHO: Geneva, Switzerland, 2014.
2. Albani, V.; Butler, L.T.; Traill, W.B.; Kennedy, O.B. Fruit and vegetable intake: Change with age across childhood and adolescence. *Br. J. Nutr.* **2017**, *117*, 759–765. [CrossRef] [PubMed]
3. World Health Organization (WHO). *Fruit and Vegetable Promotion Initiative—A Meeting Report*; WHO: Geneva, Switzerland, 2003.

4. Touyz, L.M.; Wakefield, C.E.; Grech, A.M.; Quinn, V.F.; Costa, D.S.J.; Zhang, F.F.; Cohn, R.J.; Sajeev, M.; Cohen, J. Parent-targeted home-based interventions for increasing fruit and vegetable intake in children: A systematic review and meta-analysis. *Nutr. Rev.* **2018**, *76*, 154–173. [CrossRef] [PubMed]

5. Pem, D.; Jeewon, R. Fruit and Vegetable Intake: Benefits and Progress of Nutrition Education Interventions-Narrative Review Article. *Iran. J. Public Health* **2015**, *44*, 1309–1321. [PubMed]

6. Hodder, R.K.; O'Brien, K.M.; Stacey, F.G.; Wyse, R.J.; Clinton-McHarg, T.; Tzelepis, F.; James, E.L.; Bartlem, K.M.; Nathan, N.K.; Sutherland, R.; et al. Interventions for increasing fruit and vegetable consumption in children aged five years and under. *Cochrane Database Sys. Rev.* **2018**, *5*, sCD008552. [CrossRef]

7. Vereecken, C.; Pedersen, T.P.; Ojala, K.; Krølner, R.; Dzielska, A.; Ahluwalia, N.; Giacchi, M.; Kelly, C. Fruit and vegetable consumption trends among adolescents from 2002 to 2010 in 33 countries. *Eur. J. Public Health* **2015**, *25*, 16–19. [CrossRef] [PubMed]

8. Roberts, C. Chapter 7: Fruit and vegetable consumption. In *Health Survey for England 2013*, 1st ed.; Craig, R., Mindell, J., Eds.; NHS Digital: Leeds, UK, 2013. Available online: http://content.digital.nhs.uk/catalogue/PUB16076/HSE2013-Ch7-fru-veg-com.pdf (accessed on 1 March 2019).

9. Rasmussen, M.; Krølner, R.; Klepp, K.I.; Lytle, L.; Brug, J.; Bere, E.; Due, P. Determinants of fruit and vegetable consumption among children and adolescents: A review of the literature. Part I: Quantitative studies. *Int. J. Behav. Nutr. Phys. Act.* **2006**, *3*, 22. [CrossRef] [PubMed]

10. Krølner, R.; Rasmussen, M.; Brug, J.; Klepp, K.I.; Wind, M.; Due, P. Determinants of fruit and vegetable consumption among children and adolescents: A review of the literature. Part II: Qualitative studies. *Int. J. Behav. Nutr. Phys. Act.* **2011**, *8*, 112. [CrossRef]

11. Lautenschlager, L.; Smith, C. Beliefs, knowledge, and values held by inner-city youth about gardening, nutrition, and cooking. *Agric. Hum. Values* **2007**, *24*, 245–258. [CrossRef]

12. Thurber, K.A.; Banwell, C.; Neeman, T.; Dobbins, T.; Pescud, M.; Lovett, R.; Banks, E. Understanding barriers to fruit and vegetable intake in the Australian Longitudinal Study of Indigenous Children: A mixed-methods approach. *Public Health Nutr.* **2016**, *20*, 832–847. [CrossRef]

13. Ard, J.D.; Fitzpatrick, S.; Desmond, R.A.; Sutton, B.S.; Pisu, M.; Allison, D.B.; Franklin, F.; Baskin, M.L. The impact of cost on the availability of fruits and vegetables in the homes of schoolchildren in Birmingham, Alabama. *Am. J. Public Health* **2007**, *97*, 367–372. [CrossRef]

14. Zeinstra, G.G.; Koelen, M.A.; Kok, F.J.; de Graaf, C. Cognitive development and children's perceptions of fruit and vegetables; a qualitative study. *Int. J. Behav. Nutr. Phys. Act.* **2007**, *4*, 30. [CrossRef]

15. Draxten, M.; Fulkerson, J.A.; Friend, S.; Flattum, C.F.; Schow, R. Parental role modeling of fruits and vegetables at meals and snacks is associated with children's adequate consumption. *Appetite* **2014**, *78*, 1–7. [CrossRef]

16. Guzek, D.; Głąbska, D.; Lange, E.; Jezewska-Zychowicz, M. A Polish Study on the Influence of Food Neophobia in Children (10–12 Years Old) on the Intake of Vegetables and Fruits. *Nutrients* **2017**, *9*, 563. [CrossRef]

17. Scaglioni, S.; De Cosmi, V.; Ciappolino, V.; Parazzini, F.; Brambilla, P.; Agostoni, C. Factors Influencing Children's Eating Behaviours. *Nutrients* **2018**, *10*, 706. [CrossRef]

18. Yee, A.Z.; Lwin, M.O.; Ho, S.S. The influence of parental practices on child promotive and preventive food consumption behaviors: A systematic review and meta-analysis. *Int. J. Behav. Nutr. Phys. Act.* **2017**, *14*, 47. [CrossRef]

19. Hingle, M.; Beltran, A.; O'Connor, T.; Thompson, D.; Baranowski, J.; Baranowski, T. A model of goal directed vegetable parenting practices. *Appetite* **2011**, *58*, 444–449. [CrossRef]

20. Groele, B.; Głąbska, D.; Gutkowska, K.; Guzek, D. Mother's Fruit Preferences and Consumption Support Similar Attitudes and Behaviors in Their Children. *Int. J. Environ. Res. Public Health* **2018**, *15*, 2833. [CrossRef]

21. Cheff, R.; Roche, B. *Considerations for Compensating Research Participants Fairly & Equitably*; Wellesley Institute: Toronto, ON, Canada, 2018; pp. 1–11.

22. Livingstone, M.B.; Robson, P.J. Measurement of dietary intake in children. *Proc. Nutr. Soc.* **2000**, *59*, 279–293. [CrossRef]

23. Oliveria, S.A.; Ellison, R.C.; Moore, L.L.; Gillman, M.W.; Garrahie, E.J.; Singer, M.R. Parent-child relationships in nutrient intake: The Framingham Children's Study. *Am. J. Clin. Nutr.* **1992**, *56*, 593–598. [CrossRef]

24. World Health Organization (WHO). *Diet, Nutrition and the Prevention of Chronic Diseases*; Report of a Joint FAO/WHO Expert Consultation; Technical Report Series, No. 916; WHO: Geneva, Switzerland, 2003.
25. McDonald, J.H. *Handbook of Biological Statistics*, 3rd ed.; Sparky House Publishing: Baltimore, MD, USA, 2014; pp. 254–260.
26. Korinek, E.V.; Bartholomew, J.B.; Jowers, E.M.; Latimer, L.A. Fruit and vegetable exposure in children is linked to the selection of a wider variety of healthy foods at school. *Mater. Child. Nutr.* **2013**, *11*, 999–1010. [CrossRef]
27. Chung, L.M.Y.; Fong, S.S.M. Appearance alteration of fruits and vegetables to increase their appeal to and consumption by school-age children: A pilot study. *Health Psychol. Open* **2018**, *5*. [CrossRef]
28. Guzek, D.; Głąbska, D.; Mellová, B.; Zadka, K.; Żywczyk, K.; Gutkowska, K. Influence of Food Neophobia Level on Fruit and Vegetable Intake and Its Association with Urban Area of Residence and Physical Activity in a Nationwide Case-Control Study of Polish Adolescents. *Nutrients* **2018**, *10*, 897. [CrossRef]
29. Fildes, A.; van Jaarsveld, C.H.; Wardle, J.; Cooke, L. Parent-administered exposure to increase children's vegetable acceptance: A randomized controlled trial. *J. Acad. Nutr. Diet.* **2014**, *114*, 881–888. [CrossRef]
30. Remington, A.; Añez, E.; Croker, H.; Wardle, J.; Cooke, L. Increasing food acceptance in the home setting: A randomized controlled trial of parent-administered taste exposure with incentives. *Am. J. Clin. Nutr.* **2012**, *95*, 72–77. [CrossRef]
31. Holley, C.E.; Haycraft, E.; Farrow, C. 'Why don't you try it again?' A comparison of parent led, home based interventions aimed at increasing children's consumption of a disliked vegetable. *Appetite* **2015**, *87*, 215–222. [CrossRef] [PubMed]
32. Corsini, N.; Slater, A.; Harrison, A.; Cooke, L.; Cox, D.N. Rewards can be used effectively with repeated exposure to increase liking of vegetables in 4–6-year-old children. *Public Health Nutr.* **2013**, *16*, 942–951. [CrossRef]
33. Cooke, L. The importance of exposure for healthy eating in childhood: A review. *J. Hum. Nutr. Diet.* **2007**, *20*, 294–301. [CrossRef]
34. Johnson, S.L.; Goodell, L.S.; Williams, K.; Power, T.G.; Hughes, S.O. Getting my child to eat the right amount. Mothers' considerations when deciding how much food to offer their child at a meal. *Appetite* **2015**, *88*, 24–32. [CrossRef] [PubMed]
35. Savage, J.S.; Fisher, J.O.; Birch, L.L. Parental influence on eating behavior: Conception to adolescence. *J. Law Med. Ethics* **2007**, *35*, 22–34. [CrossRef]
36. Koh, G.A.; Scott, J.A.; Woodman, R.J.; Kim, S.W.; Daniels, L.A.; Magarey, A.M. Maternal feeding self-efficacy and fruit and vegetable intakes in infants. Results from the SAIDI study. *Appetite* **2014**, *81*, 44–51. [CrossRef] [PubMed]
37. Wadolowska, L.; Slowinska, M.A.; Pabjan-Adach, K.; Przybylowicz, K.; Niedzwiedzka, E. The Comparison of Food Eating Models of Mothers and Their Daughters. *Pak. J. Nutr.* **2007**, *6*, 381–386. [CrossRef]
38. Wadolowska, L.; Ulewicz, N.; Sobas, K.; Wuenstel, J.W.; Slowinska, M.A.; Niedzwiedzka, E.; Czlapka-Matyasik, M. Dairy-Related Dietary Patterns, Dietary Calcium, Body Weight and Composition: A Study of Obesity in Polish Mothers and Daughters, the MODAF Project. *Nutrients* **2018**, *10*, 90. [CrossRef]
39. Sobas, K.; Wadolowska, L.; Slowinska, M.A.; Czlapka-Matyasik, M.; Wuenstel, J.; Niedzwiedzka, E. Like Mother, Like Daughter? Dietary and Non-Dietary Bone Fracture Risk Factors in Mothers and Their Daughters. *Iran. J. Public Health* **2015**, *44*, 939–952. [PubMed]
40. Głąbska, D.; Guzek, D.; Mellová, B.; Zadka, K.; Żywczyk, K.; Gutkowska, K. The National After-School Athletics Program Participation as a Tool to Reduce the Risk of Obesity in Adolescents after One Year of Intervention: A Nationwide Study. *Int. J. Environ. Res. Public Health* **2019**, *16*, 405. [CrossRef] [PubMed]
41. Osera, T.; Tsutie, S.; Kobayashi, M.; Kurihara, N. Relationship of Mothers' Food Preferences and Attitudes with Children's Preferences. *Food Nutr. Sci.* **2012**, *3*, 1–6. [CrossRef]
42. Sutherland, L.A.; Beavers, D.P.; Kupper, L.L.; Bernhardt, A.M.; Heatherton, T.; Dalton, M.A. Like parent, like child: Child food and beverage choices during role playing. *Arch. Pediatr. Adolesc. Med.* **2008**, *162*, 1063–1069. [CrossRef]
43. Campbell, K.J.; Crawford, D.A.; Hesketh, K.D. Australian parents' views on their 5–6-year-old children's food choices. *Health Promot. Int.* **2007**, *22*, 11–18. [CrossRef]

44. Campbell, K.J.; Crawford, D.A.; Salmon, J.; Carver, A.; Garnett, S.P.; Baur, L.A. Associations between the home food environment and obesity-promoting eating behaviors in adolescence. *Obesity* **2007**, *15*, 719–730. [CrossRef]

45. Nepper, M.J.; Chai, W. Parents' barriers and strategies to promote healthy eating among school-age children. *Appetite* **2016**, *103*, 157–164. [CrossRef]

46. Pearson, N.; Biddle, S.J.; Gorely, T. Family correlates of fruit and vegetable consumption in children and adolescents: A systematic review. *Public Health Nutr.* **2009**, *12*, 267–283. [CrossRef]

47. Zysk, W.; Głąbska, D.; Guzek, D. Role of Front-of-Package Gluten-Free Product Labeling in a Pair-Matched Study in Women with and without Celiac Disease on a Gluten-Free Diet. *Nutrients* **2019**, *11*, 398. [CrossRef]

48. Gutkowska, K.; Czarnecki, J.; Głąbska, D.; Guzek, D.; Batóg, A. Consumer perception of health properties and of other attributes of beef as determinants of consumption and purchase decisions. *Rocz. Panstw. Zakl. Hig.* **2018**, *69*, 413–419. [CrossRef]

49. Olewnik-Mikołajewska, A.; Guzek, D.; Głąbska, D.; Gutkowska, K. Consumer behaviors towards novel functional and convenient meat products in Poland. *J. Sens. Stud.* **2016**, *31*, 193–205. [CrossRef]

50. Castro, I.A.; Majmundar, A.; Williams, C.B.; Baquero, B. Customer Purchase Intentions and Choice in Food Retail Environments: A Scoping Review. *Int. J. Environ. Res. Public Health* **2018**, *15*, 2493. [CrossRef]

51. Horning, M.L.; Fulkerson, J.A.; Friend, S.E.; Story, M. Reasons Parents Buy Prepackaged, Processed Meals: It Is More Complicated Than "I Don't Have Time". *J. Nutr. Educ. Behav.* **2016**, *49*, 60–66. [CrossRef]

52. Beltran, A.; O'Connor, T.M.; Hughes, S.O.; Thompson, D.; Baranowski, J.; Nicklas, T.A.; Baranowski, T. Parents' Qualitative Perspectives on Child Asking for Fruit and Vegetables. *Nutrients* **2017**, *9*, 575. [CrossRef]

53. Russell, C.G.; Worsley, A.; Liem, D.G. Parents' food choice motives and their associations with children's food preferences. *Public Health Nutr.* **2015**, *18*, 1018–1027. [CrossRef] [PubMed]

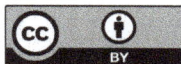

nutrients

MDPI

Article

Evaluation of the Effect of a Growing up Milk Lite vs. Cow's Milk on Diet Quality and Dietary Intakes in Early Childhood: The Growing up Milk Lite (GUMLi) Randomised Controlled Trial

Amy L. Lovell [1,*], Tania Milne [2], Yannan Jiang [3], Rachel X. Chen [3], Cameron C. Grant [4,5,6] and Clare R. Wall [1]

[1] Discipline of Nutrition and Dietetics, Faculty of Medical and Health Sciences, University of Auckland, Auckland 1142, New Zealand; c.wall@auckland.ac.nz
[2] Faculty of Medical and Health Sciences, University of Auckland, Auckland 1142, New Zealand; t.milne@auckland.ac.nz
[3] Department of Statistics, Faculty of Science, University of Auckland, Auckland 1142, New Zealand; y.jiang@auckland.ac.nz (Y.J.); rachel.chen@auckland.ac.nz (R.X.C.)
[4] Department of Paediatrics: Child and Youth Health, University of Auckland, Grafton 1023, New Zealand; cc.grant@auckland.ac.nz
[5] Centre for Longitudinal Research He Ara ki Mua, University of Auckland, Auckland 1743, New Zealand
[6] General Paediatrics, Starship Children's Hospital, Auckland District Health Board, Auckland, Auckland 1142, New Zealand
* Correspondence: a.lovell@auckland.ac.nz; Tel.: +64-9-3739785

Received: 29 December 2018; Accepted: 15 January 2019; Published: 20 January 2019

Abstract: Summary scores provide an alternative approach to measuring dietary quality. The Growing Up Milk-Lite (GUMLi) Trial was a multi-centre, double-blinded, randomised controlled trial of children randomised to receive a reduced protein GUM (GUMLi) or unfortified cow's milk (CM). In a secondary analysis of the GUMLi Trial, we used the Probability of Adequate Nutrient Intake (PANDiet) to determine the nutritional adequacy of the diets of participating children living in Auckland. The PANDiet was adapted to the New Zealand Nutrient Reference Values and data from four 24 h Recalls (24HR) collected at months 7, 8, 10, and 11 post-randomisation were used. Differences between randomised groups (GUMLi vs. CM) of the PANDiet and its components were made. Eighty-three Auckland participants were included in the study (GUMLi $n = 41$ vs. CM $n = 42$). Total PANDiet scores were significantly higher in the GUMLi group ($p < 0.001$), indicating better overall nutrient adequacy and diet quality. Dietary intakes of children in both groups met the recommendations for fat, total carbohydrates and most micronutrients; however, protein intakes exceeded recommendations. Consumption of GUMLi was associated with higher nutritional adequacy, with an increased likelihood of meeting nutrient requirements; however, the impact of the family diet and GUMLi on dietary diversity requires further evaluation.

Keywords: diet quality; PANDiet index; early childhood; nutritional adequacy; nutrient intake quality; growing up milk

1. Introduction

Early food habits, practices, and dietary patterns develop rapidly within the first two years of life [1,2]; with evidence that diet quality may decline as children age [3]. Evaluating diet quality in paediatric populations is of increasing interest, however, due to a paucity of evidence-based dietary guidelines for children under two, combining these multidimensional behaviours into a single meaningful measure remains a challenge [4].

Diet quality can be determined using nutrient, food, or food and nutrient-based indices [5]. Index scores are determined 'a priori', using dietary guidelines, recommended nutrient intakes, or current nutrition knowledge of optimal dietary patterns [6–9]. The resulting numeric representation of dietary quality or nutrient adequacy can be used as a nutritional benchmark in identifying relationships between the whole-of-diet and later health [6,7,10,11]. Nutrient-based measures of diet quality reflect adequacy of nutrient intake, however, require detailed dietary assessment, additional analyses and statistical modelling before a final score is calculated [5,6]. In contrast, food-based indices provide an indirect measure of nutrient and non-nutrient interactions, where a score is easily calculated based on awarding points for fulfilling certain criteria [5,6]. The Probability of Adequate Nutrient Intake (PANDiet) score is a complete, nutrient-based diet quality index, employing probabilistic calculations of nutrient adequacy [12]. The index has been evaluated in French [12], US [12] adult populations and a UK [13] paediatric population and has shown to be a useful tool in assessing diet quality at the population level [12].

There is limited research on the contribution of milk to the diets of children under two [14–16], specifically, whether Growing Up Milks (GUM) provide a nutritional advantage compared to standard cow's milk (CM) [17]. Simulation data have shown that replacing CM with GUM resulted in protein intakes more in line with recommendations, reduced saturated fatty acid (SFA) intake and increased likelihood of adequate intakes of vitamin D and iron [17,18]. We aimed to evaluate the dietary quality of the Auckland children participating in the GUMLi Trial aged 18- to 23-months, using an adapted PANDiet index and determine nutritional adequacy according to intervention allocation.

2. Materials and Methods

2.1. Study Design and Participants

This is a secondary analysis of data collected as part of the GUMLi trial. Briefly, the GUMLi trial was a multi-centre, double blinded, randomised controlled trial performed in Auckland, New Zealand (*n* = 108) and Brisbane, Australia (*n* = 52) from 2015 to 2017. One hundred and sixty healthy children aged one were randomised 1:1 to receive unfortified cow's milk (CM) or a reduced protein GUM (GUMLi), fortified with iron, vitamin D, pre- and probiotics (Danone Pty Ltd., Auckland, New Zealand) until the age of two. GUMLi had a reduced energy and protein content compared to commercial GUM on the market, 60 kcal/100 mL vs. 71 kcal/100 mL and 1.7 g/100 mL protein vs. 2.2 g/100 mL. An energy-matched, non-fortified cow's milk was used as an active control, with a protein content of 3.1 g/100 mL. The primary trial outcome evaluated the effect of consuming GUMLi versus unfortified CM as part of a whole diet for 12-months on body composition at two years of age [19]. Secondary outcomes included dietary intake (food frequency questionnaire or 24 h), micronutrient status, and cognitive development.

The study received ethical approval from the Health and Disability Ethics Committee of the Ministry of Health, New Zealand (14/NTB/152), and the University of Queensland Medical Research Ethics Committee, Brisbane, Australia (2014001318). The GUMLi Trial was registered with the Australian New Zealand Clinical Trials Registry, reference number: ACTRN12614000918628. Written informed consent was obtained from all participants. At month six post-randomisation, primary caregivers were invited to complete four record-assisted twenty-four-hour recalls (24 h). Of the 108 Auckland participants, 83 (77%) completed four 24 h. Four (4%) opted out of the study (but continued with the main trial), eleven (10 %) withdrew from the main trial and nine (8%) took part, but did not complete four 24 h. Only 14 (27%) participants from Brisbane completed four 24 h, therefore, the decision was made not to include them in the analysis.

2.2. Dietary Intakes

A dietitian collected dietary data over the phone using record-assisted 24HRs between months 6 to 11 post-randomisation, according to a standardised procedure [20]. Four 24 h were collected per participant on randomly allocated days (three weekdays and one weekend day). The record-assisted 24HR differed from standard 24HRs, as caregivers recoded their child's intake over the pre-defined 24-h period preceding the phone call. This methodology was used in a pilot validation study for the New Zealand Children's Nutrition Survey [21] and the Australian Children's Nutrition and Physical Activity Survey (CNPAS) [22,23]. A 'Foods fed by other adults' form, adapted from the Feeding Infants and Toddlers study (FITS) [24,25] was used to record intake if the child was in the care of another adult i.e., day-care. Use of dietary supplements, homemade recipes, and portion sizes (household measures or gram weight) were recorded. A food model booklet, reproduced with permission from CNPAS was used to assist with describing serving sizes [22,23]. Breastfeeding was recorded as time (minutes) and quantity estimated using a conversion factor of 10 mL/min, max 10 min [26,27]. All 24HR were double-checked to identify mistakes, missing foods, or clarify recipes. A dietetics student entered the data into Foodworks® (version 9, Xyris Software, Pty Ltd., Australia) and checked for completeness. Nutritional data were derived from the FOODfiles 2016 database [28] and nutritional profiles of commercial toddler foods sourced from companies or nutrient information panels.

2.3. Assessment of Nutrient Intakes with Nutrient Reference Values

Nutrient intakes were compared to the Australian and New Zealand Nutrient Reference Values (NRVs) [29]. Prevalence of inadequate intakes were assessed using the cut-off point method for nutrients with an Estimated Average Requirement (EAR) value [30]. This method has previously been shown to produce realistic estimates of the prevalence of inadequate dietary intakes [30]. The EAR, derived by the Institute of Medicine (IoM) was used for vitamin D (10 μg/day) [31].

2.4. Assessment of Diet Quality Using the PANDiet Score

The development and design of the PANDiet score has been reported in detail elsewhere [12,32]. Briefly, the PANDiet provides a measure of diet quality through the probability of having adequate nutrient intake, ranging from 0–100, where the higher the score, the better the diet quality and nutrient adequacy [12,32]. The PANDiet is an average of the Adequacy and Moderation sub-scores, which rely on the calculation of probability of adequacy for 25 nutrients and consider duration of dietary assessment, day-to-day variability, nutrient reference values, inter-variability of intake, and mean nutrient intakes [12,32]. The Adequacy sub-score calculates the probability that usual nutrient intake is above a reference value and the Moderation sub-score calculates the probability that the usual nutrient intake meets requirements and does not exceed a reference value [12,33]. Using the original methods [12], the PANDiet score calculation for protein and micronutrients was adjusted using the Australian and New Zealand NRVs and inter-variability for children one- to three years of age [29]. There are no recommendations for total fat, poly-unsaturated fatty acids (PUFA) and carbohydrate in children under two. Therefore, as seen in Verger et al. [32], we used the reference values set by the European Food Safety Authority (EFSA) [34], Nordic recommendations for SFA and non-milk extrinsic sugars (NMES) [35] and the IoM upper limit for protein [36]. The risk of excessive intakes were assessed using a penalty value system [12], using the upper limit as a reference [29] (Table S1).

Participants were classified according to their randomisation into the trial and allocation to receive GUMLi or CM. The trial analysis was conducted based on the assumption that the PANDiet index was suitable to use as an outcome measure and the difference between randomised groups, if observed, would indicate an effect of the intervention.

2.5. Statistical Analysis

A sample size of 64 participants in each arm is required to have 80% power at 5% significant level (two-sided) to detect a 0.5 SD difference in body fat percent (primary outcome) between the two arms at the end of the 12-month intervention. Statistical analyses were performed using SAS version 9.4 (SAS Institute Inc., Cary, NC, USA). Baseline characteristics were summarised by treatment group (GUMLi vs. CM) using descriptive statistics. Continuous variables were reported as mean and standard deviation (SD) and categorical variables described as frequencies and percentages. The characteristics of the Auckland sub-group included in this study (N = 83) were compared to those in the Auckland cohort who did not participate (N = 25). Chi-Square test or Fisher's Exact test were used for categorical variables, and the Kruskal-Wallis test or two-sample t-test was used for continuous variables. The impact of the intervention on energy and nutrient intakes were evaluated at each 24HR time point (month 7, 8, 10, and 11 post-randomisation), using random effect mixed models with an autoregressive covariance structure on repeated measures. The fixed effects model included participant sex, treatment group, time point and its interaction with the treatment group. Model-adjusted mean differences between nutrient intakes of both groups and 95% confidence intervals (95% CI) were reported at each time point, with associated p-values. The impact of the intervention on the overall PANDiet score, sub-scores and components using all 24 h data were evaluated using linear regression models adjusting for sex. Model-adjusted mean differences between two groups were estimated and tested. All statistical tests were two-sided with a statistical significance of $p < 0.05$. As a secondary analysis, missing data was not imputed and no adjustment for multiple comparisons were considered.

3. Results

One hundred and eight Auckland children participated in the main GUMLi trial. Of these, 83 (77%) were included in this sub-study, with no significant differences between GUMLi and CM groups for any baseline characteristics (Table 1), therefore, it was assumed that any differences in PANDiet scores would be attributed to the intervention milk. No statistical differences were observed between the Auckland participants included in the analysis (N = 83) and those excluded (N = 25), except for maternal educational attainment (80% vs. 60%; p = 0.047) (Table S2). GUMLi and CM composition are presented in Table S3. Both milks were energy-matched per 100 mL, however compared to CM, GUMLi was lower in SFA and protein, with higher carbohydrate and dietary fibre, and nutritionally significant amounts of iron and vitamin D (cholecalciferol).

Table 1. Child and maternal characteristics of the Auckland cohort (N = 83) included in the PANDiet cohort.

Baseline Demographics	Study Group Intervention (N = 41) n (%)	Control (N = 42) n (%)	p-Value *
Child's sex			0.062
Boy	19 (46)	28 (67)	
Girl	22 (54)	14 (33)	
Other children in the family			0.222
No	16 (39)	22 (52)	
Yes	25 (61)	20 (48)	
Day care attendance			0.893
No	25 (61)	25 (60)	
Yes	16 (39)	17 (40)	
Breastfed at baseline			0.415
No	27 (66)	24 (57)	
Yes	14 (34)	18 (43)	
Mother's Ethnicity			0.903
Māori	8 (20)	6 (14)	
Pacific	0 (0)	1 (2)	
Asian	3 (7)	2 (5)	
European	23 (56)	26 (62)	
Other	7 (17)	7 (17)	
Mother's Age, years (mean ± SD)	32 ± 5	32 ± 4	0.874
Mother's BMI, kgm^2 (mean ± SD)	26 ± 5	27 ± 6	0.916

Table 1. *Cont.*

Baseline Demographics	Study Group Intervention (N = 41) n (%)	Control (N = 42) n (%)	p-Value *
Mother's Highest Level of Education			0.589
No school qualifications	0(0)	0(0)	
Primary	2 (5)	0 (0)	
Secondary	5 (12)	7 (17)	
Tertiary	33 (80)	33 (79)	
Other	1 (2)	2 (5)	
Mother's Employment Status			0.082
Full-time caregiver	14 (34)	15 (36)	
Full-time paid employment	5 (12)	13 (31)	
Part-time paid employment	14 (34)	13 (31)	
Receiving a benefit	1 (2)	0 (0)	
Unemployed, no benefit	3 (7)	0 (0)	
Other	4 (10)	1 (2)	
Smoking			
Current smoking	1 (2)	1 (2)	1.000
Smoking before pregnancy	5 (12)	2 (5)	0.432
Smoking during pregnancy	1 (2)	0 (0)	0.494

* Unadjusted *p*-values, Chi-square test or Fisher's Exact test is used to test the difference between groups for categorical variables; the Kruskal-Wallis test or two-sample *t*-test is used to compare the medians/means between groups for continuous variables.

3.1. Evaluation of Nutrient Intakes

Mean (SD) daily nutrient intakes at the four 24HR time points are displayed in Table 2, according to GUMLi or CM group. For the purpose of table length, only nutrients with significant relationships at any time point are displayed. A full table is presented in Table S4. There were no differences between groups at any time point for energy, sodium, PUFA, vitamin A, vitamin B-6, folate, magnesium, and selenium. Children in the GUMLi group had significantly higher intakes of vitamin C and iron across all time points, and children in the CM group had significant higher intakes of riboflavin and potassium.

Table 2. Nutrient intake among Auckland children (N = 83) from 18 and 23 months of age (month 7–11 post randomisation) [1,2].

Nutrients	Usual Intake Values Intervention (N = 41) Mean (SD)	Control (N = 42) Mean (SD)	Adjusted Difference (95%CI)	p *
Energy (kcal)				
Month 07	1135.92 (294.19)	1122.34 (187.51)	36.61 (−93.18, 166.41)	0.579
Month 08	1114.07 (277.52)	1246.07 (378.83)	−108.96 (−238.76, 20.84)	0.100
Month 10	1128.31 (383.78)	1068.61 (291.44)	82.74 (−47.05, 212.54)	0.210
Month 11	1190.24 (288.14)	1118.93 (283.21)	94.34 (−35.45, 224.14)	0.154
Carbohydrate (g)				
Month 07	142.45 (40.53)	127.44 (36.36)	18.26 (−0.25, 36.76)	0.053
Month 08	138.50 (38.12)	144.65 (56.59)	−2.90 (−21.41, 15.61)	0.758
Month 10	138.25 (45.72)	123.41 (41.01)	18.09 (−0.42, 36.59)	0.055
Month 11	145.81 (41.01)	126.61 (43.06)	22.45 (3.94, 40.96)	0.018 *
Total fat (g)				
Month 07	38.49 (13.70)	43.91 (11.34)	−4.69 (−11.04, 1.65)	0.146
Month 08	37.76 (14.79)	46.21 (16.22)	−7.72 (−14.07, −1.37)	0.017 *
Month 10	39.53 (17.61)	40.34 (13.50)	−0.08 (−6.42, 6.27)	0.981
Month 11	43.99 (15.81)	43.75 (13.59)	0.97 (−5.38, 7.32)	0.764
Saturated fat (g)				
Month 07	18.98 (7.37)	21.16 (5.98)	−1.96 (−5.27, 1.34)	0.243
Month 08	18.11 (7.41)	22.16 (8.16)	−3.83 (−7.14, −0.53)	0.023 *
Month 10	19.46 (8.88)	19.73 (7.77)	−0.05 (−3.35, 3.26)	0.977
Month 11	20.93 (8.11)	21.00 (6.84)	0.15 (−3.16, 3.45)	0.930
NMES (g)				
Month 07	45.46 (18.22)	42.02 (17.88)	4.33 (−5.27, 13.93)	0.375
Month 08	45.90 (19.00)	49.01 (30.16)	−2.22 (−11.83, 7.38)	0.649
Month 10	40.13 (23.17)	39.00 (19.24)	2.03 (−7.58, 11.63)	0.678
Month 11	48.53 (25.02)	39.29 (21.47)	10.14 (0.54, 19.74)	0.039 *
Protein (g)				
Month 07	46.07 (17.15)	50.13 (10.13)	−3.26 (−9.65, 3.13)	0.316
Month 08	46.09 (14.01)	56.47 (17.08)	−9.58 (−15.97, −3.19)	0.004 *
Month 10	46.45 (18.34)	44.33 (12.51)	2.92 (−3.47, 9.31)	0.369
Month 11	44.59 (14.36)	47.48 (13.13)	−2.09 (−8.48, 4.30)	0.520

Table 2. *Cont.*

Nutrients	Usual Intake Values		Adjusted Difference (95%CI)	p *
	Intervention (N = 41) Mean (SD)	Control (N = 42) Mean (SD)		
Thiamin (mg)				
Month 07	1.50 (0.63)	1.19 (0.84)	0.34 (0.03, 0.64)	0.030 *
Month 08	1.54 (0.56)	1.29 (0.72)	0.28 (−0.02, 0.59)	0.069
Month 10	1.35 (0.70)	1.03 (0.82)	0.36 (0.05, 0.66)	0.022 *
Month 11	1.36 (0.68)	0.99 (0.64)	0.40 (0.10, 0.71)	0.010 *
Riboflavin (mg)				
Month 07	1.82 (0.64)	2.12 (0.64)	−0.29 (−0.56, −0.02)	0.037 *
Month 08	1.71 (0.54)	2.30 (0.77)	−0.58 (−0.85, −0.30)	<0.0001 *
Month 10	1.66 (0.50)	2.07 (0.67)	−0.39 (−0.66, −0.11)	0.006 *
Month 11	1.63 (0.61)	2.11 (0.57)	−0.47 (−0.74, −0.20)	0.001 *
Niacin (mg)				
Month 07	19.97 (7.25)	17.79 (4.64)	2.49 (−0.12, 5.09)	0.061
Month 08	20.63 (5.18)	20.09 (7.30)	0.85 (−1.75, 3.45)	0.521
Month 10	19.34 (6.64)	15.80 (5.87)	3.84 (1.24, 6.45)	0.004 *
Month 11	19.09 (5.31)	17.28 (5.39)	2.11 (−0.49, 4.71)	0.112
Vitamin B12 (µg)				
Month 07	2.36 (1.12)	2.78 (1.09)	−0.41 (−0.91, 0.09)	0.108
Month 08	2.25 (1.30)	3.17 (1.55)	−0.91 (−1.41, −0.41)	0.0004 *
Month 10	2.14 (0.94)	2.57 (0.93)	−0.42 (−0.92, 0.07)	0.095
Month 11	2.03 (0.91)	2.58 (1.15)	−0.55 (−1.05, −0.05)	0.031 *
Vitamin C (mg)				
Month 07	104.00 (44.39)	45.38 (37.36)	57.38 (35.76, 79.01)	<0.0001 *
Month 08	99.95 (39.44)	50.22 (54.71)	48.48 (26.86, 70.11)	<0.0001 *
Month 10	92.84 (34.62)	50.54 (65.97)	41.05 (19.43, 62.68)	0.0002 *
Month 11	92.51 (48.54)	58.80 (61.49)	32.47 (10.85, 54.10)	0.003 *
Vitamin D (µg)				
Month 07	6.02 (6.57)	3.23 (3.18)	2.80 (1.07, 4.53)	0.002 *
Month 08	4.73 (2.70)	3.59 (4.00)	1.16 (−0.57, 2.89)	0.188
Month 10	5.17 (2.76)	2.92 (2.49)	2.27 (0.54, 4.00)	0.011 *
Month 11	4.86 (3.44)	3.73 (4.75)	1.15 (−0.58, 2.88)	0.194
Calcium (mg)				
Month 07	901.26 (268.15)	898.06 (287.37)	8.15 (−113.76, 130.06)	0.895
Month 08	808.31 (257.94)	943.49 (314.09)	−130.24 (−252.15, −8.33)	0.036 *
Month 10	899.34 (284.54)	836.03 (251.58)	68.25 (−53.65, 190.16)	0.271
Month 11	830.41 (284.29)	891.05 (280.79)	−55.70 (−177.60, 66.21)	0.369
Zinc (mg)				
Month 07	6.75 (2.76)	6.11 (1.51)	0.71 (−0.22, 1.64)	0.133
Month 08	6.64 (2.24)	6.85 (2.65)	−0.13 (−1.07, 0.80)	0.776
Month 10	6.44 (2.45)	5.37 (1.74)	1.14 (0.21, 2.07)	0.017 *
Month 11	6.42 (1.77)	5.45 (1.69)	1.04 (0.11, 1.97)	0.029 *
Phosphorus (mg)				
Month 07	1023.06 (284.32)	1004.05 (202.02)	33.99 (−83.88, 151.87)	0.571
Month 08	966.96 (257.85)	1106.43 (293.65)	−124.49 (−242.36, −6.62)	0.039 *
Month 10	984.67 (335.64)	930.98 (252.54)	68.68 (−49.20, 186.55)	0.252
Month 11	989.53 (278.71)	988.18 (262.19)	16.33 (−101.54, 134.20)	0.785
Potassium (mg)				
Month 07	1666.69 (703.04)	1962.08 (433.28)	−283.10 (−528.37, −37.83)	0.024 *
Month 08	1537.51 (481.42)	2232.75 (761.17)	−682.95 (−928.21, −437.68)	<0.0001 *
Month 10	1406.79 (493.64)	1861.05 (503.26)	−441.97 (−687.24, −196.70)	0.001 *
Month 11	1512.12 (526.22)	1987.09 (511.40)	−462.67 (−707.94, −217.40)	0.000 *
Iron (mg)				
Month 07	10.62 (3.36)	6.23 (2.82)	4.58 (3.31, 5.85)	<0.0001 *
Month 08	10.80 (2.96)	6.90 (2.75)	4.10 (2.83, 5.37)	<0.0001 *
Month 10	9.83 (2.89)	5.64 (3.07)	4.38 (3.11, 5.65)	<0.0001 *
Month 11	10.26 (3.24)	5.24 (2.35)	5.21 (3.93, 6.48)	<0.0001 *
Copper (mg)				
Month 07	0.62 (0.32)	0.6 (0.24)	0.04 (−0.08, 0.15)	0.524
Month 08	0.6 (0.26)	0.68 (0.35)	−0.06 (−0.18, 0.05)	0.255
Month 10	0.63 (0.28)	0.5 (0.21)	0.15 (0.04, 0.26)	0.010 *
Month 11	0.6 (0.18)	0.53 (0.18)	0.09 (−0.02, 0.2)	0.115
Iodine (µg)				
Month 07	64.08 (23.15)	52.65 (24.78)	11.80 (0.49, 23.11)	0.041 *
Month 08	63.58 (29.84)	55.72 (21.88)	8.22 (−3.09, 19.54)	0.154
Month 10	60.53 (27.92)	53.13 (26.95)	7.77 (−3.55, 19.08)	0.178
Month 11	65.92 (30.56)	53.53 (21.06)	12.76 (1.45, 24.07)	0.027

* $p < 0.05$. [1] Repeated measures mixed model with an autoregressive covariance structure, adjusting for sex.
[2] Only nutrients with significant relationships at any of the four time points are displayed.

Compared with New Zealand NRVs [29], intakes of most nutrients were adequate, i.e., median intake (average all four 24 h) ≥ nutrient reference value across both groups Figure 1. Nutrients with median intakes below reference values in both groups were vitamin D, potassium, copper, and iodine.

Group A: Cow's Milk

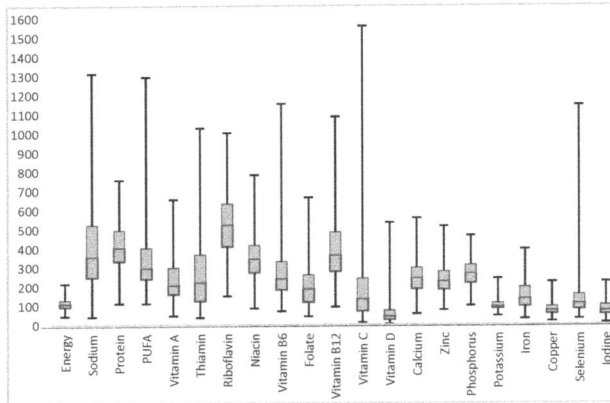

Group B: GUMLi

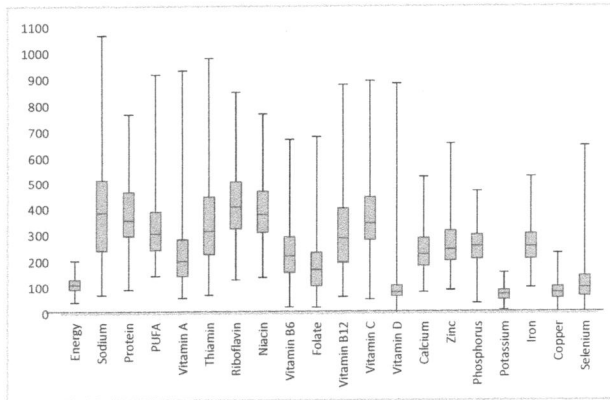

Figure 1. Intake of energy and nutrients as a percentage of New Zealand reference values (28) in 18- to 23-month-old children from the Auckland cohort participating in the GUMLi trial (median (—), interquartile range (box; 25th and 75th percentiles), minimum and maximum value). GUMLi = Growing Up Milk—Lite.

3.2. PANDiet Scores According to Intake of GUMLi or CM

Mean PANDiet score, sub-scores and individual components are displayed in Table 3. After adjusting for sex, children in the GUMLi group had significantly higher PANDiet scores and Adequacy scores compared to the CM group (adjusted mean difference +3.11 and +4.17, respectively). There was no difference in the Moderation sub score and energy intake between groups. Of note, the Adequacy sub-score was 2.5 and 2.6 times greater than the Moderation sub-score in the GUMLi and CM group, respectively, indicating poor adherence to the recommendations for avoiding excessive nutrient intakes.

There were no differences in component of the Moderation sub-score, except for total fat and total carbohydrates, where the CM group had a higher probability of avoiding excessive total fat intake and the GUMLi group had a higher probability of avoiding excessive total carbohydrate intake. The GUMLi group tended to have higher probability of avoiding excessive protein intake (not significant). The mean probabilities for avoiding excessive intakes were low for sodium (≤ 0.03),

SFA (≤0.10) and NMES (≤0.23) in this population. There were no differences between groups in components of the Adequacy sub-score, except for total fat, thiamin, vitamin C, vitamin D, iron, and iodine where the GUMLi group had a higher probability of having adequate intakes for these nutrients, and vitamin B12 where the CM group had a higher probability of having an adequate intake.

Table 3. PANDiet scores, sub-scores, and individual components, among Auckland children (*N* = 83) from 18 and 23 months of age (month 7–11 post randomisation) [1,2].

Score	Intervention (*N* = 41) Mean (SD)	Control (*N* = 42) Mean (SD)	Adjusted Difference (95% CI)	*p*-Value *
PANDiet [3]	52.9 (3.07)	50.12 (3.97)	3.11 (1.56, 4.67)	0.0001 *
Moderation sub-score	29.82 (6.47)	27.77 (6.58)	2.06 (−0.87, 4.99)	0.1660
Protein	0.41 (0.50)	0.33 (0.48)	0.08 (−0.14, 0.30)	0.4747
Total Fat	0.10 (0.30)	0.48 (0.51)	−0.40 (−0.59, −0.22)	<0001 *
Total Carbohydrate	0.85 (0.36)	0.55 (0.50)	0.33 (0.14, 0.53)	0.0011 *
SFA	0.10 (0.16)	0.06 (0.12)	0.05 (−0.01, 0.11)	0.1231
NMES	0.16 (0.22)	0.23 (0.28)	−0.08 (−0.19, 0.03)	0.1699
Sodium	0.03 (0.14)	0.02 (0.04)	0.01 (−0.03, 0.06)	0.5832
Adequacy sub-score	75.98 (4.98)	72.46 (5.88)	4.17 (1.82, 6.51)	0.0007 *
Protein	0.99 (0.03)	1.00 (0.001)	−0.01 (−0.01, 0.002)	0.1697
Total Carbohydrate	0.98 (0.03)	1.00 (0.00)	−0.02 (−0.07, 0.03)	0.4293
Total Fat	1.00 (0.00)	0.86 (0.35)	0.14 (0.03, 0.26)	0.0140 *
PUFA	0.15 (0.19)	0.18 (0.23)	−0.01 (−0.10, 0.08)	0.7975
Vitamin A	0.96 (0.08)	0.98 (0.02)	−0.02 (−0.05, 0.001)	0.0560
Thiamin	1.00 (0.005)	0.94 (0.09)	0.06 (0.03, 0.09)	0.0001 *
Riboflavin	1.00 (0.001)	1.00 (0.0003)	−0.0003 (−0.001, 0.00)	0.0853
Niacin	1.00 (0.00001)	1.00 (0.0005)	0.0001 (0.00, 0.0002)	0.1819
Vitamin B6	0.00 (0.00)	0.00 (0.00)	0.00 (0.00,0.00)	0.9775
Folate	0.89 (0.18)	0.91 (0.21)	−0.01 (−0.10, 0.07)	0.7717
Vitamin B12	0.99 (0.02)	1.00 (0.01)	−0.01 (−0.02, −0.003)	0.0081 *
Vitamin C	1.00 (0.01)	0.71 (0.32)	0.30 (0.20, 0.40)	<0001 *
Vitamin D	0.43 (0.34)	0.19 (0.31)	0.25 (0.10, 0.39)	0.0011 *
Calcium	0.99 (0.02)	1.00 (0.02)	−0.002 (−0.01, 0.01)	0.7227
Magnesium	0.99 (0.02)	1.00 (0.004)	−0.005 (−0.01, 0.002)	0.1826
Zinc	1.00 (0.003)	0.99 (0.02)	0.01 (−0.0002, 0.01)	0.0585
Phosphorus	1.00 (0.01)	1.00 (0.002)	−0.001 (−0.003, 0.0005)	0.1323
Potassium	1.00 (0.002)	1.00 (1E−6)	−0.0003 (−0.001, 0.0002)	0.1998
Iron	1.00 (0.01)	0.78 (0.32)	0.25 (0.16, 0.35)	<0001 *
Copper	0.34 (0.30)	0.27 (0.27)	0.10 (−0.03, 0.23)	0.1203
Selenium	0.57 (0.37)	0.70 (0.28)	−0.09 (−0.23, 0.06)	0.2314
Iodine	0.46 (0.28)	0.29 (0.24)	0.18 (0.06, 0.30)	0.0035 *

NMES, Non-milk Extrinsic Sugars; PANDiet, The Probability of Adequate Nutrient Intake score; PUFA, Poly0unsaturated Fatty Acids; SFA, Saturated Fatty Acids. * *p* < 0.05. [1] Linear regression model, adjusting for sex. [2] All the PANDiet component scores range from 0 to 1, where 1 represents a 100% probability that the intake is adequate according to a reference value. [3] Combined data from all four 24HR were used to calculate the overall PANDiet score and adequacy and moderation sub-scores, which ranged from 0 to 100. The higher the score or sub-scores, the better the nutrient adequacy of the diet.

4. Discussion

Using the PANDiet index, we have evaluated the diet quality and nutritional adequacy of 18-to−23-month-old Auckland children participating in the GUMLi Trial, according to GUMLi or CM consumption. This is the first study to use data from a randomised controlled trial to measure the impact of a dietary intervention, such as GUM on diet quality using a nutrient-based index, such as the PANDiet score. Total PANDiet scores were significantly higher in the GUMLi group, indicating better overall nutrient adequacy and diet quality. Nutrient intakes of children in both groups met recommendations for fat, total carbohydrates and most micronutrients; however, protein sodium, NMES, and SFA intakes exceeded recommendations. Whilst average total energy intakes were similar, the children consuming GUMLi had higher probabilities of having adequate intakes of vitamin C, vitamin D and iron, and were less likely to have insufficient intakes of vitamin D. Further analysis of food group consumption, adherence to dietary guidelines, or nutrient densities would elucidate whether the GUMLi intervention had an impact on dietary diversity, as an inverse relationship between dietary diversity and formula intake has previously been reported in 12- to 16-month-old Australian children [16].

4.1. Diet Quality and PANDiet Scores According to GUMLi or CM Allocation

GUM has been shown to improve intakes of iron, vitamin C, vitamin D, and PUFA's during the dietary transition from a milk-based intake to a 'family diet' in cross-sectional, observational studies [14–16,37]. The PANDiet has previously been evaluated in 12- to 18-month-old-children in the U.K. according to GUM or commercial infant foods (CIF) consumption [32]. Consuming GUM was associated with greater nutritional adequacy with a mean PANDiet score of 74.1 compared to children who did not consume GUM or CIF (difference of +7.2 points) [32]. A much smaller difference of +2.78 was observed in our sample, where consuming GUMLi was associated with greater nutritional adequacy. More recently, the difference in PANDiet scores for 'at risk children with Diabetic mothers' and 'not at risk' children in the BABYDIET study was similar at +2.4 points (65.9 and 68.3, respectively) [13].

It is important to note the effect of differences in national nutrient recommendations on PANDiet calculations and resultant scores. In the present study, the PANDiet score calculation was adjusted according to Australia and New Zealand NRVs where available [29], and if not, the reference values determined by Verger et al. [32] who used nutrient recommendations for UK children 12- to 36-months-of-age [34,35,38]. The greatest variation in recommendations were for selenium and folate, where the New Zealand NRVs are 1.7–2.4 times higher than the UK, (folate: 120 µg vs. 50 µg and selenium: 20 µg vs. 11.5 µg). The probability of adequate would be higher than the current calculation if we used the UK recommendations in our sub-score calculation. As all probabilities of adequacy are equally weighted, higher component scores will contribute to a higher total Adequacy sub-score and resultant PANDiet score [12].

In this population, the quality of both fat and carbohydrates are of concern. Children had low probabilities for avoiding excessive intakes for SFA ($\leq$0.10) and low probabilities for having adequate PUFA intakes (<0.20). An altered ratio of total and SFA has been described in two other studies, and is an important consideration, given the role of PUFA's in cognitive and visual development [37,39]. At each time point in the study, NMES exceeded the recommendations (>11% EI). Similar intakes were observed in a nationally representative sample of one- to four-year-old Irish children, where mean NMES intakes exceeded recommendations at 12% energy intake (EI) and increased with age [40].

4.2. Strengths and Limitations

The PANDiet provides an accurate measure of diet quality at an individual and population level through assessing global nutrient adequacy, and is strengthened by the use of a probabilistic calculation of nutrient adequacy, as previously described [12]. The index was designed to be as exhaustive as possible, and describes the role that different foods/food groups have in contributing to diet quality, at the nutrient level [12]. Our analysis is strengthened by the use of New Zealand NRVs to assess nutrient adequacy in the New Zealand context, however, because of this, cross-national comparisons of the PANDiet score are limited. Previous studies have used large, observational cohorts, where each subject has one PANDiet score calculated at a single time point, using multiple measures of dietary assessment [12,32,33]. For the present study, dietary data were collected on one day per month, over four months; therefore, month-to-month variation was considered in the PANDiet calculation. Using a record-assisted 24HR, allowed inclusion of children in the care of other adults (i.e., at day care), however, the reliance on parent and other adult-reported measures may lead to an increase in misreporting or social desirability bias. Mother's in our sample were older and highly educated, which may have affected total PANDiet scores. The ethnicity distribution in our sample was not considered representative of the Auckland population; therefore, no differences between ethnicities were evaluated. The validity of the PANDiet index was not evaluated for RCT data, therefore, further evaluation of the PANDiet in a larger, more representative cohort of New Zealand children under two is recommended to determine whether the PANDiet has predictive validity with respect to longitudinal health outcomes.

Nutrients **2019**, *11*, 203

5. Conclusions

The consumption of GUMLi was associated with higher nutritional adequacy of the diets of children 18- to 23-months-of-age defined by PANDiet score, with increased likelihood of meeting nutrient requirements. However, consumption of GUMLi did not guarantee 100% nutrient adequacy. GUMLi consumers still had excessive protein intakes, but were more likely to have carbohydrate and SFA intakes that were in line with recommendations and improved iron and vitamin D intakes. Although GUMLi had a positive effect on index scores, consumption toward the latter half of the second year of life may not have the same impact as during early childhood as previously reported in younger children according to GUM consumption [32]. This may be because in the latter part of the second year of life, children are more likely to be following a family diet of varying quality, with a reduced reliance on fortified milks. Suggesting that other dietary strategies to promote a healthy diet through optimising nutrient intake could also result in more favourable dietary intake profiles, rather than solely concentrating on milk [41], however, further research is required on the consequences of consuming GUMLi on overall dietary diversity.

Supplementary Materials: The following are available online at http://www.mdpi.com/2072-6643/11/1/203/s1, Table S1. PANDiet for Australian and New Zealand children aged from 18 to 23 months: components, reference values and inter-individual variability, Table S2. Nutritional composition of CM and GUMLi per 100 mL of prepared product, Table S3. Characteristics of the Auckland cohort included versus excluded in the PANDiet analysis, Table S4. Nutrient intake among Auckland children (*N* = 83) from 18 to 23 months of age (month 7–11 post randomisation)

Author Contributions: Conceptualisation: C.R.W. and C.C.G.; methodology: A.L.L. and C.R.W.; formal analysis: Y.J. and R.X.C.; data curation: A.L.L. and T.M.; writing—original draft preparation: A.L.L.; writing—review and editing: A.L.L., C.R.W., and C.C.G.; project administration: A.L.L. and T.M.; funding acquisition: C.R.W. and C.C.G.

Funding: The GUMLi Trial received an investigator-initiated grant from Danone Nutricia Research. The funder had no role in the study design, data collection, analysis, and interpretation of the study. There are no restrictions or delays on the timely publication of the results of the trial.

Acknowledgments: The authors thank E.O. Verger for his assistance in calculating and interpreting the PANDiet index.

Conflicts of Interest: C.R.W. has received honoraria for presentations and consultations from Danone, Nutricia, Pfizer, and Fonterra. C.C.G. has received honoraria for consultations from Fonterra. A.L.L. states no conflict of interest. T.M. states no conflict of interest. Y.J. states no conflict of interest. R.X.C. states no conflict of interest. The funders had no role in the design of the study; in the collection, analyses, or interpretation of data; in the writing of the manuscript; or in the decision to publish the results.

References

1. Northstone, K.; Emmett, P.M. Are dietary patterns stable throughout early and mid-childhood? A birth cohort study. *Br. J. Nutr.* **2008**, *100*, 1069–1076. [CrossRef] [PubMed]
2. Morgan, J. Nutrition for toddlers: The foundation for good health—2. Current problems and ways to overcome them. *J. Fam. Health Care* **2005**, *15*, 85–88. [PubMed]
3. Golley, R.K.; Hendrie, G.A.; McNaughton, S.A. Scores on the Dietary Guideline Index for Children and Adolescents Are Associated with Nutrient Intake and Socio-Economic Position but Not Adiposity—3. *J. Nutr.* **2011**, *141*, 1340–1347. [CrossRef] [PubMed]
4. Ruel, M.T.; Menon, P. Child feeding practices are associated with child nutritional status in Latin America: Innovative uses of the demographic and health surveys. *J. Nutr.* **2002**, *132*, 1180–1187. [CrossRef] [PubMed]
5. Kant, A.K. Indexes of overall diet quality: A review. *J. Am. Diet. Assoc.* **1996**, *96*, 785–791. [CrossRef]
6. Marshall, S.; Burrows, T.; Collins, C.E. Systematic review of diet quality indices and their associations with health-related outcomes in children and adolescents. *J. Hum. Nutr. Diet.* **2014**, *27*, 577–598. [CrossRef]
7. Wirt, A.; Collins, C.E. Diet quality—What is it and does it matter? *Public Health Nutr.* **2009**, *12*, 2473–2492. [CrossRef]
8. Waijers, P.M.; Feskens, E.J.; Ocké, M.C. A critical review of predefined diet quality scores. *Br. J. Nutr.* **2007**, *97*, 219–231. [CrossRef]

123

9. Hu, F.B. Dietary pattern analysis: A new direction in nutritional epidemiology. *Curr. Opin. Lipidol.* **2002**, *13*, 3–9. [CrossRef]

10. Lazarou, C.; Newby, P.K. Use of dietary indexes among children in developed countries. *Adv. Nutr.* **2011**, *2*, 295–303. [CrossRef]

11. Smithers, L.G.; Golley, R.K.; Brazionis, L.; Emmett, P.; Northstone, K.; Lynch, J.W. Dietary patterns of infants and toddlers are associated with nutrient intakes. *Nutrients* **2012**, *4*, 935–948. [CrossRef] [PubMed]

12. Verger, E.O.; Mariotti, F.; Holmes, B.A.; Paineau, D.; Huneau, J. Evaluation of a diet quality index based on the probability of adequate nutrient intake (PANDiet) using national French and US dietary surveys. *PLoS ONE* **2012**, *7*, e42155. [CrossRef] [PubMed]

13. Schoen, S.; Jergens, S.; Barbaresko, J.; Nöthlings, U.; Kersting, M.; Remer, T.; Stelmach-Mardas, M.; Ziegler, A.G.; Hummel, S. Diet quality during infancy and early childhood in children with and without risk of type 1 diabetes: A DEDIPAC study. *Nutrients* **2017**, *9*, 48. [CrossRef] [PubMed]

14. Ghisolfi, J.; Fantino, M.; Turck, D.; de Courcy, G.P.; Vidailhet, M. Nutrient intakes of children aged 1–2 years as a function of milk consumption, cows' milk or growing-up milk. *Public Health Nutr.* **2013**, *16*, 524–534. [CrossRef]

15. Walton, J.; Flynn, A. Nutritional adequacy of diets containing growing up milks or unfortified cow's milk in Irish children (aged 12–24 months). *Food Nutr. Res.* **2013**, *57*, 21836. [CrossRef] [PubMed]

16. Byrne, R.; Magarey, A.; Daniels, L. Food and beverage intake in Australian children aged 12–16 months participating in the NOURISH and SAIDI studies. *Aust. N. Z. J. Public Health* **2014**, *38*, 326–331. [CrossRef] [PubMed]

17. Vandenplas, Y.; De Ronne, N.; Van De Sompel, A.; Huysentruyt, K.; Robert, M.; Rigo, J.; Scheers, I.; Brasseur, D.; Goyens, P. A Belgian consensus-statement on growing-up milks for children 12–36 months old. *Eur. J. Pediatr.* **2014**, *173*, 1365–1371. [CrossRef]

18. Eussen, S.R.; Pean, J.; Olivier, L.; Delaere, F.; Lluch, A. Theoretical impact of replacing whole cow's milk by young-child formula on nutrient intakes of UK young children: Results of a simulation study. *Ann. Nutr. Metab.* **2015**, *67*, 247–256. [CrossRef] [PubMed]

19. Wall, C.R.; Hill, R.J.; Lovell, A.L.; Matsuyama, M.; Milne, T.; Grant, C.C. A Multi-Centre, Double Blind, Randomised, Placebo Controlled Trial to Evaluate the Effect of Consuming Growing Up Milk. 'Lite' on Body Composition in Children Aged 12–23 Months. Available online: https://www.anzctr.org.au/Trial/Registration/TrialReview.aspx?id=366785 (accessed on 29 December 2018).

20. Blanton, C.A.; Moshfegh, A.J.; Baer, D.J.; Kretsch, M.J. The USDA Automated Multiple-Pass Method accurately estimates group total energy and nutrient intake. *J. Nutr.* **2006**, *136*, 2594–2599. [CrossRef]

21. Watson, P. *Development & Pretesting of Methodologies for the Children's Nutrition Survey: Validation Report: A Report to the Ministry of Health. Report Three*; Institute of Food, Nutrition and Human Health, Massey University: Palmerston North, NZ, USA, 2003.

22. Coblac, L.; Bowen, J.; Burnett, J.; Syrette, J.; Dempsey, J.; Balle, S.; Wilson, C.; Flight, I.; Good, N.; Saunders, I. *Australian National Children's Nutrition and Physical Activity Survey: Main Findings*; Australian Bureau of Statistics: Canberra, Australia, 2008.

23. User Guide. *Australian National Children's Nutrition and Physical Activity Survey*; Commonwealth Scientific Industrial Research Organisation: Canberra, Australia, 2010.

24. Briefel, R.R.; Reidy, K.; Karwe, V.; Devaney, B. Feeding infants and toddlers study: Improvements needed in meeting infant feeding recommendations. *J. Am. Diet. Assoc.* **2004**, *104* (Suppl. 1), 31. [CrossRef]

25. Devaney, B.; Kalb, L.; Briefel, R.; Zavitsky-Novak, T.; Clusen, N.; Ziegler, P. Feeding infants and toddlers study: Overview of the study design. *J. Am. Diet. Assoc.* **2004**, *104* (Suppl. 1), 8. [CrossRef] [PubMed]

26. Emmett, P.; North, K.; Noble, S. Types of drinks consumed by infants at 4 and 8 months of age: A descriptive study. *Public Health Nutr.* **2000**, *3*, 211–217. [CrossRef] [PubMed]

27. Lennox, A.; Sommerville, J.; Ong, K.; Henderson, H.; Allen, R. *Diet and Nutrition Survey of Infants and Young Children*; Department of Health and Food Standards Agency: London, UK, 2013.

28. Institute for Plant & Food Research Limited, Ministry of Health. *New Zealand Food composition Database: New Zealand FOODfiles*; Institute for Plant & Food Research Limited, Ministry of Health: Wellington, New Zealand, 2016.

29. National Health and Medical Research Council. *Nutrient Reference Values for Australia and New Zealand Including Recommended Dietary Intakes*; National Health and Medical Research Council: Canberra, Australia, 2006.

30. Carriquiry, A.L. Assessing the prevalence of nutrient inadequacy. *Public Health Nutr.* **1999**, *2*, 23–34. [CrossRef] [PubMed]

31. Institute of Medicine. *Dietary Reference Itakes for Calcium and Vitamin, D*; Institute of Medicine: Washington, DC, USA, 2011.

32. Verger, E.O.; Eussen, S.; Holmes, B.A. Evaluation of a nutrient-based diet quality index in UK young children and investigation into the diet quality of consumers of formula and infant foods. *Public Health Nutr.* **2016**, *19*, 1785–1794. [CrossRef] [PubMed]

33. Verger, E.O.; Eussen, S.; Holmes, B.A. Diet quality and nutritional adequacy of young children in the UK according to their consumption of young child formula and commercial infant food. *Proc. Nutr. Soc.* **2015**, *74*, E250. [CrossRef]

34. Agostoni, C.V.; Berni Canani, R.; Fairweather Tait, S.; Heinonen, M.; Korhonen, H.; La Vieille, S.; Marchelli, R.; Martin, A.; Naska, A.; Neuhäuser Berthold, M.; et al. Scientific Opinion on nutrient requirements and dietary intakes of infants and young children in the European Union: EFSA Panel on Dietetic Products, Nutrition and Allergies (NDA). *EFSA J.* **2013**, *11*, 1–103.

35. Nordic Council of Ministers. *Nordic Nutrition Recommendations 2012: Integrating Nutrition and Physical Activity*; Nordic Council of Ministers: Copenhagen, Denmark, 2014.

36. Institute of Medicine (US); Panel on Macronutrients, Institute of Medicine (US). *Standing Committee on the Scientific Evaluation of Dietary Reference Intakes. Dietary Reference Intakes for Energy, Carbohydrate, Fiber, Fat, Fatty Acids, Cholesterol, Protein, and Amino Acids*; Institute of Medicine: Washington, DC, USA, 2005.

37. Hilbig, A.; Drossard, C.; Kersting, M.; Alexy, U. Nutrient adequacy and associated factors in a nationwide sample of German toddlers. *J. Pediatr. Gastroenterol. Nutr.* **2015**, *61*, 130–137. [CrossRef] [PubMed]

38. Panel on Dietary Reference Values of the Committee on Medical Aspects of Food Policy. *Dietary Reference Values for Food Energy and Nutrients for the United Kingdom: Report of the Panel on Dietary Reference Values of the committee On Medical Aspects of Food Policy*; HM Stationery Office: Richmond, UK, 1991.

39. Butte, N.F.; Fox, M.K.; Briefel, R.R.; Siega-Riz, A.M.; Dwyer, J.T.; Deming, D.M.; Reidy, K.C. Nutrient intakes of US infants, toddlers, and preschoolers meet or exceed dietary reference intakes. *J. Am. Diet. Assoc.* **2010**, *110*, S37. [CrossRef] [PubMed]

40. Walton, J.; Kehoe, L.; McNulty, B.A.; Nugent, A.P.; Flynn, A. Nutrient intakes and compliance with nutrient recommendations in children aged 1–4 years in Ireland. *J. Hum. Nutr. Diet.* **2017**, *30*, 665–676. [CrossRef] [PubMed]

41. Hojsak, I.; Bronsky, J.; Campoy, C.; Domellöf, M.; Embleton, N.; Fidler Mis, N.; Hulst, J.; Indrio, F.; Lapillonne, A.; Mølgaard, C.; et al. Young Child Formula: A Position Paper by the ESPGHAN Committee on Nutrition. *J. Pediatr. Gastroenterol. Nutr.* **2018**, *66*, 177–185. [CrossRef] [PubMed]

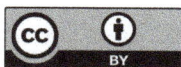

nutrients

Review

Design, Development and Construct Validation of the Children's Dietary Inflammatory Index

Samira Khan [1,2], Michael D. Wirth [1,2,3,4], Andrew Ortaglia [3], Christian R. Alvarado [1,3], Nitin Shivappa [1,2,3], Thomas G. Hurley [1,2] and James R. Hebert [1,2,3,*]

[1] Statewide Cancer Prevention and Control Program (CPCP), Arnold School of Public Health, University of South Carolina, 915 Greene Street, Columbia, SC 29208, USA; khans@mailbox.sc.edu (S.K.); wirthm@mailbox.sc.edu (M.D.W.); alvarac@email.sc.edu (C.R.A.); shivappa@mailbox.sc.edu (N.S.); thurley@mailbox.sc.edu (T.G.H.)

[2] Connecting Health Innovations, LLC, Columbia, SC 29201, USA; skhan@chi-llc.net (S.K.); mwirth@chi-llc.net (M.D.W.); nshivappa@chi-llc.net (N.S.); thurley@chi-llc.net (T.G.H.)

[3] Epidemiology and Biostatistics, Arnold School of Public Health, University of South Carolina, 915 Greene Street, Columbia, SC 29208, USA; ORTAGLIA@mailbox.sc.edu

[4] College of Nursing, University of South Carolina, Columbia, SC 29208, USA

[*] Correspondence: jhebert@mailbox.sc.edu or jhebert@chi-llc.net; Tel: +1-803-576-5666

Received: 28 June 2018; Accepted: 24 July 2018; Published: 30 July 2018

Abstract: Objective: To design and validate a literature-derived, population-based Children's Dietary Inflammatory Index (C-DII)^{TM}. Design: The C-DII was developed based on a review of literature through 2010. Dietary data obtained from children in 16 different countries were used to create a reference database for computing C-DII scores based on consumption of macronutrients, vitamins, minerals, and whole foods. Construct validation was performed using quantile regression to assess the association between C-reactive protein (CRP) concentrations and C-DII scores. Data Sources: All data used for construct validation were obtained from children between six and 14 years of age (n = 3300) who participated in the U.S. National Health and Nutrition Examination Survey (NHANES) (2005–2010). Results: The C-DII was successfully validated with blood CRP concentrations in this heterogeneous sample of 3300 children from NHANES (52% male; 29% African American, 25% Mexican American; mean age 11 years). The final model was adjusted for sex, age, race, asthma, body mass index (BMI), and infections. Children in level 3 (i.e., quartiles 3 and 4 combined) of the C-DII (i.e., children with the most pro-inflammatory diets) had a CRP value 0.097 mg/dL higher than that in level 1 (i.e., quartile 1) for CRP values at the 75th percentile of CRP using quantile regression (p < 0.05). Conclusion: The C-DII predicted blood CRP concentrations among children 6–14 years in the NHANES. Further construct validation with CRP and other inflammatory markers is required to deepen understanding of the relationship between the C-DII and markers of inflammation in children.

Keywords: diet; inflammation; children's-dietary inflammatory index

1. Introduction

Inflammation is regulated in the body through a variety of processes that involve intercellular signaling via well-characterized cytokine and chemokine messengers [1–4]. An acute inflammatory response is necessary for normal physiologic functioning, including response to infectious disease agents [5–9]. This acute inflammatory response is characterized by an increase in vascular permeability and blood flow accompanied by the accumulation of inflammatory mediators, fluid, and leukocytes. Acute inflammatory responses are time-limited and require negative feedback signaling between pro-inflammatory cytokines that turn on the response and anti-inflammatory cytokines that signal acute inflammatory responses to cease [10,11]. Because of the unique nutritional needs of children,

Nutrients 2018, *10*, 993; doi:10.3390/nu10080993   126   www.mdpi.com/journal/nutrients

and because it is imperative to deal with enteric and other infections, to which children are especially vulnerable, much of the initial focus of the field of immunology was on children and childhood nutrition [9,12].

In contrast to acute inflammation, chronic systematic inflammation results when negative feedback does not occur (or is either incomplete or inefficient) [10,13]. The chronic phase is characterized by a specific cellular immune response along with specific humoral responses [14,15]. In addition to its role in regulating acute inflammatory responses, diet also has been implicated in regulating chronic inflammation [16,17].

The Dietary Inflammatory Index (DII®) was developed to classify human dietary patterns on a continuous scale from anti-inflammatory to pro-inflammatory [18]. Although the original DII could predict changes in C-reactive protein (CRP) levels, a newer version of the DII was developed that reflected an update in the review of peer-reviewed articles by adding those published from 2007 to 2010 and a refined scoring algorithm [19]. Subsequently, the new DII has been construct validated in nine studies against inflammatory biomarkers in different populations and under varying conditions [20–26].

In the process of publishing the new DII, we observed that the relationship between total caloric intake and DII score is highly idiosyncratic across populations, and by body size. For example, in most populations, DII scores decrease with increasing caloric intake [27–29]. This observation led, in part, to development of the Energy Density-DII (E-DII) and then to the Children's Dietary Inflammatory Index (C-DII™). In addition, the world standard database used for the DII includes data on dietary parameters only from adults, and not all the parameters that comprise the DII (e.g., alcohol intake) are appropriate to include when evaluating children's dietary intake. With these limitations in mind, we set out to create a "world" standard database of food parameters that could be used to calculate C-DII scores among children. At the same time, it was understood that construct validation of the C-DII was necessary. Therefore, we also sought to conduct a construct validation to test the relationship between C-DII scores and levels of an inflammatory biomarker, CRP. We hypothesized that children with more pro-inflammatory diets (i.e., higher C-DII scores) will have higher values of CRP compared to children with lower C-DII scores.

This paper describes the development of the C-DII and the relationship between C-DII scores and blood concentrations of CRP in a nationally representative sample of children.

2. Methods

2.1. C-DII^{TM} Development

To develop the C-DII, methods similar to those used to develop the current version of the DII were employed [19]. First, the "inflammatory effect scores", which were derived from an extensive literature search to develop the DII, were still applicable and therefore used for the development of the C-DII. The Dietary Inflammatory Index (DII®) was developed to classify human dietary patterns on a continuous scale from anti-inflammatory to pro-inflammatory [18]. Although the original DII could predict changes in CRP levels, a newer version of the DII was developed that reflected an update in the review of peer-reviewed articles by adding those published from 2007 to 2010 and a refined scoring algorithm [19]. Subsequently, the new DII has been construct validated in nine studies against inflammatory biomarkers in different populations and under varying conditions [20–26]. This work entailed a literature review of 1943 articles that was conducted to identify food parameters which are associated with six inflammatory biomarkers: Interleukin-1beta (IL-1β), interleukin-4 (IL-4), interleukin-6 (IL-6), interleukin-10 (IL-10), tumor necrosis factor-alpha (TNF-α), and CRP. By contrast with the constrained list of the six inflammatory biomarkers, the list of dietary parameters was open. For each article reviewed, a score was assigned for each food parameter based on its effect on inflammation. A '+1' was assigned if the effect of the parameter was pro-inflammatory, a '−1' was assigned if the effect of the parameter was anti-inflammatory; and '0' was assigned if the effect of the parameter was neutral. Each food parameter for which a finding existed was assigned a score for each article separately [19]. Published articles were weighted by study design, with highest weight assigned to experimental studies in humans and the lowest weight assigned to cell culture experiments. Based on the weights, pro- or anti-inflammatory fractions were calculated for each food parameter. Next, the overall inflammatory effect score specific to each food parameter was calculated by subtracting the anti-inflammatory fraction from pro-inflammatory fraction [19].

The food parameters used to calculate C-DII scores are: vitamin A, thiamine, riboflavin, niacin, vitamin B6, folic acid, vitamin B12, vitamin D, vitamin C, vitamin E, beta carotene, energy, carbohydrates, fiber, total fat, saturated fat, mono-unsaturated fatty acid (MUFA), poly-unsaturated fatty acid (PUFA), cholesterol, protein, alcohol, iron (Fe), magnesium (Mg), selenium (Se), and zinc (Zn).

Developing a Composite Database Representing a Diversity of Children's Diets

Dietary intakes from a wide range of diverse populations from different countries representing six continents were used to construct a composite database for the C-DII. The methodology used was virtually identical to that employed for developing the DII for adults. Data collection began in August 2016 and ended in May 2017. Using the National Library of Medicine database (Medline), we identified 35 different published papers with sample size over 200 with children's diet data collected using either a food frequency questionnaire (FFQ) or diet recalls. Overall, data were collected from 16 different countries representing diverse diets from six different continents.

Dietary data for creating a global database were collected from three different sources: (1) datasets (*n* = 11) received directly from the study principal investigators (from collaborations during DII development); (2) from published articles (*n* = 3); (3) National Health and Nutrition Examination (NHANES) Survey reports (*n* = 2). We sent emails to the authors of the 35 published articles with sample size >200 to obtain consent to use data. After three attempts to obtain consent to use data, we finalized a list of the articles from which we could extract dietary data for the global database. The decision was based on the availability of macro and micronutrients presented in the tables in the articles for children age 6–14 years.

The world database used for the C-DII contains dietary information from the following countries (and sources): (i) USA—the NHANES data set 2005–2011 [30]; (ii) Australia—mean values were taken from the National Nutrition Survey report of 1999 [31]; (iii) Japan—means were taken from the National Nutrition Survey Report [32]; (iv) Korea—mean values were taken from the Korean National Health and Nutrition Examination Survey (KNHANES); (v) Spain, (vi) Belgium, (vii) Greece, (viii) Germany, (ix) France, (x) Italy, (xi) Sweden, and (xii) Austria—means were taken from the Healthy Lifestyle in Europe by Nutrition in Adolescence (HELENA) study [33]; (xiii) Venezuela—means were taken from an article published by Bernal et al. [34]; (xiv); United Arab Emirates—means were taken from an article published by Ali et al. [35]; and (xvi) Chile—means were taken from an article published by Liberona et al. [36].

Missing food parameters for countries included in the database were left blank, and the overall mean and standard deviation were calculated using only data from the datasets that had information on that specific food parameter. For example, the mean and standard deviation for vitamin A were calculated using 13 countries because South Africa, Venezuela, and Chile did not have information on that food parameter. Some sources of data provided mean intake values separately for males and females or for different age groups within the range of 6–14 years; in such cases, the values were averaged. For example, the data from the United Emirates, gathered from the article by Ali et al. [35], had children separated by sex, and by age group: 6–8, 9–13, and 14–18 years. In this case, the values were averaged first between age groups for each sex, and then averaged between males and females. The list of 25 food parameters and the information regarding each country (present or missing for each food parameter) is presented in Supplementary Table S1.

Individual estimates of consumption were standardized to a global database of children's dietary intake, in a manner analogous to methods used to compute adult DII scores. As children's diet differs from the adult diet, one difference between the DII and the C-DII is that the C-DII identified only 25 food parameters, compared to the 45 used in scoring of the adult DII.

2.2. Calculation of the Children's Dietary Inflammatory Index

Calculation of the C-DII is based on the dietary intake data that are related to the regionally representative world database. These values become multipliers to express an individual child's exposure relative to the 'standard global mean' as a Z-score. This is done by subtracting the 'standard mean' from the reported amount and dividing this value by the global standard deviation. This Z-score is then converted to a proportion to avoid 'right skewing'. A symmetrical distribution was achieved with values centered on 0 (null) and bounded between −1 (maximally anti-inflammatory) and +1 (maximally pro-inflammatory), by doubling each proportion and then subtracting '1'. This centered proportion score is then multiplied by the 'overall food parameter-specific inflammatory effect score'. In the final step, 'food parameter-specific DII scores' are added to create the 'overall C-DII score' for an individual child. This approach eliminates the problem of non-comparability of units because the Z-scores and centered proportion scores are independent of the units of measurement [19]. This technique is the same as that used previously in the development of the DII [19]. Additionally, the C-DII, just like recent developments in the DII, can be calculated per 1000 calories consumed to take into account differing amounts of energy consumption between people.

2.3. Validation Study: NHANES Study Population

The NHANES survey examines a nationally representative sample of about 10,000 persons each year, and it employees a complex, multistage probability sampling design and generates weights to create a nationally representative dataset of the US population. More detailed information about the NHANES methods and protocols can be found on the Centers for Disease Control and Prevention (CDC)—National Center for Health Statistics website [37].

The proposed study population was restricted to children age 6–14 years (primary inclusion criterion) from the NHANES dataset (2005–2010) who had complete dietary data, demographics, and blood results, including CRP. There were 3445 children with CRP information and 145 were removed due to missing information. The final sample for analysis included data from 3300 children.

2.4. Dietary Assessment

NHANES 24-h dietary recall data were used to calculate C-DII scores. These data were collected through in-person interviews conducted by trained dietary interviewers fluent in English and Spanish. These staff members and the USDA's Food Survey Research Group were responsible for the dietary data collection, maintenance of the databases, and data processing. The food parameters from the NHANES data set included carbohydrates, protein, fat, fiber, fatty acids, vitamins (A, B1, B2, B6, B12, C, D, E), iron, magnesium, zinc, selenium, folic acid and beta carotene. To account for total energy intake, the C-DII was calculated per 1000 calories of food consumed.

2.5. CRP Data

The blood samples for CRP determination were processed, stored and analyzed at the University of Washington, Seattle, WA, using Behring Nephelometer for quantitative CRP determination (NHANES 2009–2010 data documentation, 2011). The blood specimens for children aged 3 years and older were collected in a mobile examination clinic by using regular or serum-separator vacutainers, and specimens were kept frozen at $< -20\,^\circ\text{C}$ if testing was not done within 24 h of specimen collection. The serum or plasma was separated from the cells within 60 min of collection; recommended sample volume for assay is 1.0 mL. Specimens are stored in glass or plastic vials and kept tightly sealed. The lower detection limit for CRP was 0.02 ng/mL.

2.6. Study Population and Covariates

Study covariates included demographic characteristics, such as age, sex, race, body mass index (BMI kg/m^2), ethnicity, self-reported asthma, and infection at the time of data collection. Subjects with missing information on any of these variables were removed from the analysis.

2.7. Statistical Analyses

The statistical software SAS 9.4® (SAS Institute, Cary, NC, USA) and R 3.4.3® (The R Foundation, Vienna, Austria) were used for analyses. For descriptive analysis, we report continuous variables with means and standard deviation (SD) and categorical variables using frequencies and percentage across C-DII quartiles. Chi Square tests were performed for descriptive statistics of categorical covariates across C-DII quartiles, and Analysis of Variance (ANOVAs) were used for the continuous covariates (See Table 1 for a list of covariates).

Table 1. Participants' characteristics across quartiles of the children's dietary inflammatory index (C-DII) among 3300 children. NHANES, 2005–2012.

	C-DII Quartiles				
	1st	2nd	3rd	4th	
Participant Characteristics	(−3.99, −0.04)	(−0.05, 1.14)	(1.14, 2.07)	(2.08, 4.39)	*p*-value [a]
Age (years)					<0.0001
	10.0 ± 3.0	11.0 ± 3.0	11.0 ± 3.0	11.0 ± 3.0	
Sex					0.29
Male	411 (48.52)	430 (51.62)	413 (49.64)	409 (51.9)	
Female	436 (51.48)	403 (48.38)	419 (50.36)	379 (48.1)	
Race					<0.0001
Non-Hispanic Black	180 (21.25)	212 (25.45)	223 (26.8)	229 (29.06)	
Non-Hispanic White	224 (26.45)	228 (27.37)	229 (27.52)	251 (31.85)	
Mexican American	323 (38.13)	267 (32.05)	262 (31.49)	198 (25.13)	
Other	120 (14.17)	126 (15.13)	118 (14.18)	110 (13.96)	
Body mass index (tertiles) [b,c,d]					0.19
I	705 (83.43)	682 (82.17)	671 (81.04)	640 (81.42)	
II	82 (9.7)	103 (12.41)	101 (12.2)	84 (10.69)	
III	58 (6.69)	45 (5.42)	56 (6.76)	62 (7.89)	
Asthma [e]					0.01
Yes	128 (15.11)	134 (16.13)	145 (17.45)	155 (19.7)	
No	719 (84.89)	697 (83.87)	686 (82.55)	632 (80.3)	
Infection [e]					0.06
Yes	252 (27.39)	237 (25.76)	225 (24.46)	206 (22.39)	
No	571 (24.72)	579 (25.06)	595 (25.76)	565 (24.46)	

[a] *p* Value for Chi-square test; [b] BMI (kg/m^2): Category I Under or Normal weight (i.e., <25 kg/m^2); [c] BMI (kg/m^2): Category II Overweight (i.e., ≥25 kg/m^2 and <30 kg/m^2); [d] BMI (kg/m^2): Category III Obese (i.e., ≥30 kg/m^2); [e] Asthma and Infection are self-reported; Column percentages may not equal 100% due to rounding. Stratum total may not equal column totals due to missing data. For categorical covariates, frequencies (%) were presented, and chi-square tests were used to derive *p*-values. For continuous covariates, means and standard deviations were presented, and ANOVAs were used to derive *p*-values.

The C-DII scores were expressed as quartiles, and CRP weighted percentiles were used for analysis (see Table 2 for percentile details). For this analysis, we combined quartiles 3 and 4 of the C-DII because the ranges in values for these quartiles were somewhat narrow and, together, represented the most pro-inflammatory diets. Also, combining these two quartiles provided a larger sample size for the comparison of interest, therefore, providing more statistical power. For these analyses, C-DII scores were expressed as three levels, with 1 = quartile 1 (anti-inflammatory); 2 = quartile 2 (neutral); and 3 = quartiles 3 + 4 (most pro-inflammatory). For all comparative analyses, C-DII quartile 1 was used as the reference. Categorizing the C-DII initially into quartiles was done because the DII is typically analyzed using quartiles, and C-DII follows strategies and methodologies used to assess and validate the DII [22,24].

Table 2. The quantile regression coefficients for children's dietary inflammatory index treated categorically with 3 levels (level 1 is the reference level) adjusted for sex, age, race, asthma, BMI and infection, NHANES, 2005–2012 *.

| | Weighted CRP Levels | | | | | | | | | | | |
| | 25th Percentile | | | 50th Percentile | | | 75th Percentile | | | 90th Percentile | | |
	Est.	SE	95% CI	Est.	SE	95% CI	Est.	SE	95% CI	Est.	SE	95% CI
C-DII Level												
2 (Quartile 2)	0.014	0.009	(−0.004, 0.032)	† 0.045	0.020	(0.005, 0.085)	† 0.113	0.055	(0.005, 0.221)	0.233	0.192	(−0.144, 0.609)
3 (Quartiles 3 + 4)	0.017	0.009	(−0.001, 0.035)	† 0.054	0.023	(0.009, 0.099)	† 0.097	0.041	(0.016, 0.177)	0.157	0.142	(−0.122, 0.436)

CRP, C-reactive protein. * Tabulated data are: The quantile regression coefficients (Est.), standard errors (SE) and 95% confidence intervals (CI). † Indicates a significant value (at $\alpha = 0.05$).

Quantile regression was used to assess the association between C-DII levels and weighted CRP, treated as the dependent variable, across adjusted CRP percentiles (25th, 50th, 75th and 90th) after controlling for sex, age, race, asthma, BMI, and infections. "R" version 3.43 was used for the quantile regression analysis, with the survey package extended to accommodate quantile regression, accounting for the NHANES complex survey design using standard errors calculated via replicate weights [38].

Quantile regression has the advantage of allowing the examination of relationships across the entire CRP distribution, allowing for a comprehensive evaluation of the association between C-DII and CRP. Quantile regression coefficients are interpreted similarly to mean regression coefficients except that a quantile regression coefficient indicates the change in the value at the modeled percentile, not the mean, of the dependent variable. For example, consider a categorical predictor such as C-DII classified by quartile, with the lowest C-DII quartile being the reference level. A coefficient estimate of 0.1 mg/L for the second quartile of C-DII in the quantile regression model for the 90th percentile would indicate that the 90th percentile of CRP is estimated to be 0.1 mg/L greater for children in the second C-DII quartile as compared to children in the first C-DII quartile after controlling for other covariates in the model (See Figure 1 for a depiction).

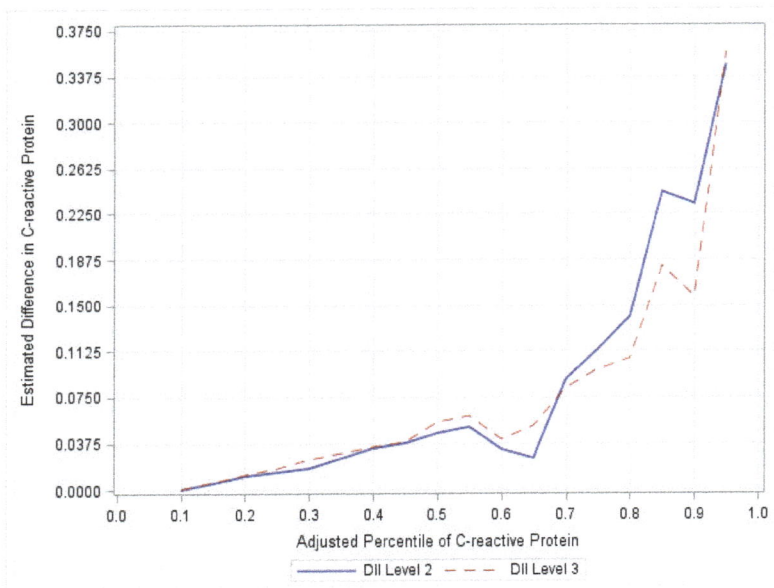

Figure 1. Plot of regression coefficients (C-DII and CRP). The magnitude of the differences in CRP increases at the upper percentiles up to the 85th percentile. CRP for children in C-DII group 2 as compared to C-DII group 1 at the 85th percentile is over 5 times the difference in CRP at the median, NHANES, 2005–2012.To reinforce the validity of our study, a logistic regression was performed using dichotomized CRP as the dependent variable (designated as high risk if CRP $\geq$ 0.50 mg/L or low risk <0.50 mg/dL) using a median cut-point. The odds of a CRP value $\geq$ 0.50 mg/L were obtained for those in C-DII level 3 compared to level 1, controlling for sex, age, race, asthma, BMI, and infections.

3. Results

Characteristics of children from the NHANES database (2005–2010 two-year cycles) whose data were used to validate C-DII scores are presented in Table 1. Weighted mean CRP value (n = 3193) was 0.84 mg/dL (standard error (SE) = 0.03). C-DII mean score was +0.99 (SE = 0.05), with values ranging from a maximally anti-inflammatory value of −3.98 to a maximally pro-inflammatory value of +4.39. Participants in quartile 1 had the least inflammatory scores (−3.98 to −0.04) and children in upper quartiles 3 and 4 had the most pro-inflammatory diet (2.07 to 4.39). The majority (≈82%) of the children in all quartiles were normal weight. More children in upper quartiles 3 and 4 reported asthma (17.4% and 19.7%, respectively) ($p < 0.01$) compared to lower quartiles (15.1% and 16.1%).

Significant differences in CRP were observed at the adjusted 50th and 75th percentiles for both groups, that is levels 2 (quartile 2) and 3 (quartiles 3 + 4 combined). Differences in CRP for children in C-DII level 2 as compared to C-DII level 1 were 0.045 and 0.113 mg/dL at the 50th and 75th percentiles, respectively. Similarly, differences in CRP for children in C-DII level 3 as compared to C-DII level 1 were 0.054 and 0.097 mg/dL at the 50th and 75th percentiles, respectively (see Table 2). The estimates for the association of C-DII on the adjusted 25th, 50th, 75th and 90th percentile CRP values are shown in Table 2.

For both C-DII levels 2 and 3, the magnitude of the estimated impact of C-DII tended to increase with increasing CRP percentiles. The magnitude of the differences in CRP between C-DII level 3 and 1 increase up to the 85th percentile. The estimated difference in CRP for children in C-DII level 2, as compared to C-DII level 3, at the 85th percentile is over 5 times the difference in CRP at the median (see Figure 1). The regression coefficients at the 90th percentile did not reach the nominal cut-point for statistical significance because the standard errors also increased, which tends to occur at the upper tail of the distribution.

Based on the logistic regression results, children in C-DII levels 2 and 3 had increased odds of having a CRP value above 0.50 mg/L. Specifically, children in C-DII level 2 (which equates to quartile 2) had 22% increased odds (95% confidence intervals (CI) = 0.94–1.59) of a CRP value above 0.50 mg/L compared to children in C-DII level 1. However, this did not achieve statistical significance. Children in C-DII level 3 (which equates to C-DII quartiles 3 and 4) had statistically significant 38% increased odds of an elevated CRP compared to children in C-DII level 1 (odds ratio (OR) = 1.38, 95% CI = 1.11–1.71, data not tabulated).

We also conducted sensitivity analyses, limiting the data set to observations for children without asthma and without an infection (as suggested by the reviewer) (Supplementary Table S2). This deletion of 1239 observations, or about 40% of the previous unweighted sample size, reduced the sample size from 3112 to 1873. There was no change in the direction of any regression coefficient. The only noteworthy difference between analyses is that the coefficient for the 90th percentile for CDII quartile 3 became statistically significant. Due to the significant reduction in the total number of observations, the appropriateness of the NHANES supplied survey weights becomes questionable.

4. Discussion

Results from this study showed that: (1) We were able to construct a global reference database for C-DII analogous to what we had done for the DII; and (2) Results from the construct validation indicated that the resulting C-DII scores were associated with CRP values among children 6 to 14 years of age in the NHANES data set. Analyses were performed to examine the association between three levels of the C-DII and the complete distribution of CRP using quantile regression. The major finding from these analyses is that CRP levels differ across the levels of the C-DII and the association of the C-DII is not constant across the CRP distribution. Specifically, we found that in level 2 of the C-DII there was significant increase in levels of CRP at the 50th, 55th, 70th, 75th, 80th, and 85th percentiles. This also is consistent with previous studies that have shown that quantile regression allows for the examination of outcomes at multiple levels, and is not influenced by outliers or skewness of the dependent variable [39]. Results in level 3 of the C-DII, representing the 3rd and 4th C-DII quartiles were more strongly in support of our hypothesis. Increased levels of the C-DII are associated with an increase in levels of CRP which is a risk factor for obesity and chronic disease.

Obesity is a pro-inflammatory state and childhood obesity is strongly associated with chronic inflammation and is on the rise [40–42]. It is known that obese children often become obese adults [43] and are more likely to suffer from insulin resistance [44], high blood pressure, unhealthy levels of serum lipids, and increased cardiovascular disease (CVD) risk [45]. This obesity epidemic is the result of specific changes in our environment and health-related behaviors [46,47]. High-calorie, inexpensive foods have become widely available and are heavily advertised [47,48]. Therefore, it is important to develop tools that can help monitor children's diet to tackle childhood obesity and its important correlate, inflammation.

Diet plays an essential role in the regulation of chronic inflammation [18,49–51]. Western diets rich in red meat, high-fat, sugar, dairy products, and refined grains have been associated with higher levels of CRP and other inflammatory markers [52,53]. Several studies have investigated individual food items such as meat or individual nutrients, such as vitamin C, and have observed associations with inflammation [54–59]. However, it is important to note that nutrients and individual foods are rarely consumed alone in a diet. Therefore, a nutrient or individual food effect may not be independent of the effect of other nutrients in the diet. Until recently, no dietary index was developed to predict inflammatory potential of whole diet; i.e., not just individual items or nutrients. Few research studies have investigated the effects of dietary indices such as the Healthy Eating Index (HEI), and Mediterranean Diet scores [60,61]. Therefore, there was a need to develop a comprehensive tool that can help children and their parents make healthier food choices that, in turn, can help reduce the risk of chronic diseases by directly influencing inflammation and preventing, or at least greatly limiting, weight gain.

The DII was developed and validated against inflammatory markers in adult populations and has been associated with a range of outcomes including cancer, metabolic syndrome, and asthma [19,62–65]. An important component of the DII calculation is the standardization of food parameter intake estimates to a "global" database of intake for the food parameters [19]. Furthermore, in developing the DII we identified eleven food consumption data sets from different parts of the world to represent a range of dietary intakes, which was used as the 'reference' database [19]. However, DII use among younger individuals (e.g., 6–14 year olds) is limited because of the "global" database used for this index. There are several barriers that prevent use of the current DII among children. The "global" standard database includes only adult dietary intakes and not all of the food parameters that comprise the DII (e.g., alcohol) may be appropriate for children dietary intake. Furthermore, we could not obtain data on garlic from any dataset we collected for the global database. Therefore, we developed C-DII, which can provide guidance for improving diets among children, and in combating obesity. Childhood obesity has been on the rise in the US, and obese children are more likely to become obese adults who experience risk factors associated with chronic disease risk [40–43,45]. Therefore, it is imperative that we create tools to monitor dietary patterns that can contribute to fluctuations in inflammation levels in the body resulting in obesity and chronic diseases [50,66]. To address this need, we developed the C-DII, which is based on the scoring algorithm of the DII.

A necessary step in the process was to identify dietary data collected in children from around the world. A total of 16 such data sets were obtained that included the US NHANES [30], the Korean NHANES [67], HELENA study (in ten European cities in Greece, Germany, Belgium, France, Hungary, Italy, Sweden, Austria, and Spain) [33], and a dataset from South Africa [68] that helped create the "world" database for C-DII.

The C-DII represents an innovative tool for evaluating the inflammatory potential of children's diet and it can be applied to any child population in which dietary information of sufficient quality has been gathered. The C-DII is not limited to data from 24-h recalls but can be used with a wide range of dietary data from various sources, including children-appropriate food frequency questionnaires (FFQ). The C-DII can be used to establish intervention strategies regarding an individual child's dietary goals to reduce inflammation and the risk of various health conditions [19].

This study has several strengths. It is the first study to develop and validate an index to explore the inflammatory potential of children's diet based on a global database. Second, it provided a unique opportunity to assess the inflammatory potential of diet in relation to CRP in a nationally representative sample. Third, it was possible to control for several confounding factors such as age, sex, race, BMI, and infection, and asthma.

Despite its strengths, there were several limitations to this study including a relative paucity of robust and reliable data on child nutrition. Regular public health surveillance of child nutrition occurs infrequently around the world, and few research studies have collected children dietary data, so to find reliable sources for these data was challenging, and not all datasets provided 100% complete dietary data. Additionally, we were limited by the availability of dietary data (i.e., a single 24-h dietary recall) in the NHANES.

5. Conclusions

Results indicate that the C-DII predicts CRP among children aged 6 to 14 years, and it appears that the C-DII is more strongly predictive of CRP among the higher levels CRP compared to lower levels of CRP. The C-DII can be used as a means for informing primary prevention and for educating physicians and other providers, parents and children on the importance of a healthy diet to reduce chronic disease rates and to enhance feelings of well-being and to improve quality of life. Further construct validation is required to deepen the understanding of the relationship between the C-DII and markers of inflammation in children. Additionally, more research should be focused on the role of diet in inflammation-related conditions in children.

Supplementary Materials: The following are available online at http://www.mdpi.com/2072-6643/10/8/993/s1, Table S1: Food Parameters available in different countries, Table S2: Shows the quantile regression coefficients for children's Dietary Inflammatory Index treated categorically with 3 levels (level 1 is the reference level) adjusted for sex, age, race, and BMI, NHANES, 2005–2012.

Author Contributions: N.S., M.D.W. and S.K. were involved in the design of the C-DII, analyzed the data and collaborated with J.R.H. in writing the original draft of the paper. C.R.A. provided data management and critical input in revising drafts of the paper. T.G.H. was involved in the design of the C-DII, provided data management expertise, and helped in writing the paper. A.O. was involved in analyzing the data, provided high-level statistical expertise and had input in writing the paper. J.R.H. devised the initial dietary inflammatory index concept, guided the design of all phases of developing the C-DII and took the lead in writing the paper.

Funding: This study was supported by the United States Department of Agriculture (USDA 12011784). A. Ortaglia and T. Hurley were not supported by this grant. The United States Department of Agriculture had no role in the design, analysis or writing of this article.

Acknowledgments: The authors wish to thank Seul Ki Choi, who helped with the KNHANES data, and Jumpei Kodama, who helped with the Japanese NHANES data.

Conflicts of Interest: CDII is a product of Connecting Health Innovations, a company planning to develop computer and smart phone applications for counseling and dietary intervention in children. Nitin Shivappa and Michael Wirth are employees of CHI, and James Hebert owns controlling interest in CHI.

References

1. Neumann, P.A.; Koch, S.; Hilgarth, R.S.; Perez-Chanona, E.; Denning, P.; Jobin, C.; Nusrat, A. Gut commensal bacteria and regional Wnt gene expression in the proximal versus distal colon. *Am. J. Pathol.* **2014**, *184*, 592–599. [CrossRef] [PubMed]
2. Shehzad, A.; Ha, T.; Subhan, F.; Lee, Y.S. New mechanisms and the anti-inflammatory role of curcumin in obesity and obesity-related metabolic diseases. *Eur. J. Nutr.* **2011**, *50*, 151–161. [CrossRef] [PubMed]
3. Maihöfner, C.; Charalambous, M.P.; Bhambra, U.; Lightfoot, T.; Geisslinger, G.; Gooderham, N.J. Expression of cyclooxygenase-2 parallels expression of interleukin-1beta, interleukin-6 and NF-kappaB in human colorectal cancer. *Carcinogenesis* **2003**, *24*, 665–671. [CrossRef] [PubMed]
4. McCullough, L.E.; Miller, E.E.; Calderwood, L.E.; Shivappa, N.; Steck, S.E.; Forman, M.R.; Mendez, M.A.; Maguire, R.; Fuemmeler, B.F.; Kollins, S.H.; et al. Maternal inflammatory diet and adverse pregnancy outcomes: Circulating cytokines and genomic imprinting as potential regulators? *Epigenetics* **2017**, *12*, 688–697. [CrossRef] [PubMed]
5. Chandra, R.K. Immunodeficiency in undernutrition and overnutrition. *Nutr. Rev.* **1981**, *39*, 225–231. [CrossRef] [PubMed]

6.   Chandra, R.K.; Tejpar, S. Diet and immunocompetence. *Int. J. Immunopharmacol.* **1983**, *5*, 175–180. [CrossRef]

7.   Chandra, R.K. Nutrition, immunity, and infection: Present knowledge and future directions. *Lancet* **1983**, *1*, 688–691. [PubMed]

8.   Kortman, G.A.; Mulder, M.L.; Richters, T.J.; Shanmugam, N.K.; Trebicka, E.; Boekhorst, J.; Timmerman, H.M.; Roelofs, R.; Wiegerinck, E.T.; Laarakkers, C.M.; et al. Low dietary iron intake restrains the intestinal inflammatory response and pathology of enteric infection by food-borne bacterial pathogens. *Eur. J. Immunol.* **2015**, *45*, 2553–2567. [CrossRef] [PubMed]

9.   Jones, K.D.; Thitiri, J.; Ngari, M.; Berkley, J.A. ; Childhood malnutrition: Toward an understanding of infections, inflammation, and antimicrobials. *Food Nutr. Bull.* **2014**, *35*, S64–S70. [CrossRef] [PubMed]

10.   Elenkov, I.J.; Iezzoni, D.G.; Daly, A.; Harris, A.G.; Chrousos, G.P. Cytokine dysregulation, inflammation and well-being. *Neuroimmunomodulation* **2005**, *12*, 255–269. [CrossRef] [PubMed]

11.   Kiecolt-Glaser, J.K.; Derry, H.M.; Fagundes, C.P. Inflammation: Depression fans the flames and feasts on the heat. *Am. J. Psychiatry* **2015**, *172*, 1075–1091. [CrossRef] [PubMed]

12.   Hebert, J.R. Growth monitoring: The "G" in GOBI FFF. In *Child Health and Survival: The UNICEF GOBI FFF Program*; Cash, R., Keusch, G.T., Lamstein, J., Eds.; Croom Helm: London, UK, 1987; pp. 11–20.

13.   Mathe, E.; Nguyen, G.H.; Funamizu, N.; He, P.; Moake, M.; Croce, C.M.; Hussain, S.P. Inflammation regulates microRNA expression in cooperation with p53 and nitric oxide. *Int. J. Cancer* **2012**, *131*, 760–765. [CrossRef] [PubMed]

14.   Larsen, J.M. The immune response to *Prevotella bacteria* in chronic inflammatory disease. *Immunology* **2017**, *151*, 363–374. [CrossRef] [PubMed]

15.   Kagnoff, M.F. Immunology of the intestinal tract. *Gastroenterology* **1993**, *105*, 1275–1280. [CrossRef]

16.   Saita, E.; Kondo, K.; Momiyama, Y. Anti-inflammatory diet for atherosclerosis and coronary artery disease: Antioxidant foods. *Clin. Med. Insights Cardiol.* **2014**, *8*, 61–65. [CrossRef] [PubMed]

17.   Ramallal, R.; Toledo, E.; Martinez, J.A.; Shivappa, N.; Hébert, J.R.; Martínez-González, M.A.; Ruiz-Canela, M. Inflammatory potential of diet, weight gain, and incidence of overweight/obesity: The SUN cohort. *Obesity* **2017**, *25*, 997–1005. [CrossRef] [PubMed]

18.   Cavicchia, P.P.; Steck, S.E.; Hurley, T.G.; Hussey, J.R.; Ma, Y.; Ockene, I.S.; Hébert, J.R. A new dietary inflammatory index predicts interval changes in high-sensitivity c-reactive protein. *J. Nutr.* **2009**, *139*, 2365–2372. [CrossRef] [PubMed]

19.   Shivappa, N.; Steck, S.E.; Hurley, T.G.; Hussey, J.R.; Hébert, J.R. Designing and developing a literature-derived population-based dietary inflammatory index. *Public Health Nutr.* **2014**, *17*, 1689–1696. [CrossRef] [PubMed]

20.   Shivappa, N.; Steck, S.E.; Hurley, T.G.; Hussey, J.R.; Ma, Y.; Ockene, I.S.; Tabung, F.; Hébert, J.R. A population-based dietary inflammatory index predicts levels of c-reactive protein (CRP) in the SEASONS Study. *Public Health Nutr.* **2014**, *17*, 1825–1833. [CrossRef] [PubMed]

21.   Shivappa, N.; Hebert, J.R.; Rietzschel, E.R.; De Buyzere, M.L.; Langlois, M.; Debruyne, E.; Marcos, A.; Huybrechts, I. Associations between dietary inflammatory index and inflammatory markers in the Asklepios Study. *Br. J. Nutr.* **2015**, *113*, 665–671. [CrossRef] [PubMed]

22.   Shivappa, N.; Wirth, M.D.; Hurley, T.G.; Hébert, J.R. Association between the Dietary Inflammatory Index (DII) and telomere length and C-reactive protein from the National Health and Nutrition Examination Survey-1999-2002. *Mol. Nutr. Food Res.* **2016**, *61*, 1600630. [CrossRef] [PubMed]

23.   Tabung, F.K.; Steck, S.E.; Zhang, J.; Ma, Y.; Liese, A.D.; Agalliu, I.; Hingle, M.; Hou, L.; Hurley, T.G.; Jiao, L.; et al. Construct validation of the dietary inflammatory index among postmenopausal women. *Ann. Epidemiol.* **2015**, *25*, 398–405. [CrossRef] [PubMed]

24.   Wirth, M.D.; Shivappa, N.; Davis, L.; Hurley, T.G.; Ortaglia, A.; Drayton, R.; Blair, S.N.; Hébert, J.R. Construct validation of the Dietary Inflammatory Index among African Americans. *J. Nutr. Health Aging* **2017**, *21*, 487–491. [CrossRef] [PubMed]

25.   Vahid, F.; Shivappa, N.; Hekmatdoost, A.; Hebert, J.R.; Davoodi, S.H.; Sadeghi, M. Association between Maternal Dietary Inflammatory Index (DII) and Abortion in Iranian Women and Validation of DII with Serum Concentration of Inflammatory Factors: Case-Control Study. *Appl. Physiol. Nutr. Metab.* **2017**, *42*, 511–516. [CrossRef] [PubMed]

26. Boden, S.; Wennberg, M.; Van Guelpen, B.; Johansson, I.; Lindahl, B.; Andersson, J.; Shivappa, N.; Hebert, J.R.; Nilsson, L.M. Dietary inflammatory index and risk of first myocardial infarction; a prospective population-based study. *Nutr. J.* **2017**, *16*, 21. [CrossRef] [PubMed]

27. Ge, I.; Rudolph, A.; Shivappa, N.; Flesch-Janys, D.; Hébert, J.R.; Chang-Claude, J. Dietary inflammation potential and postmenopausal breast cancer risk in a German case-control study. *Breast* **2015**, *24*, 491–496. [CrossRef] [PubMed]

28. Peres, L.C.; Bandera, E.V.; Qin, B.; Guertin, K.A.; Shivappa, N.; Hebert, J.R.; Abbott, S.E.; Alberg, A.J.; Barnholtz-Sloan, J.; Bondy, M.; et al. Dietary Inflammatory Index and Risk of Epithelial Ovarian Cancer in African American Women. *Int. J. Cancer* **2017**, *140*, 535–543. [CrossRef] [PubMed]

29. Harmon, B.E.; Wirth, M.D.; Boushey, C.J.; Wilkens, L.R.; Draluck, E.; Shivappa, N.; Steck, S.E.; Hofseth, L.; Haiman, C.A.; Le Marchand, L.; et al. The Dietary Inflammatory Index Is Associated with Colorectal Cancer Risk in the Multiethnic Cohort. *J. Nutr.* **2017**, *147*, 430–438. [CrossRef] [PubMed]

30. *2005–2011 National Health and Nutrition Examination Survey (NHANES)*; Centers for Disease Control and Prevention, US Department of Health and Human Services: Hyattsville, MD, USA, 2011.

31. Commonwealth Scientific Industrial Research Organisation (CSIRO). *2007 Australian National Children's Nutrition and Physical Activity Survey: Main Findings*; Australian Bureau of Statistics, Australian Government Publishing Service: Canberra, Australia, 2008.

32. Ministry of Health, Labour and Welfare, Tokyo, Japan. National Health and Nutrition Survey, Continuous through Sept 2017. Available online: http://www.mhlw.go.jp/bunya/kenkou/kenkou_eiyou_chousa.html (accessed on 26 July 2018).

33. Shivappa, N.; Hebert, J.R.; Marcos, A.; Diaz, L.E.; Gomez, S.; Nova, E.; Michels, N.; Arouca, A.; González-Gil, E.; Frederic, G.; et al. Association between dietary inflammatory index and inflammatory markers in the HELENA study. *Mol. Nutr. Food Res.* **2017**, *61*, 1600707. [CrossRef] [PubMed]

34. Bernal, J.; Lorenzana, A. Dietary diversity and associated factors among beneficiaries of 77 child care centers: Central Regional, Venezuela. *Arch. Latinoam. Nutr.* **2003**, *53*, 52–58.

35. Ali, H.; Ng, S.; Zaghloul, S.; Harrison, G.G.; Qazaq, H.S.; El Sadig, M.; Yeatts, K. ; High proportion of 6 to 18-year-old children and adolescents in the United Arab Emirates are not meeting dietary recommendations. *Nutr. Res.* **2013**, *33*, 447–456. [CrossRef] [PubMed]

36. Liberona, Y.; Castillo, O.; Engler, V.; Villarroel, L.; Rozowski, J. Nutritional profile of schoolchildren from different socio-economic levels in Santiago, Chile. *Public Health Nutr.* **2010**, *14*, 142–149. [CrossRef] [PubMed]

37. US Centers for Disease Control and Prevention (CDC), National Center for Health Statistics. National Health and Nutrition Examination Survey. Atlanta, GA, USA. Available online: https://www.cdc.gov/nchs/nhanes/index.htm (accessed on 26 July 2018).

38. Lumley, T. *Complex. Surveys: A Guide to Analysis Using R*; John Wiley & Sons: Hoboken, NJ, USA, 2010.

39. Bottai, M.; Frongillo, E.A.; Sui, X.; O'Neill, J.R.; McKeown, R.E.; Burns, T.L.; Liese, A.D.; Blair, S.N.; Pate, R.R. Use of Quantile Regression to Investigate the Longitudinal Association between Physical Activity and Body Mass Index. *Obesity* **2014**, *22*, E149–E156. [CrossRef] [PubMed]

40. Ogden, C.L.; Carroll, M.D.; Curtin, L.R.; McDowell, M.A.; Tabak, C.J.; Flegal, K.M. Prevalence of overweight and obesity in the United States, 1999–2004. *JAMA* **2006**, *295*, 1549–1555. [CrossRef] [PubMed]

41. Ogden, C.L.; Carroll, M.D.; Curtin, L.R.; Lamb, M.M.; Flegal, K.M. Prevalence of high body mass index in US children and adolescents, 2007–2008. *JAMA* **2010**, *303*, 242–249. [CrossRef] [PubMed]

42. Ogden, C.L.; Carroll, M.D.; Kit, B.K.; Flegal, K.M. Prevalence of Childhood and Adult Obesity in the United States, 2011–2012. *JAMA* **2014**, *311*, 806–814. [CrossRef] [PubMed]

43. Freedman, D.S.; Khan, L.K.; Serdula, M.K.; Dietz, W.H.; Srinivasan, S.R. The relation of childhood BMI to adult adiposity: The Bogalusa Heart Study. *Pediatrics* **2005**, *115*, 22–27. [CrossRef] [PubMed]

44. Nathan, B.M.; Moran, A. Metabolic complications of obesity in childhood and adolescence: More than just diabetes. *Curr. Opin. Endocrinol.* **2008**, *15*, 21–29. [CrossRef] [PubMed]

45. Sen, S.; Rifas-Shiman, S.L.; Shivappa, N.; Wirth, M.D.; Hebert, J.R.; Gold, D.R.; Gillman, M.W.; Oken, E. Associations of prenatal and early life dietary inflammatory potential with childhood adiposity and cardiometabolic risk in Project Viva. *Pediatr. Obes.* **2018**, *13*, 292–300. [CrossRef] [PubMed]

46. Nielsen, S.J.; Siega-Riz, A.M.; Popkin, B.M. Trends in energy intake in U.S. between 1977 and 1996: Similar shifts seen across age groups. *Obes. Res.* **2002**, *10*, 370–378. [CrossRef] [PubMed]

47. Nielsen, S.J.; Popkin, B.M. Patterns and trends in food portion sizes, 1977–1998. *JAMA* **2003**, *289*, 450–453. [CrossRef] [PubMed]

48. Nielsen, S.J.; Popkin, B.M. Changes in beverage intake between 1977 and 2001. *Am. J. Prev. Med.* **2004**, *27*, 205–210. [CrossRef] [PubMed]

49. Cui, X.; Jin, Y.; Singh, U.P.; Chumanevich, A.A.; Harmon, B.; Cavicchia, P.; Hofseth, A.B.; Kotakadi, V.; Poudyal, D.; Stroud, B.; et al. Suppression of DNA damage in human peripheral blood lymphocytes by a juice concentrate: A randomized, double-blind, placebo-controlled trial. *Mol. Nutr. Food Res.* **2012**, *56*, 666–670. [CrossRef] [PubMed]

50. Giugliano, D.; Ceriello, A.; Esposito, K. The effects of diet on inflammation: Emphasis on the metabolic syndrome. *J. Am. Coll. Cardiol.* **2006**, *48*, 677–685. [CrossRef] [PubMed]

51. Porrata-Maury, C.; Hernandez-Triana, M.; Rodriguez-Sotero, E.; Vilá-Dacosta-Calheiros, R.; Hernández-Hernández, H.; Mirabal-Sosa, M.; Campa-Huergo, C.; Pianesi, M. Medium- and short-term interventions with ma-pi 2 macrobiotic diet in type 2 diabetic adults of Bauta, Havana. *J. Nutr. Metab.* **2012**, *2012*, 856342. [CrossRef] [PubMed]

52. Hickling, S.; Hung, J.; Knuiman, M.; Divitini, M.; Beilby, J. Are the associations between diet and C-reactive protein independent of obesity? *Prev. Med.* **2008**, *47*, 71–76. [CrossRef] [PubMed]

53. Lopez-Garcia, E.; Schulze, M.B.; Manson, J.E.; Meigs, J.B.; Albert, C.M.; Rifai, N.; Willett, W.C.; Hu, F.B. Consumption of (*n*-3) fatty acids is related to plasma biomarkers of inflammation and endothelial activation in women. *J. Nutr.* **2004**, *134*, 1806–1811. [CrossRef] [PubMed]

54. Bertran, N.; Camps, J.; Fernandez-Ballart, J.; Arija, V.; Ferre, N.; Tous, M.; Simo, D.; Murphy, M.M.; Vilella, E.; Joven, J. Diet and lifestyle are associated with serum C-reactive protein concentrations in a population-based study. *J. Lab. Clin. Med.* **2005**, *145*, 41–46. [CrossRef] [PubMed]

55. Esmaillzadeh, A.; Kimiagar, M.; Mehrabi, Y.; Azadbakht, L.; Hu, F.B.; Willett, W.C. Fruit and vegetable intakes, C-reactive protein, and the metabolic syndrome. *Am. J. Clin. Nutr.* **2006**, *84*, 1489–1497. [CrossRef] [PubMed]

56. King, D.E.; Mainous, A.G., III; Geesey, M.E.; Woolson, R.F. Dietary magnesium and C-reactive protein levels. *J. Am. Coll. Nutr.* **2005**, *24*, 166–171. [CrossRef] [PubMed]

57. Ma, Y.; Griffith, J.A.; Chasan-Taber, L.; Olendzki, B.C.; Jackson, E.; Sanek, E.J., III; Li, W.; Pagoto, S.L.; Hafner, A.R.; Ockene, I.S. Association between dietary fiber and serum C-reactive protein. *Am. J. Clin. Nutr.* **2006**, *83*, 760–766. [CrossRef] [PubMed]

58. Viscogliosi, G.; Cipriani, E.; Liguori, M.L.; Marigliano, B.; Saliola, M.; Ettorre, E.; Andreozzi, P. Mediterranean dietary pattern adherence: Associations with prediabetes, metabolic syndrome, and related microinflammation. *Metab.. Syndr. Relat. Disord.* **2013**, *11*, 210–216. [CrossRef] [PubMed]

59. Wannamethee, S.G.; Lowe, G.D.; Rumley, A.; Bruckdorfer, K.R.; Whincup, P.H. Associations of vitamin C status, fruit and vegetable intakes, and markers of inflammation and hemostasis. *Am. J. Clin. Nutr.* **2006**, *83*, 567–574. [CrossRef] [PubMed]

60. Boynton, A.; Neuhouser, M.L.; Wener, M.H.; Wood, B.; Sorensen, B.; Chen-Levy, Z.; Kirk, E.A.; Yasui, Y.; Lacroix, K.; McTiernan, A. Associations between healthy eating patterns and immune function or inflammation in overweight or obese postmenopausal women. *Am. J. Clin. Nutr.* **2007**, *86*, 1445–1455. [CrossRef] [PubMed]

61. Serrano-Martinez, M.; Palacios, M.; Martinez-Losa, E.; Lezaun, R.; Maravi, C.; Prado, M.; Martínez, J.A.; Martinez-Gonzalez, M.A. A Mediterranean dietary style influences TNF-alpha and VCAM-1 coronary blood levels in unstable angina patients. *Eur. J. Nutr.* **2005**, *44*, 348–354. [CrossRef] [PubMed]

62. Wirth, M.D.; Burch, J.; Shivappa, N.; Violanti, J.M.; Burchfiel, C.M.; Fekedulegn, D.; Andrew, M.E.; Hartley, T.A.; Miller, D.B.; Mnatsakanova, A.; et al. Association of a dietary inflammatory index with inflammatory indices and metabolic syndrome among police officers. *J. Occup. Environ. Med.* **2014**, *56*, 986–989. [CrossRef] [PubMed]

63. Shivappa, N.; Bosetti, C.; Zucchetto, A.; Serraino, D.; La Vecchia, C.; Hébert, J.R. Dietary inflammatory index and risk of pancreatic cancer in an Italian case-control study. *Br. J. Nutr.* **2015**, *113*, 292–298. [CrossRef] [PubMed]

64. Hebert, J.R.; Shivappa, N.; Tabung, F.K.; Steck, S.E.; Wirth, M.D.; Hurley, T.G. On the use of the dietary inflammatory index in relation to low-grade inflammation and markers of glucose metabolism in the Cohort study on Diabetes and Atherosclerosis Maastricht (CODAM) and the Hoorn study. *Am. J. Clin. Nutr.* **2014**, *99*, 1520. [CrossRef] [PubMed]

65. Wood, L.G.; Shivappa, N.; Berthon, B.S.; Gibson, P.G.; Hebert, J.R. Dietary inflammatory index is related to asthma risk, lung function and systemic inflammation in asthma. *Clin. Exp. Allergy* **2015**, *45*, 177–183. [CrossRef] [PubMed]

66. Saneei, P.; Hashemipour, M.; Kelishadi, R.; Esmaillzadeh, A. The Dietary Approaches to Stop Hypertension (DASH) diet affects inflammation in childhood metabolic syndrome: A randomized cross-over clinical trial. *Ann. Nutr. Metab.* **2014**, *64*, 20–27. [CrossRef] [PubMed]

67. Shim, Y.J.P.H. Reanalysis of 2007 Korean National Health and Nutrition Examination Survey (2007 KNHANES) Results by CAN-Pro 3.0 Nutrient Database. *Korean J. Nutr.* **2009**, *42*, 577–595. [CrossRef]

68. Oldewage-Theron, W.; Kruger, R. The association between diet quality and subclinical inflammation among children aged 6–18 years in the Eastern Cape, South Africa. *Public Health Nutr.* **2017**, *20*, 102–111. [CrossRef] [PubMed]

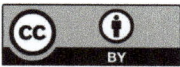

nutrients

MDPI

Article

Development of a Quality Score for the Home Food Environment Using the Home-IDEA2 and the Healthy Eating Index-2010

Sarah K. Hibbs-Shipp [1], Richard E. Boles [2], Susan L. Johnson [2], Morgan L. McCloskey [1], Savannah Hobbs [1] and Laura L. Bellows [1,*]

[1] Department of Food Science and Human Nutrition, Colorado State University, Fort Collins, CO 80523, USA; sarah.hibbs-shipp@colostate.edu (S.K.H.-S.); morgan.mccloskey@colostate.edu (M.L.M.); savannah.hobbs@colostate.edu (S.H.)
[2] Department of Pediatrics, University of Colorado Anschutz Medical Campus, Aurora, CO 80045, USA; Richard.boles@ucdenver.edu (R.E.B.); Susan.Johnson@ucdenver.edu (S.L.J.)
* Correspondence: laura.bellows@colostate.edu; Tel.: +1-970-491-1305

Received: 10 January 2019; Accepted: 4 February 2019; Published: 12 February 2019

Abstract: The home food environment (HFE) is an important factor in the development of food preferences and habits in young children, and the availability of foods within the home reflects dietary intake in both adults and children. Therefore, it is important to consider the holistic quality of the HFE. The purpose of this study was to apply the Healthy Eating Index (HEI; a measure of diet quality in conformance to the Dietary Guidelines for Americans) algorithm to the Home-IDEA2, a valid and reliable food inventory checklist, to develop a Home-IDEA2 HEI Score. After an initial score was developed, it was psychometrically tested for content, criterion, and construct validity. Content validity testing resulted in 104 foods being retained. Internal criterion testing demonstrated that 42 foods (40%) changed component scores by >5%; however, no single food changed a total Home-IDEA2 HEI score by >5%. Testing of hypothetical HFEs resulted in a range of scores in the expected directions, establishing sensitivity to varied HFEs. This study resulted in a validated methodology to assess the overall quality of the HFE, thus contributing a novel approach for examining home food environments. Future research can test interventions modifying the HFE quality to improve individual dietary intake.

Keywords: home food environment; Healthy Eating Index; dietary quality; validation; psychometric

1. Introduction

In recent years, dietary research has expanded to assess not only the foods eaten, but also the context in which the food is eaten (e.g., at home versus away from home) [1–3] and where the food was obtained (e.g., fast-food [4], sit down restaurant [5], convenience store [6,7], grocery store [8,9], school/cafeteria [10], or vending machine [9]) [11,12]. One of these areas of expanding research is the home food environment (HFE), which provides context for individual and family dietary intake [13]. The HFE has received increasing attention as an important factor in the development of food preferences and habits in children, as a contributor to obesogenic environments, and as a modifiable factor for nutritional interventions, especially those targeting childhood obesity [13–15].

The HFE is influenced by factors that include food purchasing and preparation decisions, food availability, and food accessibility [16,17]. The HFE impacts children's diet not only through examples of eating habits, but also through the actual foods that are readily available and accessible in the home [18,19]. The availability of foods within the home has been shown to reflect intake in both adults and children, and as such, provides a potential dietary intervention point [3]. Intervention targets for improving children's dietary behaviors should focus on the availability and accessibility of a spectrum of foods, including increasing healthful foods as well as reducing foods and beverages that are energy-dense and nutrient poor [20].

This increasing recognition of the environmental context of dietary intake has led to a large increase in the number of tools available for assessing a given environment with regard to availability of foods. Often HFE tools were designed to fit the researchers' immediate questions and were brief, focused on only one aspect of food availability—such as high-fat foods, sugar-sweetened beverages, or fruits & vegetables—and had limited psychometric testing performed [21]. Small food sets and a lack of a complete listing of foods in most HFE assessments has limited researchers' abilities to examine the totality of the HFE and its contributions to dietary quality.

The Home Inventory to Describe Eating and Activity (Home-IDEA2) is one such assessment that has been found to be valid and reliable in assessing food, activity, and electronic home environments among low-income minority parents of preschoolers [22]. The Home-IDEA2 is a semi-comprehensive checklist designed to assess the foods present in the home at a single point in time. It includes foods sourced from the Allowable Foods List from the US Special Supplemental Nutrition Program for Women, Infants, and Children (WIC Program), the Block Food Frequency Questionnaire, and the modified Harvard Food Frequency Questionnaire (FFQ), allowing for application to diverse households.

Given the relationship between the HFE and dietary intake, it is important to consider the HFE beyond the presence and absence of individual foods, and examine the holistic quality of the entire HFE. The Healthy Eating Index (HEI), developed by the National Cancer Institute, is the method of choice in the US for assessing dietary quality [23]. The HEI is a formalized approach that includes rules and analysis algorithms allowing for effective comparisons in the overall quality of foods across different levels of the food supply [23,24]. HEI algorithms have been applied to the US food supply level [25], the community food environment (e.g., food assistance program offerings [26], supermarket sales circulars [27], menu offerings [4], corner stores [28], grocery purchases [29], by multiple food purchase locations [30]), and at the individual food intake level (e.g., comparing diet cost to diet quality [31], comparing different dietary patterns [32–35], and evaluating differences in mortality outcomes by diet quality [36]). To date, the HEI algorithm has been applied to the HFE in one recent study [37], which demonstrates a need for more rigorous validation and psychometric testing. Application of the HEI to the HFE provides a unique way of assessing overall quality of the HFE, and allows for direct comparison to dietary intake quality, thus providing the potential for further insights into the relationship between the HFE, dietary intake, and health outcomes.

For this study, the Home-IDEA2 was used as an instrument to apply the HEI algorithm to assess the quality of the HFE. Specific objectives were to (1) develop an initial Home-IDEA2 HEI Score, and (2) psychometrically test the Home-IDEA2 HEI Score for content, criterion, and construct validity.

2. Materials and Methods

2.1. Development of an Initial Home-IDEA2 Healthy Eating Index Score

2.1.1. Application of the HEI Algorithm to the Home-IDEA2

The Healthy Eating Index (HEI) is updated to conform to each edition of the Dietary Guidelines for Americans (DGA), with the HEI-2010 [23] reflecting diet patterning in conformance with the 2010-DGAs [38]. The HEI-2010 was used, as the HEI-2015 was not yet available during the development of the Home-IDEA2 HEI Score. Briefly, the HEI-2010 scores 12 dietary components for a total score ranging from 0–100 (Table 1), with total scores less than 51 categorized as 'poor,' 51–80 as 'needs improvement,' and greater than 80 as 'good' [39]. The HEI has been applied to other food supply levels using three steps: (1) identification of a set of foods, (2) determination of the amount of each dietary constituent associated with each food in the set, and (3) deriving ratios to score each HEI component using developed algorithms [40].

Table 1. Healthy Eating Index-2010 components and scoring standards.

HEI-2010 Components	Maximum Points	Standard for Maximum Score (per 1000 kcal) [a]	Standard for Minimum Score of Zero (per 1000 kcal) [a]
Adequacy			
Total Fruit [b]	5	≥0.8 cup equiv. (102 g)	No Fruit
Whole Fruit [c]	5	≥0.4 cup equiv. (51 g)	No Whole Fruit
Total Vegetables [d]	5	≥1.1 cup equiv. (141 g)	No Vegetables
Greens & Beans [d]	5	≥0.2 cup equiv. (26 g)	No Dark Green Vegetables or Beans/Peas
Whole Grains	10	≥1.5 oz equiv. (42 g)	No Whole Grains
Dairy [e]	10	≥1.3 cup equiv. (166 g)	No Dairy
Total Protein Foods [f]	5	≥2.5 oz equiv. (71 g)	No Protein Foods
Seafood & Plant Proteins [f,g]	5	≥0.8 oz equiv. (23 g)	No Seafood or Plant Proteins
Fatty Acid Ratio [h]	10	(PUFAs + MUFAs)/SFA ≥2.5	(PUFAs + MUFAs)/SFA ≤1.2
Moderation			
Refined Grains	10	≤1.8 oz equiv. (~51.0 g)	≥4.3 oz equiv. (122 g)
Sodium	10	≤1.1 g	≥2.0 g
Empty Calories [i]	20	≤19% of energy	≥50% of energy
Total Score [j]	100		

Adapted from the National Cancer Institute's HEI-2010 Components & Scoring Standards Table [41]. (Development of the scoring rubric has been previously described in detail [42]. [a] Amounts between the minimum and maximum scores are scored proportionately. [b] Includes 100% fruit juice. [c] Includes all forms except juice. [d] Includes any beans and peas not counted as total protein foods. [e] Includes all milk products, such as fluid milk, yogurt, and cheese, and fortified soy beverages. [f] Beans and peas are included here (and not with vegetables) when the total protein foods standard is otherwise not met. [g] Includes seafood, nuts, seeds, and soy products (other than beverages), as well as beans and peas counted as total protein foods. [h] Ratio of poly- and monounsaturated fatty acids (PUFAS and MUFAS) to saturated fatty acids (SFAs): (PUFAs + MUFAs)/SFA. [i] Calories from solid fats, alcohol, and added sugars; threshold for counting alcohol is >13 g/1000 kcal. [j] The Center for Nutrition Policy and Promotion categorizes total scores as poor (less than 51), needs improvement (51–80), and good (greater than 80) [39]. Abbreviations: HEI: Healthy Eating Index; equiv., equivalents; oz., ounces; g., grams.

The Home-IDEA2 (the self-report checklist that participants complete regarding availability of select food items in the home) includes 108 food items that represent a wide variety of potential types of foods in the home. For example, there are single-items, such as "apple," that represent all types of raw apples (Granny Smith, Macintosh, Red Delicious). There are also composite items that represent a "category" of similar items, such as "citrus fruits" representing oranges, tangerines, mandarins, grapefruit, lemons, limes, etc. All items, whether single or composite, are completed in terms of "Yes/No" availability in the home. No information is obtained as to how much of these items are in the home, rather, the presence or absence of the listed foods is assessed.

The Home-IDEA2 was chosen as the basis for developing a HFE quality score using the HEI for four reasons: (1) the high feasibility for individuals to complete the survey [22], (2) the included foods are relevant to socioeconomically, racially/ethnically, and geographically diverse families with young children [43,44], (3) it has been psychometrically validated [22,44], and (4) it has demonstrated positive associations with dietary intake for a broad range of foods ranging from healthy and less healthy foods in families with young children [43]. In order to apply the HEI to the Home-IDEA2, USDA's Center for Nutrition Policy and Promotion's recommended processes were modified to include the HFE, and a 3 step process was followed (Figure 1) [40]. Because all foods in the Home-IDEA2 are listed generically and without amounts, a 'representative' food identifying a specific food code that links to the Food and Nutrition Database for Dietary Studies (FNDDS) and a representative food amount for each Home-IDEA2 item needed to be assigned to apply nutrient values before ratios and HEI score components could be derived.

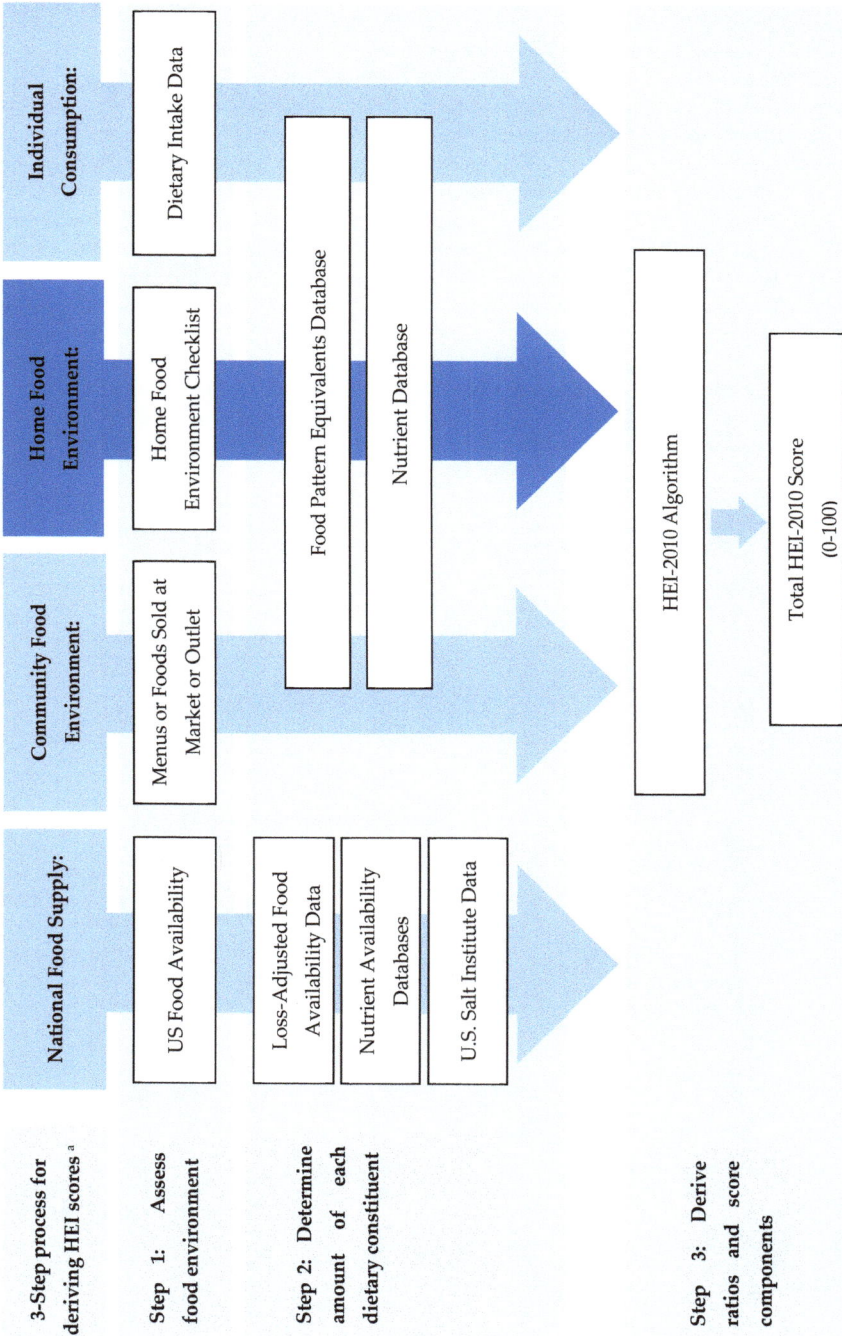

Figure 1. Three step process for deriving Healthy Eating Index (HEI) scores across different levels of the food system. [a] Figure adapted from Calculating HEI Scores at Different Levels, the HEI scoring illustration [45].

2.1.2. Representative Foods

The representative foods and food amounts for the Home-IDEA2 items were sourced from the FoodAPS, a national survey of 4826 ethnically and income-diverse U.S. households conducted by the USDA Economic Research Service (ERS) and Food and Nutrition Service (FNS) between April 2012 and January 2013 [46]. The publicly available, de-identified, food-at-home dataset was used for this study (faps_fahnutrients, downloaded 26 January 2017) [46]. A multi-part process was employed to identify a representative food for each Home-IDEA2 item. First, a keyword search within the FoodAPS file was conducted for foods that matched each Home-IDEA2 item. Next, four investigators with expertise in nutrition and psychometric testing evaluated the identified foods for face validity with Home-IDEA2 items and reasonableness for low-income, multi-ethnic households. These foods were discussed by the research team until consensus was achieved. Last, remaining options were evaluated for key nutrients/nutrient categories (e.g., sodium, whole fruit, whole grains) theorized to load into the HEI-2010 algorithm, with the food closest to the mean or median of the key nutrients/nutrient categories selected as the 'representative' food for each Home-IDEA2 item. Table 2 outlines key considerations for the selection of the representative food for citrus fruits.

Table 2. Sample considerations for the selection of the representative food for Home-IDEA2 Category of citrus fruits.

Potential Representative Food Item	HEI Component Score	Presence in Households [a]	Availability, Consumption and Other Considerations	Selection Decision
Oranges	Whole fruit; Total fruit	Common	*Availability:* Year-round; *Consumed:* As whole fruit	Selected (food code 61119010)
Clementines (Cuties®)	Whole fruit; Total fruit	Common	*Availability:* Seasonal; *Consumed:* As whole fruit	Not selected due to seasonality
Mandarins	Whole fruit; Total fruit; SOFAAS (added sugars)	Common	*Availability:* Seasonal (fresh); Year Round (packaged); *Consumed:* As whole fruit; *Other:* Packed in juice and syrup; contains added sugars	Not selected due to contribution of added sugars
Grapefruit	Whole fruit; Total fruit; SOFAAS (added sugars)	Less common	*Availability:* Seasonal (fresh); Year Round (packaged); *Consumed:* As whole fruit; *Other:* Packed in juice and syrup; contains added sugars	Not selected due low presence in households and contribution of added sugars
Tangerine	Whole fruit; Total fruit	Less common	*Availability:* Seasonal; *Consumed:* As whole fruit	Not selected due to low presence in households and seasonality
Lemons	Whole fruit; Total fruit	Common	*Availability:* Year-round; *Consumed:* Not typically eaten in whole as fruit	Not selected because not typically consumed as whole fruit
Limes	Whole fruit; Total fruit	Common	*Availability:* Year-round; *Consumed:* Not typically eaten in whole as fruit	Not selected because not typically consumed as whole fruit

[a] Presence in households was determined based on frequencies from Home-IDEA2 administered with a low-income, minority population (unpublished data). Abbreviations: HEI: Healthy Eating Index; Home-IDEA: Home Inventory Describing Eating and Activity; SoFAAS: Solid Fats, Alcohol, Added Sugars.

2.1.3. Food Amounts

For each representative food, food amounts were then selected. Within the FoodAPS dataset, the mean, median, and mode of available total edible gram weights were calculated for each representative food. Next, an internet search for standard consumer package sizes was performed. Calculated weights were adjusted to reflect reasonable package sizes for consistency across foods (e.g., milk varieties (whole, 2%, 1% skim, chocolate) were normalized to 1 gallon (3.8 L), cheese varieties (regular, low-fat) were normalized to 1 pound (454 g), meat varieties (chicken, beef) were normalized to 2 pounds (908 g), and for realistic purchase quantities (e.g., vegetable oil was reduced from 1 gallon (3.8 L) to 32 ounces (1 L)).

2.1.4. Ratios and HEI Score Components

The nutritional content for the representative foods and selected food amounts were merged with the Home-IDEA2 to create the Home-IDEA2 HEI Score database. The Home-IDEA2 captures a snapshot of the home at a single point in time, similar to a single dietary recall for one person; therefore, the HEI algorithm selected was "Calculating an individual's HEI-2010 score, using FPED, and one day of 24HR recall" [47]. Two nutrient files were created, mirroring the layout of individual dietary intake nutrient analysis files obtained from the Automated Self-Administered 24-h Recall System (ASA24), the INFMYPHEI (Items/Individuals Foods and Pyramid Equivalents Data), and TNMYPHEI (Total/Daily Total Nutrient and Pyramid Equivalents Data) files [48]. The algorithm was then applied to the Home-IDEA2 HEI Score database to generate HEI component and total scores.

2.2. Psychometric Testing on the Home-IDEA2 HEI Score

Extensive validation and psychometric testing was performed to test the functionality of the Home-IDEA2 HEI Score. Face validity was assessed throughout the selection of the representative foods and food amounts. Decisions were made to match the intention of Home-IDEA2 items and to control for foods that might reasonably be found in participants' homes. Content, internal criterion, and construct validity were also tested (Table 3).

Table 3. Development and initial validation of Home-IDEA2 HEI Score.

	Validity Measure	Research Question	Analysis Strategy
Objective 1: Develop an initial Home-IDEA2 HEI Score	Face	Do the representative food items and amounts selected represent the intent of each Home-IDEA2 item? Would the representative foods be reasonably found in the target population homes?	Expert review of representative foods and food amounts, including comparison to standard consumer packaging sizes
Objective 2: Psychometric Testing of Home-IDEA2 HEI Score	Content	Do the representative foods feed into the HEI component and total scores as theorized?	Iterative runs of the HEI-2010 algorithm on the Home-IDEA2 HEI Score Database; each food was removed individually and changes in scores were visually examined
	Criterion	Are there any individual representative foods that impact HEI component or total scores more substantially than other foods?	Iterative runs of the HEI-2010 algorithm on the Home-IDEA2 HEI Score Database; each food was removed individually and changes in scores were visually examined
	Construct	Does the Home-IDEA2 HEI Score identify different home food environments?	Test the Home-IDEA2 HEI Score on five sample Home-IDEA2 checklists representing varying diet patterns (CACFP, DASH, vegetarian, moderately processed, highly processed)

2.2.1. Content and Criterion Validity

Content and internal criterion validity were examined through over 300 rounds of iterative testing in the application of the HEI algorithm to the Home-IDEA2 HEI Score database. Iterative testing involved the removal of each food from the Home-IDEA2 HEI Score database to determine if the representative food was loading into the component scores as theorized (content validity), and to test the individual and cumulative group contributions of each food to component and total scores (internal criterion validity). The effect size was calculated by the percent change in both the component and total score after the removal of each individual food item from the total pattern. Due to the patterning nature of the HEI algorithm, it was necessary to test for inappropriately high effects of individual representative food loadings on component and total scores.

2.2.2. Construct Validity

Construct validity was assessed with five sample Home-IDEA2 checklists that were created to represent various diet patterns ranging from minimally healthful (theorized low HEI score) to very healthful (theorized high HEI score). These patterns included a highly processed pattern, a moderately processed pattern, a vegetarian pattern with minimal processed foods, and two dietary patterns that were used as evidence-based referent groups: the DASH diet [49], and a pattern based on the Dietary Guidelines for Americans (DGA) [50]. To test adherence to the DGA, a Child and Adult Care Food Program (CACFP) weekly menu was used to create the sample checklist. These food patterns were selected to examine sensitivity, and to evaluate if our tool and the resulting quality score would produce different scores for different home food environments. All analyses were conducted using SAS (version 9.4; SAS Institute Inc., Cary, NC, USA). The HEI-2010 algorithm was provided by the National Cancer Institute [40].

3. Results

3.1. Development of an Initial Home-IDEA2 HEI Score

In the process of determining representative foods from the FoodAPS, two Home-IDEA2 items were eliminated. "Unprepared mixes" was eliminated due to the complexity of options available, which did not allow for an accurate selection of a single representative food, and there were no options for "tortilla, other" outside of corn or flour, which were already captured as individual food items. In the process of determining food amounts, two additional Home-IDEA2 items were removed due to a lack of total edible gram (TEG) weights (rice cakes), and a TEG weight that had no comparable consumer purchase size (deer—the TEG from the FoodAPS database represented an entire deer carcass), leaving 104 foods in the Home-IDEA2 HEI Score database.

3.2. Psychometric Testing on the Home-IDEA2 HEI Score

3.2.1. Content and Criterion Validity

In testing content validity, results from iterative testing showed that two foods (those representing chocolate/candy and unsweetened cereal) did not load into component scores as initially hypothesized. Therefore, changes were made to the representative foods initially selected for chocolate/candy and unsweetened cereal to correct component score loading and maintain the original intent of the food within the Home-IDEA2. Inconsistent effects in component outcomes were also observed for processed food items and cooking oils/fats. Food amounts were adjusted to create similar effect sizes on component scores within each food category (e.g., fruits, processed foods, grains, cooking oils).

Iterative testing was then repeated to confirm changes in effect sizes for component and total scores. Internal criterion validity was demonstrated, as each representative food had larger percentage effect sizes in the relevant component score(s) than in the total score (Table 4). Five foods—ramen, brown rice, broccoli, grapes, and vegetable oil—were highlighted, as they were the foods in the

Home-IDEA2 HEI Score database that had the largest impact in a given component score: e.g., Sodium, Whole Grain, Whole Fruit, and Fatty Acid Ratios, respectively. Despite larger changes to component scores, there was no single food that resulted in a change of greater than 5% to the total score. For example, the absence of broccoli from a household yielded a 21.1% negative change to the Greens and Beans component score, but only a negative 1.2% change to the total score. Of the 104 foods in the Home-IDEA2 HEI Score database, 42 affected a change of at least 5% in one or more component scores when removed from analysis. Of those 42 foods, 13 affected a 10–20% change, with 2 affecting over a 20% change (broccoli: −21.1% change in Greens and Beans; vegetable oil: −31.1% change in Fatty Acid Ratio). This demonstrated internal criterion validity with regard to the intent of the algorithm (i.e., component scores represent individual food contribution, whereas the total score represents the overall patterning) [24].

Table 4. Criterion validity testing: percent (%) change values for HEI-2010 components and total score when specified food was removed from the Home-IDEA2 HEI Score database for 5 example foods.

HEI-2010 Component	Percent (%) Change [a]				
	Ramen	Brown Rice	Broccoli	Grapes	Vegetable Oil
Adequacy					
Total Fruit	2.0	0.7	0.1	−5.3	5.5
Whole Fruit	3.3	1.2	0.1	−10.7	5.1
Total Vegetables	2.0	0.7	−3.8	0.3	5.4
Greens and Beans	0.7	0.3	−21.1	0.1	2.0
Whole Grains	2.2	−7.3	0.1	0.3	5.9
Dairy	2.6	0.9	0.1	0.3	7.0
Total Protein Foods	3.0	1.1	0.1	0.4	8.2
Seafood and Plant Proteins	0.0	0.0	0.0	0.0	0.0
Fatty Acid Ratio	4.2	-0.1	0.0	0.0	−31.1
Moderation					
Refined Grains	5.4	−1.4	−0.1	−0.5	−10.5
Sodium	11.4	−1.7	0.0	−0.6	−12.7
SoFAAS Calories	1.5	−0.9	-0.1	−0.3	−7.0
Total Score	3.4	−0.9	−1.2	−0.9	−4.2

[a] Percent change was calculated relative to the maximum score for each component category, so the values presented are normalized to accurately reflect the correct weighting across categories. For example, if there was a change of 0.05 in a component with a maximum score of 5, the relative percent change is 1.0%, whereas a maximum score of 10 yields a percent change of 0.5%. Positive percent change values indicate that the component or total score has increased (become more aligned with the 2010 DGAs). Negative percent change values indicate that the component or total score has decreased (become less aligned with the 2010 DGAs). Abbreviations: HEI: Healthy Eating Index; Home-IDEA: Home Inventory Describing Eating and Activity; DGA: Dietary Guidelines for Americans; SoFAAS: Solid Fats, Alcohol, Added Sugars.

3.2.2. Construct Validity

The analyses of the five sample HFEs resulted in a range of scores in the expected directions for both component and total scores (Table 5). The highest total scores (out of 100) resulted from the minimally processed/vegetarian (93.8) and DASH (88.9) HFEs and are classified as 'good' (total score >80) according to the Center for Nutrition Policy and Promotion's standardized guidelines for HEI scores [39]. The CACFP HFE resulted in a nearly 'good' score, 78.9, with low scores for the seafood and plant proteins and fatty acid ratio components, as CACFP menus used to create the sample HFE did not include any food items that would contribute to the seafood and plant protein component. Moreover, while the CACFP menus contained substantial dairy (contributing saturated fatty acids to the denominator), they did not include foods that contained MUFAs and PUFAs (the numerator) for the fatty acid ratio component. All other component scores, excluding sodium, were maximized by the CACFP environment, thus indicating a high ability to detect adherence to the DGAs within the bounds of using the Home-IDEA2. The moderately and highly processed HFEs scored lower for most component scores and generated lower total scores (in the 'needs improvement' category and close to 'poor') than the more healthful HFEs, suggesting measurement sensitivity to different patterns in the anticipated directions.

Table 5. Construct validity: five sample home food environments and resulting HEI-2010 component and total scores.

HEI-2010 Components	Maximum Points	Sample Home Food Environments					
		Home-IDEA2 (All Foods Present)	Highly Processed	Moderately Processed	Minimally Processed, Vegetarian	DASH	CACFP
Adequacy							
Total Fruit	5	2.9	2.0	3.0	4.4	3.3	5.0
Whole Fruit	5	4.7	3.7	4.1	5.0	3.6	5.0
Total Vegetables	5	2.8	2.0	3.4	5.0	5.0	5.0
Greens & Beans	5	1.1	2.1	0.0	5.0	5.0	5.0
Whole Grains	10	6.2	0.5	0.5	10.0	8.0	10.0
Dairy	10	7.4	6.1	4.4	4.4	4.0	9.1
Total Protein Foods	5	4.3	4.7	4.3	5.0	5.0	5.0
Seafood & Plant Proteins	5	5.0	5.0	2.6	5.0	5.0	0.0
Fatty Acid Ratio	10	8.1	6.5	10.0	10.0	10.0	0.0
Moderation							
Refined Grains	10	6.2	0.8	5.0	10.0	10.0	10.0
Sodium	10	8.9	6.9	7.7	10.0	10.0	6.4
Empty Calories	20	17.6	15.7	20.0	20.0	20.0	18.4
Total Score [a]	100	75.2	56.0	64.9	93.8	88.9	78.9

[a] The Center for Nutrition Policy and Promotion categorizes total scores as poor (less than 51), needs improvement (51–80), and good (greater than 80) [39]. Abbreviations: HEI: Healthy Eating Index; DASH, Dietary Approaches to Stop Hypertension; CACFP, Child and Adult Care Food Program.

To further examine construct validity, broccoli was included in all five sample HFE patterns; broccoli is the only vegetable in the Home-IDEA2 HEI Score database that contributed to the Greens and Beans component. The Highly Processed sample HFE had non-maximum scores for the Greens and Beans component, whereas the Minimally Processed household, DASH household, and CACFP households scored the maximum of 5. This demonstrated that the presence of a single food within the total patterning of a given household may result in a range of scores within a component.

4. Discussion

In this study, a HFE quality score was developed by applying the HEI to the Home-IDEA2, a validated assessment of the HFE. The development process used to produce the Home-IDEA2 HEI Score mirrored those employed for the HEI-2010 [24] and, therefore, utilized a validated method in which an index of dietary quality was quantitatively applied to foods available in the home environment. Because the HFE is a significant target for efforts focused on prevention of childhood obesity, enhancing researchers' ability to measure multiple environmental correlates, including availability, accessibility, and quality of foods, is critical to understanding children's food behaviors and dietary intake.

Having a comprehensive measure of HFE overall quality in addition to dietary intake quality provides a more complete picture of how the HFE may impact dietary intake at the pattern level, thus aligning HFE research with current trends in dietary intake research examining dietary patterning in addition to individual food groups or nutrients [51–54]. Further, having a validated Home-IDEA2 HEI Score provides several important opportunities for researchers. The Home-IDEA2 HEI Score can be used not only to easily summarize food quality in the home, but to measure the overall quality of the home food environment as an intervention target. Similarly, the score could be used in a larger cohort study for assessing the associations between the quality of the HFE and health outcomes.

Extensive steps were taken to validate the Home-IDEA2 HEI Score at each step of the development process. Examining the relative percent change of individual foods to component and total scores confirmed that the vast majority of representative foods had negligible impact on the total score when considered individually. Because the HEI is designed to measure overall patterning, this was critical, as it demonstrated that no individual food had the power to significantly impact the total score. It should be noted that changes in the presence or absence of foods may reflect changes in the overall categorization of a home's Home-IDEA2 HEI Score as poor (less than 51), needs improvement (51–80), or good (greater than 80) [39]. For example, as Ramen induced a 3.4% change to the total score, it is feasible that a home's overall Home-IDEA2 HEI Score might move above or below these prescribed categories. Construct validity was demonstrated through testing of five sample HFEs, which revealed both total and component scores in the expected directions. Similarly, this analysis resulted in a range of total scores for each of the five sample HFEs (56.0–93.8), indicating that scores ranged from nearly all three standardized HEI rating quality categories: poor, needs improvement, and good [39].

The process of applying the HEI algorithm to the Home-IDEA2 revealed opportunities for improvement of the checklist. First, the Home-IDEA2 was not designed with the HEI in mind, thus, the retrospective application of the HEI identified gaps in the food items included in the checklist. The Home-IDEA2 was unbalanced, with a greater variety and higher number of more healthful foods feeding into the HEI components that make up the adequacy score, compared with fewer options for less healthful/processed food items that contribute to the HEI components contributing to the moderation score. This is highlighted by the Home-IDEA HEI score (Table 5) of 75.2 (out of 100) when all foods were checked as present in the home. Ideally, when both healthful (adequacy) and unhealthful (moderation) foods are adequately represented, the total HEI score should be lower. Future iterations of the checklist should include more options of moderation foods. Similarly, future versions of the Home-IDEA should be designed with the HEI in mind and include multiple food types that represent HEI components (so that the presence of one food, like broccoli, does not create a perfect component score). Further understanding of how the presence or absence of these foods in the home might affect the Home-IDEA2 HEI Score, and whether or not equal representation is given to all food components of the HEI, is warranted.

While the HEI is designed to measure adherence to the U.S. Dietary Guidelines, algorithms for other dietary patterns, such as the DASH diet, the Mediterranean diet, the Alternative HEI, and country/region specific dietary guidelines, could be applied in a similar manner as the HEI to the Home-IDEA2. The process of applying a dietary pattern algorithm to the HFE to develop a quality score has the potential to be replicated to encompass culturally specific eating patterns, or could be used to compare and contrast HFE across countries/regions. Culturally tailoring the Home-IDEA2 or the application of the dietary pattern algorithms to different HFE assessment tools would require content, criterion, and construct validity testing to ensure that the tool and the algorithm were reflecting the intent of the dietary pattern appropriately.

There were limitations and strengths to this study. As mentioned, the predetermined list of foods reduced participant and researcher burden, but the Home-IDEA2 is not all-inclusive and may place limits on capturing the full diversity of foods in the home. The Home-IDEA2 is similar to a single dietary recall for one person, and as such, is subject to the same limitations, such as substantial day-to-day variability. While the checklist has been validated and successfully used in low-income, multi-ethnic families with young children [43,44], food items cover a large portion of foods frequently consumed by all Americans, and future research with other audiences is warranted. The food categories of the Home-IDEA2 were assigned representative foods for nutrient content and food amount using the FoodAPS database, a nationally representative database of U.S. households. However, it should be noted that the selection of representative foods (face validity) was completed by the experts in nutrition and psychometric testing, and, therefore, the subjectivity of these selections is a limitation. Finally, the development and validation procedures for the Home-IDEA2 HEI Score were modeled after USDA recommendations. Extensive validation procedures and psychometric testing were used to ensure that the Home-IDEA2 HEI Score was functioning as intended.

5. Conclusions

The ability to assess the quality of the foods in the home holistically via the application of an HEI score allows for a more complete view of the HFE, and provides a useful form of measurement to future observational and intervention studies working to gain a fuller understanding of the HFE. Previous literature has shown the importance of understanding and measuring the HFE, because of the predictive ability of the availability of food in the home to the types of foods that children eat [16–18]. This study adds to the literature a psychometrically tested and thoroughly validated measure. While this study used an existing instrument, future modifications to the Home-IDEA2 are needed to address the aforementioned limitations, to improve sensitivity and enhance the ability to accurately measure the overall quality of the HFE with a constrained number of food items. The ability to quantify HFE quality in a valid way provides researchers with a methodology to holistically assess families and children's food environments, which may contribute to a greater understanding of dietary intake and, ultimately, health outcomes.

Author Contributions: Conceptualization, S.K.H.-S., R.E.B., S.L.J., and L.L.B.; Methodology, S.K.H.-S., R.E.B., S.L.J., M.L.M., S.H., L.L.B.; Formal Analysis, S.K.H.-S.; Writing—original draft preparation, S.K.H.-S., M.L.M., S.H., L.L.B.; Writing—review and editing, S.K.H.-S., R.E.B., S.L.J., M.L.M., S.H., L.L.B.; Project Administration, S.K.H.-S., R.E.B., L.L.B.; Funding Acquisition, L.L.B., S.L.J., R.E.B.

Funding: This protocol was jointly funded by the Colorado Agricultural Experiment Station (USDA Hatch funds) Grant Number COL00640, the Colorado State University School of Public Health Faculty Seed Grant, and the Agriculture and Food Research Initiative Grant number 2015-68001-23240 from the U.S. Department of Agriculture, National Institute of Food and Agriculture. The data management portion of this project was supported by NIH/NCRR Colorado CTSI Grant Number UL1 RR025780.

Acknowledgments: The authors would like to acknowledge John Hurdle and Philip Brewster at the University of Utah for their guidance in the development of the Home-IDEA2 HEI Score.

Conflicts of Interest: The authors declare no conflict of interest. The funders had no role in the design of the study; in the collection, analyses, or interpretation of data; in the writing of the manuscript, or in the decision to publish the results.

References

1. Altman, M.; Cahill Holland, J.; Lundeen, D.; Kolko, R.P.; Stein, R.I.; Saelens, B.E.; Welch, R.R.; Perri, M.G.; Schechtman, K.B.; Epstein, L.H.; et al. Reduction in food away from home is associated with improved child relative weight and body composition outcomes and this relation is mediated by changes in diet quality. *J. Acad. Nutr. Diet.* **2015**, *115*, 1400–1407. [CrossRef] [PubMed]

2. Kant, A.K.; Whitley, M.I.; Graubard, B.I. Away from home meals: Associations with biomarkers of chronic disease and dietary intake in American adults, NHANES 2005–2010. *Int. J. Obes. (Lond.)* **2015**, *39*, 820–827. [CrossRef] [PubMed]

3. Couch, S.C.; Glanz, K.; Zhou, C.; Sallis, J.F.; Saelens, B.E. Home food environment in relation to children's diet quality and weight status. *J. Acad. Nutr. Diet.* **2014**, *114*, 1569–1579. [CrossRef] [PubMed]

4. Kirkpatrick, S.I.; Reedy, J.; Kahle, L.L.; Harris, J.L.; Ohri-Vachaspati, P.; Krebs-Smith, S.M. Fast-food menu offerings vary in dietary quality, but are consistently poor. *Public Health Nutr.* **2013**, *17*, 924–931. [CrossRef] [PubMed]

5. Powell, L.M.; Nguyen, B.T. Fast-food and full-service restaurant consumption among children and adolescents: Effect on energy, beverage, and nutrient intake. *JAMA Pediatr.* **2013**, *167*, 14–20. [CrossRef] [PubMed]

6. Stern, D.; Ng, S.W.; Popkin, B.M. The nutrient content of US household food purchases by store type. *Am. J. Prev. Med.* **2016**, *50*, 180–190. [CrossRef] [PubMed]

7. Cavanaugh, E.; Mallya, G.; Brensinger, C.; Tierney, A.; Glanz, K. Nutrition environments in corner stores in Philadelphia. *Prev. Med.* **2013**, *56*, 149–151. [CrossRef]

8. Caspi, C.E.; Pelletier, J.E.; Harnack, L.; Erickson, D.J.; Laska, M.N. Differences in healthy food supply and stocking practices between small grocery stores, gas-marts, pharmacies and dollar stores. *Public Health Nutr.* **2016**, *19*, 540–547. [CrossRef]

9. Aggarwal, A.; Monsivais, P.; Cook, A.J.; Drewnowski, A. Positive attitude toward healthy eating predicts higher diet quality at all cost levels of supermarkets. *J. Acad. Nutr. Diet.* **2014**, *114*, 266–272. [CrossRef]

10. Driessen, C.E.; Cameron, A.J.; Thornton, L.E.; Lai, S.K.; Barnett, L.M. Effect of changes to the school food environment on eating behaviours and/or body weight in children: A systematic review. *Obes. Rev.* **2014**, *15*, 968–982. [CrossRef]

11. Drewnowski, A.; Rehm, C.D. Energy intakes of US children and adults by food purchase location and by specific food source. *Nutr. J.* **2013**, *12*, 59. [CrossRef] [PubMed]

12. Poti, J.M.; Slining, M.M.; Popkin, B.M. Where are kids getting their empty calories? Stores, schools, and fast-food restaurants each played an important role in empty calorie intake among US children during 2009–2010. *J. Acad. Nutr. Diet.* **2014**, *114*, 908–917. [CrossRef] [PubMed]

13. Rosenkranz, R.R.; Dzewaltowski, D.A. Model of the home food environment pertaining to childhood obesity. *Nutr. Rev.* **2008**, *66*, 123–140. [CrossRef] [PubMed]

14. Boles, R.E.; Yun, L.; Hambidge, S.J.; Davidson, A. Influencing the Home Food and Activity Environment of Families of Preschool Children Receiving Home-Based Treatment for Obesity. *Clin. Pediatr.* **2015**, *54*, 1387–1390. [CrossRef] [PubMed]

15. Bekelman, T.A.; Bellows, L.L.; Johnson, S.L. Are Family Routines Modifiable Determinants of Preschool Children's Eating, Dietary Intake, and Growth? A Review of Intervention Studies. *Curr. Nutr. Rep.* **2017**, *6*, 1–19. [CrossRef]

16. Gebremariam, M.K.; Vaqué-Crusellas, C.; Andersen, L.F.; Stok, F.M.; Stelmach-Mardas, M.; Brug, J.; Lien, N. Measurement of availability and accessibility of food among youth: A systematic review of methodological studies. *Int. J. Behav. Nutr. Phys. Act.* **2017**, *14*, 22. [CrossRef] [PubMed]

17. Pearson, N.; Biddle, S.J.; Gorely, T. Family correlates of fruit and vegetable consumption in children and adolescents: A systematic review. *Public Health Nutr.* **2009**, *12*, 267–283. [CrossRef] [PubMed]

18. Neumark-Sztainer, D.; Wall, M.; Perry, C.; Story, M. Correlates of fruit and vegetable intake among adolescents: Findings from Project EAT. *Prev. Med.* **2003**, *37*, 198–208. [CrossRef]

19. Cullen, K.W.; Baranowski, T.; Owens, E.; Marsh, T.; Rittenberry, L.; Moor, C.D. Availability, Accessibility, and Preferences for Fruit, 100% Fruit Juice, and Vegetables Influence Children's Dietary Behavior. *Health. Educ. Behav.* **2003**, *30*, 615–626. [CrossRef]

20. Santiago-Torres, M.; Adams, A.K.; Carrel, A.L.; LaRowe, T.L.; Schoeller, D.A. Home food availability, parental dietary intake, and familial eating habits influence the diet quality of urban Hispanic children. *Child. Obes.* **2014**, *10*, 408–415. [CrossRef]

21. Pinard, C.A.; Yaroch, A.L.; Hart, M.H.; Serrano, E.L.; McFerren, M.M.; Estabrooks, P.A. Measures of the home environment related to childhood obesity: A systematic review. *Public Health Nutr.* **2012**, *15*, 97–109. [CrossRef] [PubMed]

22. Boles, R.E.; Burdell, A.; Johnson, S.L.; Gavin, W.J.; Davies, P.L.; Bellows, L.L. Home food and activity assessment. Development and validation of an instrument for diverse families of young children. *Appetite* **2014**, *80*, 23–27. [CrossRef] [PubMed]

23. Guenther, P.M.; Casavale, K.O.; Reedy, J.; Kirkpatrick, S.I.; Hiza, H.A.; Kuczynski, K.J.; Kahle, L.L.; Krebs-Smith, S.M. Update of the Healthy Eating Index: HEI-2010. *J. Acad. Nutr. Diet.* **2013**, *113*, 569–580. [CrossRef] [PubMed]

24. Guenther, P.M.; Kirkpatrick, S.I.; Reedy, J.; Krebs-Smith, S.M.; Buckman, D.W.; Dodd, K.W.; Casavale, K.O.; Carroll, R.J. The Healthy Eating Index-2010 is a valid and reliable measure of diet quality according to the 2010 Dietary Guidelines for Americans. *J. Nutr.* **2014**, *144*, 399–407. [CrossRef] [PubMed]

25. Miller, P.E.; Reedy, J.; Kirkpatrick, S.I.; Krebs-Smith, S.M. The United States Food Supply Is Not Consistent with Dietary Guidance: Evidence from an Evaluation Using the Healthy Eating Index-2010. *J. Acad. Nutr. Diet.* **2015**, *115*, 95–100. [CrossRef] [PubMed]

26. Byker, C.; Smith, T. Food assistance programs for children afford mixed dietary quality based on HEI-2010. *Nutr. Res.* **2015**, *35*, 35–40. [CrossRef] [PubMed]

27. Jahns, L.; Scheett, A.J.; Johnson, L.K.; Krebs-Smith, S.M.; Payne, C.R.; Whigham, L.D.; Hoverson, B.S.; Kranz, S. Diet Quality of Items Advertised in Supermarket Sales Circulars Compared to Diets of the US Population, as Assessed by the Healthy Eating Index-2010. *J. Acad. Nutr. Diet.* **2016**, *116*, 115–122. [CrossRef] [PubMed]

28. He, M.; Tucker, P.; Irwin, J.D.; Gilliland, J.; Larsen, K.; Hess, P. Obesogenic neighbourhoods: The impact of neighbourhood restaurants and convenience stores on adolescents' food consumption behaviours. *Public Health Nutr.* **2012**, *15*, 2331–2339. [CrossRef] [PubMed]

29. Appelhans, B.M.; French, S.A.; Tangney, C.C.; Powell, L.M.; Wang, Y. To what extent do food purchases reflect shoppers' diet quality and nutrient intake? *Int. J. Behav. Nutr. Phys. Act.* **2017**, *14*, 46. [CrossRef]

30. Wilson, M.; Krebs-Smith, S.; Reedy, J.; Story, M.; Britten, P.; Juan, W. Diet Quality, Measured Using the Healthy Eating Index-2010, Varies by Source Where Food is Obtained in the United States. *FASEB J.* **2016**, *30*, 409.6.

31. Rehm, C.D.; Monsivais, P.; Drewnowski, A. Relation between diet cost and Healthy Eating Index 2010 scores among adults in the United States 2007–2010. *Prev. Med.* **2015**, *73*, 70–75. [CrossRef]

32. Clarys, P.; Deliens, T.; Huybrechts, I.; Deriemaeker, P.; Vanaelst, B.; De Keyzer, W.; Hebbelinck, M.; Mullie, P. Comparison of Nutritional Quality of the Vegan, Vegetarian, Semi-Vegetarian, Pesco-Vegetarian and Omnivorous Diet. *Nutrients* **2014**, *6*, 1318. [CrossRef] [PubMed]

33. Wang, D.D.; Leung, C.W.; Li, Y.; Ding, E.L.; Chiuve, S.E.; Hu, F.B.; Willett, W.C. Trends in dietary quality among adults in the united states, 1999 through 2010. *JAMA Intern. Med.* **2014**, *174*, 1587–1595. [CrossRef] [PubMed]

34. Harmon, B.E.; Boushey, C.J.; Shvetsov, Y.B.; Ettienne, R.; Reedy, J.; Wilkens, L.R.; Le Marchand, L.; Henderson, B.E.; Kolonel, L.N. Associations of key diet-quality indexes with mortality in the Multiethnic Cohort: The Dietary Patterns Methods Project. *Am. J. Clin. Nutr.* **2015**, *101*, 587–597. [CrossRef] [PubMed]

35. Liese, A.D.; Krebs-Smith, S.M.; Subar, A.F.; George, S.M.; Harmon, B.E.; Neuhouser, M.L.; Boushey, C.J.; Schap, T.E.; Reedy, J. The Dietary Patterns Methods Project: Synthesis of Findings across Cohorts and Relevance to Dietary Guidance. *J. Nutr.* **2015**, *145*, 93–402. [CrossRef] [PubMed]

36. Reedy, J.; Krebs-Smith, S.M.; Miller, P.E.; Liese, A.D.; Kahle, L.L.; Park, Y.; Subar, A.F. Higher Diet Quality Is Associated with Decreased Risk of All-Cause, Cardiovascular Disease, and Cancer Mortality among Older Adults. *J. Nutr.* **2014**, *144*, 881–889. [CrossRef] [PubMed]

37. Kong, A.; Schiffer, L.; Antonic, M.; Braunschweig, C.; Odoms-Young, A.; Fitzgibbon, M. The relationship between home-and individual-level diet quality among African American and Hispanic/Latino households with young children. *Int. J. Behav. Nutr. Phys. Act.* **2018**, *15*, 5. [CrossRef] [PubMed]

38. U.S. Department of Health & Human Services and U.S. Department of Agriculture. Dietary Guidelines for Americans: 2015–2020. Available online: http://health.gov/dietaryguidelines/2015/guidelines/ (accessed on 27 September 2017).

39. Basiotis, P.P.; Carlson, A.; Gerrior, S.A.; Juan, W.Y.; Lino, M. The Healthy Eating Index: 1999–2000. U.S. Department of Agriculture, Center for Nutrition Policy and Promotion, 2002. Available online: https://www.cnpp.usda.gov/sites/default/files/healthy_eating_index/HEI99-00report.pdf (accessed on 7 February 2019).

40. National Institutes for Health and National Cancer Institute: HEI Tools for Researchers. Available online: https://epi.grants.cancer.gov/hei/calculating-hei-scores.html (accessed on 11 February 2019).

41. National Institutes for Health and National Cancer Institute: Developing the Healthy Eating Index. Available online: https://epi.grants.cancer.gov/hei/developing.html#f1a (accessed on 11 February 2019).

42. Guenther, P.M.; Reedy, J.; Krebs-Smith, S.M.; Reeve, B.B.; Basiotis, P.P. Development and evaluation of the healthy eating index-2005. *J. Am. Diet. Assoc.* **2008**, *108*, 1896–1901. [CrossRef] [PubMed]

43. Boles, R.E.; Johnson, S.L.; Burdell, A.; Davies, P.L.; Gavin, W.J.; Bellows, L.L. Home food availability and child intake among rural families identified to be at-risk for health disparities. *Appetite* **2019**, *34*, 135–141. [CrossRef] [PubMed]

44. Bellows, L.L.; Boles, R.E.; Hibbs-Shipp, S.K.; Burdell, A.; Johnson, S.L. Development of a Comprehensive Checklist to Capture Food, Physical Activity and Sedentary Devices in the Home Environment: The Home Inventory Describing Eating and Activity (Home-IDEA2). *J. Nutr. Educ. Behav.* **2019**, in press. [CrossRef] [PubMed]

45. National Institutes for Health and National Cancer Institute: Research Uses of the HEI; HEI Scoring Illustration. Available online: https://epi.grants.cancer.gov/hei/uses.html#differentlevels (accessed on 11 February 2019).

46. United States Department of Agriculture and Economic Research Service. FoodAPS: National Household Food Acquisition and Purchase Survey. Available online: https://www.ers.usda.gov/foodaps (accessed on 26 April 2017).

47. National Institutes for Health and National Cancer Institute: Healthy Eating Index SAS Code. Available online: https://epi.grants.cancer.gov/hei/tools.html (accessed on 11 February 2019).

48. National Institutes for Health and National Cancer Institute: ASA24 Researcher Website. Available online: https://asa24.nci.nih.gov/researchersite/ (accessed on 11 February 2019).

49. Dash Diet Eating Plan. The Dash Diet Eating Plan, Dash Diet Recipes. Available online: https://www.nhlbi.nih.gov/files/docs/public/heart/new_dash.pdf (accessed on 6 October 2017).

50. U.S. Department of Health and Human Services and U.S. Department of Agriculture. 2010–2015. Dietary Guidelines for Americans. December 2010. Available online: https://health.gov/dietaryguidelines/2010/ (accessed on 30 January 2019).

51. Hu, F.B. Dietary pattern analysis: A new direction in nutritional epidemiology. *Curr. Opin. Lipidol.* **2002**, *13*, 3–9. [CrossRef] [PubMed]

52. Jacobs, D.R.; Steffen, L.M. Nutrients, foods, and dietary patterns as exposures in research: A framework for food synergy. *Am. J. Clin. Nutr.* **2003**, *78*, 508S–513S. [CrossRef] [PubMed]

53. Jannasch, F.; Kröger, J.; Schulze, M.B. Dietary Patterns and Type 2 Diabetes: A Systematic Literature Review and Meta-Analysis of Prospective Studies. *J. Nutr.* **2017**, *147*, 1174–1182. [CrossRef] [PubMed]

54. Cespedes, E.M.; Hu, F.B.; Tinker, L.; Rosner, B.; Redline, S.; Garcia, L.; Hingle, M.; Van Horn, L.; Howard, B.V.; Levitan, E.B.; et al. Multiple healthful dietary patterns and type 2 diabetes in the Women's Health Initiative. *Am. J. Epidemiol.* **2016**, *183*, 622–633. [CrossRef] [PubMed]

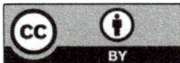

nutrients

MDPI

Article

Pediatric-Adapted Liking Survey (PALS): A Diet and Activity Screener in Pediatric Care

Kayla Vosburgh [1], Sharon R. Smith [2], Samantha Oldman [1], Tania Huedo-Medina [1] and Valerie B. Duffy [1,*]

[1] Department of Allied Health Sciences, University of Connecticut, Storrs, CT 06269, USA
[2] CT Children's Medical Center, University of Connecticut School of Medicine, Hartford, CT 06106 2, USA
*   Correspondence: valerie.duffy@uconn.edu; Tel.: +1-860-486-1997

Received: 18 June 2019; Accepted: 16 July 2019; Published: 18 July 2019

Abstract: Clinical settings need rapid yet useful methods to screen for diet and activity behaviors for brief interventions and to guide obesity prevention efforts. In an urban pediatric emergency department, these behaviors were screened in children and parents with the 33-item Pediatric-Adapted Liking Survey (PALS) to assess the reliability and validity of a Healthy Behavior Index (HBI) generated from the PALS responses. The PALS was completed by 925 children (average age = 11 ± 4 years, 55% publicly insured, 37% overweight/obese by Body Mass Index Percentile, BMI-P) and 925 parents. Child–parent dyads differed most in liking of vegetables, sweets, sweet drinks, and screen time. Across the sample, child and parent HBIs were variable, normally distributed with adequate internal reliability and construct validity, revealing two dimensions (less healthy—sweet drinks, sweets, sedentary behaviors; healthy—vegetables, fruits, proteins). The HBI showed criterion validity, detecting healthier indexes in parents vs. children, females vs. males, privately- vs. publicly-health insured, and residence in higher- vs. lower-income communities. Parent's HBI explained some variability in child BMI percentile. Greater liking of sweets/carbohydrates partially mediated the association between low family income and higher BMI percentile. These findings support the utility of PALS as a dietary behavior and activity screener for children and their parents in a clinical setting.

Keywords: dietary screener; obesity prevention; sweet preference; children; diet quality

1. Introduction

The worldwide childhood overweight/obesity prevalence ranges from 22 to 24% [1]. Obesity in U.S. children is estimated at 17%, including 5.8% extreme obesity (BMI ≥ 120% of the 95th percentile) [2]. Obesity prevention requires a multi-sector approach [3], including screening, brief interventions and referrals between clinical and community sectors [4]. As the pediatric emergency department (PED) is utilized for non-urgent care [5], it should be part of this multi-sector approach [6–9] to reach low-income children who often have unhealthy dietary behaviors and lack access to primary care [6]. Brief obesity interventions have been successfully accomplished in the PED [7]. Clinicians need rapid, yet useful tools to screen behaviors for patient-centered interventions to promote healthy behaviors [10]. As parent involvement is critical [11], these tools should capture parent and child behaviors.

Conventional dietary assessment asks children or parents to recall food/beverage intake (e.g., 24-h recall,) or usual intake frequency [12,13], which is time intensive, often involves misreporting [14], and may cause defensive parent response and low-compliance in a clinical setting [15]. Screening usual consumption by asking likes/dislikes offers a feasible alternative. Recall of liking is quicker and cognitively simpler than behavioral recall with potentially less parent unease. Reported food liking correlates with reported intake [16–18], biomarkers of intake and/or adiposity in children [18] and adults [19–21]. The Pediatric-adapted Liking Survey (PALS) is fast, has a high response rate in the PED, with good-to-excellent clinical-to-home test–retest reliability [22]. Furthermore, results from an assessment of children's preference for food and physical activity (PA) can guide program planning [23]. Health promotion across the socio-ecological framework needs to develop healthy food and PA preferences in children [24].

The present study further develops PALS [22] to address needs in clinical settings. One need is to screen dietary behaviors in children and their parents (i.e., child–parent dyads) with comparable methods. The dietary patterns of children and parents can show weak-to-moderate resemblance [25]. The second is to assess dietary behaviors toward food/beverage groups and diet healthiness (i.e., diet quality). Few studies have examined diet quality in child–parent dyads [26]. We have shown that liking survey responses can form a reliable and valid diet quality index that explains significant variation in markers of nutritional status and health in preschoolers [18] and adults [21,27]. Diet quality indexes improve the understanding of diet-health relationships [28], inform interventions [29] and monitoring [30] in children. From analysis of three cycles of U.S. National Health and Nutrition Examination Survey (NHANES), diet quality among children is low, showing socio-economical and race/ethnic disparities [31]. The third need is to feasibly screen PA and sedentary behaviors in child–parent dyads. PA encouragement is key as children age, especially targeting those of economic disadvantage [32]. As questionnaires inform PA assessment [33], we enhanced the PALS [22] with physical and sedentary activities as well as additional foods.

Our specific objective was to screen both children's and parent's food and activity liking and to assess the reliability and validity of a Healthy Behavior Index (HBI) generated from the liking responses. Measures of reliability and validity followed that for the Healthy Eating Index [34], including the ability of the HBI to detect differences between child and parent, by the child's age and gender, proxies of the family's economic status, and the child's Body Mass Index Percentile (BMI-P). Finally, we examined models of interaction between income and food liking to explain variability in the child's BMI-P.

2. Materials and Methods

2.1. Participants

This observational study enrolled a convenience sample of 5 to 17-year-old children who sought medical care at the Connecticut Children's Medical Center's PED in Hartford, CT. The sample size was to capture diversity in the child to address the study aims and allow for multivariate analysis within a diverse sample. Children were excluded from participating if they had a history of severe behavioral/mental health conditions, were non-English speaking, or too ill to participate. Institutional Review Boards approved this study. To participate, parents/guardians signed informed consent, and children ages 7 and older signed an assent. Of those consenting to participate and meeting the inclusion criteria, 93% completed the protocol. The final sample, collected from March 2013 to April 2016, included 925 child–parent dyads who were diverse in child age, race/ethnicity, and family economic status (Table 1).

Table 1. Characteristics of children seeking medical care in a Pediatric Emergency Department.

	n = 925	%
Age (Avg. 10.9 years)		
5–<9 year	356	38
9–<13 year	257	28
13–17 year	312	34
Sex		
Male	463	50.1
Female	462	49.9
Race/Ethnicity		
Caucasian	357	38.6
Black	133	14.4
Hispanic	344	37.2
Other	91	9.8
Insurance		
Private	382	41.3
Public	507	54.8
Self pay	16	1.7
Other	20	2.2
Income Level *,a		
<$21,432	26	2.8
$21,433–41,186	288	31.1
$41,187–68,212	245	26.5
$68,213–112,262	313	33.8
≥$112,263	29	3.1
Food Insecurity *,b		
Greatest risk	574	62.1
Higher than average risk	102	11
Lower than average risk	134	14.5
Lowest risk	99	10.7

* Percentages ≠ 100 due to missing data (<3%); [a] Based on zip code analysis using U.S. Census Bureau data from the 2010–2014 American Community Survey 5-Year Estimates (U.S. Census Bureau. 2010–2014 American Community Survey 5-year estimates: Income in the past 12 months (in 2014 inflation-adjusted dollars)). American FactFinder: Community Facts Website. factfinder.census.gov/faces/nav/jsf/pages/index.xhtml. Accessed May 30, 2019.); [b] Based on data from the Zwick Center for Food and Resource Policy and the Cooperative Extension System at the University of Connecticut [35].

2.2. Study Procedure and Measures

Data collection took place in the patient's exam room. Research assistants enrolled patients, confirmed the inclusion/exclusion criteria, collected the child's address, age, gender, race/ethnicity, type of health insurance, and history of chronic medical condition (e.g., asthma, diabetes).

The community of family residence by zip code was reported by the parent/caregiver which served beyond type of health insurance as another proxy of family income and level of food insecurity. Median household income by zip code, reported by the U.S. Census Bureau, 2010–2014 American Community Survey 5-Year Estimates, was used to determine the family's income level. A Connecticut ranking of town food security (based on economic and social characteristics, access to food retailers, utilization of public food assistance) was used to assess participants' risk of food insecurity [35].

Pediatric-Adapted Liking Survey (PALS): Both child and parent/guardian were asked to complete the PALS, a food and activity liking/disliking survey, based on their own likes and dislikes (average completion time was <4 min). This three-page, paper/pencil PALS consisted of 33 food items and activities, represented with both pictures and words as described previously [22]. Participants reported their level of liking/disliking, marking a perpendicular line anywhere along the scale with seven faces labeled as "love it," "really like it," "like it," "it's ok," "dislike it," "really dislike it," and "hate it." Distance was measured from the scale center (0; "he/she thinks it's okay") to the participant's marking (±100; "he/she loves/hates it"). Children and parents/caregivers also could mark "never tried/done."

The Healthy Behavior Index (HBI) was conceptually constructed based on the 2015 Dietary Guidelines [36], with a single index similar to the Healthy Eating Index (HEI) and following our previously validated, liking-based diet quality indices [18,21] with the addition of PA and screen time (sedentary behavior). Foods and activities were sorted into conceptual groups and multiplied by weights consistent with the Dietary Guidelines [18,21,27]: vegetables (+3), fruits (+2), protein (+2), sweets (−3), sugary drinks (−3), fiber (+2), salty (−2), dairy (+2), PA (+2) and screen time (−3). The final HBI was the average of weighted groups that formed an internally reliable, normally distributed index: vegetables, fruits, protein, sweets, sugary drinks, and screen time. Higher indexes indicated healthier behaviors.

Measured and Self-Reported Adiposity: The child's height was measured by trained research assistants (cm; portable Stadiometer, Seca®) and weight was obtained from the electronic health record (kg; platform medical scale) to calculate Body Mass Index (BMI). Age-and-sex specific BMI-Ps were calculated with the with the online calculator [37], with the child's exact age (based on birth and measurement dates) and the U.S. Centers for Disease Control 2000 growth charts to assign underweight <5th, healthy weight 5th–<85th, overweight 85th–<95th, or obese ≥95th percentile [38]. Parents/caregivers and children self-reported the child's body size using a sex-specific, 7-point drawing [39] for categorization (underweight <2, healthy weight 2 to <5, overweight 5 to 6, obese ≥ 6).

2.3. Data Analysis

Data were analyzed using SPSS statistical software (version 22.0) with the Process v3.1 (afhayes@processmacro.org) with a significance criterion of $p < 0.05$. Descriptive statistics were used to compare BMI-P against national statistics and contrast measured versus self-rated body size. All variables were evaluated for distribution, normality and central tendency. Table 2 describes the assessment of reliability and validity of the HBI. Analysis of covariance included controlling for demographic variables (age, gender, race/ethnicity, income, as appropriate) as indicated in the results section. Direct relationships between parent and child HBI and adiposity were examined with standard multiple linear regression analysis while controlling for demographic variables and child's liking of PA. Additionally, multivariate modeling was used to assess associations between food liking, proxies of family income and food insecurity, and child BMI-P.

Table 2. Tests to assess the internal reliability and validity of the Healthy Behavior Index (HBI) [34].

Question	Test Statistic
Reliability	
How internally consistent is the total index?	Cronbach's Alpha
What are the relationships among the index components?	Pearson's *r* correlations between each component
Which components have the most influence on the total index?	Pearson's *r* correlations between each component and the total index
Construct and Concurrent Criterion Validity	
Does the index score foods and behaviors based on those recommended by the 2015 Dietary Guidelines?	Descriptive statistics
Does the index allow for sufficient variation in scores among individual?	Measures of central tendency, histogram, normality testing (Kolmogorov-Smirnov)
What is the underlying structure of the index (i.e., > 1 dimension)?	Principal component analysis and plot; derived factors to explain >50% of variance
Does the index distinguish between groups with known differences (i.e., concurrent criterion validity)?	Descriptive statistics, ANOVA with post-hoc analysis, ANCOVA, multiple regression analysis between demographic characteristics, PA liking and child's BMI-P

3. Results

Overall, 37.4% of children were classified as overweight or obese by BMI-P (Table 3), which was comparable to the U.S. average of 36.6% of children aged 5 to <18 years old [2]. Children ages 9 to 13 years old had higher rates of overweight (21%) and obesity (25.3%) than any other age group. Extreme obesity in children ages 6–11 and 12–19 years old was 7 and 9.5%, respectively, and exceeded U.S. averages of 4.3 and 9.1%, respectively [2]. Independent of age and gender, a higher BMI-P was seen in children covered by public health insurance (70.02 ± 1.26 SEM) than by private health insurance (62.64 ± 1.52) (F(1,916) = 14.231, *p* < 0.001). In similar analyses, higher BMI-P was seen in children from families who reported residency in communities with lower income (compressing the highest and low income levels (F(2,894) = 5.583, *p* < 0.005) and greater risk of food insecurity (F(3,901) = 3.574, *p* = 0.014). Among overweight children, nearly half of children (47.6%) and parents (49.7%) self-reported being a lower body size than measured; among obese children, most children (94.8%) and parents (84.4%) also self-reported being a lower body size than measured.

Table 3. Body Mass Index (BMI) percentiles by age and gender of children who were patients at a pediatric emergency department (PED).

	5–<18 Years		5–<9 Years		9–<13 Years		13–<18 Years	
	Count	% *	Count	% *	Count	% *	Count	% *
5th–<85th percentile								
Male	275	29.7	102	28.7	74	28.8	99	31.7
Female	277	29.9	110	30.9	59	23.0	108	34.6
Total	552	59.6	212	59.6	133	51.8	207	66.3
85th–<95th percentile								
Male	68	7.4	22	6.2	31	12.1	15	4.8
Female	82	8.9	27	7.6	23	8.9	32	10.3
Total	150	16.2	49	13.8	54	21.0	47	15.1
≥95th percentile								
Male	105	11.4	48	13.5	35	13.6	22	7.1
Female	91	9.8	28	7.9	30	11.7	33	10.6
Total	196	21.2	76	21.4	65	25.3	55	17.7

* Percentages ≠ 100 due to missing data (Percent of total sample size, *n* = 925; <2% missing). Underweight (<5th percentile) not shown due to small sample size (*n* = 19, avg. age = 9.7 years, mean BMI percentile = 1.52 and SD = 1.33).

3.1. Relative Comparison of Parent and Child Food and Activity Liking

Across the sample (Figure 1), parents averaged the highest preference for fruits and PA, while children reported the highest preference for sweets and screen time (e.g., watching TV, playing video games, listening to music). Children reported lower liking for fiber-rich foods and vegetables compared with parent reporting. Variance within food/activity groups was highest for children's liking of healthier groups (vegetables, fruit, proteins), and parental liking of the less healthy groups (sweets drinks and sweets) (Table 4). For children and parents, the least liked items had the highest variability in ratings. By effect sizes, the magnitude of difference between child–parent dyads was largest for vegetables, sweet drinks, screen time, and sweets.

Following our previous study [18], three groups of children were identified from the relative liking for sweets versus a pleasurable non-food: greater liking of screen time than sweets; equal liking; greater liking of sweets than screen time. From ANCOVA controlling for age and gender, children with higher affinity for screen time than sweets had significantly higher BMI-P [F(2, 873) = 4.022, *p* < 0.05] than children with higher affinity for sweets than screen time.

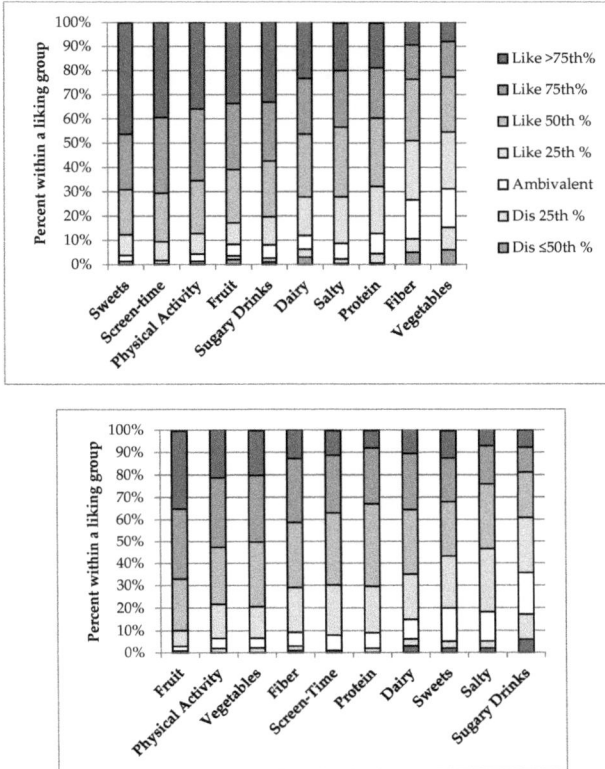

Figure 1. Liking of food/beverage and activity groups (left to right as most to least liked) in children (top graph) and parents (bottom graph), shown as percent within a food or activity group as liking (above the white neutral rating) and disliking (below the white neutral rating), with the darker the shading indicating stronger the liking or disliking.

Table 4. Variance and estimated effect sizes of child ($n = 925$) and parent ($n = 925$) survey-reported liking of foods and activities.

	Child			Parent			Effect Size
	Mean	SD	Variance	Mean	SD	Variance	Cohen's d
Vegetables	19.5	40.5	1636.6	48.4	30.6	938.3	0.8 *
Fruits	56.9	33.1	1098.0	60.5	27.4	749.7	0.1
Protein	40.9	35.3	1242.7	37.9	27.9	778.6	0.1
Sweet drinks	55.0	33.3	1108.7	14.1	39.6	1565.5	1.1 *
Screen time	64.3	26.5	701.6	39.9	27.7	768.0	0.9 *
Sweets	64.4	31.2	974.2	31.0	36.3	1317.7	1.0 *
Fiber	23.6	38.4	1476.7	41.6	30.6	936.4	0.5
Salty	44.1	32.1	1028.4	28.3	30.6	933.4	0.5
PA	59.5	29.8	888.1	49.3	30.7	940.4	0.3
Dairy	45.6	36.7	1346.3	35.5	34.6	1198.1	0.3

* Large effect size.

3.2. Internal Reliability of the HBI

The parent and child HBI approached acceptable internal reliability ($\alpha = 0.646$ versus 0.613, respectively). Children and parents who reported high liking of sweets also reported significantly higher liking of screen time and sugary drinks, as well as lower liking (disliking) for vegetables (all Spearman's rho's, $p < 0.01$). Child and parent HBI were highly influenced by liking of vegetables, sugary drinks, and sweets (Pearson's r between ±0.47 and 0.71, $p < 0.01$).

3.3. Construct Validity of the HBI

The child and parent HBI were normally distributed (Figure 2), with the parent's distribution towards the higher indexes. Although weak, child and parent HBI were significantly correlated ($r = 0.219$, $p < 0.01$), with similar correlation across all groups making up the HBI.

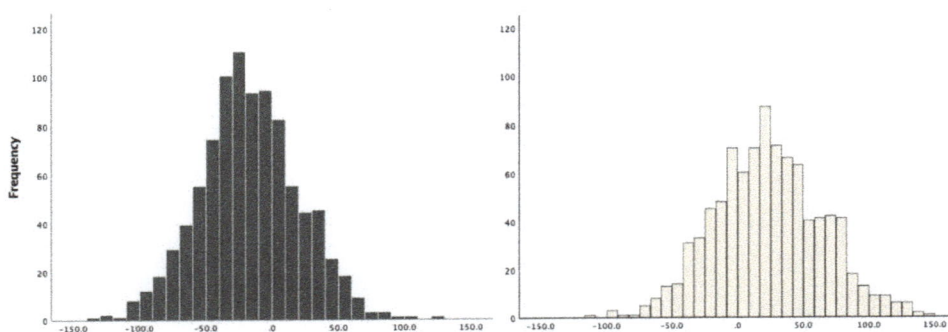

Figure 2. Histograms showing normal distributions of HBI in children (5–17 years old; left) and parents (right).

Principal component analysis (PCA) of the child HBI revealed two underlying dimensions—less healthy (screen time, sugary drinks, sweets) and healthy (vegetables, fruits, protein), which accounted for 57.2% of total variance. The PCA for the parents as well as child demographic and BMI-P categories (shown in Table 2) produced similar results for less healthy and healthy dimensions and >50% total variance explained, supporting a consistent underlying structure of the HBI.

3.4. Concurrent Criterion Validity of the HBI

The comparison of mean differences in child HBI via ANOVA, with post-hoc tests as appropriate, revealed significant effects of gender (males < females), health insurance type (public < private), race/ethnicity (Hispanic/Latino and Black/African American < White), income levels (determined through zip code analysis; low income < high income), and risk of food insecurity (high risk < low risk) (Table 5). Similar findings were seen for child or parent HBI. Greater age was correlated with healthier behaviors ($r = 0.239$, $p = 0.000$) as seen in females and males. In an income by race/ethnicity ANCOVA controlling for age and gender, income category was the sole significant contributor to child HBI ($p < 0.001$), with only a trend for an interaction with race/ethnicity ($p = 0.09$). In a gender by race ANCOVA, controlling for age, there were significant main effects on child HBI ($p = 0.008$ and 0.014, respectively), but no significant interaction effects. In summary, children who were older, white, female, covered by private insurance, and from communities with higher income and lower risk for food insecurity had the highest or healthiest HBI.

No significant differences in child HBI were found with BMI-P categories. However, a multiple linear regression model predicting child BMI-P from parent HBI, gender, insurance, and child liking for PA was significant among children of healthy weight (between 10th and 85th BMI-P). Significant predictors of higher child BMI-P were seen among lower parent HBI ($\beta = -0.11$, $p < 0.05$) and higher child liking of PA ($\beta = 0.15$, $p < 0.005$).

Table 5. Analysis of variance for mean child and parent Healthy Behavior Index (HBI) by child's demographics, community food environment, and adiposity.

Characteristic *	Child				Parent			
	Mean HBI	*n*	SD	*p*-Value	Mean HBI	*n*	SD	*p*-Value
Gender								
Male	−53.8	449	40.1	0.002 **	13.0	449	44.8	0.280
Female	−45.3	439	43.0		16.2	439	43.9	
Race/Ethnicity								
White	−41.1	341	42.3	0.000 **	23.0	341	43.1	<0.001 **
Af. Amer./Black	−55.2	129	39.3	0.006 †	10.1	129	43.3	0.023 †
Hispanic/Latino	−55.5	330	40.7	0.000 †	8.7	330	44.2	<0.001 †
Insurance Type								
Private	−44.0	364	40.4	0.001 **	23.7	364	41.3	<0.001 **
Public	−53.7	490	41.9		7.3	490	45.0	
Income Level								
$21,433–41,186	−58.9	277	40.9	0.000 **	4.8	277	45.2	<0.001 *
$41,187–68,212	−47.4	234	41.5	0.015 a	14.7	234	41.3	0.075
$68,213–112,262	−41.8	301	41.0	0.000 a	24.4	301	42.3	<0.001 a
Food Insecurity								
Greatest risk	−54.2	552	40.9	0.000 **	7.8	552	43.5	<0.001 **
>than avg. risk	−46.1	99	42.1	0.272	19.7	99	46.4	0.058
<than avg. risk	−40.7	125	39.0	0.005 b	27.9	125	39.9	<0.001 b
Lowest risk	−36.8	97	44.6	0.001 b	27.3	97	42.3	<0.001 b
BMI Percentile								
Normal weight	−49.6	523	40.7		14.8	523	44.3	
Overweight	−46.6	149	42.4	0.716 ^	12.0	149	40.7	0.767 ^
Obese	−49.0	189	42.7	0.984 ^	15.1	189	44.5	0.996 ^
Overall	−49.4	908	42.1	—	14.5	904	43.9	—

* Characteristics of child, not parent; the overall number is less than 925 due to missing data; ** Overall significant result, $p < 0.05$; † Significant result, $p < 0.05$, compared to white; a Significant result, $p < 0.05$, compared to lower income level ($21,43 3–41,186); b Significant result, $p < 0.05$, compared to those at greatest risk for food insecurity; ^ *p*-value compared to normal weight.

Due to the interactions between health insurance (proxy of family income), parent liking and BMI-P, the possibility that parent-liking mediates the relationship between health insurance and child BMI-P was examined. Of several models tested, parent liking for carbohydrate-rich foods (average of salty, sweet drinks, fiber, sweets groups; Cronbach's $\alpha = 0.74$), was most explanatory, particularly in younger children (5 to 9 years old). Shown in Figure 3, higher parent liking of these foods explained some of the correlation between public insurance and higher child BMI-P ($Z = 1.954$, $p = 0.05$; bootstrap lower level confidence interval = 0.2239, bootstrap upper level confidence interval = 3.6938).

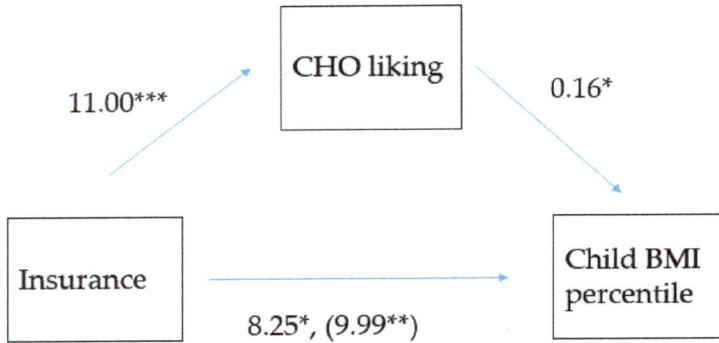

Figure 3. Model of the association between health insurance as a proxy of family income (dichotomous variable, where 1 = private; 2 = public) and the child's Body Mass Index Percentile (BMI-P), mediated by the parent's liking of carbohydrate-rich foods among 925 in children seen in an urban pediatric emergency department. * $p \leq 0.05$; ** $p \leq 0.01$; *** $p \leq 0.005$. The (coefficient in the parenthesis) represents the association between insurance and BMI-P before parent liking was added to the model, indicating that parent liking partially mediated the insurance and BMI-P relationship (indirect coefficient = 1.954, $p = 0.05$).

4. Discussion

Clinical settings need brief measures to screen children's behaviors in a method that is acceptable to families, has reasonable utility, can guide child and family-centered messages to encourage healthy behaviors, and can inform interventions for the prevention of obesity, particularly in at-risk groups. The present observational study recruited children and families from an urban, pediatric emergency department (PED) to assess children's and parents' liking of foods and activities with the Pediatric-Adapted Liking Survey (PALS) and test the reliability and validity of a Healthy Behavior Index (HBI), constructed from their PALS responses. The study sample of 925 child–parent dyads was diverse in race/ethnicity and >50% low-income, with children ranging in age from 5 to 17 years old, and with rates of overweight and obesity at or exceeding that for the U.S. The PALS is a novel diet and activity screener that showed good acceptability in this clinical setting and diverse sample. It was easily completed by children and parents and identified expected differences (children reporting a greater affinity for sugary foods/beverages and screen time, but lower affinity for vegetables than parents). The HBI neared adequate internal reliability and had normal distribution across both parents and children. For validity, the HBI measured two themes (healthy and less healthy), supporting its construct validity, and detected expected differences in healthy behaviors between groups, supporting its criterion validity. Healthier indexes were seen in females versus males, older versus younger children, parent versus child, families on private versus public insurance, and those living in higher income/food secure versus lower income/food insecure communities. For Body Mass Index Percentile (BMI-P), a higher parent-reported HBI was associated with lower percentiles across children who fell in the healthy range (between the 10th and 85th percentiles). In sub-analysis, part of the association between higher child BMI-P among families on public health insurance (i.e., lower income) was explained by greater parent liking of carbohydrate/sweet foods and beverages.

Simple indices with low participant and practitioner burden, such as the PALS and generated HBI, can be useful in a clinical setting [40] and to assess changes in response to interventions for children and families [30]. The indexes emphasize that positive health arises from moderating less healthy behaviors and encouraging those that are healthier. As the most effective obesity prevention programs for children involve the family [11], clinicians could begin conversations based on similarities and differences between child and parent dietary/activity likes and dislikes [41]. Parents influence the child's consumption of healthy and less healthy foods through controlling their availability, modeling consumption of these foods, and setting norms and attitudes toward healthy eating [42]. In the present study, child–parent dyads differed most for liking of sweets and sugary beverages. This agrees with a large multi-center study of families, which found stronger associations between parents and children for healthy rather than unhealthy foods [43]. Children prefer higher level of sweets than adults, linked to physical growth and energy need during development [44]. As higher added sugar consumption associates with poor diet quality and excess adiposity [45], families can look to healthier sweet options including fruit and fruit-based desserts. Parenting behaviors of restricting less healthy foods, using foods as a punishment or reward, or pressuring children to eat are ineffective at improving healthy eating behaviors [42]. Child–parent dyads also differed significantly in vegetable liking. Clinicians can encourage parents to show explicit liking of healthier foods [42], including tasting and consuming a variety of vegetables, involving children in cooking, supporting school meal participation, and family mealtime. Parents and children differed significantly in liking screen time yet were closer in liking for PA. Parent's liking and knowledge about screen time is significantly related to levels of screen time activity in children, which supports screen time interventions that target the child and the parent [46]. Parent modeling and support, including co-activity, can improve PA in children [47]. As preferences, attitudes and believes of parents are important predictors of PA that is performed with parents and children together [48], clinicians could probe beyond the PALS screening to identify which activities are enjoyed by both the child and parent and ways to facilitate and encourage family-based PA.

The indexes derived from the PALS showed good variability across the sample with acceptable internal reliability and validity. Although Cronbach's alpha for the HBI fell below the traditionally accepted value of $\alpha = 0.70$, this may be expected due to the complex nature of measuring diet quality, and therefore may not be a required characteristic [34]. Additionally, the child and parent HBI had a similar multi-dimensional structure of healthy (fruits, vegetables, protein) and less healthy (sweets, sweet drinks, and screen time) items. The HBI showed concurrent criterion validity through distinguishing between groups with known differences. Our results and others have found higher diet quality and health behavior indexes among females [49]. However, our findings that older children had higher diet quality and health behavior indexes differed from others, which found the opposite age relationship [50,51]. The present study found that white children reported higher diet quality and health behaviors than Hispanics/Latinos, consistent with an analysis of 2003–2004 U.S. NHANES [50], yet no significant difference was found between Blacks/African Americans and Hispanics/Latinos [50]. Finally, by using proxies of family income from community demographics, lower HBIs were found among children from families with lower income, receiving public medical insurance, and living in communities at high risk for food insecurity, consistent with multiple studies [50–52]. Our results are comparable to previous work that find healthier diet quality and behaviors among parents than their children [53].

The value of diet quality and health indexes is the ability to associate with health outcomes [40]. The present study found a significant but weak association between healthier parent HBI and lower BMI-P in healthy weight children. However, the child-reported HBI did not associate significantly with BMI-P. The association between indexes of diet quality or health behaviors and adiposity in recent scientific literature has been inconsistent. In cross-sectional studies, it has ranged from better diet quality and higher adiposities among children [54], to no significant association [55–57] or lack of consistent association [58], to healthier diet patterns in those who were overweight or obese [59]. Other studies only report demographic differences in diet quality in children and not the diet quality–adiposity association [60,61]. However, a large prospective study in children found significant associations with less healthy diet quality and increased adiposity over time [62]. Regarding activity, obese children have higher reported screen time and lower PA than do non-obese children from a systematic review, but the differences are small [63]. In the present study, the lack of significant association between the child-reported HBI and BMI-P may reflect a higher level of misreporting among overweight/obese children. Weight status has been shown to influence dietary reports by children, with heavier children being more likely to misreport due to social pressures and expectations [64]. It also may be important to examine dietary components to improve the diet quality and lower energy intakes, such as sugary beverages [65], fruits and vegetables [57] or, as in the present study, carbohydrate/sweet foods. Additionally, improvements in diet quality have been associated with improvements in body composition across an intensive diet and lifestyle intervention for overweight/obese adolescents [66]. According to a critical review, improvements in diet quality are required to improve cardiometabolic health, including obesity [67].

We found a positive association between child-reporting liking of PA and BMI-P, which is consistent with finding that obese children were more likely to report taking part in healthy behaviors [68]. Obese children are more likely to have been informed of their weight status by a physician [68], despite their perception of lower body size than what is measured in this study and others [69]. In the present study, children reported a high liking for screen time. Higher liking of screen time activities in children has been shown to associated with greater screen time behaviors [46]. Excessive screen time has been linked to lower diet quality [70], increased rates of obesity and negative health conditions [71]. When compared to liking for sweets, we found that children with a relatively higher affinity for screen time than sweets had significantly higher BMI-P than those who preferred sweets to screen time. Examining these relative rankings could help tailor messages to support healthy behavior and healthy weight. Parental encouragement has shown positive longitudinal effects on PA in adolescents [72].

Despite the findings of the present study, the question remains whether it is useful to ask parents and children to self-report their diet and PA behaviors. Furthermore, can asking likes or dislikes of foods/beverages and activities be reflective enough of usual behaviors to serve as a screener to guide a dialogue between health professionals, children and families? Screeners are short instruments to, for example, distinguish between healthier versus less healthy behaviors. Behavioral screeners need to be useful but not overly burdensome or cause families to become defensive [15]. All self-reported measures have the potential for reporting bias yet supply important information despite the emergence of dietary intake biomarkers [73]. If over time, for example, we eat what we like and avoid what we do not, reported liking reflects a pattern of what was consumed, but cannot capture total energy intake. Taste and food preference drive consumption. Food preference and intake are used interchangeably in nutrition literature [74,75] and food preference provides a proxy of consumption for examining health outcomes [76]. Survey-reported preference or liking correlates with self-reported intake in children [18,77] and adults [16,19,27,78–80], as well as with biomarkers of dietary intake and/or adiposity in children [18] and adults [19–21]. Similar to the present study, liking survey responses can be formed into an index of diet quality that explains variability in carotenoid status in preschoolers [18] and cardiovascular disease risk factors and BMI [21,27] in adults. However, food preference or liking can show marginal [19] or non-significant [81,82] associations with self-reported intake or BMI. Discrepancy in reported liking and intake does not imply that reported liking is inaccurate, and instead may reflect dietary restraint (intake is less than liking) in adults [19,27,83] and parents who are trying to limit their children's consumption of less healthy foods [18]. Conversely, individuals who are trying to improve their diet healthiness may consume a food that is not well liked [18,27].

Encounters between health professionals and families can motivate attention to and action towards improving a child's healthy behaviors for obesity prevention [84]. Improvements in the healthiness of a child's diet is promoted when both parents and children prefer the same food/beverage [85]. The PALS in the present study has previously identified patterns of food preferences that are associated with parent feeding practices [86]. Having children and parents self-evaluate their food and activity liking can act as a stepping stone to introduce a conversation regarding healthy behaviors and to identify goals and areas for change. Even if children are not overweight or obese at the time of the assessment, their behaviors may put them at future health risk. It is important to address and improve pleasure from healthy eating to achieve healthier dietary behaviors [17,87,88] and tailor nutrition education messages [89]. Preliminary work from our group has shown that doing the PALS online is acceptable in children and parents, is reported to stimulate self-reflection on diet and activity behaviors, can generate immediate tailored feedback on diet quality and healthy behaviors [90]. Preferences can change, including in response to marketing of unhealthy foods [91] as well as with interventions to improve preference for healthy foods [92–95] and decrease preference for less healthy foods [83,96].

This study had both strengths and weaknesses. The PED can be an acceptable setting to screen health behaviors related to obesity risk and for brief interventions, particularly because it provides health care to high-risk populations, such as low-income, minority families [6–9]. Additionally, this study utilized the PALS diet and activity screener, which was acceptable to both children and parents, with testing of reliability and validity using multiple statistical techniques and criteria [34,97]. The PALS was similar in structure and methods to our previous study in preschoolers, which was parent-reported, validated against reported dietary intake, a biomarker of carotenoid status and BMI-P [18,98]. As a limitation, only one measure of dietary behaviors was assessed without a more complete evaluation of PA behaviors. Since obesogenic dietary behaviors involve both hedonic responses to pleasurable foods and appetite, the PALS could be supplemented with constructs of appetite and satiety [99]. Previous work by our group has shown increased precision in making diet-health associations by combining the liking survey with multiple measures of dietary behaviors [18]. Because the intent was to screen for dietary and PA, the present study did not include a biomarker of nutritional status or a device to measure PA. Furthermore, the HBI did not explain BMI-P across children with lowest to highest percentiles, but only among children of healthy BMI-P. Detecting associations between child adiposity, dietary patterns and behaviors may require longitudinal study designs [100]. Further, BMI-P may not be the most useful measure of adiposity for a racially/ethnically diverse sample of children and adolescents [101].

5. Conclusions

Pediatric clinical and translational research settings need rapid yet useful ways to screen for health behaviors to inform brief interventions, referrals, and obesity prevention programs. A simple liking survey provides an acceptable and useful screener of diet and activity behaviors in child–parent dyads. The survey took less than 4 min to complete on average and had a high participation rate. Liking for foods and activities was formed into a healthy behavior index that had acceptable internal reliability and good variability across children and parents. Healthier behavior indexes were seen in children from income-disadvantaged families and those from less food secure communities. Liking for less healthy foods explained some of the association between low family income and higher child BMI percentile. Health care providers could use the liking survey responses to initiate conversations with children and parents and to encourage healthy diet and physical activity behaviors. The PALS can be performed as a paper/pencil survey, but for future direction, also can be performed online with theory-based health promotion messages delivered to the children and parents based on response algorithms [90,102]. PALS responses across groups of child–parent dyads can inform broader nutrition education programming and messages, such as in the nutrition education arm of the U.S. Supplemental Nutrition Assistance Program (SNAP-Ed) [103].

Author Contributions: S.R.S. and V.B.D. conceived and designed the study; K.V. and S.O. oversaw the experimental methods; K.V., S.O., T.H.-M. and V.B.D. conducted the statistical analyses; K.V., S.O., T.H.-M. and V.B.D. interpreted the data; K.V., S.O. and V.B.D. wrote the manuscript; all authors reviewed the manuscript.

Funding: This research was funded by USDA National Institute of Food and Agriculture, Hatch project 1001056. The funders had no role in the study design, the data collection and the analysis, decision to publish, or the preparation of the manuscript.

Conflicts of Interest: The authors declare no conflict of interest. The funders had no role in the design of the study; in the collection, analyses, or interpretation of data; in the writing of the manuscript, or in the decision to publish the results.

References

1. Ng, M.; Fleming, T.; Robinson, M.; Thomson, B.; Graetz, N.; Margono, C.; Mullany, E.C.; Biryukov, S.; Abbafati, C.; Abera, S.F.; et al. Global, regional, and national prevalence of overweight and obesity in children and adults during 1980–2013: A systematic analysis for the Global Burden of Disease Study 2013. *Lancet* **2014**, *384*, 766–781. [CrossRef]

2. Ogden, C.L.; Carroll, M.D.; Lawman, H.G.; Fryar, C.D.; Kruszon-Moran, D.; Kit, B.K.; Flegal, K.M. Trends in obesity prevalence among children and adolescents in the United States, 1988–1994 Through 2013–2014. *JAMA* **2016**, *315*, 2292–2299. [CrossRef]

3. Institute of Medicine. *Accelerating Progress in Obesity Prevention: Solving the Weight of the Nation*; The National Academies Press: Washington, DC, USA, 2012; Available online: http://www.nationalacademies.org/hmd/Reports/2012/Accelerating-Progress-in-Obesity-Prevention.aspx (accessed on 1 June 2019).

4. Division of Nutrition, Physical Activity, and Obesity, National Center for Chronic Disease Prevention and Health Promotion. Childhood Obesity Research Demonstration (CORD) 1.0. Available online: https://www.cdc.gov/obesity/strategies/healthcare/cord1.html (accessed on 1 June 2019).

5. Kubicek, K.; Liu, D.; Beaudin, C.; Supan, J.; Weiss, G.; Lu, Y.; Kipke, M.D. A profile of nonurgent emergency department use in an urban pediatric hospital. *Pediatr. Emerg. Care* **2012**, *28*, 977–984. [CrossRef] [PubMed]

6. Chandler, I.; Rosenthal, L.; Carroll-Scott, A.; Peters, S.M.; McCaslin, C.; Ickovics, J.R. Adolescents who visit the emergency department are more likely to make unhealthy dietary choices: An opportunity for behavioral intervention. *J. Health Care Poor Underserv.* **2015**, *26*, 701–711. [CrossRef] [PubMed]

7. Haber, J.J.; Atti, S.; Gerber, L.M.; Waseem, M. Promoting an obesity education program among minority patients in a single urban pediatric Emergency Department (ED). *Int. J. Emerg. Med.* **2015**, *8*, 38. [CrossRef]

8. Prendergast, H.M.; Close, M.; Jones, B.; Furtado, N.; Bunney, E.B.; Mackey, M.; Marquez, D.; Edison, M. On the frontline: Pediatric obesity in the emergency department. *J. Natl. Med. Assoc.* **2011**, *103*, 922–925. [CrossRef]

9. Vaughn, L.M.; Nabors, L.; Pelley, T.J.; Hampton, R.R.; Jacquez, F.; Mahabee-Gittens, E.M. Obesity screening in the pediatric emergency department. *Pediatr. Emerg. Care* **2012**, *28*, 548–552. [CrossRef]

10. Brown, C.L.; Halvorson, E.E.; Cohen, G.M.; Lazorick, S.; Skelton, J.A. Addressing childhood obesity: opportunities for prevention. *Pediatr. Clin. North Am.* **2015**, *62*, 1241–1261. [CrossRef]

11. Gori, D.; Guaraldi, F.; Cinocca, S.; Moser, G.; Rucci, P.; Fantini, M.P. Effectiveness of educational and lifestyle interventions to prevent paediatric obesity: Systematic review and meta-analyses of randomized and non-randomized controlled trials. *Obes. Sci. Pract.* **2017**, *3*, 235–248. [CrossRef]

12. National Cancer Institute, Division of Cancer Control and Population Sciences. Register of Validated Short Dietary Assessment Instruments. Available online: https://epi.grants.cancer.gov/diet/shortreg/ (accessed on 1 June 2019).

13. National Collaborative on Childhood Obesity Research. Available online: http://www.nccor.org/nccor-tools/measures/ (accessed on 1 June 2019).

14. Bel-Serrat, S.; Julian-Almarcegui, C.; Gonzalez-Gross, M.; Mouratidou, T.; Bornhorst, C.; Grammatikaki, E.; Kersting, M.; Cuenca-Garcia, M.; Gottrand, F.; Molnar, D.; et al. Correlates of dietary energy misreporting among European adolescents: The healthy lifestyle in Europe by nutrition in adolescence (HELENA) study. *Br. J. Nutr.* **2016**, *115*, 1439–1452. [CrossRef]

15. Arheiam, A.; Albadri, S.; Laverty, L.; Harris, R. Reasons for low adherence to diet-diaries issued to pediatric dental patients: A collective case study. *Patient Prefer. Adher.* **2018**, *12*, 1401–1411. [CrossRef] [PubMed]

16. Tuorila, H.; Huotilainen, A.; Lähteenmäki, L.; Ollila, S.; Tuomi-Nurmi, S.; Urala, N. Comparison of affective rating scales and their relationship to variables reflecting food consumption. *Food Qual. Prefer.* **2008**, *19*, 51–61. [CrossRef]

17. Lanfer, A.; Knof, K.; Barba, G.; Veidebaum, T.; Papoutsou, S.; de Henauw, S.; Soos, T.; Moreno, L.A.; Ahrens, W.; Lissner, L. Taste preferences in association with dietary habits and weight status in European children: Results from the IDEFICS study. *Int. J. Obes. (Lond.)* **2012**, *36*, 27–34. [CrossRef]

18. Sharafi, M.; Perrachio, H.; Scarmo, S.; Huedo-Medina, T.B.; Mayne, S.T.; Cartmel, B.; Duffy, V.B. Preschool-adapted liking survey (PALS): A brief and valid method to assess dietary quality of preschoolers. *Child. Obes.* **2015**, *11*, 530–540. [CrossRef] [PubMed]

19. Duffy, V.B.; Lanier, S.A.; Hutchins, H.L.; Pescatello, L.S.; Johnson, M.K.; Bartoshuk, L.M. Food preference questionnaire as a screening tool for assessing dietary risk of cardiovascular disease within health risk appraisals. *J. Am. Diet Assoc.* **2007**, *107*, 237–245. [CrossRef] [PubMed]

20. Pallister, T.; Sharafi, M.; Lachance, G.; Pirastu, N.; Mohney, R.P.; MacGregor, A.; Feskens, E.J.; Duffy, V.; Spector, T.D.; Menni, C. Food preference patterns in a UK twin cohort. *Twin Res. Hum. Genet.* **2015**, *18*, 793–805. [CrossRef] [PubMed]

21. Sharafi, M.; Duffy, V.B.; Miller, R.J.; Winchester, S.B.; Sullivan, M.C. Dietary behaviors of adults born prematurely may explain future risk for cardiovascular disease. *Appetite* **2016**, *99*, 157–167. [CrossRef] [PubMed]

22. Smith, S.; Johnson, S.; Oldman, S.; Duffy, V. Pediatric-adapted liking survey: Feasible and reliable dietary screening in clinical practice. *Caries Res.* **2018**, *53*, 153–159. [CrossRef]

23. Vaidya, A.; Oli, N.; Krettek, A.; Eiben, G. Preference of food-items and physical activity of peri-urban children in Bhaktapur. *J. Nepal Health Res. Counc.* **2017**, *15*, 150–158. [CrossRef]

24. Beckerman, J.P.; Alike, Q.; Lovin, E.; Tamez, M.; Mattei, J. The development and public health implications of food preferences in children. *Front. Nutr.* **2017**, *4*, 66. [CrossRef]

25. Wang, Y.; Beydoun, M.A.; Li, J.; Liu, Y.; Moreno, L.A. Do children and their parents eat a similar diet? Resemblance in child and parental dietary intake: Systematic review and meta-analysis. *J. Epidemiol. Community Health* **2011**, *65*, 177–189. [CrossRef] [PubMed]

26. Lipsky, L.M.; Haynie, D.L.; Liu, A.; Nansel, T.R. Resemblance of diet quality in families of youth with type 1 diabetes participating in a randomized controlled behavioral nutrition intervention trial in Boston, MA (2010–2013): A secondary data analysis. *J. Acad. Nutr. Diet.* **2019**, *119*, 98–105. [CrossRef] [PubMed]

27. Sharafi, M.; Rawal, S.; Fernandez, M.L.; Huedo-Medina, T.B.; Duffy, V.B. Taste phenotype associates with cardiovascular disease risk factors via diet quality in multivariate modeling. *Physiol. Behav.* **2018**, *194*, 103–112. [CrossRef] [PubMed]

28. Nicklas, T.A.; Morales, M.; Linares, A.; Yang, S.J.; Baranowski, T.; De Moor, C.; Berenson, G. Children's meal patterns have changed over a 21-year period: The Bogalusa heart study. *J. Am. Diet. Assoc.* **2004**, *104*, 753–761. [CrossRef] [PubMed]

29. Alzaben, A.S.; MacDonald, K.; Robert, C.; Haqq, A.; Gilmour, S.M.; Yap, J.; Mager, D.R. Diet quality of children post-liver transplantation does not differ from healthy children. *Pediatr. Transpl.* **2017**, *21*. [CrossRef] [PubMed]

30. Wilson, T.A.; Liu, Y.; Adolph, A.L.; Sacher, P.M.; Barlow, S.E.; Pont, S.; Sharma, S.; Byrd-Williams, C.; Hoelscher, D.M.; Butte, N.F. Behavior modification of diet and parent feeding practices in a community—Vs. primary care-centered intervention for childhood obesity. *J. Nutr. Educ. Behav.* **2018**, *51*, 150–161. [CrossRef] [PubMed]

31. Thomson, J.L.; Tussing-Humphreys, L.M.; Goodman, M.H.; Landry, A.S. Diet quality in a nationally representative sample of American children by sociodemographic characteristics. *Am. J. Clin. Nutr.* **2019**, *109*, 127–138. [CrossRef] [PubMed]

32. Craike, M.; Wiesner, G.; Hilland, T.A.; Bengoechea, E.G. Interventions to improve physical activity among socioeconomically disadvantaged groups: An umbrella review. *Int. J. Behav. Nutr. Phys. Act.* **2018**, *15*, 43. [CrossRef]

33. King, A.C.; Powell, K.E.; Members, A.C. 2018 Physical Activity Guidelines Advisory Committee Scientific Report. Available online: https://health.gov/paguidelines/second-edition/report/ (accessed on 18 June 2019).

34. Guenther, P.M.; Kirkpatrick, S.I.; Reedy, J.; Krebs-Smith, S.M.; Buckman, D.W.; Dodd, K.W.; Casavale, K.O.; Carroll, R.J. The healthy eating index-2010 is a valid and reliable measure of diet quality according to the 2010 dietary guidelines for Americans. *J. Nutr.* **2014**, *144*, 399–407. [CrossRef]

35. Rabinowitz, A.N.; Martin, J. Community food security in Connecticut: An evaluation and ranking of 169 towns; Zwick Center Outreach Report. 2012. Available online: https://ideas.repec.org/p/ags/ucozfr/154264.html (accessed on 18 June 2019).

36. U.S. Department of Health and Human Services; U.S. Department of Agriculture. *2015–2020 Dietary Guidelines for Americans*, 8th ed.; U.S. Department of Health and Human Services: Washington, DC, USA; U.S. Department of Agriculture: Washington, DC, USA, 2015. Available online: http://health.gov/dietaryguidelines/2015/guidelines/ (accessed on 1 June 2019).

37. Centers for Disease Control and Prevention. Healthy Weight. BMI Percentile Calculator for Child and Teen. Available online: https://www.cdc.gov/healthyweight/bmi/calculator.html (accessed on 14 July 2019).

38. Centers for Disease Control and Prevention. About Child & Teen BMI. Available online: https://www.cdc.gov/healthyweight/assessing/bmi/childrens_bmi/about_childrens_bmi.html# interpreted%20the%20same%20way (accessed on 14 July 2019).

39. Collins, M.E. Body figure perceptions and preferences among preadolescent children. *Int. J. Eat. Disord.* **1991**, *10*, 199–208. [CrossRef]

40. Marshall, S.; Burrows, T.; Collins, C.E. Systematic review of diet quality indices and their associations with health-related outcomes in children and adolescents. *J. Hum. Nutr. Diet.* **2014**, *27*, 577–598. [CrossRef] [PubMed]

41. Hebestreit, A.; Intemann, T.; Siani, A.; De Henauw, S.; Eiben, G.; Kourides, Y.A.; Kovacs, E.; Moreno, L.A.; Veidebaum, T.; Krogh, V.; et al. Dietary patterns of European children and their parents in association with family food environment: results from the I. family study. *Nutrients* **2017**, *9*, 126. [CrossRef] [PubMed]

42. Yee, A.Z.; Lwin, M.O.; Ho, S.S. The influence of parental practices on child promotive and preventive food consumption behaviors: A systematic review and meta-analysis. *Int. J. Behav. Nutr. Phys. Act.* **2017**, *14*, 47. [CrossRef] [PubMed]

43. Bogl, L.H.; Silventoinen, K.; Hebestreit, A.; Intemann, T.; Williams, G.; Michels, N.; Molnar, D.; Page, A.S.; Pala, V.; Papoutsou, S.; et al. Familial resemblance in dietary intakes of children, adolescents, and parents: Does dietary quality play a role? *Nutrients* **2017**, *9*, 892. [CrossRef] [PubMed]

44. Mennella, J.A.; Bobowski, N.K.; Reed, D.R. The development of sweet taste: From biology to hedonics. *Rev. Endocr. Metab. Disord.* **2016**, *17*, 171–178. [CrossRef]

45. Wang, J.; Shang, L.; Light, K.; O'Loughlin, J.; Paradis, G.; Gray-Donald, K. Associations between added sugar (solid vs. liquid) intakes, diet quality, and adiposity indicators in Canadian children. *Appl. Physiol. Nutr. Metab.* **2015**, *40*, 835–841. [CrossRef] [PubMed]

46. Verloigne, M.; Van Lippevelde, W.; Bere, E.; Manios, Y.; Kovacs, E.; Grillenberger, M.; Maes, L.; Brug, J.; De Bourdeaudhuij, I. Individual and family environmental correlates of television and computer time in 10- to 12-year-old European children: The ENERGY-project. *BMC Public Health* **2015**, *15*, 912. [CrossRef]

47. Yao, C.A.; Rhodes, R.E. Parental correlates in child and adolescent physical activity: A meta-analysis. *Int. J. Behav. Nutr. Phys. Act.* **2015**, *12*, 10. [CrossRef]

48. Rhodes, R.E.; Lim, C. Promoting parent and child physical activity together: Elicitation of potential intervention targets and preferences. *Health Educ. Behav.* **2018**, *45*, 112–123. [CrossRef]

49. Bolton, K.A.; Jacka, F.; Allender, S.; Kremer, P.; Gibbs, L.; Waters, E.; de Silva, A. The association between self-reported diet quality and health-related quality of life in rural and urban Australian adolescents. *Aust. J. Rural Health* **2016**, *24*, 317–325. [CrossRef]

50. Hiza, H.A.; Casavale, K.O.; Guenther, P.M.; Davis, C.A. Diet quality of Americans differs by age, sex, race/ethnicity, income, and education level. *J. Acad. Nutr. Diet.* **2013**, *113*, 297–306. [CrossRef]

51. Golley, R.K.; Hendrie, G.A.; McNaughton, S.A. Scores on the dietary guideline index for children and adolescents are associated with nutrient intake and socio-economic position but not adiposity. *J. Nutr.* **2011**, *141*, 1340–1347. [CrossRef] [PubMed]

52. Andreyeva, T.; Tripp, A.S.; Schwartz, M.B. Dietary quality of Americans by Supplemental Nutrition Assistance Program participation status: A systematic review. *Am. J. Prev. Med.* **2015**, *49*, 594–604. [CrossRef]

53. Robson, S.M.; Couch, S.C.; Peugh, J.L.; Glanz, K.; Zhou, C.; Sallis, J.F.; Saelens, B.E. Parent diet quality and energy intake are related to child diet quality and energy intake. *J. Acad. Nutr. Diet.* **2016**, *116*, 984–990. [CrossRef] [PubMed]

54. Shang, L.; O'Loughlin, J.; Tremblay, A.; Gray-Donald, K. The association between food patterns and adiposity among Canadian children at risk of overweight. *Appl. Physiol. Nutr. Metab.* **2014**, *39*, 195–201. [CrossRef] [PubMed]

55. Cagiran Yilmaz, F.; Cagiran, D.; Ozcelik, A.O. Adolescent obesity and its association with diet quality and cardiovascular risk factors. *Ecol. Food Nutr.* **2019**, *58*, 207–218. [CrossRef] [PubMed]

56. Archero, F.; Ricotti, R.; Solito, A.; Carrera, D.; Civello, F.; Di Bella, R.; Bellone, S.; Prodam, F. Adherence to the Mediterranean diet among school children and adolescents living in northern Italy and unhealthy food behaviors associated to overweight. *Nutrients* **2018**, *10*. [CrossRef] [PubMed]

57. Mellendick, K.; Shanahan, L.; Wideman, L.; Calkins, S.; Keane, S.; Lovelady, C. Diets rich in fruits and vegetables are associated with lower cardiovascular disease risk in adolescents. *Nutrients* **2018**, *10*. [CrossRef] [PubMed]

58. Murakami, K. Associations between nutritional quality of meals and snacks assessed by the Food Standards Agency nutrient profiling system and overall diet quality and adiposity measures in British children and adolescents. *Nutrition* **2018**, *49*, 57–65. [CrossRef] [PubMed]

59. Xu, F.; Cohen, S.A.; Greaney, M.L.; Greene, G.W. The association between US adolescents' Weight status, weight perception, weight satisfaction, and their physical activity and dietary behaviors. *Int. J. Environ. Res. Public Health* **2018**, *15*. [CrossRef] [PubMed]

60. Lee, J.; Kubik, M.Y.; Fulkerson, J.A. Diet quality and fruit, vegetable, and sugar-sweetened beverage consumption by household food insecurity among 8- to 12-year-old children during summer months. *J. Acad. Nutr. Diet.* **2019**. [CrossRef] [PubMed]

61. Hunt, E.T.; Brazendale, K.; Dunn, C.; Boutte, A.K.; Liu, J.; Hardin, J.; Beets, M.W.; Weaver, R.G. Income, race and its association with obesogenic behaviors of U.S. children and adolescents, NHANES 2003–2006. *J. Community Health* **2019**, *44*, 507–518. [CrossRef] [PubMed]

62. Ambrosini, G.L.; Emmett, P.M.; Northstone, K.; Howe, L.D.; Tilling, K.; Jebb, S.A. Identification of a dietary pattern prospectively associated with increased adiposity during childhood and adolescence. *Int. J. Obes. (Lond.)* **2012**, *36*, 1299–1305. [CrossRef] [PubMed]

63. Elmesmari, R.; Martin, A.; Reilly, J.J.; Paton, J.Y. Comparison of accelerometer measured levels of physical activity and sedentary time between obese and non-obese children and adolescents: A systematic review. *BMC Pediatr.* **2018**, *18*, 106. [CrossRef] [PubMed]

64. Vanhelst, J.; Beghin, L.; Duhamel, A.; De Henauw, S.; Ruiz, J.R.; Kafatos, A.; Androutsos, O.; Widhalm, K.; Mauro, B.; Sjostrom, M.; et al. Do adolescents accurately evaluate their diet quality? The HELENA study. *Clin. Nutr.* **2017**, *36*, 1669–1673. [CrossRef] [PubMed]

65. Leung, C.W.; DiMatteo, S.G.; Gosliner, W.A.; Ritchie, L.D. Sugar-sweetened beverage and water intake in relation to diet quality in U.S. children. *Am. J. Prev. Med.* **2018**, *54*, 394–402. [CrossRef] [PubMed]

66. De Miguel-Etayo, P.; Moreno, L.A.; Santabarbara, J.; Martin-Matillas, M.; Azcona-San Julian, M.C.; Marti Del Moral, A.; Campoy, C.; Marcos, A.; Garagorri, J.M.; Group, E.S. Diet quality index as a predictor of treatment efficacy in overweight and obese adolescents: The EVASYON study. *Clin. Nutr.* **2019**, *38*, 782–790. [CrossRef] [PubMed]

67. Arsenault, B.J.; Lamarche, B.; Despres, J.P. Targeting overconsumption of sugar-sweetened beverages vs. overall poor diet quality for cardiometabolic diseases risk prevention: place your bets! *Nutrients* **2017**, *9*. [CrossRef] [PubMed]

68. Tovar, A.; Chui, K.; Hyatt, R.R.; Kuder, J.; Kraak, V.I.; Choumenkovitch, S.F.; Hastings, A.; Bloom, J.; Economos, C.D. Healthy-lifestyle behaviors associated with overweight and obesity in US rural children. *BMC Pediatr.* **2012**, *12*, 102. [CrossRef]

69. Sugiyama, T.; Horino, M.; Inoue, K.; Kobayashi, Y.; Shapiro, M.F.; McCarthy, W.J. Trends of child's weight perception by children, parents, and healthcare professionals during the time of terminology change in childhood obesity in the United States, 2005–2014. *Child. Obes.* **2016**, *12*, 463–473. [CrossRef] [PubMed]

70. Sisson, S.B.; Shay, C.M.; Broyles, S.T.; Leyva, M. Television-viewing time and dietary quality among U.S. children and adults. *Am. J. Prev. Med.* **2012**, *43*, 196–200. [CrossRef] [PubMed]

71. Strasburger, V.C.; Jordan, A.B.; Donnerstein, E. Health effects of media on children and adolescents. *Pediatrics* **2010**, *125*, 756–767. [CrossRef] [PubMed]

72. Bauer, K.W.; Nelson, M.C.; Boutelle, K.N.; Neumark-Sztainer, D. Parental influences on adolescents' physical activity and sedentary behavior: Longitudinal findings from Project EAT-II. *Int. J. Behav. Nutr. Phys. Act.* **2008**, *5*, 12. [CrossRef] [PubMed]

73. Labonte, M.E.; Kirkpatrick, S.I.; Bell, R.C.; Boucher, B.A.; Csizmadi, I.; Koushik, A.; L'Abbe, M.R.; Massarelli, I.; Robson, P.J.; Rondeau, I.; et al. Dietary assessment is a critical element of health research—Perspective from the partnership for advancing nutritional and dietary assessment in Canada. *Appl. Physiol. Nutr. Metab.* **2016**, *41*, 1096–1099. [CrossRef] [PubMed]

74. Garnier, S.; Vallee, K.; Lemoine-Morel, S.; Joffroy, S.; Drapeau, V.; Tremblay, A.; Auneau, G.; Mauriege, P. Food group preferences and energy balance in moderately obese postmenopausal women subjected to brisk walking program. *Appl. Physiol. Nutr. Metab.* **2015**, *40*, 741–748. [CrossRef] [PubMed]

75. Beheshti, R.; Jones-Smith, J.C.; Igusa, T. Taking dietary habits into account: A computational method for modeling food choices that goes beyond price. *PLoS ONE* **2017**, *12*, e0178348. [CrossRef] [PubMed]

76. Lee, Y.H.; Shelley, M.; Liu, C.T.; Chang, Y.C. Assessing the association of food preferences and self-reported psychological well-being among middle-aged and older adults in contemporary china-results from the china health and nutrition survey. *Int. J. Environ. Res. Public Health* **2018**, *15*. [CrossRef]

77. Fletcher, S.; Wright, C.; Jones, A.; Parkinson, K.; Adamson, A. Tracking of toddler fruit and vegetable preferences to intake and adiposity later in childhood. *Matern. Child Nutr.* **2017**, *13*. [CrossRef] [PubMed]

78. Ramsay, S.A.; Rudley, M.; Tonnemaker, L.E.; Price, W.J. A comparison of college students' reported fruit and vegetable liking and intake from childhood to adulthood. *J. Am. Coll. Nutr.* **2017**, *36*, 28–37. [CrossRef]

79. Park, H.; Shin, Y.; Kwon, O.; Kim, Y. Association of sensory liking for fat with dietary intake and metabolic syndrome in korean adults. *Nutrients* **2018**, *10*. [CrossRef]

80. Charlot, K.; Malgoyre, A.; Bourrilhon, C. Proposition for a shortened version of the leeds food preference questionnaire (LFPQ). *Physiol. Behav.* **2019**, *199*, 244–251. [CrossRef] [PubMed]

81. Potter, C.; Griggs, R.L.; Ferriday, D.; Rogers, P.J.; Brunstrom, J.M. Individual variability in preference for energy-dense foods fails to predict child BMI percentile. *Physiol. Behav.* **2017**, *176*, 3–8. [CrossRef] [PubMed]

82. Low, J.Y.Q.; Lacy, K.E.; McBride, R.L.; Keast, R.S.J. The associations between oral complex carbohydrate sensitivity, BMI, liking, and consumption of complex carbohydrate based foods. *J. Food Sci.* **2018**, *83*, 2227–2236. [CrossRef] [PubMed]

83. Ledikwe, J.H.; Ello-Martin, J.; Pelkman, C.L.; Birch, L.L.; Mannino, M.L.; Rolls, B.J. A reliable, valid questionnaire indicates that preference for dietary fat declines when following a reduced-fat diet. *Appetite* **2007**, *49*, 74–83. [CrossRef]

84. Lowenstein, L.M.; Perrin, E.M.; Berry, D.; Vu, M.B.; Pullen Davis, L.; Cai, J.; Tzeng, J.P.; Ammerman, A.S. Childhood obesity prevention: Fathers' reflections with healthcare providers. *Child. Obes.* **2013**, *9*, 137–143. [CrossRef] [PubMed]

85. Groele, B.; Glabska, D.; Gutkowska, K.; Guzek, D. Mother's fruit preferences and consumption support similar attitudes and behaviors in their children. *Int. J. Environ. Res. Public Health* **2018**, *15*. [CrossRef] [PubMed]

86. Vollmer, R.L.; Baietto, J. Practices and preferences: Exploring the relationships between food-related parenting practices and child food preferences for high fat and/or sugar foods, fruits, and vegetables. *Appetite* **2017**, *113*, 134–140. [CrossRef] [PubMed]

87. Nekitsing, C.; Hetherington, M.M.; Blundell-Birtill, P. Developing healthy food preferences in preschool children through taste exposure, sensory learning, and nutrition education. *Curr. Obes. Rep.* **2018**, *7*, 60–67. [CrossRef]

88. Marty, L.; Miguet, M.; Bournez, M.; Nicklaus, S.; Chambaron, S.; Monnery-Patris, S. Do hedonic- versus nutrition-based attitudes toward food predict food choices? A cross-sectional study of 6- to 11-year-olds. *Int. J. Behav. Nutr. Phys. Act.* **2017**, *14*, 162. [CrossRef]

89. Jalkanen, H.; Lindi, V.; Schwab, U.; Kiiskinen, S.; Venalainen, T.; Karhunen, L.; Lakka, T.A.; Eloranta, A.M. Eating behaviour is associated with eating frequency and food consumption in 6-8 year-old children: The physical activity and nutrition in children (PANIC) study. *Appetite* **2017**, *114*, 28–37. [CrossRef]

90. Duffy, V.B.; Smith, S. Leveraging Technology to Deliver Tailored SNAP-Ed Messages. Available online: https://snaped.fns.usda.gov/success-stories/leveraging-technology-deliver-tailored-snap-ed-messages (accessed on 14 July 2019).

91. Sadeghirad, B.; Duhaney, T.; Motaghipisheh, S.; Campbell, N.R.; Johnston, B.C. Influence of unhealthy food and beverage marketing on children's dietary intake and preference: A systematic review and meta-analysis of randomized trials. *Obes. Rev.* **2016**, *17*, 945–959. [CrossRef] [PubMed]

92. De Wild, V.W.T.; de Graaf, C.; Jager, G. Use of different vegetable products to increase preschool-aged children's preference for and intake of a target vegetable: A randomized controlled trial. *J. Acad. Nutr. Diet.* **2017**, *117*, 859–866. [CrossRef] [PubMed]

93. Magarey, A.; Mauch, C.; Mallan, K.; Perry, R.; Elovaris, R.; Meedeniya, J.; Byrne, R.; Daniels, L. Child dietary and eating behavior outcomes up to 3.5 years after an early feeding intervention: The NOURISH RCT. *Obesity (Silver Spring)* **2016**, *24*, 1537–1545. [CrossRef] [PubMed]

94. Cunningham-Sabo, L.; Lohse, B. Cooking with Kids positively affects fourth graders' vegetable preferences and attitudes and self-efficacy for food and cooking. *Child. Obes.* **2013**, *9*, 549–556. [CrossRef] [PubMed]

95. Wall, D.E.; Least, C.; Gromis, J.; Lohse, B. Nutrition education intervention improves vegetable-related attitude, self-efficacy, preference, and knowledge of fourth-grade students. *J. Sch. Health* **2012**, *82*, 37–43. [CrossRef] [PubMed]

96. Ebneter, D.S.; Latner, J.D.; Nigg, C.R. Is less always more? The effects of low-fat labeling and caloric information on food intake, calorie estimates, taste preference, and health attributions. *Appetite* **2013**, *68*, 92–97. [CrossRef]

97. Carbonneau, E.; Bradette-Laplante, M.; Lamarche, B.; Provencher, V.; Begin, C.; Robitaille, J.; Desroches, S.; Vohl, M.C.; Corneau, L.; Lemieux, S. Development and validation of the food liking questionnaire in a French-Canadian population. *Nutrients* **2017**, *9*, 1337. [CrossRef]

98. Scarmo, S.; Henebery, K.; Peracchio, H.; Cartmel, B.; Lin, H.; Ermakov, I.V.; Gellermann, W.; Bernstein, P.S.; Duffy, V.B.; Mayne, S.T. Skin carotenoid status measured by resonance Raman spectroscopy as a biomarker of fruit and vegetable intake in preschool children. *Eur. J. Clin. Nutr.* **2012**, *66*, 555–560. [CrossRef]

99. Freitas, A.; Albuquerque, G.; Silva, C.; Oliveira, A. Appetite-related eating behaviours: An overview of assessment methods, determinants and effects on children's weight. *Ann. Nutr. Metab.* **2018**, *73*, 19–29. [CrossRef]

100. Fernandez-Alvira, J.M.; Bammann, K.; Eiben, G.; Hebestreit, A.; Kourides, Y.A.; Kovacs, E.; Michels, N.; Pala, V.; Reisch, L.; Russo, P.; et al. Prospective associations between dietary patterns and body composition changes in European children: The IDEFICS study. *Public Health Nutr.* **2017**, *20*, 3257–3265. [CrossRef]

101. Weber, D.R.; Moore, R.H.; Leonard, M.B.; Zemel, B.S. Fat and lean BMI reference curves in children and adolescents and their utility in identifying excess adiposity compared with BMI and percentage body fat. *Am. J. Clin. Nutr.* **2013**, *98*, 49–56. [CrossRef] [PubMed]

102. Oldman, S. Improving Diet & Physical Activity Behaviors through Tailored Mhealth Messages: Application to Childhood Obesity Prevention in a Pediatric Emergency Department. Master's Thesis, Health Promotion Sciences, University of Connecticut, Mansfield, CT, USA, 2018.

103. U.S. Department of Agriculture. SNAP-Ed Connection. Available online: https://snaped.fns.usda.gov/ (accessed on 14 July 2019).

![nutrients logo] *nutrients* MDPI

Article

Parents' Reports of Preschoolers' Diets: Relative Validity of a Food Frequency Questionnaire and Dietary Patterns

Liisa Korkalo [1,†], Henna Vepsäläinen [1,*,†], Carola Ray [2], Essi Skaffari [1], Reetta Lehto [2],
Helena Henrietta Hauta-alus [3], Kaija Nissinen [4], Jelena Meinilä [2,5], Eva Roos [2,6] and
Maijaliisa Erkkola [1]

[1]   Department of Food and Nutrition, University of Helsinki, P.O. Box 66, 00014 Helsinki, Finland;
      liisa.korkalo@helsinki.fi (L.K.); essi.skaffari@helsinki.fi (E.S.); maijaliisa.erkkola@helsinki.fi (M.E.)
[2]   Folkhälsan Research Center, Topeliuksenkatu 20, 00250 Helsinki, Finland; carola.ray@folkhalsan.fi (C.R.);
      reetta.lehto@folkhalsan.fi (R.L.); jelena.meinila@folkhalsan.fi (J.M.); eva.roos@folkhalsan.fi (E.R.)
[3]   Children's Hospital, Pediatric Research Center, University of Helsinki and Helsinki University Hospital,
      Biomedicum 2 C, P.O. Box 705, 00020 HUS Helsinki, Finland; helena.hauta-alus@helsinki.fi
[4]   Seinäjoki University of Applied Sciences, Kampusranta 11, 60101 Seinäjoki, Finland; kaija.nissinen@seamk.fi
[5]   Department of Obstetrics and Gynecology, University of Helsinki and Helsinki University Hospital,
      P.O. Box 22, 00014 Helsinki, Finland
[6]   Department of Public Health, University of Helsinki, P.O. Box 20, 00014 Helsinki, Finland
*   Correspondence: henna.vepsalainen@helsinki.fi; Tel.: +358-44-358-1467
†   These authors contributed equally to this work.

Received: 3 December 2018; Accepted: 9 January 2019; Published: 13 January 2019

Abstract: The accurate assessment of food consumption is crucial in nutritional studies. Since modern nutrition science has become more interested in diet as a whole, studies validating food frequency questionnaires (FFQs) and exploratory dietary patterns are needed. We aimed at examining the relative validity of a 47-item FFQ against three-day food records among three- to six-year-old Finnish children, as well as investigating the consistency of the dietary patterns derived using the principal component analysis (PCA), with food record and FFQ data as inputs. We conducted the PCA without forcing the food record data to match the FFQ items. Altogether, 75% or more of the participants were classified into the same or adjacent quarter of vegetables and fruits as well as sugary food consumption. Furthermore, the intake of folate and vitamin C increased linearly in the quarters of vegetable and fruit consumption, as did the intake of sucrose in quarters of sugary food consumption. Three fairly similar dietary patterns were identified from food records and FFQ data. Concerning the patterns, more than 70% of the participants were classified into the same or adjacent quarter. However, the Spearman correlation coefficients between the respective pattern scores were low (0.25–0.33). The FFQ showed acceptable validity when ranking food group consumption compared to food records. Additionally, the FFQ-derived dietary patterns were consistent with those derived using food record data.

Keywords: validation study; dietary assessment methods; food diary; cross-classification; children; whole diet; preschool; DAGIS Study

1. Introduction

As food consumption cannot be measured objectively, researchers must rely on self-reported methods, such as food records, dietary recalls, or food frequency questionnaires (FFQs). FFQs are often used in large, epidemiological studies because of their cost-effectiveness and relatively low respondent burden [1,2]. Children under the age of 7 years are not able to report their own food consumption, and thus, the acquisition of dietary information is dependent on parents, other guardians, or early childhood educators, for instance [3]. Therefore, the accuracy of dietary assessment in children is dependent on the adults' ability to reliably and validly report the children's food consumption. The relative validity of an FFQ can be investigated by comparing the food consumption data obtained using an FFQ with the data obtained using a separate dietary assessment method. Food records are a good method for estimating the relative validity of an FFQ, because the two methods do not share the main sources of errors [4], but other reference methods, such as 24-hour recalls or plasma biomarkers, have also been used in studies validating FFQs among children [5].

Traditionally, validation studies have compared the consumption frequency of certain foods or food groups (e.g., fruits and vegetables, or beverages) or calculated nutrient intakes (e.g., calcium or energy intake) derived using two separate methods (see, for example, [6–10]). However, data-driven dietary patterns that are indicative of a person's whole diet have become popular in nutritional epidemiology [11]. One of the most frequently used methods to derive dietary patterns is principal component analysis (PCA), which is based on intercorrelations between food items [12,13]. The extraction of dietary patterns using PCA requires, however, multiple subjective decisions, such as the selection of dietary variables, to be included in the analysis [14]. Furthermore, the dietary assessment method used to measure food consumption may affect the extracted patterns. Thus, the validation of PCA-derived dietary patterns is beneficial.

Data-driven dietary patterns are thought to reflect the usual food consumption of the participants. Thus, FFQs, which also describe food consumption in general, have mostly been used as inputs in the dietary pattern analysis. Since the late 1990s, several studies have compared FFQ-based dietary patterns with patterns derived from food record data among adults [15–21]. Only two studies have compared FFQ- and food-record-based patterns among children [22,23]. However, the studies have matched each food in the food records with an FFQ item, possibly resulting in artificially increased correlation coefficients [20].

The objective of the current study was two-fold, namely: (1) to study the relative validity of a non-quantitative 47-item FFQ against a three-day food record (reference method) of preschool children by evaluating the ability of the FFQ to rank individuals in the same order according to food consumption as compared to the reference method, and (2) to study the consistency of the data-driven dietary patterns derived by PCA using two sources (food record and FFQ) of data. Our study broadly looked at the validity by examining both the direct (comparison of food consumption to food consumption) and indirect (comparison of food consumption to nutrient intake) validity of the FFQ, as well as the relative validity of the dietary patterns. However, we only measured food consumption outside of preschool.

2. Materials and Methods

2.1. Study Participants

Increased Health and Wellbeing in Preschools (DAGIS) is a research project that aims to diminish socio-economic differences in preschool children's energy balance-related behaviors in Finland (www.dagis.fi). As a part of the larger project, a cross-sectional study was conducted between September 2015 and April 2016, and the details of the sampling process are described in open access format [24]. In short, the cross-sectional study was conducted in eight municipalities. Altogether, 86 communal preschools (56% of those invited) consented to participate. These preschools operated from Monday to Friday and served three meals per day—breakfast, lunch, and an afternoon snack. Preschools operating 24 hours per day were not included in the sample. From the consenting preschools, all of the children in the target age of three to six years (*n* = 3592) and their families were invited to participate through an invitation letter. Children in preschools with a low participation rate (≤30% in each of the preschool groups for three to six year-olds) were excluded. The final sample consisted of 864 children (24% of those invited) from 66 preschools. A parent or legal guardian of each participating child provided written informed consent. The University of Helsinki Ethical review board in humanities and social and behavioral sciences reviewed the study on 24 February 2015, and found the study ethically acceptable (Statement 6/2015).

2.2. FFQ

We designed a short FFQ for measuring children's food consumption during the previous week outside of preschool hours. The FFQ was developed to assess the children's dietary quality in general, and specific attention was paid to capturing the consumption patterns of vegetables and fruits as well as sugary foods and beverages. The FFQ included 47 food items divided under seven headings, as follows: vegetables, fruits, and berries; dairy products; fish; meat and eggs; cereal products; drinks; and others (i.e., sweets and snacks). The questionnaire was available in both official languages of Finland (Finnish and Swedish) and in English; the English version of the FFQ is available online [25]. A shortened, 25-item version of the FFQ has been tested for reproducibility with mostly moderate or good intraclass correlation coefficients [26].

The participating families received a letter including the FFQ, a three-day food record, and detailed instructions by post. The instructions were to fill in the FFQ first and the three-day food record later, on pre-set dates. The time between the two methods was roughly one week. In the FFQ, the respondent (parent or legal guardian) reported how many times during the past week the child had consumed different foods outside preschool. We intentionally restricted the FFQ to not cover foods and drinks consumed during the preschool hours because the parents would not have been able to reliably report these foods. The time spent at preschool may vary from child to child as well as from day to day, and therefore, we did not specify which meals should be included or excluded in the FFQ. The FFQ included the following three answer columns: "not at all", 'times per week", and "times per day". The instruction was to either tick the "not at all" box or to write a number in one of the other columns. If two or more FFQ items were missing, nutritionists contacted the families and the missing items were completed if possible.

2.3. Three-Day Food Record Data

The study group assigned the exact dates (two weekdays and one weekend day) for each family to fill in the food record. These three days were not always consecutive days. In some cases, when the pre-set dates were unsuitable for the family, the parents contacted the study group and the dates were renegotiated. The instruction was to record all of the foods and beverages consumed by the child during the three days, except for consumption at preschool. We provided the families with a children's food picture book, specifically designed for use in this project, to assist in portion size estimation [27,28]. The parents estimated portion sizes by using the food picture book or household measures, by weighing, or from package labels. The instruction was to list all of the ingredients of the composite dishes. For prepacked products, the exact brand and product name was to be given. Preschool personnel filled in a separate food record during preschool hours, but these data were not used in the analyses of this paper.

The larger DAGIS project had a specific focus on vegetables and fruits as well as sugary food consumption [29]; therefore, these food groups were given special attention in the food record checking process. Nutritionists checked all of the food records. If there were shortcomings in the information concerning vegetables, fruits, and berries, or sugar-containing foods or beverages, the nutritionists made follow-up phone calls or emailed the parents to complete missing details of these foods. As an example, if the parent had forgotten to record the type of yoghurt product, we asked if it was a natural yoghurt or sugar-sweetened yoghurt. Nutritionists entered the food record data using AivoDiet dietary software (version 2.2.0.0, Aivo Oy, Turku, Finland). AivoDiet software included the Fineli Food Composition Database Release 16 (2013). New food items were added into the database when necessary. The database includes recipes for typical Finnish mixed dishes. For each individual meal, the nutritionists either used a suitable recipe found in the database or created a new recipe according to parents' reports. During data entry, each meal was tagged with a code indicating the place of consumption, which enabled us to remove the foods eaten at preschool from the analyses.

To compare the food consumption frequencies during the three-day food record period with the food consumption frequencies reported in the FFQ, we listed every food code used in the food record data and assigned them to the corresponding FFQ row(s). The food record data used in the analyses of this paper included a total of 2421 individual food codes (food items or mixed dishes). Each mixed dish food code was assigned to no more than three rows, according to the main ingredients. For example, a meat soup, which included carrots and potatoes, was assigned to the rows "red meat", "potatoes", and "cooked and canned vegetables". Out of the 2421 food codes, 1714 codes were assigned to one FFQ row, 228 codes to two FFQ rows, and 96 codes to three FFQ rows. The rest (i.e., 383 codes) represented foods not covered by the FFQ, and these were not assigned to any FFQ rows. These codes included, for example, spices, savory pastries, and fat spreads.

2.4. Comparison of the FFQs and Food Records

For the comparison of the FFQs and food records, we used data from all of the children with their FFQs filled in with no more than six missing rows out of the 47 rows, and three days of complete data in the food record ($n = 756$). The number of families who filled in the FFQs for these children was 674; 594 families had one child in the sample, 78 families had two children in the sample, and two families had three children in the sample. The majority ($n = 747$; 99%) of these children were in the target age group of three to six years old, but seven children were two years old and two were seven years old. The differences in the age and sex distribution between the children included in the analysis and the children excluded from the analysis because of missing food consumption information ($n = 108$) were tested using the Student's t-test and Chi-Squared test.

To test how well the FFQ was able to rank individuals in the same categories of food consumption frequency when compared to the reference method (food record), each child was assigned to one of four categories created according to the quartiles of the distribution. Note that we only considered food consumption outside of preschool hours. The categories were cross-tabulated, and the percentages in the same, same or adjacent, and opposite quarters were calculated. We also calculated the proportions of non-consumers and the weekly and daily consumers according to the FFQ. For foods with a high proportion of non-consumers, the majority of the participants were automatically assigned to the first category and the data were assigned into only two or three categories in total. This was true for both methods. Thus, some cells in the cross-tabulations remained empty.

To evaluate whether the food consumption frequency, as measured by the FFQ, was associated with the intake of key nutrients, as calculated from the three-day food records that indicate the consumption of specific types of foods, the mean intakes of selected nutrients were computed according to the consumption categories of selected food groups from the FFQs. We selected the food groups that the DAGIS project has a specific focus on (i.e., vegetables and fruit, and sugary foods and beverages). The consumption frequency was evaluated against the folate and vitamin C (vegetable and fruit consumption) and sucrose intake (sugary foods and beverages). In addition, we evaluated milk, which is typically consumed daily by Finnish preschoolers, against calcium intake. The food group frequency categories were created by summing the responses of the selected FFQ rows. Missing values were treated as zeros when summing the responses. We then categorized the food group consumption frequencies into quarters. Trend analysis was performed using linear regression. The food consumption frequency quarter was treated as a continuous predictor variable, and the nutrient intakes were square root transformed.

2.5. Comparison of Dietary Patterns

In order to identify the existing dietary patterns in the sample, we conducted separate PCAs using (1) the FFQ food groups and (2) food record data (all of the items consumed outside preschool) as inputs. All of the children with complete FFQ data ($n = 758$; 88% of all of the DAGIS participants) were included in the FFQ-based PCA, in which all of the 47 FFQ food items were used as input variables (see [30] for more details). For the food-record-based analysis, the food record codes were collapsed into 64 food groups based on the nutritional similarity of the foods. All of the children with food record data from three days and with no more than six missing FFQ rows ($n = 756$) were included in the analysis. Of these food groups, we excluded 17 because of low consumption (mean consumption less than 10 g in three days). Due to having no nutritional value and inconsistencies in reporting, we further excluded water from the analysis. Similarly, a mixed group containing foods that could not easily be classified into any of the existing food groups (e.g., spices, spice sauces, meal replacement products, and other miscellaneous foods) was excluded. Thus, the consumption of 45 food groups (g/day) were used as inputs in the food-record-based PCA (see Supplementary Table S1 for included and excluded food groups). IBM SPSS Statistics versions 22 (IBM Corp., Armonk, NY, USA) and 25 (IBM Corp., Armonk, NY, USA) were used in the PCA.

Based on the eigenvalues (minimum value of at least 1.5), scree plots, and interpretability of the components, we chose three components for the FFQ-based analysis and five components for the food-record-based analysis. The analyses were then rerun with forced three- or five-component solutions, respectively. The components were rotated with an orthogonal Varimax transformation, and standardized component scores for all of the components were calculated for each participant. Thus, the obtained component scores represented how closely the food consumption of each participant mirrored each of the empirically derived dietary patterns. The children with complete data for both methods ($n = 705$; 93% of those included in the comparison of FFQs and food records) were included in the dietary pattern analysis comparison. We used Spearman correlation coefficients to compare the FFQ- and food-record-based dietary pattern scores. In addition, we categorized the FFQ- and food-record-based dietary pattern scores into quarters and calculated the proportion of participants classified into the same quarter, same or adjacent quarter, or grossly misclassified into opposite quarters.

3. Results

The majority of the children ($n = 742$; 98%) had food record data for two weekdays and one weekend day, as planned. The rest ($n = 14$; 2%) had food record data for one weekday and two weekend days. A preschool day was defined as a day when the child ate at least one meal at preschool, and most children had food record data for two preschool days ($n = 621$; 82%). Others had either one ($n = 108$; 14%) or no preschool days ($n = 27$; 4%) included in the three-day food record. The children included in the current analysis did not differ from the excluded children in terms of age (Student's *t*-test $p = 0.89$) or gender (Chi-Squared test $p = 0.51$).

3.1. Comparison of FFQs and Food Records

Table 1 shows the proportions of participants classified into same, same or adjacent, and opposite quarters, using the two dietary assessment methods. Depending on the FFQ food item, 60%–96% of the participants were classified into the same or adjacent quarter. The proportion of participants classified into the same or adjacent quarter were 72%–80% for vegetables and fruits (fresh fruit; fresh vegetables; cooked and canned vegetables; peas, beans, lentils, and soya). The respective proportions for sugary treats (ice cream; chocolate; sweets; cakes, cupcakes, sweet rolls, Danish pastries, pies, and other sweet pastries; sweet biscuits and cereals bars) were 70%–81%, whereas the consumption of sugary everyday foods (flavored yoghurt; puddings; sugar-sweetened cereals and muesli; berry, fruit, and chocolate porridge with added sugar; berry and fruit soups with added sugar) were classified into the same or adjacent quarter in 71%–87% of participants. Regarding the consumption of sugary beverages (soft drinks; flavored and sweetened milk- and plant-based drinks; sugar-sweetened juice drinks), 69%–78% of the participants were classified into the same or adjacent quarter. The proportion of participants grossly misclassified was 10% or less for vegetables and fruits as well as for sugary foods. Of the individual food items, flavored nuts, almonds, and seeds; whole milk and sour milk; berry, fruit, and chocolate porridge; and reduced-sugar soft juices and soft drinks were most similarly reported, with 85% or more of the participants classified into the same quarter. Canned and frozen fruits, eggs, reduced-sugar soft juices and soft drinks, and dried fruit and berries were the least accurately classified, with 15%–22% of the participants grossly misclassified into opposite quarters.

Table 1. Comparison of food consumption frequencies of foods eaten outside preschool measured with a seven-day food frequency questionnaire (FFQ) and a three-day food record in the Increased Health and Wellbeing in Preschools (DAGIS) study (2015–2016, *n* = 756).

Food Item	*n*	Consumption Frequency according to FFQ, % of Participants			Comparison of the Two Methods, % of Participants		
		Not at All	Less than Daily	Daily	In the Same Quarter	In the Same or Adjacent Quarter	Grossly Misclassified Into Opposite Quarters
Vegetables, fruit and berries							
Fresh vegetables	754	2	29	69	35	76	7
Cooked and canned vegetables [1]	753	25	59	16	35	73	9
Potatoes (in all its forms)	755	3	85	13	30	72	6
Peas, beans, lentils, and soya	754	70	29	1	68	72	13
Fresh fruit	756	2	47	51	38	80	3
Canned and frozen fruit	754	80	20	0.4	78	78	22
Berries	752	30	63	7	41	70	7
Dried fruit and berries	756	58	41	1	61	64	15
Commercial baby foods and smoothies (no added sugar)	755	75	23	1	75	77	14
Berry and fruit soups (with added sugar)	754	64	34	2	66	71	10
Dairy products							
Skimmed milk and sour milk	752	51	6	43	71	96	0.9
1% fat milk, semi-skimmed milk, and sour milk	755	46	8	46	63	94	0.3
Whole milk and sour milk	753	89	7	4	90	90	10
Low-fat cheese (less than 20% fat)	751	60	26	14	59	71	10
High-fat cheese (20% or more fat)	755	33	40	27	50	81	5
Flavored and sweetened milk- and plant-based drinks	755	55	38	7	60	76	12
Natural yoghurt and quark (also plant-based products)	755	63	33	3	67	72	14
Flavored yoghurt and quark (also plant-based products)	754	23	61	16	49	83	3
Puddings	755	67	32	1	69	72	14
Ice cream	754	41	58	1	37	81	10
Fish, meat, and eggs							
Fish dishes and fish products	754	20	79	0.4	29	73	6
Red meat (beef, pork, lamb and mutton, and game)	754	3	91	6	33	65	12
White meat (poultry)	756	13	84	3	35	70	7
Cold cuts	750	35	46	20	43	74	9
Sausages, frankfurters, and luncheon meats	754	23	71	6	31	72	8
Eggs	755	39	60	1	47	71	21
Cereal products							
Brown rice and pasta	755	39	59	2	45	70	12
White rice and pasta	755	30	69	2	33	70	9
Rye bread, crispbread, and thin rye crackers	755	13	55	32	45	75	9
Multigrain bread and wholemeal bread	754	18	59	24	36	74	8
White bread	755	67	28	5	58	63	12
Sugar-sweetened cereals and muesli	754	52	44	3	52	74	10
Berry, fruit, and chocolate porridge (with added sugar)	756	91	9	1	87	87	13
Wholegrain porridge and cereals (no added sugar)	756	31	54	15	46	82	5
Sweet biscuits and cereal bars	755	29	69	2	35	70	9
Sweet pastries [2]	755	22	77	0.3	27	71	6
Drinks							
Sugar-sweetened juice drinks	752	24	68	8	37	69	8
Fruit juice (no added sugar)	754	54	39	6	58	79	9
Soft drinks (with added sugar)	756	72	28	0.1	72	78	7
Reduced sugar juices and soft drinks	755	87	12	1	85	85	15

Table 1. *Cont.*

Food Item	n	Consumption Frequency according to FFQ, % of Participants			Comparison of the Two Methods, % of Participants		
		Not at All	Less than Daily	Daily	In the Same Quarter	In the Same or Adjacent Quarter	Grossly Misclassified Into Opposite Quarters
Others							
Chocolate	754	35	64	1	33	78	13
Sweets	756	16	83	1	20	78	14
Added sugar, honey, or syrup [3]	754	59	35	6	62	69	9
Jams, marmalades, and sweetened spreads	755	67	30	3	66	73	9
Plain nuts, almonds, and seeds	754	72	25	3	78	80	11
Flavored nuts, almonds, and seeds (e.g., salted nuts)	755	91	9	0	91	91	9
Crisps and popcorn	756	48	52	0.4	45	60	10

Items in the table are in the same order as in the FFQ (available at https://helda.helsinki.fi/handle/10138/235382). [1] As a side dish or as an ingredient in a dish. [2] Cakes, cupcakes, sweet rolls, Danish pastries, pies, and other sweet pastries. [3] for example, in porridge, tea, berries, yoghurt, or quark.

The calculated mean daily vitamin C and folate intakes increased linearly in the quarters of vegetable and fruit consumption (Table 2). Similarly, calcium intake was positively associated with milk consumption frequency, whereas sucrose intake increased in the quarters of sugary treats, sugary everyday foods, and sugary beverage consumption.

Table 2. Mean daily nutrient intake from foods consumed outside of preschool (three-day food record) according to categories of food group consumption (FFQ) in the DAGIS study (2015–2016, n = 756).

	Quarter of Food Group Consumption Frequency according to FFQ				p-Value for Trend [1]
	First	Second	Third	Fourth	
Vitamin C (mg) intake according to vegetable and fruit [2] consumption	35	47	54	61	<0.001
Folate intake (μg) according of vegetable and fruit [2] consumption	88	91	104	109	<0.001
Calcium intake (mg) according to milk [3] consumption	503	610	724	770	<0.001
Sucrose intake (g) according to sugary treats [4] consumption	26	29	29	34	<0.001
Sucrose intake (g) according to sugary everyday food [5] consumption	25	28	31	35	<0.001
Sucrose intake (g) according to sugary beverage [6] consumption	26	28	29	36	<0.001

[1] Linear regression with food consumption frequency category as a continuous predictor variable; nutrient intakes were square root transformed. [2] Sum of the FFQ rows "fresh vegetables", "cooked and canned vegetables", "peas, beans, lentils, and soya", and "fresh fruit'. [3] Sum of the FFQ rows "skimmed milk and sour milk", "1% fat milk, semi-skimmed milk, and sour milk", and "whole milk and sour milk'. [4] Sum of the FFQ rows "ice cream", "sweet biscuits and cereal bars", "cakes, cupcakes, sweet rolls, Danish pastries, pies, and other sweet pastries", "chocolate", and "sweets". [5] Sum of the FFQ rows "flavored yoghurt and quark", "puddings", "sugar-sweetened cereals and muesli", "berry, fruit and chocolate porridge (with added sugar)", and "berry and fruit soups (with added sugar)". [6] Sum of the FFQ rows "flavored and sweetened milk- and plant-based drinks", "sugar-sweetened juice drinks", and "soft drinks (with added sugar)".

3.2. Comparison of Dietary Patterns

The five food-record-based components explained altogether 19.7% of the variance in the sample (Supplementary Table S2), whereas the corresponding percentage in the FFQ-based analysis was 16.7% (for more details regarding the FFQ-based dietary patterns, please see [30]). Supplementary Table S2 also shows the loadings of foods into the components, percentage of variance explained by each component, and the eigenvalues in the food-record-based PCA. The food-record-based patterns were labelled "health-conscious", "sandwich", "sweets-and-treats", "milk, potatoes, and minced meat", and "pasta, minced meat, and fruit", based on the foods loading positively to each component. The FFQ-based patterns were named "sweets-and-treats", "health-conscious", and "vegetables-and-processed meats", and have been reported in more detail elsewhere [30]. The three strongest patterns identified using the two methods were very similar to each other, and there were relatively low, positive correlations between the pattern scores (Table 3). Regarding each of the dietary pattern scores, over 70% of the participants were classified into the same or adjacent quarter, whereas the proportion of participants classified into opposite quarters was 6%–9% for the three patterns (Table 4).

Table 3. Spearman correlation coefficients between the FFQ- and food-record-based dietary pattern scores (strongest positive correlation shown in bold).

	Food-Record-Based Dietary Patterns				
	Health-Conscious	Sandwich	Sweets-and-Treats	Milk, Potatoes and Minced Meat	Pasta, Minced Meat and Fruit
FFQ-based dietary patterns					
Sweets-and-treats	−0.19 [1]	−0.18 [1]	**0.27** [1]	0.22 [1]	−0.10 [1]
Health-conscious	**0.33** [1]	−0.05	−0.30 [1]	−0.16 [1]	0.08 [2]
Vegetables-and-processed meats	0.19 [1]	**0.25** [1]	0.16 [1]	0.08 [2]	0.11 [1]

[1] $p \leq 0.01$. [2] $p \leq 0.05$.

Table 4. The proportion of participants classified into the same, same or adjacent, or opposite quarters using the FFQ- and food-record-based dietary pattern scores.

	% of Participants Classified into the Same Quarter	% of Participants Classified into the Same or Adjacent Quarters	% of Participants Grossly Misclassified into Opposite Quarters
Sweets-and-treats patterns	34	72	7
Health-conscious patterns	35	73	6
Vegetables-and-processed meats/sandwich patterns	35	73	9

4. Discussion

The aim of the current study was to compare the food consumption frequencies and empirical dietary patterns derived with the following two methods: food records and FFQs. Regarding consumption frequencies, the percentage of participants classified into the same or adjacent quarter as measured with FFQs and food-records was 60%–96%. Considering vegetable and fruit consumption, 72%–80% of the participants were classified into the same or adjacent quarter in the current study, whereas the corresponding percentages for sugar-containing foods were 69%–87%. Furthermore, the calculated nutrient intakes for key nutrients increased linearly in the quarters of vegetable and fruit, and sugar-containing food consumption. In addition, we found dietary patterns of the same kind using FFQ and food-record food groups as input variables. To our knowledge, this is the first study to perform PCA separately based on FFQs and food records without forcing the food record food codes to match the FFQ rows, which could lead to overestimated correlation coefficients [20].

4.1. Relative Validity of the DAGIS FFQ

The percentages of participants classified into the same or adjacent quarter were the greatest for skimmed milk and sour milk (96%); 1% fat milk, semi-skimmed milk, and sour milk (94%); flavored nuts, almonds, and seeds (91%); and whole milk and sour milk (90%). In general, the food items that were used only by a small percentage of participants (less than 20% according to the FFQ) had the largest proportions of participants classified into the same or adjacent quarter. Among food items that were used by more than 20% of the participants at least once according to the FFQs, commercial baby foods and smoothies with no added sugar; plain almonds, nuts, and seeds; and soft drinks with added sugar were most similarly reported, as 77%–80% of the participants were classified into the same or adjacent quarter as measured with the FFQs and food records. By contrast, the relative validity of our FFQ to assess the consumption frequency of canned and frozen fruit, eggs, reduced sugar juices and soft drinks, and dried fruit and berries could partly be criticized, because 15%–22% of the participants were grossly misclassified into opposite quarters by the two methods. The difference in time spans (three days vs. seven days) might at least partly explain these misclassifications. In the future, it would be advisable to rephrase these items or to incorporate the foods into FFQ rows with a lower proportion of misclassification (for example, canned and frozen fruit could be incorporated into fresh fruit).

Our first aim was to compare the consumption frequencies reported using food records and FFQs. Considering vegetable and fruit consumption, 35%–68% of the participants were classified into the same quarter in the current study, whereas previous studies reported respective percentages ranging from 35%–49% for vegetable and fruit FFQ items [6,8,9]. The fact that the calculated intakes of vitamin C and folate increased linearly through the quarters of vegetable and fruit consumption frequency (Table 2) gives additional support to our finding that, compared to food records, the FFQ is able to rank the children acceptably according to food group consumption. Using a somewhat similar approach, Flood et al. reported an increasing trend in the calculated vitamin C intake for vegetable consumption, but not for fruit consumption [7].

Regarding sugary foods, the percentages of participants classified into the same quarter varied depending on the type of foods. The lowest percentages were observed for sugary treats (ice cream 37%; sweet biscuits and cereal bars 35%; sweet pastries 27%; sweets 20%; chocolate 33%). These are typically foods that are not consumed daily, and thus, their habitual consumption frequency may have been more accurately captured by the FFQ. On the other hand, as keeping a food record is known to affect food behavior [1], it may be that the parents withheld sugary treats during the three days the food records were kept. Previous studies have reported corresponding percentages ranging from 32%–37% [6,8,9]. However, the wide variation in food groupings between the studies limits the comparison. In the current study, 49%–87% of the participants were classified into the same quarter with regard to sugary everyday foods (berry and fruit soups; flavored yoghurt and quark; puddings; sugar-sweetened cereals and muesli; berry, fruit, and chocolate porridge), whereas the corresponding range for sugary beverages (flavored and sweetened milk- and plant-based drinks; sugar-sweetened juice drinks; soft drinks) was 37%–72%. The calculated sucrose intake increased linearly in the quarters of sugary treats, sugary everyday foods, and sugary beverages, suggesting a good indirect validity.

4.2. Relative Validity of the Dietary Patterns

Currently, explorative or data-driven dietary patterns are used frequently in modern nutrition science [11]. The dietary pattern approach has many advantages. First, the patterns provide us with a broader conception of food consumption and can add to our understanding of dietary behavior [31]. Second, the pattern approach is free of a priori assumptions concerning, for example, healthful diets, and describes the actual parallel presence of different patterns in the diets of the participants [12]. PCA is one of the most frequently used methods for dietary pattern analysis, and usually FFQ data are used as inputs for the analysis. The validity of the FFQs used to derive dietary patterns is often under study, but only a few studies have investigated the relative validity of the resulting dietary patterns among children [22,23].

To our knowledge, this is the first study to compare dietary patterns derived using two dietary assessment methods, without forcing the input variables to be similar (i.e., matching the foods from the food records into FFQ rows). The matching of the food items has resulted in the exclusion of a large number of foods that cannot be matched to each of the FFQ rows. For example, in a sample of middle-aged and elderly Swedish women, as much as 54% of the foods in the food records were excluded from the analyses [18]. Using this approach, the validity of the patterns is likely to be better than the actual validity [20].

In the present study, we found three quite similar dietary patterns using two dietary assessment methods (FFQs and food records). The pattern scores were correlated as statistically significantly, but the correlation coefficients were relatively low (0.25–0.33) [32]. Previous studies have reported correlations ranging from 0.32–0.74 among adults [15–20], and the correlations have been of the same order among adolescents [22] and toddlers [23]. Our lower correlation coefficients are probably due to not matching the foods from the food records to the FFQ rows. Instead, we conducted the PCA separately, using FFQ rows and food record data as inputs. Thus, we believe that the correlation coefficients in this study reflect the validity of the dietary patterns more realistically. However, more than 70% of the participants were classified into the same or adjacent quarter, according to the dietary pattern scores. Hence, it seems that despite the low correlation coefficients, the two dietary assessment methods can provide fairly similar dietary patterns and rank the participants similarly based on the dietary pattern scores.

4.3. Strengths and Limitations

The present study had several strengths. First, we had a large sample size of preschool-aged children and their parents as participants. Second, we used both direct (cross-classification) and indirect (calculated nutrient intakes) measures to assess the validity of the DAGIS FFQ. Furthermore, we investigated the relative validity of the dietary patterns using both food record data and FFQ rows as inputs. As we did not match the foods in the food records to the FFQ rows for this analysis, we were able to examine the similarity of the derived patterns without artificially overestimating the correlation coefficients. We believe that our approach provided us a more realistic and comprehensive view of the validity of the FFQ.

Our study used food records as the reference method for dietary assessment. However, it is crucial to consider the design of the study critically. FFQs are designed to measure the usual consumption of foods, whereas food records capture only the foods eaten during a few days [1]. Thus, three-day food records may underestimate the consumption of certain foods, such as sugar-containing treats or fish, and FFQs may be able to assess the consumption of these foods more accurately. As dietary patterns are thought to reflect the usual consumption of foods and beverages, FFQs could be thought of as a more accurate assessment method for less frequently used foods. In the present study, the FFQ measured food consumption during the previous week. Thus, the time span did not vary considerably between the two methods (seven days vs. three days), suggesting that the two methods can be meaningfully compared. As our FFQ only measured foods eaten outside of preschool hours, it does not represent the whole diet of the children. Thus, to make the two methods comparable, we excluded foods eaten at preschool from the reference method (three-day food record). However, should the FFQ be used in other studies, it must be noted that the relative validity has only been investigated concerning the foods eaten outside of preschool hours.

As measuring food consumption is not straightforward and every method has its own pitfalls, our measurements were not free of error. It is possible that some foods are most accurately measured using food records, whereas for other foods, the most accurate method might be FFQ. Thus, it must be kept in mind that whenever we are "validating" an FFQ, we are, in fact, just comparing it with another, equally (although differently) biased dietary assessment method, and not the true food consumption, which we unfortunately are unable to assess. Furthermore, the participating families in the DAGIS study were highly educated (in nearly 70% of the families, the highest educational level was bachelor's degree or higher [24]). As the socio-economic status of the family may be associated with misreporting [33], the results of this study may have to be generalized with caution.

5. Conclusions

The FFQ designed for the DAGIS study can rank participants acceptably. Special attention was paid to vegetables and fruits, and sugar-containing foods. The indirect measures of validity (mean intake of selected nutrients in quarters of the consumption) supported the aforementioned conclusion. In addition, three fairly similar dietary patterns were identified using both food-record and FFQ data as inputs, and the percentage of participants classified into the same or adjacent quarters were acceptable. Thus, we conclude that the DAGIS FFQ is a valid measure for vegetable and fruit as well as sugary food consumption. In addition, the DAGIS FFQ can be used to derive dietary patterns that are consistent with those derived using food record data.

Supplementary Materials: The following are available online at http://www.mdpi.com/2072-6643/11/1/159/s1: Table S1: Food groups included and excluded in the food-record-based analysis and their mean consumption among 3–6 year-olds in the DAGIS study (2015–2016, *n* = 756); Table S2: Characteristics of the five food-record-based dietary patterns identified among 3–6 year-olds in the DAGIS study (2015–2016).

Author Contributions: Conceptualization, L.K., H.V., E.R. and M.E.; methodology, L.K., H.V., C.R., R.L., H.H.H.-a., K.N., J.M., E.R. and M.E.; formal analysis, L.K. and H.V.; investigation, C.R., E.S., R.L. and K.N.; data curation, L.K., H.V., E.S., R.L. and K.N.; writing (original draft preparation), L.K. and H.V.; writing (review and editing), C.R., E.S., R.L., H.H.H.-a., K.N., J.M., E.R. and M.E.; visualization, L.K. and H.V.; supervision, E.R. and M.E.; project administration, M.E.; funding acquisition, E.R. and M.E.

Funding: This research was funded by the Folkhälsan Research Center, the University of Helsinki, The Ministry of Education and Culture in Finland, The Ministry of Social Affairs and Health, The Academy of Finland (Grants: 285439, 287288, 288038), The Juho Vainio Foundation, the Signe and Ane Gyllenberg Foundation, The Finnish Cultural Foundation/South Ostrobothnia Regional Fund, the Päivikki and Sakari Sohlberg foundation, the Medicinska Föreningen Liv och Hälsa, the Finnish Foundation for Nutrition Research, and the Finnish Food Research Foundation.

Acknowledgments: The authors thank the preschools, the preschool personnel, and the families for their participation in the DAGIS study, as well as the staff for data collection.

Conflicts of Interest: Liisa Korkalo is a board member of the company TwoDads. The authors declare no other conflict of interest.

References

1. Slimani, N.; Freisling, H.; Illner, A.; Huybrechts, I. Methods to determine dietary intake. In *Nutrition Research Methodologies*, 1st ed.; Lovegrove, J.A., Hodson, L., Sharma, S., Lanham-New, S.A., Eds.; John Wiley & Sons Ltd.: Chichester, UK, 2015.
2. Willett, W. Food frequency methods. In *Nutritional Epidemiology*, 3rd ed.; Willett, W., Ed.; Oxford University Press: New York, NY, USA, 2013.
3. Livingstone, M.B.E.; Robson, P.J. Measurement of dietary intake in children. *Proc. Nutr. Soc.* **2000**, *59*, 279–293. [CrossRef] [PubMed]
4. Willett, W.; Lenart, E. Reproducibility and validity of food frequency questionnaires. In *Nutritional Epidemiology*, 3rd ed.; Willett, W., Ed.; Oxford University Press: New York, NY, USA, 2013.
5. Kolodziejczyk, J.; Merchant, G.; Norman, G. Reliability and validity of child/adolescent food frequency questionnaires that assess foods and/or food groups. *J. Pediatr. Gastroenterol. Nutr.* **2012**, *55*, 4–13. [CrossRef] [PubMed]
6. Buch-Andersen, T.; Pérez-Cueto, F.J.A.; Toft, U. Relative validity and reproducibility of a parent-administered semi-quantitative FFQ for assessing food intake in Danish children aged 3-9 years. *Public Health Nutr.* **2016**, *19*, 1184–1194. [CrossRef] [PubMed]
7. Flood, V.M.; Wen, L.M.; Hardy, L.L.; Rissel, C.; Simpson, J.M.; Baur, L.A. Reliability and validity of a short FFQ for assessing the dietary habits of 2-5-year-old children, Sydney, Australia. *Public Health Nutr.* **2014**, *17*, 498–509. [CrossRef] [PubMed]
8. Huybrechts, I.; De Backer, G.; De Bacquer, D.; Maes, L.; De Henauw, S. Relative validity and reproducibility of a food-frequency questionnaire for estimating food intakes among Flemish preschoolers. *Int. J. Environ. Res. Public Health* **2009**, *6*, 382–399. [CrossRef] [PubMed]

9. Klohe, D.M.; Clarke, K.K.; George, G.C.; Milani, T.J.; Hanss-Nuss, H.; Freeland-Graves, J. Relative validity and reliability of a food frequency questionnaire for a triethnic population of 1-year-old to 3-year-old children from low-income families. *J. Am. Diet Assoc.* **2005**, *105*, 727–734. [CrossRef] [PubMed]

10. Marshall, T.A.; Eichenberger, G.J.M.; Broffitt, B.; Stumbo, P.J.; Levy, S.M. Relative validity of the Iowa Fluoride Study targeted nutrient semi-quantitative questionnaire and the block kids' food questionnaire for estimating beverage, calcium, and vitamin D intakes by children. *J. Am. Diet Assoc.* **2008**, *108*, 465–472. [CrossRef]

11. Mozaffarian, D.; Rosenberg, I.; Uauy, R. History of modern nutrition science—Implications for current research, dietary guidelines, and food policy. *BMJ* **2018**, *361*, k2392. [CrossRef]

12. Newby, P.K.; Tucker, K.L. Empirically derived eating patterns using factor or cluster analysis: A review. *Nutr. Rev.* **2004**, *62*, 177–203. [CrossRef]

13. Willett, W. Issues in analysis and presentation of dietary data. In *Nutritional Epidemiology*, 3rd ed.; Willett, W., Ed.; Oxford University Press: New York, NY, USA, 2013.

14. Martínez, M.E.; Marshall, J.R.; Sechrest, L. Invited commentary: Factor analysis and the search for objectivity. *Am. J. Epidemiol.* **1998**, *148*, 17–19. [CrossRef]

15. Beck, K.L.; Kruger, R.; Conlon, C.A.; Heath, A.M.; Coad, J.; Matthys, C.; Jones, B.; Stonehouse, W. The relative validity and reproducibility of an iron food frequency questionnaire for identifying iron-related dietary patterns in young women. *J. Acad. Nutr. Diet* **2012**, *112*, 1177–1187. [CrossRef]

16. Crozier, S.R.; Inskip, H.M.; Godfrey, K.M.; Robinson, S.M. Dietary patterns in pregnant women: A comparison of food-frequency questionnaires and 4 d prospective diaries. *Br. J. Nutr.* **2008**, *99*, 869–875. [CrossRef] [PubMed]

17. Hu, F.B.; Rimm, E.; Smith-Warner, S.A.; Feskanich, D.; Stampfer, M.J.; Ascherio, A.; Sampson, L.; Willett, W.C. Reproducibility and validity of dietary patterns assessed with a food-frequency questionnaire. *Am. J. Clin. Nutr.* **1999**, *69*, 243. [CrossRef] [PubMed]

18. Khani, B.R.; Ye, W.; Terry, P.; Wolk, A. Reproducibility and validity of major dietary patterns among Swedish women assessed with a food-frequency questionnaire. *J. Nutr.* **2004**, *134*, 1541–1545. [CrossRef] [PubMed]

19. Nanri, A.; Shimazu, T.; Ishihara, J.; Takachi, R.; Mizoue, T.; Inoue, M.; Tsuqane, S. Reproducibility and validity of dietary patterns assessed by a food frequency questionnaire used in the 5-year follow-up survey of the Japan Public Health Center-Based Prospective Study. *J. Epidemiol.* **2012**, *22*, 205–215. [CrossRef] [PubMed]

20. Okubo, H.; Murakami, K.; Sasaki, S.; Kim, M.K.; Hirota, N.; Notsu, A.; Fukui, M.; Date, C. Relative validity of dietary patterns derived from a self-administered diet history questionnaire using factor analysis among Japanese adults. *Public Health Nutr.* **2010**, *13*, 1080–1089. [CrossRef] [PubMed]

21. Togo, P.; Heitmann, B.L.; Sørensen, T.I.; Osler, M. Consistency of food intake factors by different dietary assessment methods and population groups. *Br. J. Nutr.* **2003**, *90*, 667–678. [CrossRef]

22. Ambrosini, G.L.; O'Sullivan, T.A.; de Klerk, N.H.; Mori, T.A.; Beilin, L.J.; Oddy, W.H. Relative validity of adolescent dietary patterns: A comparison of a FFQ and 3 d food record. *Br. J. Nutr.* **2011**, *105*, 625–633. [CrossRef] [PubMed]

23. Mills, V.C.; Skidmore, P.M.; Watson, E.O.; Taylor, R.W.; Fleming, E.A.; Heath, A.L. Relative validity and reproducibility of a food frequency questionnaire for identifying the dietary patterns of toddlers in New Zealand. *J. Acad. Nutr. Diet* **2015**, *115*, 551–558. [CrossRef] [PubMed]

24. Lehto, E.; Ray, C.; Vepsäläinen, H.; Korkalo, L.; Lehto, R.; Kaukonen, R.; Suhonen, E.; Nislin, M.; Nissinen, K.; Skaffari, E.; et al. Increased Health and Wellbeing in Preschools (DAGIS) Study—differences in children's energy balance-related behaviors (EBRBs) and in long-term stress by parental educational level. *Int. J. Environ. Res. Public Health* **2018**, *15*, 2313. [CrossRef] [PubMed]

25. Vepsäläinen, H. Food Environment and Whole-Diet in Children—Studies on Parental Role Modelling and Food Availability. Ph.D. Thesis, University of Helsinki, Helsinki, Finland, June 2018.

26. Määttä, S.; Vepsäläinen, H.; Lehto, R.; Erkkola, M.; Roos, E.; Ray, C. Reproducibility of preschool and guardian reports on energy balance-related behaviors and their correlates in Finnish preschool children. *Children* **2018**, *5*, 144. [CrossRef] [PubMed]

27. Nissinen, K.; Sillanpää, H.; Korkalo, L.; Roos, E.; Erkkola, M. *Annoskuvakirja Lasten Ruokamäärien Arvioinnin Avuksi*, 1st ed.; Unigrafia: Helsinki, Finland, 2016.

28. Nissinen, K.; Korkalo, L.; Vepsäläinen, H.; Mäkiranta, P.; Koivusilta, L.; Roos, E.; Erkkola, M. Accuracy in the estimation of children's food portion sizes against the food picture book: Do parents and early educators estimate portions with similar accuracy? *J. Nutr. Sci.* **2018**, *7*, e35. [CrossRef] [PubMed]

29. Määttä, S.; Lehto, R.; Nislin, M.; Ray, C.; Erkkola, M.; Sajaniemi, N.; Roos, E. Increased health and well-being in preschools (DAGIS): Rationale and design for a randomized controlled trial. *BMC Public Health* **2015**, *15*, 402. [CrossRef] [PubMed]

30. Vepsäläinen, H.; Korkalo, L.; Mikkilä, V.; Lehto, R.; Ray, C.; Nissinen, K.; Skaffari, E.; Fogelholm, M.; Koivusilta, L.; Roos, E.; et al. Dietary patterns and their associations with home food availability among Finnish pre-school children: A cross-sectional study. *Public Health Nutr.* **2018**, *21*, 1232–1242. [CrossRef] [PubMed]

31. Hu, F.B. Dietary pattern analysis: A new direction in nutritional epidemiology. *Curr. Opin. Lipidol.* **2002**, *13*, 3–9. [CrossRef] [PubMed]

32. Hinkle, D.E.; Jurs, S.G.; Wiersma, W. *Applied Statistics for the Behavioral Sciences*, 5th ed.; Houghton Mifflin Company: Boston, MA, USA, 2003.

33. Börnhorst, C.; Huybrechts, I.; Ahrens, W.; Eiben, G.; Michels, N.; Pala, V.; Molnár, D.; Russo, P.; Barba, G.; Bel-Serrat, S.; et al. Prevalence and determinants of misreporting among European children in proxy-reported 24 h dietary recalls. *Br. J. Nutr.* **2013**, *109*, 1257–1265. [CrossRef] [PubMed]

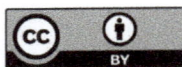

nutrients

MDPI

Article

Dietary Patterns in Primary School are of Prospective Relevance for the Development of Body Composition in Two German Pediatric Populations

Maike Wolters [1,†,*], Gesa Joslowski [2,†], Sandra Plachta-Danielzik [3], Marie Standl [4], Manfred J. Müller [3], Wolfgang Ahrens [1] and Anette E. Buyken [2,5]

[1] Leibniz Institute for Prevention Research and Epidemiology—BIPS, Department: Epidemiological Methods and Etiologic Research, Achterstr. 30, 28359 Bremen, Germany; ahrens@leibniz-bips.de
[2] IEL—Nutritional Epidemiology, University of Bonn, DONALD Study, Heinstück 11, 44225 Dortmund, Germany; gesa.joslowski@gmx.de (G.J.); anette.buyken@uni-paderborn.de (A.E.B.)
[3] Institute of Human Nutrition and Food Science, Christian-Albrechts University, 24118 Kiel, Germany; s.plachta-danielzik@kompetenznetz-ced.de (S.P.-D.); mmueller@nutrfoodsc.uni-kiel.de (M.J.M.)
[4] Institute of Epidemiology I, Helmholtz Zentrum München—German Research Center for Environmental Health, D-85764 Neuherberg, Germany; marie.standl@helmholtz-muenchen.de
[5] Institute of Nutrition, Consumption and Health, Faculty of Natural Science, University Paderborn, 33098 Paderborn, Germany
*   Correspondence: wolters@leibniz-bips.de; Tel.: +49-421-218-56-845
†   These authors contributed equally to this work.

Received: 5 September 2018; Accepted: 27 September 2018; Published: 5 October 2018

Abstract: This study performed comparative analyses in two pediatric cohorts to identify dietary patterns during primary school years and examined their relevance to body composition development. Nutritional and anthropometric data at the beginning of primary school and two or four years later were available from 298 and 372 participants of IDEFICS-Germany (Identification and prevention of Dietary-induced and lifestyle-induced health Effects In Children and infants Study) and the KOPS (Kiel Obesity Prevention Study) cohort, respectively. Principal component analyses (PCA) and reduced rank regression (RRR) were used to identify dietary patterns at baseline and patterns of change in food group intake during primary school years. RRR extracted patterns explaining variations in changes in body mass index (BMI), fat mass index (FMI), and waist-to-height-ratio (WtHR). Associations between pattern adherence and excess gain in BMI, FMI, or WtHR (>75th percentile) during primary school years were examined using logistic regression. Among PCA patterns, only a change towards a more Mediterranean food choice during primary school years were associated with a favorable body composition development in IDEFICS-Germany ($p < 0.05$). In KOPS, RRR patterns characterized by a frequent consumption of fast foods or starchy carbohydrate foods were consistently associated with an excess gain in BMI and WtHR (all $p < 0.005$). In IDEFICS-Germany, excess gain in BMI, FMI, and WtHR were predicted by a frequent consumption of nuts, meat, and pizza at baseline and a decrease in the consumption frequency of protein sources and snack carbohydrates during primary school years (all $p < 0.01$). The study confirms an adverse impact of fast food consumption on body composition during primary school years. Combinations of protein and carbohydrate sources deserve further investigation.

Keywords: body composition; primary school; dietary pattern; principal component analysis; reduced rank regression; prevention

1. Introduction

Most Western societies report the highest prevalence of overweight/obesity among children and adolescents at the end of primary school [1,2]. Thus, primary school years are now regarded as a further window of opportunity when interventions targeting development or the reversal of becoming overweight or obese are particularly warranted [3–8].

Upon entry into primary school, many aspects of a child's daily routine change, which may all contribute to the lower remission of overweight during primary school years as compared to pre-school years. Importantly, nutritional behavior may change substantially and these changes may best be captured by dietary pattern analysis, which allows insights into the joint relevance of multiple dietary components for overweight development. Yet, to date, few studies examined the prospective relevance of dietary patterns for the development of body composition [9–15] and most of these were performed among adolescents [10,11,13]. In addition, such analyses should often consider BMI only [10–12], which is, however, only a proxy measure of adiposity. Consideration of more adiposity-specific measures such as fat mass or waist circumference is, therefore, warranted [16–19].

Additionally, patterns of dietary change during primary school years may be of relevance for an unfavorable development of body composition during this period. In a previous analysis, we observed that both the selection of unfavorable carbohydrate sources (more white bread, less pulses, and whole grain bread) at the beginning of primary school and an increased consumption of processed savory food during primary school years were related to adverse changes in BMI and fat mass during primary school years in a sample of German school children participating in the DONALD Study (Dortmund Nutritional and Longitudinally Designed Study) [9]. These patterns were identified by using reduced rank regression (RRR) to identify dietary patterns best explaining variation in changes of body composition during primary school years. Ideally, these dietary patterns should be applied to another cohort so as to confirm their relevance for German pediatric populations in general. In practice, this is, however, not possible because of different dietary assessment methods used in different studies (e.g., German pediatric cohort studies often assess consumption frequency only, i.e., use food propensity questionnaires [20]). Comparative analysis based on a different dietary assessment method but using a similar analytic approach is, therefore, a feasible alternative approach. Similar dietary patterns identified with this analytical approach would be highly informative for the formulation of preventive and interventional strategies targeted at primary school age children.

Therefore, the aims of the present study were to identify and describe dietary patterns at the beginning of the primary school period as well as patterns of dietary changes during the course of primary school in two German pediatric cohort studies known as the Kiel Obesity Prevention Study (KOPS) and the Identification and prevention of Dietary-induced and lifestyle-induced health Effects In Children and infants (IDEFICS)-Germany cohort. In a further step, we illustrated the impact of adherence to the identified dietary patterns on excess gain in the body mass index (BMI), fat mass index (FMI), or waist-to-height ratio (WtHR) (increases >75th percentile) during primary school years.

2. Methods

2.1. Study Populations

The study designs of the KOPS and the IDEFICS-Germany study were described previously [16,21,22]. KOPS is a cohort study to investigate determinants and preventive measures of childhood obesity. It was performed between 1996 and 2001 in the context of a school entry health examination [23,24]. A representative group of 4997 children participated in the study [24,25]. At the end of the primary school period (fourth grade), follow-up information was collected from 1764 children (35% of the original population) during examinations performed in the school setting between 2000 and 2005 [23,24]. For the present analyses, complete information on dietary habits at baseline (age 5 to 7 years) and follow-up (age 9 to 11 years) was available for 415 children. Of these, 372 had complete anthropometric data at both time points as well as information on potential confounding factors.

The IDEFICS-Germany study is a multicenter study designed to investigate and prevent diet-related and lifestyle-related disorders among European children (aged 2–9.9 years at baseline). The present analysis is based on data of the German subsample. In 2007/2008, 2066 children were recruited from kindergartens and schools in Germany. Anthropometric measurements were performed at baseline and at the two-year follow-up and dietary and lifestyle questionnaires were administered. A total of 993 children had complete dietary data at baseline and follow-up. Of these, 312 children provided dietary data at the beginning of primary school (i.e., age 5 to 7 years) and at least two years later. Complete anthropometric measurements at baseline and follow-up and data on potential covariates were available for 298 children included in the analyses.

This study was conducted according to the guidelines laid down in the Declaration of Helsinki and all procedures involving human subjects were approved by the local ethics committee in Kiel and the ethics review board of the University of Bremen written informed consent was obtained from the parents or legal caregivers of all children.

2.2. Nutritional Assessment

In KOPS, dietary intake was assessed using a 24 item food propensity questionnaire (FPQ) based on the WHO MONICA FFQ (food frequency questionnaire) adapted to children [26] (see Table S1). It was completed by the parents or primary caregiver who provided dietary information over the last six months. The FPQ—i.e., an FFQ inquiring consumption frequencies but not the amounts consumed was validated against a seven day diet record in 24 and 61 5–7 and 9–11 year old children, respectively [27]. Consumption frequencies were asked from mutually exclusive alternatives: never or less than once a week, 1 to 2 times per week, and 3 to 6 times per week or daily.

The Children's Eating Habits Questionnaire (CEHQ) was used to assess dietary intake in the IDEFICS-Germany study [28]. This reproducible and validated instrument [28–30] inquiring the consumption frequency of 43 foods and beverages (see Table S2) was completed by parents or other caregivers. Frequencies of consumption during the past month were asked from mutually exclusive alternatives: never or less than once a week, 1 to 3 times per week, 4 to 6 times per week, once per day, twice per day, and three or more times per day.

2.3. Anthropometric Measurements and Calculations

Anthropometric measurements in KOPS were performed by trained nutritionists and physicians [25]. Weight and height were measured to the nearest of 0.1 kg and 0.5 cm with a calibrated electronic scale and a stadiometer (Seca, Hamburg, Germany). Waist circumference was measured midway between the lowest rib and the top of the iliac crest at the end of gentle expiration with an inelastic tape. A bioelectrical impedance analysis (BIA) was performed by using a terapolar bio-impedance analyzer (BIA 2000-C, Data Input, Frankfurt/M, Germany) and fat mass was calculated with an algorithm developed in Kiel using air-displacement plethysmography as the reference method [16,31].

In IDEFICS-Germany, anthropometric measurements included weight, height, BIA, and waist circumference. Children were barefoot and wore only underwear and a T-shirt. Weight measurements to the nearest 0.1 kg and BIA were carried out using an electronic scale (Tanita BC 420 SMA, Tanita Europe GmbH, Sindelfingen, Germany). Height was measured using a telescopic height measuring instrument (Seca 225 stadiometer, Hamburg, Germany) to the nearest 0.1 cm. Fat mass was calculated with an algorithm derived from BIA [32]. Waist circumference was measured using an inelastic Seca 200 tape (Seca, Hamburg, Germany) according to World Health Organization Standards [33].

For both study samples, BMI was calculated from measured height and weight (weight (kg)/height^2 (m^2)). FMI and FFMI were calculated relating fat mass and fat free mass (weight—fat mass) to height^2 (m^2). For WtHR (waist circumference(m)/height(cm), a simple practical non-invasive tool reflecting visceral fat of a value >0.5 was considered to indicate excessive upper body fat accumulation [34]. Since absolute measures are considered a better alternative than z-scores when assessing adiposity changes [35], the response variables were the changes in BMI, FMI, and WtHR between the end and the beginning of the primary school period. Being overweight was defined according to the International Obesity Task Force criteria [36].

2.4. Statistical Methods

To facilitate comparison to the findings from the DONALD study, the statistical approach in the present analysis was analogous to that in Diethelm et al. [9]. Dietary patterns at the beginning of the primary school period and patterns of changes during primary school years were derived by two different empirical methods: PCA and RRR. Intake frequencies were standardized by using z-scores (by age group and sex (mean = 0, SD = 1)). Due to the extracted dietary patterns being similar for boys and girls in both cohorts, the data were pooled for the analyses.

2.4.1. PCA

PCA analyses were conducted by using the PROC FACTOR procedure in SAS. The first PCA was conducted to identify dietary patterns at the beginning of the primary school period (PCA baseline pattern) while the second PCA identified patterns of dietary changes between the end and the beginning of the primary school period (PCA change pattern). For this purpose, changes in the intake frequencies of food groups were obtained (standardized intake frequencies at the end of the primary school period minus standardized intake frequencies at the beginning of the primary school period).

To select the baseline and change patterns to be retained in analyses, the following criteria were used: (1) eigenvalues exceeding 1 (based on the rationale that each component should explain more variance than a single variable in the data set), (2) the scree plot (a graphical presentation of the eigenvalues where a break indicates how many factors should be retained), and (3) factor interpretability [37,38]. Two baseline patterns and three change patterns were retained for further analyses. After a varimax rotation, food groups with factor loadings $\geq |0.4|$ were considered as contributing to a pattern. For each pattern, more than three food groups were retained, which is considered an adequate number for good interpretability [38]. According to the approach of simplified pattern variables, the individual PCA factor scores (resembling adherence to the respective pattern) were based solely on the sum of the unweighted standardized frequencies of food groups that were loaded high (i.e., $\geq |0.4|$) at the respective pattern [39].

2.4.2. RRR

RRR analyses were used as a second approach. RRR is commonly applied to a set of intermediary response variables presumed to link diet to the health outcome [40]. Since current scientific evidence does not substantiate strong associations between specific nutrients and body composition development, RRR was used to directly extract dietary patterns best explaining the variation of changes in BMI, FMI, and WtHR during the primary school period; i.e., the method was used in a purely exploratory way.

RRR analyses were conducted via the PROC PLS procedure in SAS (option method = RRR) [40]. The RRR extracts linear combinations (i.e., RRR patterns) of predictor variables that explain as much variation in response variables as possible. For the first RRR, standardized intake frequencies of food groups at the beginning of the primary school period were used as predictor variables. The response variables were the changes in BMI, FMI, and WtHR between the end and the beginning of the primary school period in which each was adjusted for baseline BMI, FMI, and WtHR at the beginning of the primary school period, respectively, by applying the residual method [41] (RRR baseline factors). For the second RRR, changes in standardized intake frequencies of food groups between the end and the beginning of the primary school period were used as predictor variables. Changes in BMI, FMI, and WtHR between the end and the beginning of the primary school period adjusted for the baseline body composition were, again, the response variables (RRR change factors).

The number of factors extracted by RRR from the predictor variables is always equal to the number of response variables, i.e., three factors were identified by each RRR. However, only those patterns explaining the largest amount of response variation (as indicated by a break) were retained for further analyses. As for PCA, the individual RRR factor scores were calculated, according to the simplified pattern approach [39] including all food groups with a factor loading $\geq |0.2|$.

2.4.3. Logistic Regression Analyses

The PCA and RRR factors were used as independent predictors in the logistic regression models (PROC LOGISTIC) by estimating odds ratios (ORs) with 95% confidence intervals (95% CIs) of excess gain in BMI, FMI, or WtHR during primary school years with the lower three quartiles of increases in BMI, FMI, or WtHR serving as the reference category.

By definition, RRR patterns will be predictive of changes in BMI, FMI, and WtHR during primary school years, i.e., the response variables for which they were derived. Thus, our main interest was to (i) illustrate the effect sizes of the predicted OR and (ii) to investigate whether the obtained pattern would still be predictive after adjustment for potentially confounding factors [9]. Adjusted OR for excess gain in BMI, FMI, and WtHR are categorized by tertiles of RRR or PCA factors scores of adherence. The *p*-values for a linear trend refer to logistic regression models with continuous pattern scores of adherence as the independent variable. Potentially confounding variables were initially examined separately and included in the fully adjusted model only if they modified regression coefficients of the pattern scores in the unadjusted models by $\geq$10%. To ensure comparability between the models, we included all variables that met this criterion in any of the models investigating the relationship between a dietary pattern (baseline or change patterns) and the outcomes (excess gain in BMI, FMI, or WtHR).

The following covariates inquired from the parents by self-administered questionnaires were considered as potentially confounding factors: child's birth weight, breast feeding practice, smoking during pregnancy, parental education, parental weight and height, income, the child's physical activity, and the migration background (IDEFICS only).

Differences between baseline and follow-up were tested using the Wilcoxon rank sum test for continuous variables and the Chi-square test for categorical variables. SAS procedures (SAS, version 9.2, SAS Institute Inc., Cary, NC, USA) were used for data analysis. A *p*-value <0.05 was considered statistically significant.

3. Results

The characteristics of both study samples are given in Table 1. The anthropometric characteristics of the participants stratified by the beginning and the end of primary school years are summarized in Table 2. In the KOPS sample, waist circumference, BMI, and FFMI increased during primary school years while WtHR decreased and FMI did not change. Similarly, waist circumference, BMI, FMI, and FFMI increased during primary school years in the IDEFICS-Germany sample while WtHR decreased.

3.1. Dietary Patterns

For the KOPS sample, the dietary pattern obtained by PCA and RRR are presented in Table 3. The PCA baseline pattern 1 is characterized by a frequent consumption of 'fast food' (fish fingers, curry-sausage, or lasagna) while food groups characterizing PCA baseline pattern 2 could be summarized as 'healthy' (wholegrain, vegetables, and fruits). The PCA change pattern 1 reflects an increase in the consumption frequency of fast foods while the PCA change patterns 2 and 3 reflect changes in diet towards a healthier and an unhealthier dietary pattern, i.e., an 'increase in the consumption of vegetables and fruits' and a 'change towards unhealthy carbohydrates' (increase in white bread and savory bakery goods and decrease in whole-grain bread), respectively. The RRR patterns contained more disjoint food groups than the PCA patterns. The RRR baseline pattern was labelled a 'fast food pattern' characterized by a frequent intake of lemonade, children's yogurt, and a seldom intake of whole-grain bread, cheese, curd, and yogurt. The RRR change pattern increase in frequency of fast foods and starchy carbohydrate foods was characterized by an increase in the consumption frequency of carbohydrate sources such as whole-grain bread, potatoes, and pizza as well as fish sticks while the consumption frequency of vegetables decreased.

Table 1. Characteristics of the KOPS and IDEFICS-Germany samples included in the present analyses.

	KOPS		IDEFICS-Germany	
	Median or *n*-Number	P25, P75 or Percentage	Median or *n*-Number	P25, P75 or Percentage
n (% female)	372	49.5	298	47.3
Birth and infancy				
Birth year (min–max)		1991–1996		2000–2003
Gestational age (weeks)	40	39, 40	n/a	
Birth weight < 3500 g, *n* (%)	184	49.5	113	37.9
Appropriate for gestational age, *n* (%)	276	74.2	n/a	
Fully breast fed, *n* (%) [a]	317	85.2	182	61.1
Smoking during pregnancy, *n* (%)	63	16.9	50	17.2
Family				
Maternal overweight, *n* (%) [b,c]	104	28.0	116	39.2
Paternal overweight, *n* (%) [b,c]	161	44.9	165	61.3
Parental overweight, *n* (%) [b,d]	209	56.2	205	68.8
Parental education, *n* (%) [e]	217	58.3	149	50.0
Single parenting, *n* (%) [c,f]	57	15.5	33	11.1
Low income, *n* (%) [c,g]	10	8.3	47	17.2

Numbers are medians (P25, P75) or *n*-numbers (percentages) unless otherwise indicated. [a] KOPS: defined as full breastfeeding > 0.5 months. IDEFICS-Germany: defined as full breastfeeding > 1 months vs. no breastfeeding/missing. [b] BMI $\geq$ 25 kg/m^2. [c] Missing data KOPS: paternal overweight: *n* = 13. Single parenting: *n* = 4. Low income: *n* = 10. Missing data IDEFICS-Germany: maternal overweight: *n* = 2, paternal overweight: *n* = 29, and low income: *n* = 24. [d] At least one parent is overweight. [e] At least one parent had $\geq$12 years of schooling. [f] IDEFICS-Germany: Single parenting defined as living with mother or father or 50% of the time with each mother and father. [g] KOPS: low or low/medium income level, i.e., <1,000 € per months. IDEFICS-Germany: low income level, i.e., <1,100 € per months.

Table 2. Anthropometric characteristics of the KOPS and IDEFICS-Germany samples at the beginning (baseline) and the end (follow-up) of the primary school period.

	Beginning of the Primary School Period		End of the Primary School Period		Mean Difference between End and Beginning of Primary School Period	
	Median or *n*-Number	P25, P75, or Percentage	Median or *n*-Number	P25, P75, or Percentage	Median or *n*-Number	P25, P75, or Percentage
KOPS						
n (% female)	372	49.5	372	49.5		
Age	6.2	6.0, 6.5	9.8	9.6, 10.1	3.6	3.5, 3.7
Anthropometry						
BMI (kg/m^2)	15.41	14.63, 16.31	16.85	15.55, 18.35	1.32	0.58, 2.55
Overweight, *n* (%)[a]	37	10.0	58	15.6		
FMI (kg/m^2)	3.18	2.59, 3.91	3.17	2.28, 4.31	−0.02	−0.70, 1.00
FFMI (kg/m^2)	12.31	11.68, 12.91	13.67	13.11, 14.40	1.46	0.92, 1.97
Waist circumference (cm)	54.5	52.3, 57.5	62.0	58.0, 66.0	7.0	4.0, 10.5
Waist-to-height ratio	0.46	0.44, 0.48	0.43	0.42, 0.46	−0.02	−0.04, 0.01
WtHR >0.5[b], *n* (%)	46	12.4	36	9.7		
IDEFICS-Germany						
n (% female)	298	47.3	298	47.3		
Age	6.5	5.6, 6.9	8.5	7.7, 9.0	2.0	2.0, 2.1
Anthropometry						
BMI (kg/m^2)	15.50	14.60, 16.60	16.15	14.90, 17.80	0.60	0.10, 1.30
Overweight, *n* (%) [a]	34	11.4	48	16.1		
FMI (kg/m^2)	4.33	3.68, 5.17	4.42	3.40, 5.68	0.07	−0.44, 0.73
FFMI (kg/m^2)	11.23	10.58, 11.79	11.85	11.22, 12.36	0.61	0.39, 0.82
Waist circumference (cm)	51.6	49.5, 54.1	56.5	53.3, 60.1	4.8	2.7, 6.9
Waist-to-height ratio	0.43	0.41, 0.45	0.42	0.40, 0.45	−0.01	−0.02, 0.01
WtHR >0.5 [b], *n* (%)	12	4.0	16	5.4		

The numbers are medians (P25, P75) or *n*-numbers (percentages). Differences between baseline and follow-up were tested using the Wilcoxon rank sum test for continuous variables and a Chi-square test for categorical variables. BMI, body mass index, FMI, fat-mass index, WtHR, waist-to-height ratio, [a] Derived from the age-specific and sex-specific cut-points proposed by the International Obesity Task Force [36]. [b] The cut-off >0.5 was proposed by McCarthy et al. [34] as indicated whether the amount of upper body fat accumulation is excessive and a risk to health.

Table 3. Food groups included in the PCA and RRR patterns—KOPS sample, $n = 372$.

	Included Food Groups	Factor Loading	Explained Variance in the Food Group Intake (%)
PCA pattern [a]			
PCA baseline pattern 1 ('fast food pattern')	+ Fish sticks	0.62	12.7
	+ Curry-sausage	0.62	
	+ Lasagna	0.57	
	+ Pancakes	0.55	
	+ Potato fritters	0.52	
	+ Pizza	0.51	
	+ Meat balls	0.5	
PCA baseline pattern 2 ('wholegrain, vegetables & fruits')	+ Whole-grain bread	0.66	8.1
	+ Vegetables, salad	0.65	
	+ Fruits	0.56	
	+ Cheese, curd, yogurt	0.47	
	+ Muesli	0.43	
PCA change pattern 1 ('increase in the consumption of fast food')	+Δ Meat balls	0.61	9.4
	+Δ Fish sticks	0.57	
	+Δ Lasagna	0.54	
	+Δ Pizza	0.52	
	+Δ Pancakes	0.48	
	+Δ Curry-sausage	0.44	
	+Δ Potato fritters	0.43	
PCA change pattern 2 ('increase in the consumption of vegetables and fruits')	+Δ Vegetables, salad	0.61	6.8
	+Δ Fruits	0.57	
	+Δ Meat	0.47	
	+Δ Potatoes	0.44	
PCA change pattern 3 ('change towards unhealthy carbohydrates')	+Δ White bread	0.64	6.4
	+Δ Savory bakery goods	0.49	
	−Δ Whole-grain bread	−0.51	

	Included Food Groups	Factor Loading	Explained Variance in Response Variables [b] (%)
RRR pattern [a]			
RRR baseline pattern ('fast food pattern')	− Whole-grain bread	−0.32	Changes in BMI: 9.1 Changes in FMI: 5.5 Changes in WtHR: 7.9 Total variance: 7.5
	− Cheese, curd, yogurt	−0.32	
	+ Lemonade	0.55	
	+ Children's yogurt	0.41	
	+ Potato fritters	0.27	
	+ Meat balls	0.24	
	+ Meat	0.21	
RRR change pattern ('increase in the consumption of fast foods and starchy carbohydrate foods')	+Δ Fish sticks	0.49	Changes in BMI: 7.7 Changes in FMI: 5.9 Changes in WtHR: 8.6 Total variance: 7.4
	+Δ Whole-grain bread	0.26	
	+Δ Pizza	0.21	
	+Δ Potatoes	0.2	
	−Δ Vegetables	−0.44	
	−Δ Lemonade	−0.33	
	−Δ Sweets	−0.28	
	−Δ Chocolate spread	−0.21	
	−Δ Meat balls	−0.21	

+, positive loading, −, negative loading, Δ, change, BMI, body mass index, FMI, fat-mass index, WtHR, waist-to-height ratio. [a] PCA patterns consider food groups with factor loadings $\geq |0.4|$, RRR patterns consider food groups with factor loadings $\geq |0.2|$. [b] Changes in response variables between the beginning of the primary school period (baseline) and the end of the primary school period adjusted for the baseline.

For the IDEFICS-Germany sample, dietary patterns obtained by PCA and RRR are given in Table 4. The PCA baseline pattern 1 termed 'snack pattern' was characterized by the frequent consumption of snack foods (sweet snacks, fried potatoes, croquettes, ketchup, savory snacks, and sweetened drinks) while frequent consumption of plain unsweetened yogurt or kefir, dishes of milled cereals, nuts, and pizza dominate the PCA baseline pattern 2 ('Mediterranean type pattern'). The PCA change pattern 1 termed 'change towards a Mediterranean type pattern' is dominated by increases in the consumption frequency of nuts, pasta, fresh meat, and pizza. Increases in the consumption frequency of cooked vegetables, potatoes, beans, and legumes but also sweetened drinks, butter/ margarine, and fresh fruits characterize the PCA change pattern 2 ('change towards a traditional type pattern') while the PCA change pattern 3 ('change towards a snack pattern') is dominated by increases in the consumption frequency of sweet snacks such as biscuits or pastries, candies, ice creams, and savory snack foods such as crisps or popcorn. The RRR baseline pattern was labeled 'Nuts, meat, and pizza pattern' because it is characterized by frequent intakes of nuts, fresh meats, pizza but also yogurt, jam, and honey as well as a seldom consumption of cooked vegetables, potatoes, beans, legumes, and sweetened breakfast cereals. The RRR change pattern, 'decrease in the consumption of animal protein sources and snack carbohydrates', was characterized by an increase in the consumption of 'reduced-fat products on bread' and decreases in the consumption frequency of fresh meat, savory pastries, fried or scrambled eggs, sweetened drinks, nuts, seeds, and dried fruits.

Table 4. Food groups included in the PCA and RRR patterns—IDEFICS-Germany sample, $n = 298$.

	Included Food Groups	Factor Loading	Explained Variance in Food Group Intake (%)
PCA pattern[a]			
PCA baseline pattern 1 ('snack pattern')	+ Sweet snacks (biscuits, packaged cakes, pastries, puddings)	0.57	10.3
	+ Potatoes (fried, croquettes)	0.52	
	+ Ketchup and similar	0.51	
	+ Savory snacks (Crisps, corn crisps, popcorn)	0.51	
	+ Sweetened drinks	0.45	
	+ Chocolate, candy bars	0.44	
	+ Candies, loose candies, marshmallows	0.44	
	+ Ice cream, milk, or fruit-based bars	0.43	
PCA baseline pattern 2 ('Mediterranean type pattern')	+ Plain unsweetened yogurt or kefir	0.66	6.5
	+ Dish of milled cereals	0.57	
	+ Nuts, seeds, dried fruits	0.56	
	+ Pizza as main dish	0.45	
	+ Cheese (sliced and spreadable)	0.44	
	+ Fresh meat, not fried	0.44	
	+ Plain unsweetened milk	0.42	
	+ Fresh fruits with added sugar	0.41	
	+ Water	0.41	
	+ Pasta, noodles, rice	0.41	
PCA change pattern 1 ('change towards a Mediterranean type pattern')	+Δ Nuts, seeds, dried fruits	0.6	8.9
	+Δ Pasta, noodles, rice	0.56	
	+Δ Fresh meat, not fried	0.52	
	+Δ Pizza as main dish	0.49	
	+Δ Dish of milled cereals	0.48	
	+Δ Sweet yogurt, fermented milk beverages	0.43	
	+Δ Fried meat	0.41	
PCA change pattern 2 ('change towards a traditional type pattern')	+Δ Cooked vegetables, potatoes, beans, and legumes	0.54	4.8
	+Δ Sweetened drinks	0.49	
	+Δ Butter, margarine on bread	0.48	
	+Δ Fresh fruits without added sugar	0.47	
PCA change pattern 3 ('change towards a snack pattern')	+Δ Sweet snacks (biscuits, packaged cakes, pastries, puddings)	0.65	4.5
	+Δ Candies, loose candies, marshmallows	0.58	
	+Δ Ice cream, milk, or fruit-based bars	0.52	
	+Δ Savory snacks (Crisps, corn crisps, popcorn)	0.51	
	+Δ Chocolate, candy bars	0.46	

	Included Food Groups	Factor Loading	Explained Variance in Response Variables b (%)
RRR pattern [a]			
RRR baseline pattern ('Nuts, meat, and pizza pattern')	+ Nuts, seeds, dried fruits	0.37	Changes in BMI: 11.5 Changes in FMI: 11.9 Changes in WtHR: 12.3 Total variance: 11.9
	+ Fresh meat, not fried	0.36	
	+ Pizza as main dish	0.3	
	+ Plain unsweetened yogurt or kefir	0.23	
	+ Jam, honey	0.22	
	+ Savory pastries, fritters	0.23	
	+ Dish of milled cereals	0.24	
	− Cooked vegetables, potatoes, beans, and legumes	−0.29	
	− Breakfast cereals, muesli, sweetened	−0.23	
RRR change pattern ('decrease in the consumption of protein sources and snack carbohydrates')	+Δ Reduced-fat products on bread	0.24	Changes in BMI: 14.0 Changes in FMI: 14.3 Changes in WtHR: 12.0 Total variance: 13.5
	−Δ Fresh meat, not fried	−0.36	
	−Δ Savory pastries, fritters	−0.33	
	−Δ Fried or scrambled eggs	−0.29	
	−Δ Sweetened drinks	−0.27	
	−Δ Nuts, seeds, dried fruits	−0.3	
	−Δ Dish of milled cereals	−0.24	

+, positive loading, −, negative loading, Δ, change, BMI, body mass index, FMI, fat-mass index, WtHR, waist-to-height ratio. [a] PCA patterns consider food groups with factor loadings ≥ |0.4|, RRR patterns consider food groups with factor loadings ≥ |0.2|. [b] Changes in response variables between the beginning of the primary school period (baseline) and the end of the primary school period adjusted for baseline.

3.2. Logistic Regression Analyses

In KOPS, no significant association was found between PCA baseline patterns ('fast food pattern' and 'wholegrain, vegetables & fruits') and excess gain in BMI, FMI, or WtHR during the primary school period (Table 5). Among the PCA change patterns, only the adherence to an 'increase in the consumption of fast food' was significantly associated with higher odds for an excess gain in FMI after adjustment for parental overweight, parental education, and physical activity (p_{trend} = 0.0411). However, no similar associations were seen with odds for an excess gain in BMI or WtHR.

Figure 1 shows that a closer adherence to the RRR baseline pattern ('fast food pattern') was independently related to higher odds for an excess gain in BMI (Panel A, p_{trend} = 0.0006) and WtHR (Panel C, p_{trend} = 0.0047) but not in FMI (Panel B, p_{trend} = 0.2465) during primary school in the KOPS sample. Similarly, a closer adherence to the RRR change pattern ('increase in frequency of fast foods and starchy carbohydrate foods') predicted excess gain in BMI, FMI, and WtHR during the primary school period (Panel D–F, all p_{trend} < 0.002). Overall, those in the highest tertile of adherence were at least two times more likely to have excessively gained than their counterparts in the lowest tertile of adherence.

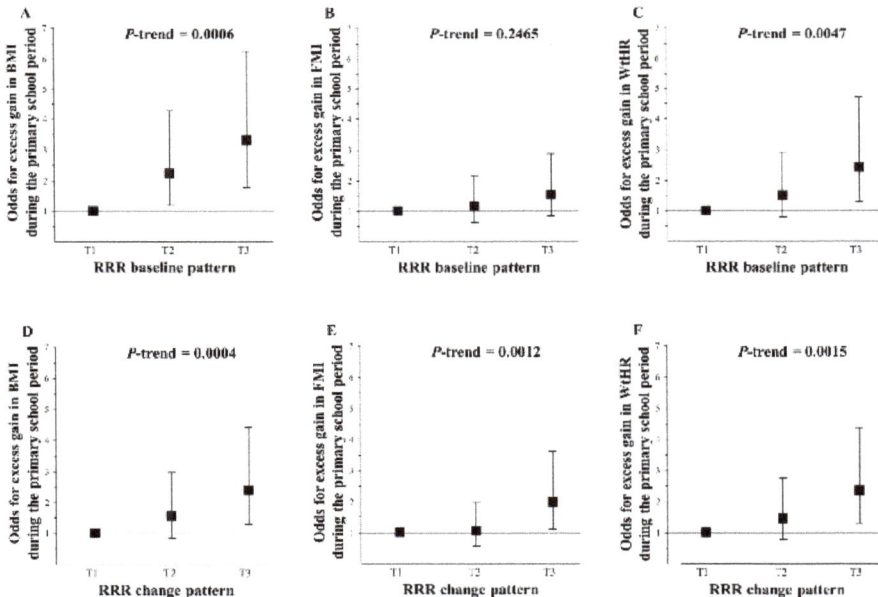

Figure 1. Odds for excess gains in BMI (panel **A** and **D**), fat-mass index (FMI, panel **B** and **E**), and waist-to-height ratio (WtHR, panel **C** and **F** during the primary school period according to tertiles of adherence to RRR baseline and change patterns ('fast food pattern' and 'increase in the consumption of fast foods and starchy carbohydrate foods', respectively)–KOPS sample (*n* = 372). Values are odd ratios (95% confidence intervals) presented in tertiles of adherence to the respective dietary pattern. Changes in body composition were adjusted for baseline body composition using the residual method. For the logistic regression analyses, the outcomes were excess gains in BMI, FMI, or WtHR defined as gains >75th percentile, adjusted for parental overweight (BMI ≥ 25 kg/m^2, yes/no), parental education (≥12 years of schooling, yes/no), and physical activity (very low, low, middle, and high). The *p*-values are based on logistic regression models with dietary pattern scores as a continuous variable. T, Tertile.

In IDEFICS-Germany, higher adherence to the PCA change pattern ('change towards a Mediterranean type pattern was associated with lower odds for excess gain in FMI, WtHR, and BMI

($p < 0.05$) (Table 6). All other PCA baseline and change patterns were not associated with changes in body composition during primary school years.

Figure 2 illustrates that both the RRR baseline and change patterns remained independently associated with substantially increased odds for excess gains in BMI, FMI, and WtHR during the primary school years in the IDEFICS-Germany sample after an adjustment for potential confounders (all $p_{\text{trend}} < 0.01$).

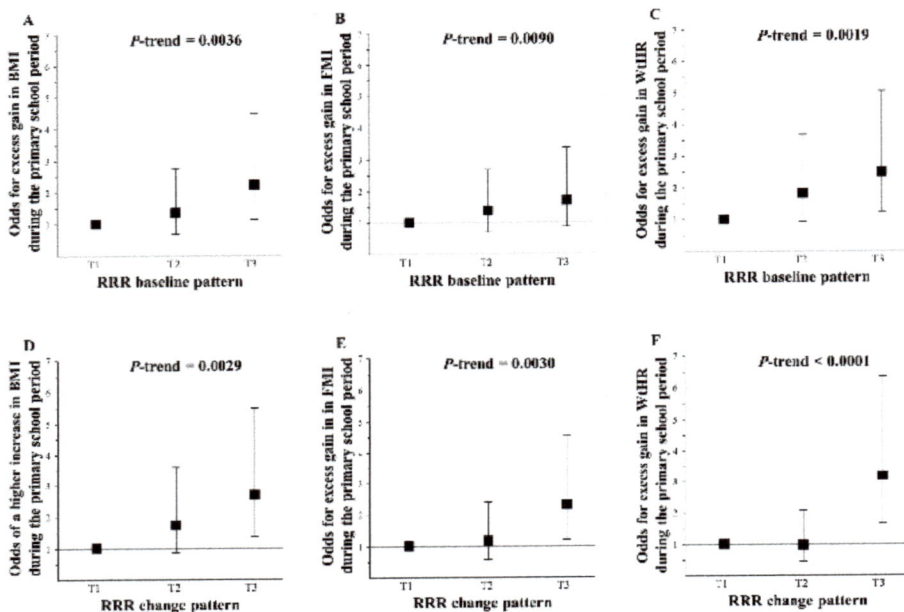

Figure 2. Odds for excess gains in BMI (panel **A** and **D**), fat-mass index (FMI, panel **B** and **E**), and waist-to-height ratio (WtHR, panel **C** and **F** during the primary school period according to tertiles of adherence to the RRR baseline and change patterns ('Nuts, meat, and pizza pattern' and 'decrease in the consumption of protein sources and snack carbohydrates', respectively)—IDEFICS-Germany sample (n = 298). Values are odd ratios (95% confidence intervals) presented in tertiles of the respective dietary pattern. Changes in body composition were adjusted for baseline body composition (BMI, FMI, or WtHR, respectively) using the residual method. For the logistic regression analyses, the outcomes were excess gains in BMI, FMI, or WtHR, which were defined as gains >75th percentile, adjusted for parental overweight (BMI $\geq$ 25 kg/m^2; yes/no), smoking during pregnancy (yes/no), and migration background (born in Germany, yes/no). Models for BMI and FMI also adjust for low income (<1.100 € per month, (no/yes/unknown): 8% of values were inputted using the missing indicator method resulting in a coding of 0, 1, and 2, respectively [42]), *p*-values based on multiple logistic regression models with dietary pattern scores as continuous variables. T, Tertile.

Table 5. Odds for excess gains in BMI, fat-mass index (FMI), or waist-to-height ratio (WtHR) [a] during the primary school period, according to tertiles of adherence to the PCA patterns—KOPS sample (n = 372).

PCA Baseline Pattern 1 ('Fast Food Pattern')

	T1	T2 OR	T2 95% CI	T3 OR	T3 95% CI	Continuous[b] OR	Continuous[b] 95% CI	p_trend[c]
BMI								
Model A	1	0.89	0.50, 1.60	1.26	0.72, 2.21	1.03	0.98, 1.09	0.2768
Model B	1	0.81	0.44, 1.49	1.00	0.55, 1.80	1.01	0.95, 1.07	0.8457
FMI								
Model A	1	0.79	0.44, 1.40	0.98	0.56, 1.73	1.02	0.97, 1.08	0.4590
Model B	1	0.67	0.37, 1.24	0.73	0.41, 1.33	0.99	0.94, 1.06	0.8556
WtHR								
Model A	1	0.59	0.32, 1.07	1.11	0.64, 1.93	1.03	0.97, 1.09	0.3318
Model B	1	0.54	0.29, 1.01	0.88	0.49, 1.57	1.00	0.95, 1.06	0.9329

PCA Baseline Pattern 2 ('Wholegrain, Vegetables & Fruits')

	T1	T2 OR	T2 95% CI	T3 OR	T3 95% CI	Continuous[b] OR	Continuous[b] 95% CI	p_trend[c]
BMI								
Model A	1	0.94	0.54, 1.64	0.60	0.33, 1.09	0.95	0.88, 1.03	0.2316
Model B	1	1.10	0.62, 1.95	0.77	0.41, 1.43	1.00	0.91, 1.08	0.9079
FMI								
Model A	1	1.20	0.69, 2.09	0.68	0.37, 1.25	0.96	0.89, 1.04	0.2859
Model B	1	1.42	0.80, 2.53	0.89	0.47, 1.67	1.00	0.92, 1.09	0.9971
WtHR								
Model A	1	0.87	0.50, 1.51	0.58	0.32, 1.05	0.96	0.89, 1.04	0.3049
Model B	1	0.97	0.55, 1.72	0.72	0.39, 1.34	1.00	0.92, 1.09	0.9676

PCA Change Pattern 1 ('Increase in the Consumption of Fast Food')

	T1	T2 OR	T2 95% CI	T3 OR	T3 95% CI	Continuous[b] OR	Continuous[b] 95% CI	p_trend[c]
BMI								
Model A	1	0.91	0.50, 1.65	1.39	0.79, 2.46	1.04	0.99, 1.10	0.1478
Model B	1	0.95	0.51, 1.75	1.49	0.83, 2.68	1.05	0.99, 1.10	0.1133
FMI								
Model A	1	1.10	0.60, 2.01	1.73	0.97, 3.07	1.05	1.00, 1.11	0.0538
Model B	1	1.19	0.64, 2.21	1.86	1.03, 3.38	1.06	1.00, 1.12	0.0411
WtHR								
Model A	1	0.76	0.42, 1.38	1.28	0.73, 2.23	1.02	0.97, 1.08	0.4498
Model B	1	0.79	0.43, 1.46	1.35	0.76, 2.40	1.02	0.97, 1.08	0.3665

PCA Change Pattern 2 ('Increase in the Consumption of Vegetables and Fruits')

	T1	T2 OR	T2 95% CI	T3 OR	T3 95% CI	Continuous[b] OR	Continuous[b] 95% CI	p_trend[c]
BMI								
Model A	1	1.01	0.57, 1.79	0.87	0.49, 1.55	1.00	0.92, 1.09	0.9687
Model B	1	1.03	0.57, 1.86	0.76	0.42, 1.39	0.98	0.90, 1.08	0.7236
FMI								
Model A	1	0.85	0.47, 1.52	1.03	0.59, 1.82	1.02	0.93, 1.11	0.7210
Model B	1	0.86	0.47, 1.57	0.92	0.51, 1.65	1.00	0.91, 1.09	0.9852
WtHR								
Model A	1	0.65	0.36, 1.17	0.91	0.52, 1.59	0.98	0.90, 1.07	0.6387
Model B	1	0.61	0.33, 1.13	0.80	0.45, 1.43	0.96	0.88, 1.05	0.3628

PCA Change Pattern 3 ('Change towards Unhealthy Carbohydrates')

	T1	T2 OR	T2 95% CI	T3 OR	T3 95% CI	Continuous[b] OR	Continuous[b] 95% CI	p_trend[c]
BMI								
Model A	1	0.83	0.47, 1.46	0.80	0.45, 1.42	0.97	0.87, 1.08	0.5265
Model B	1	0.89	0.50, 1.61	0.90	0.50, 1.63	0.99	0.88, 1.10	0.8046
FMI								
Model A	1	0.69	0.39, 1.24	0.84	0.48, 1.47	0.95	0.85, 1.06	0.3516
Model B	1	0.75	0.41, 1.35	0.96	0.53, 1.72	0.97	0.87, 1.09	0.6091
WtHR								
Model A	1	0.87	0.49, 1.52	0.67	0.37, 1.20	0.91	0.81, 1.01	0.0836
Model B	1	0.92	0.52, 1.64	0.71	0.39, 1.30	0.92	0.82, 1.03	0.1262

Values are odds ratios (95% confidence intervals) presented in tertiles of adherence to the respective dietary pattern. [a] Change in body composition was adjusted for the respective baseline value using the residual method. Odds refer to excess gains in BMI, FMI, or WtHR' defined as gains >75th percentile. [b] Continuous, i.e., per unit of pattern score. [c] Based on logistic regression models with dietary pattern scores as a continuous variable. Model A: Unadjusted. Model B: Adjusted for parental overweight (BMI $\geq$ 25 kg/m^2, yes/no), parental education ($\geq$12 years of schooling, yes/no), and physical activity (very low, low, middle, high).

Table 6. Odds for excess gains in BMI, fat-mass index (FMI), or waist-to-height ratio (WtHR) [a] during the primary school period according to tertiles of adherence to the PCA patterns—IDEFICS-Germany sample (n = 298).

		PCA Baseline Pattern 1 ("Snack Pattern")						PCA Change Pattern 1 ("Increase in the Consumption of Fast Food")					
		T2		T3		Continuous [b]			T2		T3		Continuous [b]	
	T1	OR	95% CI	OR	95% CI	OR	95% CI	p_{trend} [c]	T1	OR	95% CI	OR	95% CI	OR	95% CI	p_{trend} [c]

BMI
(Snack Pattern / Fast Food)

Row	T1	T2 OR	T2 95% CI	T3 OR	T3 95% CI	Cont OR	Cont 95% CI	p_{trend}	T1	T2 OR	T2 95% CI	T3 OR	T3 95% CI	Cont OR	Cont 95% CI	p_{trend}
BMI Model A	1	0.69	0.37, 1.29	0.52	0.27, 1.00	0.95	0.88, 1.02	0.1537	1	1.15	0.62, 2.15	0.67	0.34, 1.30	0.93	0.87, 1.00	0.0395
Model B	1	0.67	0.35, 1.26	0.47	0.23, 0.91	0.94	0.87, 1.01	0.0810	1	1.12	0.60, 2.11	0.65	0.33, 1.30	0.93	0.87, 0.99	0.0436
FMI Model A	1	1.10	0.58, 2.07	0.85	0.44, 1.63	0.99	0.92, 1.06	0.8102	1	1.21	0.65, 2.27	0.75	0.38, 1.46	0.93	0.87, 0.99	0.0454
Model B	1	1.06	0.55, 2.03	0.78	0.39, 1.52	0.98	0.91, 1.05	0.6013	1	1.05	0.55, 1.99	0.79	0.40, 1.56	0.94	0.87, 0.99	0.0490
WtHR Model A	1	1.29	0.68, 2.45	1.00	0.52, 1.94	0.99	0.92, 1.06	0.8259	1	1.04	0.55, 1.95	0.76	0.39, 1.46	0.93	0.87, 0.99	0.0409
Model B	1	1.18	0.62, 2.28	0.95	0.48, 1.87	0.98	0.92, 1.05	0.6481	1	1.04	0.55, 1.99	0.79	0.40, 1.56	0.93	0.87, 0.99	0.0490

		PCA Baseline Pattern 2 ("Mediterranean Type Pattern")						PCA Change Pattern 2 ("Change towards a Traditional Type Pattern")					
Row	T1	T2 OR	T2 95% CI	T3 OR	T3 95% CI	Cont OR	Cont 95% CI	p_{trend}	T1	T2 OR	T2 95% CI	T3 OR	T3 95% CI	Cont OR	Cont 95% CI	p_{trend}
BMI Model A	1	0.65	0.33, 1.25	0.92	0.49, 1.71	1.04	0.99, 1.09	0.1456	1	1.04	0.55, 1.99	1.06	0.55, 2.02	1.02	0.92, 1.13	0.7179
Model B	1	0.65	0.33, 1.27	0.92	0.47, 1.79	1.04	0.99, 1.11	0.1403	1	1.02	0.52, 1.98	1.06	0.54, 2.07	1.02	0.92, 1.14	0.6587
FMI Model A	1	0.96	0.51, 1.82	0.86	0.45, 1.64	1.03	0.98, 1.09	0.1957	1	1.10	0.58, 2.07	0.85	0.44, 1.63	0.99	0.89, 1.10	0.8205
Model B	1	1.00	0.52, 1.92	0.91	0.46, 1.81	1.05	0.99, 1.12	0.1073	1	1.02	0.53, 1.96	0.83	0.42, 1.63	0.99	0.89, 1.10	0.8780
WtHR Model A	1	0.62	0.32, 1.19	0.83	0.44, 1.55	1.04	0.98, 1.10	0.2349	1	0.75	0.39, 1.44	0.90	0.48, 1.70	0.95	00.86, 1.05	0.3343
Model B	1	0.60	0.31, 1.17	0.86	0.44, 1.67	1.04	0.98, 1.11	0.1764	1	0.63	0.32, 1.24	0.77	0.40, 1.50	0.94	0.85, 1.04	0.2324

	PCA Change Pattern 3 ("Change towards a Snack Pattern")					
	T1	T2 OR	T2 95% CI	T3 OR	T3 95% CI	Cont OR	Cont 95% CI	p_{trend}
BMI Model A	1	1.53	0.80, 2.99	1.41	0.73, 2.76	1.01	0.93, 1.10	0.7551
Model B	1	1.60	0.83, 3.15	1.46	0.75, 2.87	1.02	0.94, 1.11	0.6363
FMI Model A	1	1.24	0.64, 2.41	1.47	0.77, 2.83	0.98	0.90, 1.06	0.6550
Model B	1	1.27	0.65, 2.50	1.49	0.78, 2.90	0.99	0.91, 1.08	0.8546
WtHR Model A	1	1.11	0.57, 2.18	1.62	0.85, 3.11	1.03	0.95, 1.12	0.5336
Model B	1	1.17	0.59, 2.33	1.64	0.86, 3.19	1.03	0.95, 1.12	0.4342

Values are odds ratios (95% confidence intervals) presented in tertiles of adherence to the respective dietary pattern. [a] Change in body composition was adjusted for the respective baseline value using the residual method. Odds refer to excess gains in BMI, FMI, or WtHR defined as gains >75th percentile. [b] Continuous, i.e., per unit of pattern score. [c] Based on logistic regression models with dietary pattern scores as a continuous variable. Model A: Unadjusted. Model B: Adjusted for parental overweight (BMI $\geq$ 25 kg/m^2, yes/no), smoking during pregnancy (yes/no), and migration background (born in Germany, yes/no) in models for BMI and FMI additional adjustment for low income (<1.100 € per months, (no/yes/unknown): 8% of values were imputed using the missing indicator method resulting in a coding of 0, 1, and 2, respectively [42]).

4. Discussion

The present study provides new prospective evidence from two pediatric samples suggesting a relevance of dietary patterns during the primary school period identified by RRR for the development of body composition in primary school years. Our data support a potentially detrimental role of dietary patterns characterized by fast foods for BMI, FMI, and WtHR development during this critical time period. On a more exploratory level, this study also suggests that future research should shed light on the relevance of combinations of protein and carbohydrate sources for body composition development in school children.

Both PCA and RRR identified dietary patterns characterized by a preferred consumption of fast foods, which were associated with excess gains in adiposity measures both prospectively and concurrently in the KOPS cohort. Our findings are broadly in line with the ALSPAC study, which reported that an energy-dense, low-fiber, high-fat RRR dietary pattern at 7 years of age but not at 5 years of age, was predictive of fat mass at 9 years of age among UK children [14]. In addition, the preferred consumption of fast foods itself has repeatedly been related to an unfavorable body composition among children and adolescents [43–46] even though it is possible that associations with measures of obesity risk may partly reflect relations to the associated behaviors rather than the preferred consumption of these foods [47,48]. The fact that no predictive fast food pattern was identified for the IDEFICS-Germany cohort may, in part, result from differences in the focused inquiry of these foods by the employed FPQs: in KOPS, one-third of the inquired food groups (8 out of 22) referred to fast foods while only four out of 43 items in IDEFICS-Germany addressed fast foods.

Our study did also confirm a protective role of a Mediterranean type pattern identified by PCA, which was prospectively related to lower odds for excess gains in BMI, FMI, and WtHR in the German IDEFICS-Germany cohort. Similar associations have previously been reported by some [49–53] but not all [54,55] pediatric studies that were explicitly investigating the relevance of Mediterranean dietary indices or scores for body composition. Recently, a Mediterranean type diet was observed to be associated with a more favorable BMI, glucose, and lipid profile among children and adolescents presenting with components of the metabolic syndrome than a standard diet [56]. Similarly, evidence from both intervention and prospective cohort studies support benefits of Mediterranean type diets for body composition among adults [57–60].

Snacking habits have also been suggested as a potential cause contributing to the development of overweight and obesity among children. Evidence for the prospective role of a 'snacking' pattern among children is available from two prospective observational studies. In a cohort of 5-year-old to 12-year-old Columbian children, the adherence to this PCA-derived 'snacking' pattern was associated with greater increases in BMI, subscapular: triceps skinfold thickness ratio, and waist circumference over a median 2.5 year follow-up [13]. By contrast, a PCA-derived 'snacking' pattern in 2-year-old and 9.9-year-old participants of the IDEFICS-multicenter cohort was not related to a two-year BMI change [12]. In line with this, the PCA 'snack food pattern' and the 'change towards a snack pattern' identified in the IDEFICS-Germany cohort were not related to a higher BMI, FMI, or WtHR. PCA generally yields interpretable patterns, but they may not be relevant for disease outcomes because PCA is purely exploratory, which explains maximal variation in food intake [61]. In addition, PCA patterns generally tend to account for only a small amount of the total variance in food intake in pediatric populations [61–65]. Similarly, in our study, the PCA patterns accounted for only 6.4% to 12.7% and 4.5% to 10.3% of the total variance in food intake in KOPS and IDEFICS-Germany, respectively.

RRR may be more informative since it explicitly derives predictors that explain maximal variation in response variables [40,66]. In the present study, three of the RRR patterns point towards a specific relevance of combinations of unfavorable carbohydrate sources and (animal) protein sources (RRR patterns 'fast food', 'increase in the consumption of fast foods and starchy carbohydrate foods,' and 'decrease in the consumption of protein sources and snack carbohydrates.' The protein leverage hypothesis proposes that a preference for protein in combination with a decrease in the ratio of protein to carbohydrates and fat in the diet is related to excess energy intake and the risk of obesity [67,68]. The two RRR change patterns in the present study are in line with this since they suggest that either increases in (starchy) carbohydrate sources or decreases in the consumption of protein sources during primary school years were associated with an unfavorable development of body composition. Data from a large animal study conducted by the advocates of the protein leverage hypothesis revealed that a high ratio of protein to carbohydrate rather than total caloric intake was related to lower body fat content but may adversely affect cardio-metabolic health [69]. However, in adults, diets with higher plant and animal protein intake were associated with lower central adiposity [70,71] and favorable cardiometabolic markers [71]. Furthermore, in eight-year-old school children, high protein intake was positively associated with a higher fat-free mass index two years later [72]. The relevance of macronutrient ratios or of the combinations of carbohydrate and protein sources for body composition remains to be elucidated.

Despite some similarities in the identified pattern and their association with body composition development in primary school years as outlined above, the patterns differ substantially between both cohorts. Our analyses do, therefore, not confirm our initial hypothesis that similar detrimental or protective dietary patterns may be identified in the three German pediatric cohorts, i.e., DONALD, KOPS, and IDEFICS-Germany. It is likely that this largely reflects the considerable methodological differences, i.e., the different nutrition assessment methods as well as differences in the examined food groups. Comparison with other pediatric studies is further hampered by differences in the method to identify dietary patterns, e.g., the definition of high factor loadings and the fact that the simplified pattern approach is not universally applied.

To overcome some of the issues of comparability, both the criteria for sample selections and the analytical approach of the present study were similar to those previously applied in the DONALD study [9]. Additional strengths of the present study include its prospective nature, which covered the period of two and 3.6 years of primary school for IDEFICS-Germany and KOPS, respectively, with completion of one FPQ at the beginning and one at the end of the observation period as well as anthropometric examination at both points in time, which allows the analysis of changes in diet and growth. In addition, in both cohorts, FMI and WtHR—i.e., more sensitive measurements of obesity and central adiposity, respectively, were examined in addition to BMI. Nonetheless, the fact that fat mass was estimated by two different algorithms derived from the respective BIA may be seen as a limitation. In addition, changes in body composition after puberty onset are known to differ between early-maturing and late-maturing children of the same age [73]. However, puberty onset was not assessed in the studies. KOPS data stem from 2001 and one can assume that dietary behavior and other lifestyle factors may have changed in the meantime. However, results of examinations conducted in a further cohort after 10 years at school entry (2006–2008) and at the end of the primary school period (4th grade, 2010–2012) indicate that these data are still comparable [74,75]. In addition, our study is limited by the comparably small samples from the KOPS and IDEFICS-Germany cohorts. However, it has been suggested that the ratio of the sample size to the number of food groups may be more important than the absolute number of subjects [76]. We performed a number of statistical tests. Therefore, the chance may be an explanation for our findings. However, for the RRR results in particular consistency of findings across the different body composition outcomes argues against chance findings. Another limitation arises from the fact that the FPQ used in KOPS and IDEFICS-Germany did not inquire the consumption frequencies of the same food groups. Therefore, pooled analyses of the KOPS and IDEFICS-Germany samples were not possible. However, as outlined above, comparative analyses using similar analytic approaches based on the food-group specific data available from different assessment methods are desirable and were conducted.

5. Conclusions

The present study confirms an unfavorable impact of fast foods on the development of body composition during primary school years. The role of combinations of unfavorable carbohydrate sources and (animal) protein sources requires further investigation.

Supplementary Materials: The following are available online at http://www.mdpi.com/2072-6643/10/10/1442/s1, Table S1: Food groups assessed by the food propensity questionnaire (FPQ) in KOPS at baseline (*n* = 372). Table S2: Food groups assessed in IDEFICS-Germany by the Children's Eating Habits Questionnaire (CEHQ) at baseline (*n* = 298).

Author Contributions: Conceptualization, A.E.B. Data curation, M.W. and S.P.-D. Formal analysis, G.J. Funding acquisition, M.J.M., W.A., and A.E.B. Investigation, M.J.M., W.A., and A.E.B. Methodology, A.E.B and G.J. Writing-original draft, M.W. and G.J. Writing-review & editing, M.W., G.J., S.P.-D., M.S., M.J.M., W.A., and A.E.B.

Funding: This work was supported by the Kompetenznetz Adipositas (Competence Network Obesity) funded by the Federal Ministry of Education and Research (FKZ: 01GI1121A). KOPS was funded by the Deutsche Forschungsgemeinschaft (DFG Mü 5.1, 5.2, 5.3 and 5.5), WCRF, and Wirtschaftliche Vereinigung Zucker. For the IDEFICS study, we gratefully acknowledge the financial support of the European Commission within the Sixth RDT Framework Program Contract no. 016181 (Food). The publication of this article was funded by the Open Access Fund of the Leibniz Association.

Acknowledgments: The participation of all children and their families in the KOPS and IDEFICS-Germany cohort is gratefully acknowledged.

Conflicts of Interest: The authors declare no conflict of interest. The founding sponsors had no role in the design of the study, in the collection, analyses, or interpretation of data, in the writing of the manuscript, or in the decision to publish the results.

References

1. Kurth, B.M.; Schaffrath Rosario, A. [The prevalence of overweight and obese children and adolescents living in germany. Results of the german health interview and examination survey for children and adolescents (kiggs)]. *Bundesgesundheitsblatt Gesundheitsforschung Gesundheitsschutz* **2007**, *50*, 736–743. [CrossRef] [PubMed]
2. Ogden, C.L.; Carroll, M.D.; Kit, B.K.; Flegal, K.M. Prevalence of childhood and adult obesity in the united states, 2011–2012. *JAMA* **2014**, *311*, 806–814. [CrossRef] [PubMed]
3. von Kries, R.; Reulen, H.; Bayer, O.; Riedel, C.; Diethelm, K.; Buyken, A.E. Increase in prevalence of adiposity between the ages of 7 and 11 years reflects lower remission rates during this period. *Pediatr. Obes.* **2013**, *8*, 13–20. [CrossRef] [PubMed]
4. Hughes, A.R.; Sherriff, A.; Lawlor, D.A.; Ness, A.R.; Reilly, J.J. Incidence of obesity during childhood and adolescence in a large contemporary cohort. *Prev. Med.* **2011**, *52*, 300–304. [CrossRef] [PubMed]
5. Plachta-Danielzik, S.; Pust, S.; Asbeck, I.; Czerwinski-Mast, M.; Langnase, K.; Fischer, C.; Bosy-Westphal, A.; Kriwy, P.; Muller, M.J. Four-year follow-up of school-based intervention on overweight children: The kops study. *Obesity (Silver Spring)* **2007**, *15*, 3159–3169. [CrossRef] [PubMed]
6. Datar, A.; Shier, V.; Sturm, R. Changes in body mass during elementary and middle school in a national cohort of kindergarteners. *Pediatrics* **2011**, *128*, e1411–e1417. [CrossRef] [PubMed]
7. Verrotti, A.; Penta, L.; Zenzeri, L.; Agostinelli, S.; De Feo, P. Childhood obesity: Prevention and strategies of intervention. A systematic review of school-based interventions in primary schools. *J. Endocrinol. Invest.* **2014**, *37*, 1155–1164. [CrossRef] [PubMed]
8. Li, X.H.; Lin, S.; Guo, H.; Huang, Y.; Wu, L.; Zhang, Z.; Ma, J.; Wang, H.J. Effectiveness of a school-based physical activity intervention on obesity in school children: A nonrandomized controlled trial. *BMC Public Health* **2014**, *14*, 1282. [CrossRef] [PubMed]
9. Diethelm, K.; Gunther, A.L.; Schulze, M.B.; Standl, M.; Heinrich, J.; Buyken, A.E. Prospective relevance of dietary patterns at the beginning and during the course of primary school to the development of body composition. *Br. J. Nutr.* **2014**, *111*, 1488–1498. [CrossRef] [PubMed]
10. Cutler, G.J.; Flood, A.; Hannan, P.J.; Slavin, J.L.; Neumark-Sztainer, D. Association between major patterns of dietary intake and weight status in adolescents. *Br. J. Nutr.* **2012**, *108*, 349–356. [CrossRef] [PubMed]
11. Oellingrath, I.M.; Svendsen, M.V.; Brantsaeter, A.L. Tracking of eating patterns and overweight—a follow-up study of norwegian schoolchildren from middle childhood to early adolescence. *Nutr. J.* **2011**, *10*, 106. [CrossRef] [PubMed]
12. Pala, V.; Lissner, L.; Hebestreit, A.; Lanfer, A.; Sieri, S.; Siani, A.; Huybrechts, I.; Kambek, L.; Molnar, D.; Tornaritis, M.; et al. Dietary patterns and longitudinal change in body mass in european children: A follow-up study on the idefics multicenter cohort. *Eur. J. Clin. Nutr.* **2013**, *67*, 1042–1049. [CrossRef] [PubMed]

13. Shroff, M.R.; Perng, W.; Baylin, A.; Mora-Plazas, M.; Marin, C.; Villamor, E. Adherence to a snacking dietary pattern and soda intake are related to the development of adiposity: A prospective study in school-age children. *Public Health Nutr.* **2014**, *17*, 1507–1513. [CrossRef] [PubMed]

14. Johnson, L.; Mander, A.P.; Jones, L.R.; Emmett, P.M.; Jebb, S.A. Energy-dense, low-fiber, high-fat dietary pattern is associated with increased fatness in childhood. *Am. J. Clin. Nutr.* **2008**, *87*, 846–854. [CrossRef] [PubMed]

15. Emmett, P.M.; Jones, L.R.; Northstone, K. Dietary patterns in the avon longitudinal study of parents and children. *Nutr. Rev.* **2015**, *73 Suppl 3*, 207–230. [CrossRef]

16. Danielzik, S.; Pust, S.; Landsberg, B.; Muller, M.J. First lessons from the kiel obesity prevention study (KOPS). *Int. J. Obes. (Lond.)* **2005**, *29 Suppl 2*, S78–S83. [CrossRef]

17. Brambilla, P.; Bedogni, G.; Heo, M.; Pietrobelli, A. Waist circumference-to-height ratio predicts adiposity better than body mass index in children and adolescents. *Int. J. Obes. (Lond.)* **2013**, *37*, 943–946. [CrossRef] [PubMed]

18. Nagy, P.; Kovacs, E.; Moreno, L.A.; Veidebaum, T.; Tornaritis, M.; Kourides, Y.; Siani, A.; Lauria, F.; Sioen, I.; Claessens, M.; et al. Percentile reference values for anthropometric body composition indices in european children from the idefics study. *Int. J. Obes. (Lond.)* **2014**, *38 Suppl 2*, S15–S25. [CrossRef]

19. Schroder, H.; Ribas, L.; Koebnick, C.; Funtikova, A.; Gomez, S.F.; Fito, M.; Perez-Rodrigo, C.; Serra-Majem, L. Prevalence of abdominal obesity in spanish children and adolescents. Do we need waist circumference measurements in pediatric practice? *PLoS One* **2014**, *9*. [CrossRef] [PubMed]

20. Subar, A.F.; Dodd, K.W.; Guenther, P.M.; Kipnis, V.; Midthune, D.; McDowell, M.; Tooze, J.A.; Freedman, L.S.; Krebs-Smith, S.M. The food propensity questionnaire: Concept, development, and validation for use as a covariate in a model to estimate usual food intake. *J. Am. Diet. Assoc.* **2006**, *106*, 1556–1563. [CrossRef] [PubMed]

21. Muller, M.J.; Asbeck, I.; Mast, M.; Langnase, K.; Grund, A. Prevention of obesity-more than an intention. Concept and first results of the kiel obesity prevention study (KOPS). *Int. J. Obes. Relat. Metab. Disord.* **2001**, *25 (Suppl 1)*, S66–S74. [CrossRef] [PubMed]

22. Ahrens, W.; Bammann, K.; Siani, A.; Buchecker, K.; De Henauw, S.; Iacoviello, L.; Hebestreit, A.; Krogh, V.; Lissner, L.; Marild, S.; et al. The idefics cohort: Design, characteristics and participation in the baseline survey. *Int. J. Obes. (Lond.)* **2011**, *35 Suppl 1*, S3–S15. [CrossRef]

23. Von Kries, R.; Beyerlein, A.; Muller, M.J.; Heinrich, J.; Landsberg, B.; Bolte, G.; Chmitorz, A.; Plachta-Danielzik, S. Different age-specific incidence and remission rates in pre-school and primary school suggest need for targeted obesity prevention in childhood. *Int. J. Obes. (Lond.)* **2012**, *36*, 505–510. [CrossRef] [PubMed]

24. Plachta-Danielzik, S.; Landsberg, B.; Seiberl, J.; Gehrke, M.I.; Gose, M.; Kehden, B.; Muller, M.J. Longitudinal data of the kiel obesity prevention study (KOPS). *Bundesgesundheitsblatt Gesundheitsforschung Gesundheitsschutz* **2012**, *55*, 885–891. [CrossRef] [PubMed]

25. Plachta-Danielzik, S.; Landsberg, B.; Lange, D.; Seiberl, J.; Muller, M.J. Eight-year follow-up of school-based intervention on childhood overweight–the kiel obesity prevention study. *Obes Facts* **2011**, *4*, 35–43. [CrossRef] [PubMed]

26. Mast, M.; Kortzinger, I.; Konig, E.; Muller, M.J. Gender differences in fat mass of 5–7-year old children. *Int. J. Obes. Relat. Metab. Disord.* **1998**, *22*, 878–884. [CrossRef] [PubMed]

27. Pust, S. *Evaluation eines Adipositas-Präventionsprogrammes für Kinder. Ergebnisse der Kieler Adipositas-Präventionsstudie (Kops)*; Der Andere Verlag: Tönning, Lübeck, Marburg, Germany, 2006.

28. Lanfer, A.; Hebestreit, A.; Ahrens, W.; Krogh, V.; Sieri, S.; Lissner, L.; Eiben, G.; Siani, A.; Huybrechts, I.; Loit, H.M.; et al. Reproducibility of food consumption frequencies derived from the children's eating habits questionnaire used in the idefics study. *Int. J. Obes. (Lond.)* **2011**, *35 (Suppl 1)*, S61–S68. [CrossRef] [PubMed]

29. Huybrechts, I.; Bornhorst, C.; Pala, V.; Moreno, L.A.; Barba, G.; Lissner, L.; Fraterman, A.; Veidebaum, T.; Hebestreit, A.; Sieri, S.; et al. Evaluation of the children's eating habits questionnaire used in the idefics study by relating urinary calcium and potassium to milk consumption frequencies among european children. *Int. J. Obes. (Lond.)* **2011**, *35 (Suppl 1)*, S69–S78. [CrossRef] [PubMed]

30. Bel-Serrat, S.; Mouratidou, T.; Pala, V.; Huybrechts, I.; Bornhorst, C.; Fernandez-Alvira, J.M.; Hadjigeorgiou, C.; Eiben, G.; Hebestreit, A.; Lissner, L.; et al. Relative validity of the children's eating habits questionnaire-food frequency section among young european children: The idefics study. *Public Health Nutr.* **2014**, *17*, 266–276. [CrossRef] [PubMed]

31. Plachta-Danielzik, S.; Gehrke, M.I.; Kehden, B.; Kromeyer-Hauschild, K.; Grillenberger, M.; Willhoft, C.; Bosy-Westphal, A.; Muller, M.J. Body fat percentiles for german children and adolescents. *Obes Facts* **2012**, *5*, 77–90. [CrossRef] [PubMed]
32. Tyrrell, V.J.; Richards, G.; Hofman, P.; Gillies, G.F.; Robinson, E.; Cutfield, W.S. Foot-to-foot bioelectrical impedance analysis: A valuable tool for the measurement of body composition in children. *Int. J. Obes. Relat. Metab. Disord.* **2001**, *25*, 273–278. [CrossRef] [PubMed]
33. World Health Organization. Waist circumference and waist–hip ratio: Report of a who expert consultation, 8–11 December 2008. Available online: http://whqlibdoc.who.int/publications/2011/9789241501491_eng.pdf (accessed on 9 November.2017).
34. McCarthy, H.D.; Ashwell, M. A study of central fatness using waist-to-height ratios in uk children and adolescents over two decades supports the simple message-'keep your waist circumference to less than half your height'. *Int. J. Obes. (Lond.)* **2006**, *30*, 988–992. [CrossRef] [PubMed]
35. Cole, T.J.; Faith, M.S.; Pietrobelli, A.; Heo, M. What is the best measure of adiposity change in growing children: Bmi, bmi %, bmi z-score or bmi centile? *Eur. J. Clin. Nutr.* **2005**, *59*, 419–425. [CrossRef] [PubMed]
36. Cole, T.J.; Bellizzi, M.C.; Flegal, K.M.; Dietz, W.H. Establishing a standard definition for child overweight and obesity worldwide: International survey. *BMJ* **2000**, *320*, 1240–1243. [CrossRef] [PubMed]
37. Schulze, M.B.; Hoffmann, K.; Kroke, A.; Boeing, H. Dietary patterns and their association with food and nutrient intake in the european prospective investigation into cancer and nutrition (epic)-potsdam study. *Br. J. Nutr.* **2001**, *85*, 363–373. [CrossRef] [PubMed]
38. Hatcher, L. *A Step-by-Step Approach to Using the SAS System for Factor Analysis and Structural Equation Modeling*; SAS Institute: Cary, NC, USA, 2007; p. 588.
39. Schulze, M.B.; Hoffmann, K.; Kroke, A.; Boeing, H. An approach to construct simplified measures of dietary patterns from exploratory factor analysis. *Br. J. Nutr.* **2003**, *89*, 409–419. [CrossRef] [PubMed]
40. Hoffmann, K.; Schulze, M.B.; Schienkiewitz, A.; Nothlings, U.; Boeing, H. Application of a new statistical method to derive dietary patterns in nutritional epidemiology. *Am. J. Epidemiol.* **2004**, *159*, 935–944. [CrossRef] [PubMed]
41. Willett, W. *Nutritional Epidemiology*, 2nd ed.; Oxford University Press: New York, NY, USA, 1998; p. 514.
42. Haukoos, J.S.; Newgard, C.D. Advanced statistics: Missing data in clinical research-part 1: An introduction and conceptual framework. *Acad. Emerg. Med.* **2007**, *14*, 662–668. [PubMed]
43. Rosenheck, R. Fast food consumption and increased caloric intake: A systematic review of a trajectory towards weight gain and obesity risk. *Obes. Rev.* **2008**, *9*, 535–547. [CrossRef] [PubMed]
44. Braithwaite, I.; Stewart, A.W.; Hancox, R.J.; Beasley, R.; Murphy, R.; Mitchell, E.A. Fast-food consumption and body mass index in children and adolescents: An international cross-sectional study. *BMJ Open* **2014**, *4*. [CrossRef] [PubMed]
45. Whitton, C.; Ma, Y.; Bastian, A.C.; Fen Chan, M.; Chew, L. Fast-food consumers in singapore: Demographic profile, diet quality and weight status. *Public Health Nutr.* **2014**, *17*, 1805–1813. [CrossRef] [PubMed]
46. Shang, L.; O'Loughlin, J.; Tremblay, A.; Gray-Donald, K. The association between food patterns and adiposity among canadian children at risk of overweight. *Appl. Physiol. Nutr. Metab.* **2014**, *39*, 195–201. [CrossRef] [PubMed]
47. Poti, J.M.; Duffey, K.J.; Popkin, B.M. The association of fast food consumption with poor dietary outcomes and obesity among children: Is it the fast food or the remainder of the diet? *Am. J. Clin. Nutr.* **2014**, *99*, 162–171. [CrossRef] [PubMed]
48. Alexy, U.; Libuda, L.; Mersmann, S.; Kersting, M. Convenience foods in children's diet and association with dietary quality and body weight status. *Eur. J. Clin. Nutr.* **2011**, *65*, 160–166. [CrossRef] [PubMed]
49. Tognon, G.; Moreno, L.A.; Mouratidou, T.; Veidebaum, T.; Molnar, D.; Russo, P.; Siani, A.; Akhandaf, Y.; Krogh, V.; Tornaritis, M.; et al. Adherence to a mediterranean-like dietary pattern in children from eight european countries. The idefics study. *Int. J. Obes. (Lond.)* **2014**, *38 Suppl 2*, S108–S114. [CrossRef]
50. Lydakis, C.; Stefanaki, E.; Stefanaki, S.; Thalassinos, E.; Kavousanaki, M.; Lydaki, D. Correlation of blood pressure, obesity, and adherence to the mediterranean diet with indices of arterial stiffness in children. *Eur. J. Pediatr.* **2012**, *171*, 1373–1382. [CrossRef] [PubMed]
51. Schroder, H.; Mendez, M.A.; Ribas-Barba, L.; Covas, M.I.; Serra-Majem, L. Mediterranean diet and waist circumference in a representative national sample of young spaniards. *Int. J. Pediatr. Obes.* **2010**, *5*, 516–519. [CrossRef] [PubMed]

52. Martin-Calvo, N.; Chavarro, J.E.; Falbe, J.; Hu, F.B.; Field, A.E. Adherence to the mediterranean dietary pattern and bmi change among us adolescents. *Int. J. Obes. (Lond.)* **2016**, *40*, 1103–1108. [CrossRef] [PubMed]

53. Tognon, G.; Hebestreit, A.; Lanfer, A.; Moreno, L.A.; Pala, V.; Siani, A.; Tornaritis, M.; De Henauw, S.; Veidebaum, T.; Molnár, D.; et al. Mediterranean diet, overweight and body composition in children from eight european countries: Cross-sectional and prospective results from the idefics study. *Nutr. Metab. Cardiovasc. Dis.* **2014**, *24*, 205–213. [CrossRef] [PubMed]

54. Farajian, P.; Risvas, G.; Karasouli, K.; Pounis, G.D.; Kastorini, C.M.; Panagiotakos, D.B.; Zampelas, A. Very high childhood obesity prevalence and low adherence rates to the mediterranean diet in greek children: The greco study. *Atherosclerosis* **2011**, *217*, 525–530. [CrossRef] [PubMed]

55. Jennings, A.; Welch, A.; van Sluijs, E.M.; Griffin, S.J.; Cassidy, A. Diet quality is independently associated with weight status in children aged 9–10 years. *J. Nutr.* **2011**, *141*, 453–459. [CrossRef] [PubMed]

56. Velazquez-Lopez, L.; Santiago-Diaz, G.; Nava-Hernandez, J.; Munoz-Torres, A.V.; Medina-Bravo, P.; Torres-Tamayo, M. Mediterranean-style diet reduces metabolic syndrome components in obese children and adolescents with obesity. *BMC Pediatr.* **2014**, *14*, 175. [CrossRef] [PubMed]

57. Romaguera, D.; Norat, T.; Vergnaud, A.C.; Mouw, T.; May, A.M.; Agudo, A.; Buckland, G.; Slimani, N.; Rinaldi, S.; Couto, E.; et al. Mediterranean dietary patterns and prospective weight change in participants of the epic-panacea project. *Am. J. Clin. Nutr.* **2010**, *92*, 912–921. [CrossRef] [PubMed]

58. Buckland, G.; Bach, A.; Serra-Majem, L. Obesity and the mediterranean diet: A systematic review of observational and intervention studies. *Obes. Rev.* **2008**, *9*, 582–593. [CrossRef] [PubMed]

59. Shai, I.; Schwarzfuchs, D.; Henkin, Y.; Shahar, D.R.; Witkow, S.; Greenberg, I.; Golan, R.; Fraser, D.; Bolotin, A.; Vardi, H.; et al. Weight loss with a low-carbohydrate, mediterranean, or low-fat diet. *N. Engl. J. Med.* **2008**, *359*, 229–241. [CrossRef] [PubMed]

60. Bonaccio, M.; Di Castelnuovo, A.; Costanzo, S.; De Lucia, F.; Olivieri, M.; Donati, M.B.; de Gaetano, G.; Iacoviello, L.; Bonanni, A. Nutrition knowledge is associated with higher adherence to mediterranean diet and lower prevalence of obesity. Results from the moli-sani study. *Appetite* **2013**, *68*, 139–146. [CrossRef] [PubMed]

61. Michels, K.B.; Schulze, M.B. Can dietary patterns help us detect diet-disease associations? *Nutr. Res. Rev.* **2005**, *18*, 241–248. [CrossRef] [PubMed]

62. McNaughton, S.A.; Ball, K.; Mishra, G.D.; Crawford, D.A. Dietary patterns of adolescents and risk of obesity and hypertension. *J. Nutr.* **2008**, *138*, 364–370. [CrossRef] [PubMed]

63. Northstone, K.; Emmett, P.M. Are dietary patterns stable throughout early and mid-childhood? A birth cohort study. *Br. J. Nutr.* **2008**, *100*, 1069–1076. [CrossRef] [PubMed]

64. Craig, L.C.; McNeill, G.; Macdiarmid, J.I.; Masson, L.F.; Holmes, B.A. Dietary patterns of school-age children in scotland: Association with socio-economic indicators, physical activity and obesity. *Br. J. Nutr.* **2010**, *103*, 319–334. [CrossRef] [PubMed]

65. Richter, A.; Heidemann, C.; Schulze, M.B.; Roosen, J.; Thiele, S.; Mensink, G.B. Dietary patterns of adolescents in Germany—associations with nutrient intake and other health related lifestyle characteristics. *BMC Pediatr.* **2012**, *12*, 35. [CrossRef] [PubMed]

66. Weikert, C.; Schulze, M.B. Evaluating dietary patterns: The role of reduced rank regression. *Curr. Opin. Clin. Nutr. Metab. Care* **2016**, *19*, 341–346. [CrossRef] [PubMed]

67. Simpson, S.J.; Raubenheimer, D. Perspective: Tricks of the trade. *Nature* **2014**, *508*, S66. [CrossRef] [PubMed]

68. Gosby, A.K.; Conigrave, A.D.; Raubenheimer, D.; Simpson, S.J. Protein leverage and energy intake. *Obes. Rev.* **2014**, *15*, 183–191. [CrossRef] [PubMed]

69. Solon-Biet, S.M.; McMahon, A.C.; Ballard, J.W.; Ruohonen, K.; Wu, L.E.; Cogger, V.C.; Warren, A.; Huang, X.; Pichaud, N.; Melvin, R.G.; et al. The ratio of macronutrients, not caloric intake, dictates cardiometabolic health, aging, and longevity in ad libitum-fed mice. *Cell Metab.* **2014**, *19*, 418–430. [CrossRef] [PubMed]

70. Berryman, C.E.; Agarwal, S.; Lieberman, H.R.; Fulgoni, V.L., 3rd; Pasiakos, S.M. Diets higher in animal and plant protein are associated with lower adiposity and do not impair kidney function in us adults. *Am. J. Clin. Nutr.* **2016**, *104*, 743–749. [CrossRef] [PubMed]

71. Pasiakos, S.M.; Lieberman, H.R.; Fulgoni, V.L., 3rd. Higher-protein diets are associated with higher hdl cholesterol and lower bmi and waist circumference in us adults. *J. Nutr.* **2015**, *145*, 605–614. [CrossRef] [PubMed]

72. Jen, V.; Karagounis, L.G.; Jaddoe, V.W.V.; Franco, O.H.; Voortman, T. Dietary protein intake in school-age children and detailed measures of body composition: The generation r study. *Int. J. Obes. (Lond.)* **2018**. [CrossRef] [PubMed]

73. Buyken, A.E.; Bolzenius, K.; Karaolis-Danckert, N.; Gunther, A.L.; Kroke, A. Body composition trajectories into adolescence according to age at pubertal growth spurt. *Am. J. Hum. Biol.* **2011**, *23*, 216–224. [CrossRef] [PubMed]

74. Johannsen, M. *Übergewicht bei 5–7-jährigen Kindern. Analyse von Trends, Determinanten und gesundheitlichen Auswirkungen*; eine Untersuchung im Rahmen der Kieler Adipositas-Präventionsstudie (KOPS). Der Andere Verlag: Tönning, Lübeck, Marburg, Germany, 2009.

75. Gose, M.; Plachta-Danielzik, S.; Kehden, B.; Johannsen, M.; Landsberg, B.; Müller, M. Trends in incidence and determinants of overweight among 9–11-year-old children–kiel obesity prevention study (KOPS). *Obesity Facts* **2013**, *6*, 202.

76. Costello, A.B.; Osborne, J. Best practices in exploratory factor analysis: Four recommendations for getting the most from your analysis. *Pract. Assess. Res. Eval.* **2005**, *10*, 1–9.

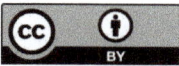

nutrients

Article

Use of vitamin and mineral supplements among adolescents living in Germany—Results from EsKiMo II

Hanna Perlitz *, Gert B.M. Mensink, Clarissa Lage Barbosa, Almut Richter, Anna-Kristin Brettschneider, Franziska Lehmann, Eleni Patelakis, Melanie Frank, Karoline Heide and Marjolein Haftenberger

Department of Epidemiology and Health Monitoring, Robert Koch Institute, 12101 Berlin, Germany; MensinkG@rki.de (G.B.M.M.); Lage-BarbosaC@rki.de (C.L.B.); RichterA@rki.de (A.R.); BrettschneiderA@rki.de (A.-K.B.); LehmannF@rki.de (F.L.); PatelakisE@rki.de (E.P.); Frank.Melanie@icloud.com (M.F.); Karoline.Heide@t-online.de (K.H.); HaftenbergerM@rki.de (M.H.)
* Correspondence: PerlitzH@rki.de; Tel.: +49-(030)-18754-2882

Received: 12 April 2019; Accepted: 24 May 2019; Published: 28 May 2019

Abstract: Dietary supplements may contribute to nutrient intake; however, actual data on dietary supplement use among adolescents living in Germany are rare. The aim of this analysis was to describe the current use of dietary supplements, its determinants, and reasons of use. Changes in supplement use over time were evaluated by comparing the results with those from EsKiMo I (2006). Data from the Eating Study as a KiGGS Module EsKiMo II (2015–2017) were used to analyze supplement intake according to sociodemographic, health characteristics, and physical exercise behavior of 12–17-year-olds (n = 1356). Supplement use during the past four weeks was assessed by a standardized computer assisted personal interview. Multivariable logistic regression was used to identify the association between supplement use and its determinants. Between 2015–2017, 16.4% (95%-CI: 13.0–19.7%) of the adolescents used dietary supplements, and its use decreased with lower levels of physical exercise and overweight. Most supplement users used only one supplement, often containing both vitamins and minerals. The most frequently supplemented nutrients were vitamin C and magnesium. The main reported reason to use supplements was 'to improve health'. Prevalence of supplement use was slightly lower in 2015-2017 than in 2006 (18.5%; 95%-CI: 15.8–21.2%). The results underline the importance of including nutrient intake through dietary supplements in nutrition surveys.

Keywords: vitamin; mineral; dietary supplements; adolescents; EsKiMo

1. Introduction

An optimal nutrient supply during the growth period of adolescence is important [1]. The majority of the population living in Germany has an adequate supply of almost all vitamins and minerals. Generally, with a balanced diet the requirements for essential nutrients will be met. However, for some nutrients, like in particular folate, iodine, and vitamin D, the nutrient status is suboptimal for large population groups in Germany. Accordingly, vitamin or mineral supplements are only recommended in Germany for medically diagnosed deficiencies or for vulnerable groups, such as infants, pregnant women, and the elderly. For adolescents, there are no recommendations for the preventive use of dietary supplements [2].

Nevertheless, sales for dietary supplements have increased in Germany and other western countries over the last decades [3,4]. The demand for supplements constituted a sale of 1.4 billion Euro in Germany in 2018 [4]. In light of the mostly adequate nutrient supply and the risks associated with an excessive intake of vitamins and nutrients, this trend should be observed critically [5].

Many studies described an increase in the use of dietary supplements, such as the National Health and Nutrition Examination Survey (NHANES) between 1971–2000 among adults [6]. The proportion of German adults who used dietary supplements during a period of seven days increased by six percent (12.3% to 18.1%) between 1997–1999 and 2008–2011 [7]. Up-to-date and representative information on supplement use among children and adolescents living in Germany is lacking. There are some studies on supplement use, but these are mainly regional and/or older studies and include different age groups. Among children and adolescents (2–18 years) who participated in the regional Dortmund Nutritional and Anthropometric Longitudinally Designed Study (DONALD) between 1986–2003, 7.5% reported the use of dietary supplements in a three-day-weighted dietary record [8]. 9.2% of children (9–12 years) from two German birth cohort studies (GINIplus and LISAplus) used dietary supplements (2005–2009) [9]. In the first representative German Eating Study as a KiGGS Module (EsKiMo) from 2006, one fifth of the adolescents (12–17 years) had used dietary supplements in the previous four weeks [10]. Current data about dietary supplement use and its determinants may help to estimate the risk of oversupply of micronutrients in specific groups. EsKiMo II, conducted from 2015 to 2017 by the Robert Koch Institute (RKI), provides recent data on the use of dietary supplements. The present analysis aims to quantify the use of vitamin and mineral supplements in association with some determinants, and to evaluate the reasons for dietary supplement use among adolescents living in Germany. A major advantage of the current analysis is the possibility to describe the change in the prevalence of dietary supplement use between 2006 and 2015–2017 by comparing results from EsKiMo I and EsKiMo II.

2. Methods

2.1. Study Design and Study Population

EsKiMo II was conducted from June 2015 until September 2017 as part of the second wave of the German Health Interview and Examination Survey for Children and Adolescents (KiGGS Wave 2). The aim of the cross-sectional EsKiMo II was to assess the dietary behavior of children and adolescents and to identify changes in food consumption in the last decade by comparison with the previous study EsKiMo I, conducted in 2006. The EsKiMo II study protocol was consented with the Federal Commissioners for Data Protection and approved by the Hannover Medical School ethics committee in June 2015 (Number 2275–2015). Written informed consent was obtained from all parents or legal guardians and participants aged 14 years and older prior to the study interviews and examinations. Details on the methodology of EsKiMo II can be found elsewhere [11–13].

Altogether, 2644 children and adolescents aged 6–17 years who took part in KiGGS Wave 2 participated in EsKiMo II (participation rate 59.4%). The current analysis is limited to 1356 adolescents aged 12–17 years, as supplement use for this age group was assessed in the same way as in EsKiMo I, which allows describing changes in supplement use between 2006 and 2015–2017. Data of 1272 adolescents who participated in EsKiMo I was included for trend analysis of vitamin and mineral supplement use over time.

2.2. Assessment of Supplement Use

Dietary supplement use was assessed using a standardized computer assisted interview within the Dietary Interview Software for Health Examination Studies DISHES [14] by trained nutritionists during home visits. The use of dietary supplements was ascertained by the following question: "Have you taken dietary supplements (like vitamins or minerals) in form of tablets, drops etc. in the last four weeks?" In case of a positive response, types (name and brand), frequencies of use, dosage form, and amounts of the supplement and reasons for using were asked. Dietary supplements were selected from a database, which was integrated in the software. This supplement database is an update from previous dietary surveys conducted in Germany by the RKI and the Max Rubner Institute. Supplements which were not included in the database were recorded as a free text with the name, brand, and dosage form.

If available, a photo of the supplement packaging was taken. Afterwards, nutrient composition of all recorded supplements was checked with the information from the package, from the internet and/or from the manufacturer, and, if necessary, updated or added in the database. Reasons for supplement use were asked by predefined categories ('to improve health', 'based on a doctor's recommendation', 'increase of physical and mental performance', 'read/heard about beneficial information', 'compensation of low fruit/vegetables consumption', 'based on a pharmacist's recommendation'), with the possibility of free texts for other reasons (more than one answer was possible).

The current analysis is limited to dietary supplements containing vitamins or minerals and considers both freely available and medically prescribed dietary supplements. Supplements containing neither vitamins nor minerals or containing vitamins or minerals in homeopathic doses were assigned to the category 'other dietary supplements' and excluded from this analysis. Protein and dietetic products were assigned to foods and not considered in this analysis. Vitamin and mineral supplements were categorized as: vitamins, minerals, and combined preparations containing both vitamin/s and mineral/s.

2.3. Assessment of Other Variables

EsKiMo II participants were visited about three to six months after participation in KiGGS Wave 2. Sociodemographic, lifestyle, and health characteristics were assessed within KiGGS Wave 2 by self-administered questionnaires completed by the parents and by the adolescents aged 11 years old and older themselves [15]. Socio-economic status (SES) was based on information about education level, occupational status, and net household income of the parents and categorized into low, medium, and high SES [16]. Attended school types were categorized as lower secondary school, upper secondary school, and other school types. Participants were defined as having a migration background, when they or at least one parent were not born in Germany or did not have the German nationality. Three categories for residence region were constructed according to federal states: north (Schleswig-Holstein, Hamburg, Lower Saxony, Bremen, Berlin, Brandenburg, Mecklenburg-Western Pomerania), middle (North Rhine-Westphalia, Hesse, Saxony, Saxony-Anhalt, Thuringia), and south (Rhineland-Palatinate, Baden-Wuerttemberg, Bavaria, Saarland). Community size was categorized as: <5000 inhabitants, 5000 to 20,000 inhabitants, 20,000 to under 100,000 inhabitants, and >100,000 inhabitants. During the personal interviews in EsKiMo II, questions about the body height and weight of the adolescents were asked. Based on this self-reported information, body mass index (BMI) (body weight in kg/body size in m^2) was calculated and assigned into age- and sex-specific BMI categories according to Kromeyer-Hauschild (underweight, normal weight, overweight) [17,18]. Furthermore, subjective health status was rated by adolescents of 11 years and older themselves in four categories, ranging from excellent to poor. Physical exercise as a specific and more intensive type of physical activity includes all kinds of sports, but without physical education at school. Questions about the usual duration (hours/minutes per week) of physical exercise were asked and replies were categorized into 'low' (less than one hour /week), 'medium' (1–3 h/week) and 'high' (more than 3 h/week).

2.4. Statistical Analysis

Prevalence of supplement use is presented according to sociodemographic and other characteristics. In addition, multivariate logistic regression was conducted to analyze the independent associations of these sociodemographic and other characteristics with supplement use. The associations were adjusted for all other variables. For supplement users, the type, number, and frequency as well as the reasons for vitamin or mineral supplement use are described. Finally, changes in the prevalence of dietary supplement use between 2006 and 2015–2017 are examined. All analyses were performed with SAS Version 9.4 (SAS Institute, Cary, NC, USA). The criterion for statistical significance was set at p-value< 0.05. A weighting factor was applied to correct for deviations from the population structure according to age (in years), sex, region (as of 31.12.2015), nationality (as of 31.12.2014), and education level of the parents (Mikrozensus 2013), as well as to consider differences in participation´s probability according to seasonality, SES of the family, and school type. In order to take the clustered design into account (with a stronger correlation of the participants within a community compared to a totally random group), the SAS survey procedures were applied. Data of 1267 adolescents from EsKiMo I are included for trend analysis. Study procedures and instruments of EsKiMo I are generally the same as for EsKiMo II and are described elsewhere [19]. Prior analyses of EsKiMo I were calculated using a weighting factor to correct for the disproportional higher number of participants from the Eastern part of Germany as well as deviations in age, sex, and nationality from the general population [10]. For the present analysis, these prevalence estimates were recalculated with a weighting factor constructed as described above and correcting deviations from the population structure of 2004. For comparison of prevalence estimates from EsKiMo I and EsKiMo II taking into account demographic changes over time, the EsKiMo I prevalence estimates were standardized to the sex- and age-structure of the population underlying the EsKiMo II data.

3. Results

In total, 16.4% of the adolescents (girls: 18.8%, boys: 14.0%) aged 12 to 17 years had used vitamin or mineral supplements in the previous four weeks (Table 1). The proportion of supplement use was similar across age groups, SES, type of school, migration background, region of residence, and community size (Table 1). Additionally, there was no association between self-assessed health status and dietary supplement use (data not shown).

The multivariable logistic regression showed that sex, weight status, and physical exercise were independent determinants of dietary supplement use. Boys use dietary supplements less frequently than girls (OR: 0.60 (0.38–0.94) and adolescents with overweight use dietary supplements less frequently compared to adolescents with normal weight (OR: 0.41 (0.21–0.79) (Table 1). The use of dietary supplements was lower for adolescents with low levels of physical exercise (OR: 0.56 (0.33–0.95) compared to those with a high level of physical exercise (Table 1).

Table 1. Associations between vitamin and/or mineral supplement use among adolescents (12–17 years) and determinants (sociodemographic characteristics, weight status, and physical exercise) in EsKiMo II (2015–2017), *n* = 1356.

Vitamin and/or Mineral Supplement Use	Prevalence [1]	Multivariate Logistic Regression Analysis [1]
	n = 1356	*n* = 1223
	% (95% CI)	adjusted OR (95% CI) [2]
Total	16.4 (13.0–19.7)	-
Sex		
Girls	18.8 (14.5–23.2)	Ref.
Boys	14.0 (9.9–18.1)	0.60 (0.38–0.94) *
Age group		
12–13 years	14.4 (10.3–18.4)	0.76 (0.46–1.26)
14–15 years	19.4 (13.2–25.5)	1.30 (0.77–2.20)
16–17 years	15.2 (10.4–20.0)	Ref.
Socio-economic status (SES) [3]		
Low	12.3 (5.4–19.2)	0.63 (0.26–1.53)
Medium	15.3 (11.7–19.0)	0.66 (0.42–1.05)
High	22.3 (16.2–28.3)	Ref
Type of school [4]		
Lower secondary school	14.5 (10.9–18.1)	0.84 (0.53–1.32)
Upper secondary school	19.2 (14.4–24.0)	Ref.
Other school types	13.4 (4.8–22.0)	1.02 (0.40–2.59)
Migration background [5]		
Yes	15.4 (6.9–23.9)	0.89 (0.48–1.67)
No	16.5 (13.2–19.9)	Ref.

Table 1. *Cont.*

Vitamin and/or Mineral Supplement Use	Prevalence [1]	Multivariate Logistic Regression Analysis [1]
Region of residence		
North	13.8 (8.5–19.0)	0.74 (0.40–1.39)
Middle	16.7 (11.7–21.6)	1.11 (0.62–1.96)
South	17.7 (11.2–24.3)	Ref.
Community size		
<5000 inhabitants	15.0 (8.5–21.5)	Ref.
5000–<20,000 inhabitants	19.9 (11.6–28.2)	1.04 (0.52–2.09)
20000–<100,000 inhabitants	16.9 (10.9–22.9)	0.83 (0.39–1.74)
≥100,000 inhabitants	13.4 (8.2–18.6)	0.76 (0.36–1.63)
Weight status		
Underweight	20.7 (11.2–30.1)	1.33 (0.73–2.41)
Normal weight	17.0 (13.1–21.0)	Ref
Overweight	9.3 (3.9–14.7)	0.41 (0.21–0.79) *
Physical Exercise		
<1 h/week	11.5 (7.2–15.9)	0.56 (0.33–0.95) *
1–3 h/week	14.8 (10.9–18.8)	0.73 (0.47–1.12)
>3 h/week	19.9 (15.0–24.9)	Ref.

[1] weighted for the German population of 2015; [2] adjusted for all other variables; [3] Socio-economic status: *n* (missing) = 19; [4] Type of school *n* (missing) = 62, including participants who already finished school; [5] migration background *n* (missing) = 9; *n* = number of subjects; OR = odds ratio; CI = confidence interval; * OR is statistical significantly different from the reference with *p*-value < 0.05.

Among the dietary supplement users, 36.9% utilize vitamin supplements, 40.8% mineral supplements, and 46.4% a combination of both vitamins and minerals (Table 2), with no differences regarding sex (data not shown). During the previous four weeks, the majority of the users had consumed only one kind of dietary supplement (72.7%), and about a quarter (27.3%) had consumed more than one (Table 2). Around 28% of the vitamin and mineral supplements were used daily (6–7 times a week) (data not shown). The most commonly used vitamin supplements contained vitamin C (43.9%), followed by vitamin D (41.1%) and vitamin B12 (30.4%). The reported mineral supplements most often contained magnesium (45.9%), zinc (28.1%), and iron (24.1%; Table 2).

Table 2. Frequency [1] of the number and type of dietary supplements used among adolescents (12–17 years) in EsKiMo II (2015–2017), *n* = 1356.

	Total	Supplement User
	n = 1356	*n* = 234
	% (95% CI)	% (95% CI)
Type of supplement [2]		
Vitamin/s	6.0 (4.3–7.7)	36.9 (29.4–44.5)
Mineral/s	6.7 (4.5–8.8)	40.8 (31.9–49.8)
Combination of vitamin/s and mineral/s	7.6 (5.5–9.7)	46.4 (38.8–54.1)
Number of supplements		
1 supplement	11.9 (9.3–14.4)	72.7 (64.8–80.6)
>1 supplement	4.5 (2.8–6.2)	27.3 (19.4–35.2)
Vitamins [1]		
Vitamin A	1.2 (0.6–1.9)	7.5 (3.7–11.9)
Thiamin	4.2 (2.7–5.7)	25.6 (17.3–34.0)
Riboflavin	4.0 (2.5–5.5)	24.2 (16.0–32.4)
Niacin	3.6 (2.1–5.1)	22.3 (14.3–30.3)
Pantothenic acid	3.3 (2.0–4.6)	20.5 (13.7–27.7)
Vitamin B6	4.2 (2.8–5.5)	25.7 (18.1–33.3)
Biotin	3.6 (2.3–5.0)	22.2 (15.7–28.6)
Folate	4.1 (2.6–5.6)	25.2 (17.6–32.8)
Vitamin B12	5.0 (3.3–6.7)	30.4 (22.1–38.7)

Nutrients **2019**, 11, 1208

Table 2. *Cont.*

	Total	Supplement User
Vitamin C	7.2 (5.4–9.0)	43.9 (35.8–52.1)
Vitamin D	6.7 (4.6–8.8)	41.1 (32.6–49.5)
Vitamin E	3.6 (2.3–5.0)	22.3 (15.1–29.6)
Vitamin K	0.9 (0.3–1.6)	5.7 (2.3–9.2)
Minerals [1]		
Calcium	3.2 (1.6–4.9)	19.8 (11.9–27.7)
Copper	1.5 (0.5–2.5)	8.9 (3.1–14.6)
Fluoride	0.4 (0.0–0.9)	2.3 (0.0–5.4)
Iron	3.9 (2.2–5.7)	24.1 (15.1–33.0)
Iodine	1.4 (0.4–2.4)	8.5 (2.7–14.4)
Potassium	0.3 (0.1–0.5)	1.9 (0.5–3.4)
Magnesium	7.5 (5.1–9.9)	45.9 (36.9–54.9)
Manganese	1.3 (0.4–2.2)	17.5 (2.6–13.0)
Molybdenum	1.3 (0.4–2.3)	8.2 (2.6–14.0)
Sodium	0.1 (0.0–0.2)	0.7 (0.0–1.5)
Phosphorus	0.4 (0.0–0.9)	2.7 (0.2–5.2)
Selenium	1.9 (0.8–2.9)	11.5 (5.6–17.4)
Zinc	4.6 (2.9–6.3)	28.1 (19.1–36.4)

[1] weighted for the German population of 2015; [2] due to multiple supplement use and multiple active components the sum of the prevalences by type of supplements or active components may deviate from the prevalence of total supplement use as displayed in Table 1; CI = confidence interval.

The most common reason for using vitamin and mineral supplements during the last four weeks was 'to improve health' (59.3%). One fifth of the participants (20.7%) reported to use supplements 'based on a doctor's recommendation', followed by 17.7% of the adolescents who reported an 'increase of physical and mental performance' as motivation. Further, less frequently reported reasons for using supplements were 'read/heard about beneficial information' (7.2%), 'compensation for low fruit/vegetables consumption' (7.2%), 'based on a pharmacist's recommendation' (3.6%). Among other reasons assessed as free text, the most often answer was 'based on KiGGS examination results' (2%) (Figure 1).

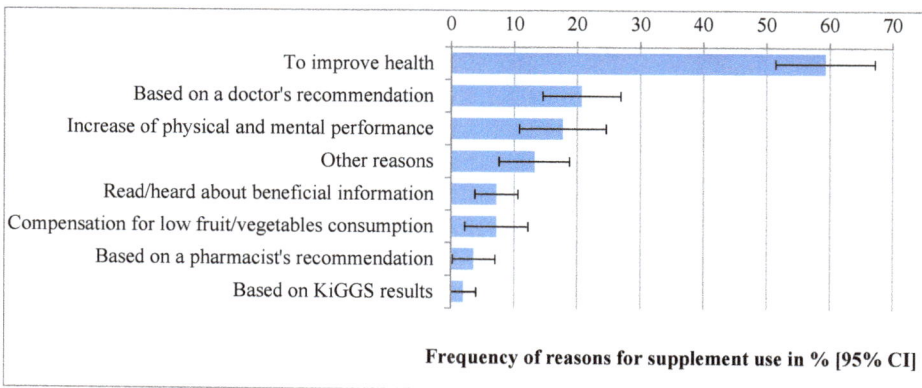

Figure 1. Prevalence and 95%-confidence intervals (CI) of reasons for dietary supplement use among adolescents (12–17 years) in EsKiMo II (2015–2017), *n* = 228 (weighted for the German population of 2015).

209

The prevalence of dietary supplement use in the previous four weeks decreased slightly, but not statistically significantly, from 18.5% to 16.4% between Eskimo I (2006) and Eskimo II (2015–2017) (Table 3).

Table 3. Trend analysis of dietary supplement use among adolescents (12–17 years) between EsKiMo I (2006) and EsKiMo II (2015–2017).

	EsKiMo I	EsKiMo I	EsKiMo II
	n = 1267 % (95% CI) Weighted for 2004	n = 1267 % (95% CI) Weighted for 2015	n = 1356 % (95% CI) Weigthed for 2015
Total	18.5 (15.8–21.2)	18.5 (15.8–21.2)	16.4 (13.0–19.7)
Girls	19.3 (15.3–23.4)	19.4 (15.3–23.5)	18.8 (14.5–23.2)
Boys	17.7 (14.3–21.1)	17.7 (14.3–21.1)	14.0 (9.9–18.1)
Type of supplement [1]			
Vitamin/s	6.2 (4.7–7.8)	6.2 (4.7–7.8)	6.0 (4.3–7.7)
Mineral/s	9.9 (7.6–12.2)	9.9 (7.6–12.3)	6.7 (4.5–8.8)
Combination of vitamin/s and mineral/s	6.1 (4.4–7.8)	6.1 (4.4–7.8)	7.6 (5.5–9.7)
Number of supplements			
1 supplement	13.6 (11.1–16.1)	13.7 (11.2–16.2)	11.9 (9.3–14.4)
>1 supplement	4.9 (3.2–6.5)	4.9 (3.2–6.5)	4.5 (2.8–6.2)

[1] due to multiple dietary supplement use and multiple active components, the sum of the prevalences by type of dietary supplements or active components may deviate from the prevalence of total dietary supplement use; CI = confidence interval.

4. Discussion

To our knowledge, no nationwide overview of recent dietary supplement use among adolescents has been presented for Germany since EsKiMo I in 2006. Our analysis show that 16.4% of the adolescents aged 12 to 17 years had used vitamin or mineral supplements in the last four weeks.

In EsKiMo II, supplement use is associated with sex, weight status, and physical exercise. Dietary supplement use was similar across age groups, SES, type of school, migration background, region of residence, community size, and subjective health status.

Comparison of our study results with other studies is difficult due to differences in methods of data collection, definitions of dietary supplements, timeframes, and age groups. In most western countries, the use of dietary supplements among children and adolescents is higher than in Germany [20–23], which is also confirmed for adults [24]. A third of the participants aged 9–18 years of the American dietary survey NHANES (2011–2014) reported dietary supplement use during the last month [20]. In an Australian study (2014–2015), 20.1% of the adolescents (10–17 years old) had used dietary supplements during the past two weeks [21].

Previous studies including children and adolescents showed inconsistent findings considering sex differences in dietary supplement use. Many studies observed no significant differences in dietary supplement use by sex [21,22,25]. Parents probably determine the supplement use for their children, which may largely explain the absence of sex differences. The German DONALD study showed a higher prevalence of dietary supplement use among boys [26]. A Polish study observed that supplement use was more common among girls [23]. Other studies observed higher supplement use among children and adolescents with underweight, which is similar to our observations [25,27,28]. Previous findings regarding the effect of physical exercise on dietary supplement use are heterogeneous and only partly comparable due to differences in data assessment and definition of physical exercise. In EsKiMo II, adolescents who reported less than one hour of physical exercise per week used less frequently dietary supplements. This finding is consistent with the results from EsKiMo I and NHANES, although different definitions for physical exercise were applied [10,27].

Previous studies were also inconsistent with regard to the effect of age on dietary supplement use. NHANES and a Korean study found a higher prevalence of dietary supplement use for younger age groups [20,22]. However, unlike our study, these studies also included children under the age of 12 years.

Other studies observed a higher prevalence of supplement use for older age groups (15–18 years; 16–18 years) [8,23]. In EsKiMo II, dietary supplement use is similar regarding SES. Previous studies consistently showed that a higher prevalence of dietary supplement use was associated with higher SES, higher education of the parents or higher household income [21,22,25,26,29]. For EsKiMo I, supplement use significantly differed by school type [10], whereas such differences were not significant for EsKiMo II, but the categories are not exactly the same. EsKiMo II did not observe differences in supplement use by migration status. The definition of migration status is very different between studies and countries, making it difficult to compare results. Although a Polish study with a small sample size observed a higher supplement use among adolescents living in bigger cities [23], dietary supplement use among adolescents was similar through different community sizes in EsKiMo II. This is similar to the results of the German Health Interview and Examination Survey (DEGS1; 2008–2011), which also observed no statistically significant differences in supplement use according to the community size and region of residence among German adults [7].

In EsKiMo II, the most frequently dietary supplements used were a combination of vitamins and minerals. Vitamin C and magnesium were the most supplemented micronutrients, similarly to results of an Australian study [21]. Other studies showed related results: in NHANES and DONALD, the most frequently dietary supplement used was also vitamin C, but the most frequent mineral supplemented was calcium and not magnesium [26,30]. A German consumer survey with adults observed similar results to EsKiMo II, with even higher prevalences for vitamin C (53%) and magnesium (59%) [31]. Vitamin C and magnesium are also the most commonly supplemented micronutrients by adults [24,31–33]. However, there are no recommendations and no need for adolescents to supplement vitamin C and magnesium [2,34].

Reasons for dietary supplements use can be diverse. Within EsKiMo II, the most commonly reported reason for vitamin or mineral supplements use was 'to improve health' (59.3%), which was also identified as the most frequent motive in previous studies (CRN Consumer survey: 58%; NHANES 2011–2014: 38.0%) [30,35]. The German NEMONIT study, for example, indicated 'prevention of nutrient deficiencies (or covering increased nutrient requirements)' (62.4%) and 'achievement or improvement of general well-being' (34.7%) as the most common motives for dietary supplement use among German adults [36]. For the participants of EsKiMo II, the recommendations of a physician were reported as the second most important reason for dietary supplements use, but this only applies to one in five adolescents (20.7%). 2% of the supplement users indicated using dietary supplements as a consequence of the personal evaluation they received after taking part on KiGGS Wave 2, from which the EsKiMo II study sample was drawn.

The prevalence of dietary supplement intake decreased slightly, but not significantly, between EsKiMo I (2006) and EsKiMo II (2015–2017). Data from the longitudinal DONALD-study among children and adolescents aged 2–18 in Germany were used to describe a time trend in dietary supplement use from 1986–2003. Supplement use peaked between 1994 and 1996 [26]. One study among adolescents in the US showed similar prevalences between 2003–2004 and 2013–2014 [37]. While former studies for adults reported an increase in dietary supplement intake [6,38], more recent results showed a stagnation in its intake and a declining trend for some particular dietary supplements [39,40]. The observed stagnation may seem surprising, considering the many lifestyle changes detected in the last decades. However, in Germany, the supply of most vitamins and minerals through natural sources meets the recommended level and this situation has not changed substantially during the last ten years.

Currently, there are no recommendations for the use of vitamin and mineral supplements among adolescents in Germany. The German Nutrition Society recommends a balanced diet to meet the requirements for essential nutrients. The use of dietary supplements is only recommended for individuals with certain medically diagnosed diseases [1]. Nevertheless, a deficit for some vitamins, such as vitamin D, folic acid, and iodine has been reported among adolescents [41]. In addition, there is a certain risk of overconsumption, in particular when more than one dose of supplements or several different supplements containing the same nutrients are consumed every day in combination with fortified foods. For the latter, the consumer is often unaware of the specific fortifications. The growing market for both product groups, including a less controllable sale and distribution over the internet, may increase the risk of side effects. Therefore, in Germany, the Federal Institute for Risk Assessment defined a recommendation for maximum levels of the amount of vitamins and minerals contained in dietary supplements [5]. Furthermore, within the observed time period, results of large randomized controlled trials could not confirm the expected additional benefits of a regular supplement intake, e.g. for vitamin D. This may have counteracted marketing and promoting activities, therefore slowing down further increases in supplement intake.

Among the strengths of our study are the representative study population and the assessment through standardized personal interviews, which took place mainly at the participant's home. Data collection of vitamin and mineral supplements was carried out using a comprehensive supplement database. For more detailed information, pictures of the dietary supplement packages were taken. The nutrient composition of all dietary supplements reported was checked. The cross-sectional design of the study can represent a limitation for certain research questions, since no direct causalities can be derived from the observed correlations. In addition, selection bias is possible due to the previous participation of the adolescents in KiGGS Wave 2. To minimize the effect of selective participation, population weights were applied to correct deviations from the German population. A further limitation could be the use of self-reported body height and weight to estimate weight status. Self-reported body weight and height of a subgroup of participants who had also taken part in physical examinations of KiGGS Wave 2 were individually compared with the measured data from KiGGS Wave 2. This comparison showed only small differences and a high correlation between the measured and self-reported data.

5. Conclusions

Almost one fifth of adolescents reported to use dietary supplements within the last four weeks; most of them took one dietary supplement. Vitamin C and magnesium were the most commonly supplemented nutrients, although predominantly no nutrient deficiency exists for these nutrients. Nevertheless, critical nutrients, such as vitamin B12 and vitamin D, were also taken frequently [34,41]. Boys, adolescents with lower physical exercise levels and with overweight were less likely to use dietary supplements. The considerable use of dietary supplements among adolescents underlines the importance of considering dietary supplements intake into account for assessing nutrient intake in nutrition surveys. Furthermore, possible oversupply should be monitored and information on the risk and benefits of specific dietary supplements should be provided to the population.

Author Contributions: G.B.M.M. conceptualized and managed the EsKiMo studies. A.R. had major contributions to the design of the studies and the conduct of EsKiMo I. H.P. and M.H. performed analyses, drafted the initial manuscript, and interpreted the data. A.-K.B., M.F., K.H., C.L.B., F.L., E.P., A.R. and G.B.M.M. reviewed and revised the manuscript. All authors were involved in the conduction and data aggregation and read and approved the final manuscript.

Funding: This work was financially supported by the German Federal Ministry of Food and Agriculture (BMEL) through the Federal Office for Agriculture and Food (BLE), grant number 2814HS004.

Acknowledgments: We would like to thank all study participants and their families, and our colleagues from the Robert Koch Institute who supported the conduction of EsKiMo II. We are especially grateful to Janet Frotscher for her support on the verification of the supplement composition data.

Conflicts of Interest: There were no conflicts of interest.

References

1. Deutsche Gesellschaft für Ernährung; Österreichische Gesellschaft für Ernährung; Schweizerische Gesellschaft für Ernährungsforschung. *Referenzwerte für die Nährstoffzufuhr*; Deutsche Gesellschaft für Ernährung (DGE), Österreichische Gesellschaft für Ernährung (ÖGE), Schweizerische Gesellschaft für Ernährung (SGE): Bonn, Germany, 2015; Volume 2.

2. Bechthold, A.; Albrecht, V.; Leschik-Bonnet, E.; Heseker, H. Beurteilung der Vitaminversorgung in Deutschland. Teil 1: Daten zur Vitaminzufuhr. *Ernährungs Umschau* **2012**, *6*, 324–336.

3. Statista, Retail Sales of Vitamins & Nutritional Supplements in the United States from 2000 to 2017 (in billion U.S. dollars). 2017. Available online: http://www.statista.com/statistics/235801/retail-sales-of-vitamins-and-nutritional-supplements-in-the-us/ (accessed on 16 November 2017).

4. Bund für Lebensmittelrecht und Lebensmittelkunde e. V. (BLL) Markt für Nahrungsergänzungsmittel in Deutschland 2018. Available online: https://www.bll.de/de/verband/organisation/arbeitskreise/arbeitskreis-nahrungsergaenzungsmittel-ak-nem/20181029-zahlen-nahrungsergaenzungsmittel-markt-2018 (accessed on 4 May 2019).

5. Weißenborn, A.; Bakhiya, N.; DeMuth, I.; Ehlers, A.; Ewald, M.; Niemann, B.; Richter, K.; Trefflich, I.; Ziegenhagen, R.; Hirsch-Ernst, K.I.; et al. Höchstmengen für Vitamine und Mineralstoffe in Nahrungsergänzungsmitteln. *J. Consum. Prot. Food Saf.* **2018**, *13*, 25–39. [CrossRef]

6. Briefel, R.R.; Johnson, C.L. Secular trends in dietary intake in the United States. *Annu. Nutr.* **2004**, *24*, 401–431. [CrossRef] [PubMed]

7. Knopf, H. Selbstmedikation mit Vitaminen, Mineralstoffen und Nahrungsergänzungsmitteln in Deutschland. *Bundesgesundheitsblatt Gesundheitsforschung Gesundheitsschutz* **2017**, *60*, 268–276. [CrossRef]

8. Sichert-Hellert, W.; Wenz, G.; Kersting, M. Vitamin Intakes from Supplements and Fortified Food in German Children and Adolescents: Results from the DONALD Study. *J. Nutr.* **2006**, *136*, 1329–1333. [CrossRef]

9. Sausenthaler, S.; Standl, M.; Buyken, A.; Rzehak, P.; Koletzko, S.; Bauer, C.P.; Schaaf, B.; Von Berg, A.; Berdel, D.; Borte, M.; et al. Regional and socio-economic differences in food, nutrient and supplement intake in school-age children in Germany: results from the GINIplus and the LISAplus studies. *Public Health Nutr.* **2011**, *14*, 1724–1735. [CrossRef]

10. Six, J.; Richter, A.; Rabenberg, M.; Hintzpeter, B.; Vohmann, C.; Ståhl, A.; Heseker, H.; Mensink, G.B.M. Supplementenkonsum bei Jugendlichen in Deutschland. *Bundesgesundheitsblatt Gesundheitsforschung Gesundheitsschutz* **2008**, *51*, 1202–1209. [CrossRef]

11. Lage Barbosa, C.; Brettschneider, A.-K.; Haftenberger, M.; Lehmann, F.; Frank, M.; Heide, K.; Patelakis, E.; Perlitz, H.; Krause, L.; Houben, R.; et al. Comprehensive assessment of food and nutrient intake of children and adolescents in Germany: EsKiMo II—The eating study as a KiGGS module. *BMC Nutr.* **2017**, *3*, 75. [CrossRef]

12. Mensink, G.B.M.; Haftenberger, M.; Brettschneider, A.-K.; Barbosa, C.L.; Perlitz, H.; Patelakis, E.; Heide, K.; Frank, M.; Lehmann, F.; Krause, L.; et al. EsKiMo II—The Eating study as a KiGGS Module in KiGGS Wave 2. *J. Health Monitoring* **2017**, *2*, 38–46.

13. Brettschneider, A.-K.; Barbosa, C.L.; Haftenberger, M.; Heide, K.; Frank, M.; Patelakis, E.; Perlitz, H.; Lehmann, F.; Richter, A.; Mensink, G.B.M. The nutrition survey EsKiMo II—Design, execution and public health policy relevance. *Ernährungs Umschau* **2018**, *65*, 80–88.

14. Mensink, G.B.M.; Haftenberger, M.; Thamm, M. Validity of DISHES 98, a computerised dietary history interview: energy and macronutrient intake. *Eur. J. Clin. Nutr.* **2001**, *55*, 409–417. [CrossRef]

15. Mauz, E.; Gößwald, A.; Kamtsiuris, P.; Hoffmann, R.; Lange, M.; von Schenck, U.; Allen, J.; Butschalowsky, H.; Frank, L.; Hölling, H.; et al. New data for action. Data collection for KiGGS Wave 2 has been completed. *J. Health Monitoring* **2017**, *2*, 2–27.

16. Lampert, T.; Hoebel, J.; Kuntz, B.; Müters, S.; Kroll, L.E. Socioeconomic status and subjective social status measurement in KiGGS Wave 2. *J. Health Monitoring* **2018**, *3*, 108–125.

17. Kromeyer-Hauschild, K.; Wabitsch, M.; Kunze, D.; Geller, F.; Geiß, H.C.; Hesse, V.; Von Hippel, A.; Jaeger, U.; Johnsen, D.; Korte, W.; et al. Perzentile für den Body-mass-Index für das Kindes- und Jugendalter unter Heranziehung verschiedener deutscher Stichproben. *Monatsschrift Kinderheilkd* **2001**, *149*, 807–818. [CrossRef]

18. Kromeyer-Hauschild, K.; Moss, A.; Wabitsch, M. Body Mass index reference values for German children, adolescents and adults. Modification of the AGA BMI reference in the age range between 15 and 18 years. *Adipositas* **2015**, *9*, 123–127.

19. Mensink, G.B.M.; Bauch, A.; Vohmann, C.; Stahl, A.; Six, J.; Kohler, S.; Fischer, J.; Heseker, H. EsKiMo—Das Ernährungsmodul im Kinder- und Jugendgesundheitssurvey (KiGGS). *Bundesgesundheitsblatt Gesundheitsforschung Gesundheitsschutz* **2007**, *50*, 902–908. [CrossRef] [PubMed]

20. Jun, S.; Cowan, A.E.; Tooze, J.A.; Gahche, J.J.; Dwyer, J.T.; Eicher-Miller, H.A.; Bhadra, A.; Guenther, P.M.; Potischman, N.; Dodd, K.W.; et al. Dietary Supplement Use among U.S. Children by Family Income, Food Security Level, and Nutrition Assistance Program Participation Status in 2011(-)2014. *Nutrients* **2018**, *10*, 1212. [CrossRef]

21. O'Brien, S.K.; Malacova, E.; Sherriff, J.L.; Black, L.J. The Prevalence and Predictors of Dietary Supplement Use in the Australian Population. *Nutrients* **2017**, *9*, 1154. [CrossRef]

22. Kang, M.; Kim, D.W.; Lee, H.; Lee, Y.J.; Jung, H.J.; Paik, H.Y.; Song, Y.J. The nutrition contribution of dietary supplements on total nutrient intake in children and adolescents. *Eur. J. Clin. Nutr.* **2016**, *70*, 257–261. [CrossRef]

23. Gajda, K.; Zielinska, M.; Ciecierska, A.; Hamulka, J. Determinants of the use of dietary supplements among secondary and high school students. *Rocz. Panstw. Zakl. Hig.* **2016**, *67*, 383–390.

24. Skeie, G.; Braaten, T.; Hjartaker, A.; Lentjes, M.; Amiano, P.; Jakszyn, P.; Pala, V.; Palanca, A.; Niekerk, E.M.; Verhagen, H.; et al. Use of dietary supplements in the European Prospective Investigation into Cancer and Nutrition calibration study. *Eur. J. Clin. Nutr.* **2009**, *63*, S226–S238. [CrossRef]

25. Bailey, R.L.; Gahche, J.J.; Thomas, P.R.; Dwyer, J.T. Why US children use dietary supplements. *Pediatr. Res.* **2013**, *74*, 737–741. [CrossRef] [PubMed]

26. Sichert-Hellert, W.; Kersting, M. Vitamin and Mineral Supplements Use in German Children and Adolescents between 1986 and 2003: Results of the DONALD Study. *Ann. Nutr. Metab.* **2004**, *48*, 414–419. [CrossRef]

27. Shaikh, U.; Byrd, R.S.; Auinger, P. Vitamin and mineral supplement use by children and adolescents in the 1999–2004 National Health and Nutrition Examination Survey: relationship with nutrition, food security, physical activity, and health care access. *Arch. Pediatr. Adolesc. Med.* **2009**, *163*, 150–157. [CrossRef] [PubMed]

28. Picciano, M.; Dwyer, J.T.; Radimer, K.L.; Wilson, D.H.; Fisher, K.D.; Thomas, P.R.; Yetley, E.A.; Moshfegh, A.J.; Levy, P.S.; Nielsen, S.J.; et al. Dietary supplement use among infants, children, and adolescents in the united states, 1999–2002. *Arch. Pediatr. Adolesc. Med.* **2007**, *161*, 978–985. [CrossRef]

29. Dwyer, J.; Nahin, R.L.; Rogers, G.T.; Barnes, P.M.; Jacques, P.M.; Sempos, C.T.; Bailey, R. Prevalence and predictors of children's dietary supplement use: The 2007 National Health Interview Survey. *Am. J. Clin. Nutr.* **2013**, *97*, 1331–1337. [CrossRef] [PubMed]

30. Bailey, R.L.; Gahche, J.J.; Miller, P.E.; Thomas, P.R.; Dwyer, J.T. Why US Adults Use Dietary Supplements. *JAMA Intern. Med.* **2013**, *173*, 355. [CrossRef]

31. Heinemann, M.; Willers, J.; Bitterlich, N.; Hahn, A. Verwendung von Nahrungsergänzungsmitteln mit Vitaminen und Mineralstoffen—Ergebnisse einer deutschlandweiten Verbraucherbefragung. *J. Verbraucherschutz Lebensmittelsicherheit* **2015**, *10*, 131–142. [CrossRef]

32. Pouchieu, C.; Andreeva, V.A.; Péneau, S.; Kesse-Guyot, E.; Lassale, C.; Hercberg, S.; Touvier, M. Sociodemographic, lifestyle and dietary correlates of dietary supplement use in a large sample of French adults: results from the NutriNet-Santé cohort study. *Br. J. Nutr.* **2013**, *110*, 1480–1491. [CrossRef] [PubMed]

33. Bailey, R.L.; Gahche, J.J.; Lentino, C.V.; Dwyer, J.T.; Engel, J.S.; Thomas, P.R.; Betz, J.M.; Sempos, C.T.; Picciano, M.F. Dietary supplement use in the United States, 2003–2006. *J. Nutr.* **2011**, *141*, 261–266. [CrossRef]

34. Lage Barbosa, C.; Brettschneider, A.K.; Haftenberger, M.; Lehmann, F.; Frank, M.; Perlitz, H.; Heide, K.; Patelakis, E.; Mensink, G.B.M. Aktueller Überblick der Ernährungssituation von Kindern und Jugendlichen in Deutschland: Ergebnisse aus EsKiMo II. Available online: https://www.dge.de/fileadmin/public/doc/wk/2019/DGE-Proc-Germ-Nutr-Soc-Vol-25-2019.pdf (accessed on 5 April 2019).

35. Dickinson, A.; Blatman, J.; El-Dash, N.; Franco, J.C. Consumer Usage and Reasons for Using Dietary Supplements: Report of a Series of Surveys. *J. Am. Nutr.* **2014**, *33*, 176–182. [CrossRef] [PubMed]

36. Frey, A.; Hoffmann, I.; Heuer, T. Characterisation of vitamin and mineral supplement users differentiated according to their motives for using supplements: results of the German National Nutrition Monitoring (NEMONIT). *Public Heal. Nutr.* **2017**, *20*, 2173–2182. [CrossRef]

37. Qato, D.M.; Alexander, G.C.; Guadamuz, J.S.; Lindau, S.T. Prevalence of Dietary Supplement Use in US Children and Adolescents, 2003–2014. *JAMA Pediatr.* **2018**, *172*, 780. [CrossRef]

38. Kim, H.J.; Giovannucci, E.; Rosner, B.; Willett, W.C.; Cho, E. Longitudinal and secular trends in dietary supplement use: Nurses' Health Study and Health Professionals Follow-Up Study, 1986–2006. *J. Acad. Nutr. Diet.* **2014**, *114*, 436–443. [CrossRef]

39. Kantor, E.D.; Rehm, C.D.; Du, M.; White, E.; Giovannucci, E.L. Trends in Dietary Supplement Use among US Adults From 1999–2012. *JAMA* **2016**, *316*, 1464–1474. [CrossRef]

Nutrients **2019**, *11*, 1208

40. Marques-Vidal, P.; Vollenweider, P.; Waeber, G. Trends in vitamin, mineral and dietary supplement use in Switzerland. The CoLaus study. *Eur. J. Clin. Nutr.* **2017**, *71*, 122–127. [CrossRef] [PubMed]
41. Mensink, G.B.M.; Heseker, H.; Stahl, A.; Richter, A.; Vohmann, C. Die aktuelle Nährstoffversorgung von Kindern und Jugendlichen in Deutschland. *Ernährungs Umschau* **2007**, *11*, 636–646.

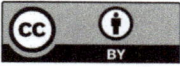

nutrients
MDPI

Article

Different Socio-Demographic and Lifestyle Factors Can Determine the Dietary Supplement Use in Children and Adolescents in Central-Eastern Poland

Ewa Sicińska *, Barbara Pietruszka, Olga Januszko and Joanna Kałuża

Department of Human Nutrition, Faculty of Human Nutrition and Consumer Sciences, Warsaw University of Life Sciences (WULS—SGGW), 159c Nowoursynowska str., 02-776 Warsaw, Poland; barbara_pietruszka@sggw.pl (B.P.); olga_januszko@sggw.pl (O.J.); joanna_kaluza@sggw.pl (J.K.)
* Correspondence: ewa_sicinska@sggw.pl; Tel.: +48-22-59-37-127

Received: 18 February 2019; Accepted: 13 March 2019; Published: 18 March 2019

Abstract: Vitamin/mineral supplement (VMS) use has become increasingly popular in children and adolescents; however, different predictors may be associated with their usage. Therefore, the aim of this study was to compare determinants of VMS use in 1578 children and adolescents. Data was collected among parents of children ($\leq$12 years old) and among adolescents (>12 years old) who attended public schools by a self-administered questionnaire. Multivariate-adjusted logistic regression models were used to estimate odds ratios (ORs) and 95% confidence intervals (95% CIs) for determining the predictors of VMS use. In children, the following determinants of VMS use were indicated: socioeconomic status (average vs. very good/good; OR: 1.69, 95% CI: 1.16–2.48), physical activity (1–5 vs. <1 h/week; OR: 1.44, 95% CI: 1.02–2.04), BMI ($\geq$25 vs. 18.5–24.9 kg/m^2; OR: 0.67, 95% CI: 0.46–0.98), and presence of chronic diseases (yes vs. no; OR: 2.32, 95% CI: 1.46–3.69). In adolescents, gender (male vs. female; OR: 0.56, 95% CI: 0.37–0.87), residential area (rural vs. urban; OR: 0.63, 95% CI: 0.40–0.99), BMI (<18.5 vs. 18.5–24.9 kg/m^2; OR: 0.35, 95% CI: 0.17–0.73), and health status (average/poor vs. at least good; OR: 1.96, 95% CI: 1.13–3.39) were factors of VMS use. In both groups, the mother's higher educational level, fortified food consumption and diet modification towards better food choices were predictors of VMS use. In conclusion, most of the predictors of VMS use were different in children and adolescents.

Keywords: adolescents; children; determinants; dietary supplements; food choice

---

1. Introduction

Dietary supplement use, especially containing vitamin/mineral supplements (VMSs), has become increasingly popular in developed countries. About half of the US adult population [1] and more than 30% of children and adolescences (<18 years old) [2] are users of these products. In Europe, depending on the country and gender, supplement use ranges from 2% to 66% in adults [3], and from 16% to 45% in children and adolescents in England, Scotland, Germany, Slovenia, and Finland [4–6]. Evidence of the benefits of using VMSs among those who eat properly are insufficient and conflicting [7]; studies have shown that the use of VMSs is usually associated with better dietary habits; however, knowledge on using supplements by adults as well as children and adolescents is insufficient [8,9]. Socio-demographic and lifestyle factors like age, sex, income, education level, health status, or physical activity may associate with dietary supplement usage [8]. Surveys on the determinants of VMS use focus mostly on adults [8], while the number of studies conducted in children (aged 2–10) [10,11] and adolescents (aged 11–19) [5,12,13] is limited, and often combine both age groups together [2,14–18]. Moreover, most of them were carried out in the US population [2,11–16]. Taking into the consideration that, in the case of children, parents decide whether to give a child a dietary supplement, while adolescents often make this decision by themselves based on advertisements, peers' or coach' recommendation [6], factors which determine the usage of dietary supplements may be different in both groups. The aim of the study was to compare socio-demographic and lifestyle determinants of VMS use in school children and adolescents in Central-Eastern Poland.

2. Materials and Methods

2.1. Study Design

The cross-sectional study was conducted in school students who attended public primary and secondary schools. The schools were selected randomly in Central-Eastern Poland based on a list of public schools in this area. The survey was conducted only in those schools of which headmasters gave consent to it. The following inclusion criteria of the students participating in the study were used: attendance to a public primary or secondary school in Central-Eastern Poland and the age of participants from 5–20 years. The exclusion criteria constituted: occurrence of a disease requiring a special diet, pregnancy or lactation (it concerned adolescents only) and incorrectly or incompletely filling in a health and lifestyle questionnaire.

The survey was conducted in accordance with the guidelines laid down by the Declaration of Helsinki. The study design and protocol were approved by the Department of Human Nutrition, Warsaw University of Life Sciences (WULS-SGGW), Poland.

2.2. Study Population and Data Collection

For the study 1200 parents of children (age 5–12 years) and 1200 adolescents (age 13–20 years) were invited to participate (Figure 1). The data was collected using the health and lifestyle questionnaire, which was distributed to parents at school meetings and to adolescents during classroom sessions. Completed questionnaires were verified by trained interviewers. A total of 1624 respondents returned the questionnaires (67.7%); however, due to incorrectly or incompletely filled in questionnaires, 46 were excluded. Finally, 1578 school students were included in the study. By completing the questionnaire, the respondents agreed to participate in the study.

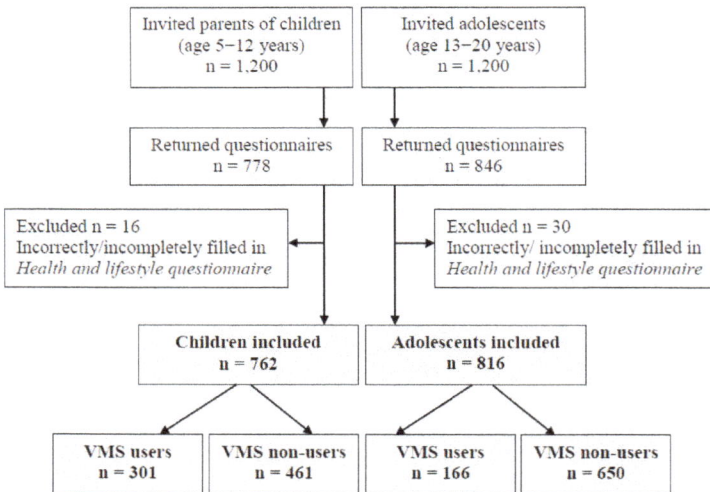

Figure 1. Flow chart of the study population. VMS: vitamin/mineral supplements. Notes: cream colour indicates study groups.

The questionnaire contained 27 questions and was composed of the following sections: socio-demographic characteristics (age, gender, place of living, mother's educational level, economic status of family); health and lifestyle status (health status, occurrence of chronic diseases, use and type of special diet, type and time spent on being physically active); eating habits (number of meals/day consumed habitually, regularity of main meal consumption, diet modification); dietary supplement usage; and voluntarily fortified foods usage. Self-reported height and weight of participants were collected and used to calculate the Body Mass Index (BMI) [19,20]. Details of the study methods have been enumerated elsewhere [21]. The questionnaire was developed and verified in an earlier study among students at the Department of Human Nutrition, WULS-SGGW, Poland [22,23].

2.3. Assessment of VMS Use

The respondents were asked about VMS taken during the year before the study as well as on the test day, about the name, and brand of dietary supplements, the usage form (i.e., pills, powder, drops etc.), and the period of application. As supplement users were considered those participants who used one or more VMSs over the 12 months before the survey. The study included short-term VMS users (from at least seven consecutive days to less than one month), medium-term users (1–3 months) and long-term users (>3 months). VMSs were categorised into: single vitamin; single mineral; multivitamin and/or mineral(s); and multicomponent supplement containing vitamin(s) and/or mineral(s) plus other ingredients including herbs or other.

When the respondents have declared VMS use, they were asked to give the reason for including these products in the diet by marking one or more predefined reasons: "Respondent's diet is poor in nutrients", "VMSs improve overall health", "VMSs are necessary when medicines are used", "VMSs were recommended by a physician", as well as they could list their own reason. When the respondents have declared not using VMSs, they were asked about the reason by marking one or more of the following statements: "Lack of effect on health improvement", "No need to use such products because of proper nutrition", "The use of VMSs can be harmful", "VMSs are too expensive", as well as they could list their own reason.

2.4. Statistical Analysis

All results were presented separately for children (≤12 years) and adolescents (>12 years). The statistically significant differences between categorical variables and VMS usage were determined using the Chi-square test. To examine the associations between VMS usage and parameters that might constitute the determinants of VMS use, the univariate (crude data) as well as multivariate-adjusted odds ratios (ORs) with 95% confidence intervals (95% CIs) were calculated using logistic regression models. The Hosmer-Lemeshow criterion was used to evaluate the models' goodness-of-fit.

The multivariate-adjusted models included potential determinants of VMS usage, i.e., age (continuous variable, years), gender (female or male), residential area (urban or rural), mother's education level (primary, high school, or university), socioeconomic status (very good/good, average, or poor), time spent on being physically active (<1, 1–5, or ≥6 h/week; not including gymnastic classes in school), BMI (<18.5, 18.5–24.9, or ≥25 kg/m²), self-reported health status (at least good, or average or poor), presence of chronic diseases (no or yes), using a special diet (no or yes), number of meals consumed per day (≤3, 4, or ≥5), consumption of fortified foods (no or yes), and intentional diet modification towards better food choices (lack of modification, excluding or including some food products, or simultaneously excluding and including some food products). Supplement non-users were the referent category for the logistic regression models. Missing data on socio-demographic and lifestyle determinants were modelled as separate categories. The statistical analyses were performed using SPSS version 23.0, and *p*-values ≤ 0.05 were considered statistically significant.

3. Results

3.1. Characteristics of the Study Population

Over the past 12 months, 29.6% of participants used VMSs, while 15.1% used VMSs on the test day. A statistically significantly higher number of children (mean age 8.6 ± 1.4 years) compared to adolescents (mean age 17.1 ± 2.1 years) used these products during the last year (39.5% vs. 20.3%, respectively; *p*-value < 0.001). In both groups, significantly more mothers of VMS users compared to non-users had a university education (Table S1). Compared to non-users, children classified as supplement users spent more time on being physically active and suffered from chronic diseases; the same tendencies were observed in adolescents. In both groups, VMS users vs. non-users declared the consumption of fortified foods more frequently, as well as modified their diet towards better food choices by intentionally including (e.g., vegetables, fruits) or/and excluding (e.g., sweets, crisps) some foods. It was observed that significantly more children who were VMS non-users than users were overweight or obese (BMI ≥ 25 kg/m^2; 33.1% vs. 23.6%, respectively); in contrast, in adolescents, more VMS non-users than users were underweight (BMI < 18.5 kg/m^2; 14.4% vs. 6.0%, respectively). A description of selected factors associated with the dietary supplement use by a part of the younger respondents, i.e., group of children aged 6–12, was also presented elsewhere [24].

3.2. Types and Duration of VMS Use and Reason for Using/Non-Using

In both groups, the most frequently used type of VMSs were multicomponent supplements containing multivitamin and/or mineral supplements with or without other ingredients, while single vitamin and single mineral were used less commonly (Table 1). As the main reasons for VMS use, parents of children and adolescents pointed out improving overall health, diet poor in nutrients, and physician recommendations. VMS non-users indicated that they did not need them because of proper nutrition. Moreover, parents of children more often than adolescents indicated as a reason not to use VMS a lack of effect on health improvement, harmful impact on health and too high of a price.

The distribution of children and adolescents using specific nutrients with vitamin/mineral supplements (VMSs) stratified by duration of use are presented in Table 2. Compared to adolescents, the number of children using vitamin supplements (A, E, D, C, B$_1$, B$_2$, niacin, B$_6$, folic acid, B$_{12}$, biotin, and pantothenic acid) was statistically significantly higher, whereas magnesium and iron supplements were consumed by a significantly lower number of children. Amongst children and adolescents, the largest number of respondents used vitamin C supplements (83.7% and 65.7%, respectively). The majority of respondents were classified as medium-term VMS users (45.8%), followed by short-term users (31.5%) and lastly long-term users (22.7%). Generally, more adolescents than children were classified as medium-term users of specific nutrients with VMSs, while children respondents were more often classified as short-term and long-term users with statistically significant differences found for vitamins C, B$_1$, B$_2$, niacin, B$_6$, B$_{12}$, and zinc.

3.3. Determinants of VMS Use in Children and Adolescents

Multivariate-adjusted odds ratios (ORs) of VMS use by socio-demographic and lifestyle factors in children and adolescents are presented in Table 3. There was found an association between mother's education level and usage of supplements in children. Compared to children of mothers with primary education, those whose mothers had high school or university education had a higher probability of dietary supplement use (OR: 2.17, 95% CI: 1.17–4.01 and OR: 2.16, 95% CI: 1.14–4.07, respectively). In comparison to respondents who assessed a familiar socioeconomic status as very good or good, children living in families with an average socioeconomic status had significantly higher odds ratios of VMS use (OR: 1.69, 95% CI: 1.16–2.48). Respondents who spent 1 to 5 h/week on being physically active (not including gymnastic classes at school) were 1.44-fold (95% CI: 1.02–2.04) more likely to be VMS users than those being physically active <1 h/week. Moreover, overweight and obese children (BMI ≥ 25 kg/m^2) were less likely to be supplement users (OR: 0.67, 95% CI: 0.46–0.98) than those with a normal BMI range (18.5–24.9 kg/m^2). An inverse statistically significant trend between BMI and usage of VMSs was observed, each 1 kg/m^2 increment in BMI was associated with a 7% (95% CI: 2–12%; p-trend = 0.008) lower probability of VMS use. Moreover, children who suffer from chronic diseases were more likely to be supplement users (OR: 2.32, 95% CI: 1.46–3.69) than those without chronic diseases. The prevalence of VMS usage was 3.79-fold (95% CI: 2.54–5.63) higher among those who were fortified product consumers vs. non-consumers. Children who intentionally modified their diet by including or excluding some food products had a 1.60-fold (95% CI: 1.01–2.53) higher probability of usage of VMS and those who simultaneously included and excluded food products had a 2.22-fold (95% CI: 1.29–3.81) higher probability of usage of VMS compared to non-consumers.

Table 1. Prevalence of specific types of vitamin/mineral supplement (VMS) use and reasons for using or non-using them by children (n = 762) and adolescents (n = 816).

Parameters	Children ≤12 years	Adolescents >12 years
	Users [a]	Users [a]
	n = 301	n = 166
	%	%
Type of VMS		
Single vitamin	20.2	25.9
Single mineral [b]	4.3	16.9
Multivitamin and/or mineral(s)	39.9	33.1
Vitamin(s)/mineral(s) + other ingredient [b]	72.1	42.8
Usage more than one VMS	13.3	12.0
Reason for using VMSs [c]		
Improve overall health	77.4	76.5
Diet poor in nutrients [b]	45.2	20.5
Physician recommendation [b]	32.2	26.5
Necessary when medicines are used [b]	10.6	4.8
Other	15.0	9.0
	Non-users	Non-users
	n = 461	n = 650
	%	%
Reason for avoidance VMSs [c]		
No need to use because of proper nutrition [b]	62.3	44.2
Lack effect on health improvement [b]	24.7	7.8
It can be harmful [b]	22.3	7.2
Too high price [b]	20.8	13.1
Other [c]	9.1	3.4

[a] supplement user—a person who used one or more VMSs over the 12 months before the survey; [b] a statistically significant difference between the group of children and adolescents; chi-square test, p-value < 0.05; [c] each respondent could select one or more answers.

Table 2. The distribution of respondents using specific nutrients with vitamin/mineral supplements (VMSs) stratified by duration of use (n = 467).

VMS Using		n (%) *	p-value	Short-Term Users 7 days–<1 month n = 147 % **	Medium-Term Users 1–3 months n = 214 % **	Long-Term Users >3 months n = 106 % **	p-value
Total [b,c]	children	301 (100)	0.012	29.9	43.9	26.2	0.048
	adolescents	166 (100)		34.3	49.4	16.3	
Vitamin A	children	215 (71.4)	<0.001	22.3	48.4	29.3	0.131
	adolescents	50 (30.1)		14.0	64.0	22.0	
Vitamin E	children	192 (63.8)	<0.001	26.0	47.4	26.6	0.236
	adolescents	51 (30.7)		19.6	60.8	19.6	
Vitamin D	children	217 (72.1)	<0.001	22.6	47.9	29.5	0.279
	adolescents	46 (27.7)		13.0	58.7	28.3	
Vitamin C [c]	children	252 (83.7)	<0.001	30.5	43.3	26.2	0.049
	adolescents	109 (65.7)		29.4	55.0	15.6	
Vitamin B_1 [a,c]	children	174 (57.8)	<0.001	24.1	46.0	29.9	0.010
	adolescents	40 (24.1)		12.5	72.5	15.0	
Vitamin B_2 [a,c]	children	189 (62.8)	<0.001	27.5	44.4	28.1	0.021
	adolescents	41 (24.7)		17.1	68.3	14.6	
Niacin [a]	children	197 (65.4)	<0.001	25.4	46.7	27.9	0.041
	adolescents	41 (24.7)		14.6	68.3	17.1	
Vitamin B_6 [a,c]	children	202 (67.1)	<0.001	26.7	46.6	26.7	0.003
	adolescents	55 (33.1)		12.7	72.7	14.6	

Table 2. *Cont.*

VMS Using		n (%) *	p-value	Short-Term Users 7 days–<1 month n = 147 % **	Medium-Term Users 1–3 months n = 214 % **	Long-Term Users >3 months n = 106 % **	p-value
Folic acid	children	138 (45.8)	<0.001	19.6	50.0	30.4	0.064
	adolescents	41 (24.7)		12.2	70.7	17.1	
Vitamin B$_{12}$ [a,c]	children	167 (55.5)	<0.001	22.8	47.3	29.9	0.016
	adolescents	40 (24.1)		12.5	72.5	15.0	
Biotin	children	127 (42.2)	<0.001	18.9	52.8	28.3	0.328
	adolescents	28 (16.9)		10.7	67.9	21.4	
Pantothenic acid	children	135 (44.9)	<0.001	25.9	48.2	25.9	0.061
	adolescents	39 (23.5)		12.8	69.2	18.0	
Calcium	children	76 (25.2)	0.900	18.4	55.3	26.3	0.828
	adolescents	41 (24.7)		21.9	56.2	21.9	
Magnesium	children	27 (9.0)	<0.001	29.6	48.1	22.3	0.532
	adolescents	44 (26.5)		18.2	56.8	25.0	
Iron	children	35 (11.6)	0.010	22.9	51.4	25.7	0.616
	adolescents	34 (20.5)		14.7	61.8	23.5	
Zinc [a,c]	children	87 (28.9)	0.210	23.0	41.4	35.6	0.015
	adolescents	39 (23.5)		12.8	69.2	18.0	

p-value was determined using the chi-square test; different letters in superscript indicate statistically significant differences between: [a] short-term and medium-term users, [b] short-term and long-term users, [c] medium-term and long-term users; * the percentage of subjects using specific nutrients was given in relation to total VMS users in children (*n* = 301) and adolescents (*n* = 166); ** percentages were calculated in relation to children or adolescents who used supplements containing specific nutrients (percentages are summarized in rows).

Table 3. Logistic regression of vitamin/mineral supplement (VMS) use by socio-demographic and lifestyle determinants in school children and adolescents.

Study Factors	Children ≤12 years (n = 762)		Adolescents >12 years (n = 816)	
	Crude	Multivariate-Adjusted	Crude	Multivariate-Adjusted
	OR (95% CI)	OR (95% CI)	OR (95% CI)	OR (95% CI)
Age (years)	0.96 (0.87–1.06)	1.01 (0.90–1.14)	0.93 (0.86–1.01)	1.15 (0.95–1.39)
P for trend	0.39	0.86	0.09	0.15
Gender				
Female	1.00	1.00	1.00	1.00
Male	0.96 (0.72–1.28)	0.94 (0.68–1.30)	0.75 (0.51–1.09)	**0.56 (0.37–0.87)**
Residential area				
Urban	1.00	1.00	1.00	1.00
Rural	1.04 (0.70–1.57)	1.43 (0.88–2.35)	0.94 (0.67–1.33)	**0.63 (0.40–0.99)**
Mother's education level				
Primary	1.00	1.00	1.00	1.00
High school	1.87 (1.10–3.18)	**2.17 (1.17–4.01)**	2.10 (0.92–4.78)	2.02 (0.85–4.79)
University	2.05 (1.23–3.40)	**2.16 (1.14–4.07)**	6.07 (2.20–16.8)	**5.19 (1.72–15.6)**
Socioeconomic status				
Very good or good	1.00	1.00	1.00	1.00
Average	1.38 (0.99–1.91)	**1.69 (1.16–2.48)**	0.76 (0.52–1.11)	0.75 (0.49–1.15)
Poor	0.64 (0.32–1.32)	1.12 (0.49–2.54)	0.59 (0.33–1.04)	0.83 (0.44–1.56)
Physical activity (h/week)				
<1	1.00	1.00	1.00	1.00
1–5	1.72 (1.26–2.36)	**1.44 (1.02–2.04)**	1.52 (1.07–2.17)	1.26 (0.85–1.86)
≥6	1.35 (0.76–2.41)	1.21 (0.63–2.32)	1.10 (0.49–2.48)	0.87 (0.36–2.13)
Body Mass Index (kg/m²)				
<18.5	0.99 (0.64–1.52)	1.10 (0.69–1.76)	0.39 (0.20–0.77)	**0.35 (0.17–0.73)**
18.5–24.9	1.00	1.00	1.00	1.00
≥25	**0.62 (0.44–0.88)**	**0.67 (0.46–0.98)**	1.14 (0.71–1.84)	0.99 (0.58–1.70)
P for trend	0.003	0.008	0.19	0.22

Table 3. *Cont.*

Study Factors	Children ≤12 years (*n* = 762)				Adolescents >12 years (*n* = 816)			
	Crude	Multivariate-Adjusted			Crude	Multivariate-Adjusted		
	OR (95% CI)	OR (95% CI)			OR (95% CI)	OR (95% CI)		
Health status								
At least good	1.00	1.00			1.00	1.00		
Average or poor	0.70 (0.37–1.32)	0.56 (0.27–1.17)			1.41 (0.89–2.24)	**1.96 (1.13–3.39)**		
Current chronic diseases								
No	1.00	1.00			1.00	1.00		
Yes	2.24 (1.52–3.31)	**2.32 (1.46–3.69)**			1.90 (0.99–3.68)	1.27 (0.61–2.66)		
Special diet								
No	1.00	1.00			1.00	1.00		
Yes	1.58 (0.88–2.83)	0.82 (0.40–1.66)			1.57 (0.96–2.58)	1.02 (0.56–1.85)		
Number of meals/day								
≤3	1.00	1.00			1.00	1.00		
4	1.38 (0.86–2.20)	1.16 (0.69–1.96)			1.52 (1.04–2.22)	1.46 (0.95–2.25)		
≥5	1.82 (1.09–3.01)	1.68 (0.96–2.95)			1.47 (0.90–2.41)	1.51 (0.86–2.65)		
Fortified food consumption								
No	1.00	1.00			1.00	1.00		
Yes	3.39 (2.35–4.89)	**3.79 (2.54–5.63)**			3.12 (2.04–4.77)	**2.54 (1.62–4.00)**		
Diet modification								
Lack of modification	1.00	1.00			1.00	1.00		
Excluding or including some foods	1.76 (1.17–2.64)	**1.60 (1.01–2.53)**			2.36 (1.51–3.70)	**2.09 (1.24–3.52)**		
Simultaneously excluding and including some foods	2.95 (1.83–4.75)	**2.22 (1.29–3.81)**			3.00 (1.85–4.87)	**3.02 (1.71–5.35)**		

Supplement user—a person who used one or more VMSs over the 12 months before the survey. Notes: bold font indicates the statistical significant results in the multivariate-adjusted analysis.

Compared to children, in adolescents, some different factors like gender or residential area were associated with VMS usage; however, some of them, like mother's education level, fortified food consumption, or diet modification towards better food choices, were overlapped with those determined for children (Table 3). VMS users vs. non-users were less likely to be male (OR: 0.56, 95% CI: 0.37–0.87) and live in rural areas (OR: 0.63, 95% CI: 0.40–0.99). In comparison to adolescents whose mothers had primary education, those with university mothers' education had a higher probability of VMS use (OR: 5.19, 95% CI: 1.72–15.6). Adolescent who were underweight (BMI < 18.5 kg/m^2) were less likely to be supplement users (OR: 0.35, 95% CI: 0.17–0.73) than those with a normal BMI (18.5–24.9 kg/m^2). In contrast to children, each 1 kg/m^2 increment in BMI was associated with a non-significant 4% (95% CI: −2–10%; p-trend = 0.22) higher probability of VMS usage. It was found that adolescents who declared average or poor health status vs. those who declared at least a good health status were more likely to be supplement users (OR: 1.96, 95% CI: 1.13–3.39). Moreover, the prevalence of VMS use was 2.54-fold (95% CI: 1.62–4.00) higher among those who were fortified food consumers vs. non-consumers; 2.09-fold (95% CI: 1.24–3.52) higher among those who intentionally included or excluded some food products; and 3.02-fold (95% CI: 1.71–5.35) higher among those who simultaneously included and excluded some food products vs. those who not modified their diet.

4. Discussion

The study showed that the majority of significant predictors of VMS use were different in children and adolescents. In children, socioeconomic status, physical activity level, BMI, and presence of chronic disease were determinants of dietary supplement use; while in adolescents, it was gender, residential area, BMI (in opposite trend compared to children), and health status. Notwithstanding, some determinants such as higher mothers' education, consumption of fortified foods, and declaration of diet modifications overlapped in both groups.

In our study, a significantly higher number of children (39.5%) compared to adolescents (20.3%) used VMSs. Similarly, in the National Health Interview Survey 2007 [2] and the National Health and Nutrition Examination Survey (NHANES) 1999–2004 [16], these products were used by more children (aged 5–11) (38.9% and 37.4%, respectively) than adolescents (12–17 years) (23.0% and 26.6%, respectively).

A higher family income was associated with a higher use of dietary supplement in studies conducted among American children and adolescent [2,10,15,16,18]. In our study, children with an average socioeconomic status compared with those with very good/good socioeconomic status had a higher probability of VMS use; however, our study was based on a self-assessment of socioeconomic status, not on exact income, which was reported in other surveys [2,10,15,18].

A higher level of parents' education was associated with an increased probability of supplement use in both examined groups. Similar observations have been reported from studies conducted in the US children and adolescent populations [2,10]. It could be explained by the increased awareness of a healthy lifestyle in people with higher education and by the fact that supplement usage is commonly considered as a pro-healthy behaviour. In fact, dietary supplements are not routinely recommended for children and adolescents who consume a varied diet. NHANES 2003–2006 results suggested that it is a controversial strategy to improve nutrient intakes [25]. Furthermore, the results of some studies indicate that unjustified supplementation may increase the total mortality risk in the population as well as incidence of specific diseases [7,26,27]. However, for certain groups, for example, children with nutritional deficiencies (e.g., vitamin D supplementation during low sunlight exposure), malabsorption or obese children in weight loss programs, VMS use could be recommended [28].

In this study, children who spent 1–5 h per week compared to those who spent <1 h/week of free time being physically active (swimming, playing football, dancing, playing tennis or other sports) had a higher probability of VMS use. Similarly, in studies conducted among American children and adolescents [11,12,14], Finnish [5] and Slovenian [6] adolescents, supplement users vs. non-users were more frequently physically active as well as less likely to watch television or video/computer games [14,15]. In American [14,15] and Korean [17] studies, overweight and obese children and adults were less likely to be supplement users. In our study, the usage of VMSs was associated with a normal BMI; children who were overweight and obese, and adolescents who were underweight had a lower probability to be supplement users.

Adolescents who declared average or poor health status and children suffering from chronic diseases compared to healthy respondents were more likely to consume VMSs. In some studies, dietary supplement use was more common in children and adolescents who used prescribed medication and among those who suffered from chronic diseases or were complaining about health [5,17]. On the contrary, in large American studies, children and adolescents who were supplement users compared to non-users more frequently declared very good or excellent health status [2,13].

Children and adolescents who were VMS users more often consumed fortified food and modified their diet towards better food choices. It was consistent with the results of other studies conducted in children and adolescents, where supplement use was associated with more healthful food choices [11], with higher diet quality score, regular consumption of some meals, low-fat foods [12,17] as well as more healthful food patterns such as higher intakes of whole grains, fruit, vegetables, and lower intakes of soft drinks, fried food, and meat [11,12,14].

We hypothesise that the differences in the determinants of dietary supplements may be a result of motivation for using these products. Parents make this decision in order to improve the nutritional habits of children, because of poor appetite or frequently occurring colds [10]; while adolescents are buying supplements by themselves, expecting a variety of effects, such as increased energy, building muscle mass or decreased weight and enhanced physical appearance, which often reflected the extensive marketing of specific dietary supplements [29]. In our study, as the main reasons for VMS use, parents of children pointed out improving children's overall health and a diet poor in nutrients; while adolescents declared improving overall health and physician recommendations. Similarly, in the American population, the main motivation of children and adolescents to use VMSs was improving overall health and preventing nutrient deficiencies [2,30].

The strengths of the present study include a large number of respondents as well as VMS users, and the detailed characteristics of participants by socio-demographic and lifestyle factors. It provided an opportunity to use the logistic regression models to determine factors significantly associated with VMS use separately in children and adolescents as well as allowed to show differences in the determinants of VMS usage between both groups. As in all observational studies, unmeasured or residual confounding cannot be disregarded. In the study, a limited number of determinants was examined; it is highly probable that some of the important factors of VMS use were not taken into account. Another limitation of this study was that the survey might not be representative for all primary and secondary school students from Central-Eastern Poland, since the study was carried out only in those schools in which the headmasters gave consent to it. Moreover, it is possible that respondents with a more health-oriented lifestyle are more likely to participate in the study. Furthermore, the methodology was not uniform; in children (5–12 years), the survey was completed by parents, while in adolescents (13–20 years) by the students themselves; this could have an effect on the outcomes.

5. Conclusions

Socio-demographic and lifestyle factors associated with VMS use may vary by age groups among school students. Children with an average socioeconomic status, who spent more free time on being physically active, with a normal body weight, and who suffered from chronic diseases, were more likely to use supplements. In adolescents, VMS users compared with non-users more often were female and lived in urban areas, less likely were underweight and assessed their health status as average or poor. In both groups, higher mothers' education, consumption of fortified food, and declaration of diet modifications towards better food choices were predictors of VMS use. Since the age of the respondents may determine different behaviours associated with the use of dietary supplements, further research should be conducted also among other age groups. Understanding the determinants affecting the use of dietary supplements in children and adolescents may identify the risk to subgroup populations of the incorrect use of dietary supplements, as well as allow the planning of appropriate public health education; therefore, further research is warranted.

Supplementary Materials: The following are available online at http://www.mdpi.com/2072-6643/11/3/658/s1. Table S1. Characteristics of children (*n* = 762) and adolescents (*n* = 816) by socio-demographic and lifestyle determinants stratified by vitamin/mineral supplement (VMS) use.

Author Contributions: Conceptualization: E.S., B.P., and J.K.; data curation: E.S. and O.J.; formal analysis: E.S. and J.K.; investigation: B.P. and J.K.; methodology: E.S. and J.K.; supervision: B.P. and J.K.; writing—original draft: E.S.; writing—review and editing: B.P. and J.K.

Funding: The research was financed by the Polish Ministry of Science and Higher Education within funds of the Faculty of Human Nutrition and Consumer Sciences, Warsaw University of Life Sciences (WULS), for scientific research.

Acknowledgments: The authors thank Katarzyna Rolf for technical support with creating the database.

Conflicts of Interest: The authors declare no conflicts of interest.

References

1. Bailey, R.L.; Gahche, J.J.; Lentino, C.V.; Dwyer, J.T.; Engel, J.S.; Thomas, P.R.; Betz, J.M.; Sempos, C.T.; Picciano, M.F. Dietary supplement use in the United States, 2003–2006. *J. Nutr.* **2011**, *141*, 261–266. [CrossRef] [PubMed]

2. Dwyer, J.; Nahin, R.L.; Rogers, G.T.; Barnes, P.M.; Jacques, P.M.; Sempos, C.T.; Bailey, R. Prevalence and predictors of children's dietary supplement use: The 2007 National Health Interview Survey. *Am. J. Clin. Nutr.* **2013**, *97*, 1331–1337. [CrossRef] [PubMed]

3. Skeie, G.; Braaten, T.; Hjartaker, A.; Lentjes, M.; Amiano, P.; Jakszyn, P.; Pala, V.; Palanca, A.; Niekerk, E.M.; Verhagen, H.; et al. Use of dietary supplements in the European Prospective Investigation into Cancer and Nutrition calibration study. *Eur. J. Clin. Nutr.* **2009**, *63*, S226–S238. [CrossRef] [PubMed]

4. Bristow, A.; Qureshi, S.; Rona, R.J.; Chinn, S. The use of nutritional supplements by 4–12 year olds in England and Scotland. *Eur. J. Clin. Nutr.* **1997**, *51*, 366–369. [CrossRef] [PubMed]

5. Mattila, V.M.; Parkkari, J.; Laakso, L.; Pihlajamaki, H.; Rimpela, A. Use of dietary supplements and anabolic-androgenic steroids among Finnish adolescents in 1991–2005. *Eur. J. Public Health* **2010**, *20*, 306–311. [CrossRef] [PubMed]

6. Sterlinko Grm, H.; Stubelj Ars, M.; Besednjak-Kocijancic, L.; Golja, P. Nutritional supplement use among Slovenian adolescents. *Public Health Nutr.* **2012**, *15*, 587–593. [CrossRef]

7. Fortmann, S.P.; Burda, B.U.; Senger, C.A.; Lin, J.S.; Whitlock, E.P. Vitamin and mineral supplements in the primary prevention of cardiovascular disease and cancer: An updated systematic evidence review for the U.S. Preventive Services Task Force. *Ann. Intern. Med.* **2013**, *159*, 824–834. [CrossRef] [PubMed]

8. Dickinson, A.; MacKay, D. Health habits and other characteristics of dietary supplement users: A review. *Nutr. J.* **2014**, *13*, 14. [CrossRef]

9. Dickinson, A.; MacKay, D.; Wong, A. Consumer attitudes about the role of multivitamins and other dietary supplements: Report of a survey. *Nutr. J.* **2015**, *14*, 66. [CrossRef]

10. Yu, S.M.; Kogan, M.D.; Gergen, P. Vitamin-mineral supplement use among preschool children in the United States. *Pediatrics* **1997**, *100*, E4. [CrossRef]

11. George, G.C.; Hoelscher, D.M.; Nicklas, T.A.; Kelder, S.H. Diet- and body size-related attitudes and behaviors associated with vitamin supplement use in a representative sample of fourth-grade students in Texas. *J. Nutr. Educ. Behav.* **2009**, *41*, 95–102. [CrossRef]

12. George, G.C.; Springer, A.E.; Forman, M.R.; Hoelscher, D.M. Associations among dietary supplement use and dietary and activity behaviors by sex and race/ethnicity in a representative multiethnic sample of 11th-grade students in Texas. *J. Am. Diet. Assoc.* **2011**, *111*, 385–393. [CrossRef]

13. Gardiner, P.; Buettner, C.; Davis, R.B.; Phillips, R.S.; Kemper, K.J. Factors and common conditions associated with adolescent dietary supplement use: An analysis of the National Health and Nutrition Examination Survey (NHANES). *BMC Complement. Altern. Med.* **2008**, *8*, 9. [CrossRef] [PubMed]

14. Reaves, L.; Steffen, L.M.; Dwyer, J.T.; Webber, L.S.; Lytle, L.A.; Feldman, H.A.; Hoelscher, D.M.; Zive, M.M.; Osganian, S.K. Vitamin supplement intake is related to dietary intake and physical activity: The Child and Adolescent Trial for Cardiovascular Health (CATCH). *J. Am. Diet. Assoc.* **2006**, *106*, 2018–2023. [CrossRef]

15. Picciano, M.F.; Dwyer, J.T.; Radimer, K.L.; Wilson, D.H.; Fisher, K.D.; Thomas, P.R.; Yetley, E.A.; Moshfegh, A.J.; Levy, P.S.; Nielsen, S.J.; et al. Dietary supplement use among infants, children, and adolescents in the United States, 1999–2002. *Arch. Pediatr. Adolesc. Med.* **2007**, *161*, 978–985. [CrossRef]

16. Shaikh, U.; Byrd, R.S.; Auinger, P. Vitamin and mineral supplement use by children and adolescents in the 1999–2004 National Health and Nutrition Examination Survey: Relationship with nutrition, food security, physical activity, and health care access. *Arch. Pediatr. Adolesc. Med.* **2009**, *163*, 150–157. [CrossRef]

17. Yoon, J.Y.; Park, H.A.; Kang, J.H.; Kim, K.W.; Hur, Y.I.; Park, J.J.; Lee, R.; Lee, H.H. Prevalence of dietary supplement use in Korean children and adolescents: Insights from Korea National Health and Nutrition Examination Survey 2007–2009. *J. Korean Med. Sci.* **2012**, *27*, 512–517. [CrossRef]

18. Jun, S.; Cowan, A.E.; Tooze, J.A.; Gahche, J.J.; Dwyer, J.T.; Eicher-Miller, H.A.; Bhadra, A.; Guenther, P.M.; Potischman, N.; Dodd, K.W.; et al. Dietary Supplement Use among U.S. Children by Family Income, Food Security Level, and Nutrition Assistance Program Participation Status in 2011–2014. *Nutrients* **2018**, *10*, 1212. [CrossRef]

19. Cole, T.J.; Bellizzi, M.C.; Flegal, K.M.; Dietz, W.H. Establishing a standard definition for child overweight and obesity worldwide: International survey. *BMJ* **2000**, *320*, 1240–1243. [CrossRef]

20. Cole, T.J.; Flegal, K.M.; Nicholls, D.; Jackson, A.A. Body mass index cut offs to define thinness in children and adolescents: International survey. *BMJ* **2007**, *335*, 194. [CrossRef]

21. Sicińska, E.; Kałuża, J.; Januszko, O.; Pietruszka, B. Comparison of factors determining voluntarily fortified food consumption between children and adolescents in Central-Eastern Poland. *J. Food Nutr. Res.* **2018**, *57*, 284–294.

22. Pietruszka, B.; Brzozowska, A. Homocysteine Serum Level in Relation to Intake of Folate, Vitamins B12, B1, B2, and B6 and MTHFR c.665C→T Polymorphism among Young Women. *Austin J. Nutr. Food Sci.* **2014**, *2*, 1052–1059.

23. Pietruszka, B. *The Effectiveness of Diet Supplementation with Folates Relative to Risk Factors for Folate Deficiencies in Young Women*; Warsaw University of Life Sciences: Warsaw, Poland, 2007; pp. 1–182.

24. Bylinowska, J.; Januszko, O.; Rolf, K.; Sicinska, E.; Kaluza, J.; Pietruszka, B. Factors influenced vitamin or mineral supplements use in a chosen group of children aged 6–12. *Rocz. Panstw. Zakl. Hig.* **2012**, *63*, 59–66. [PubMed]

25. Bailey, R.L.; Fulgoni, V.L., 3rd; Keast, D.R.; Lentino, C.V.; Dwyer, J.T. Do dietary supplements improve micronutrient sufficiency in children and adolescents? *J. Pediatr.* **2012**, *161*, 837–842. [CrossRef] [PubMed]

26. Brzozowska, A.; Kaluza, J.; Knoops, K.T.; de Groot, L.C. Supplement use and mortality: The SENECA study. *Eur. J. Nutr.* **2008**, *47*, 131–137. [CrossRef] [PubMed]

27. Kaluza, J.; Januszko, O.; Trybalska, E.; Wadolowska, L.; Slowinska, M.A.; Brzozowska, A. Vitamin and mineral supplement use and mortality among group of older people. *Przegl. Epidemiol.* **2010**, *64*, 557–563. [PubMed]

28. Kleinman, R.E. Current Approaches to Standards of Care for Children: How Does the Pediatric Community Currently Approach This Issue? *Nutr. Today* **2002**, *37*, 177–179. [CrossRef] [PubMed]

29. Dorsch, K.D.; Bell, A. Dietary supplement use in adolescents. *Curr. Opin. Pediatr.* **2005**, *17*, 653–657. [CrossRef]

30. Bailey, R.L.; Gahche, J.J.; Thomas, P.R.; Dwyer, J.T. Why US children use dietary supplements. *Pediatr. Res.* **2013**, *74*, 737–741. [CrossRef] [PubMed]

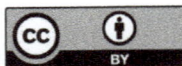

nutrients

MDPI

Article

Sugar-Sweetened Beverage Consumption and Associated Factors in School-Going Adolescents of New Caledonia

Guillaume Wattelez, Stéphane Frayon, Yolande Cavaloc, Sophie Cherrier, Yannick Lerrant and Olivier Galy *

Interdisciplinary Laboratory for Research in Education, EA 7483, University of New Caledonia,
Noumea BP R4 98851, New Caledonia; guillaume.wattelez@unc.nc (G.W.); stephanefrayon@hotmail.com (S.F.);
yolande.cavaloc@unc.nc (Y.C.); sophie.cherrier@unc.nc (S.C.); yannick.lerrant@unc.nc (Y.L.)
* Correspondence: olivier.galy@unc.nc; Tel.: +687-290-545

Received: 12 December 2018; Accepted: 30 January 2019; Published: 21 February 2019

Abstract: This cross-sectional study assessed sugar-sweetened beverage (SSB) consumption and its associations with the sociodemographic and physical characteristics, behavior and knowledge of New Caledonian adolescents. The survey data of 447 adolescents from ages 11 to 16 years were collected in five secondary public schools of New Caledonia between July 2015 and April 2016. These data included measured height and weight, SSB consumption, sociodemographic characteristics, body weight perception, physical activity, and knowledge (sugar quantity/SSB unit; energy expenditure required to eliminate a unit) and opinions about the SSB-weight gain relationship. Ninety percent of these adolescents declared regularly drinking SSBs. Quantities were associated with living environment (1.94 L·week^{-1} in urban environment vs. 4.49 L·week^{-1} in rural environment, $p = 0.001$), ethnic community (4.77 L·week^{-1} in Melanesians vs. 2.46 L·week^{-1} in Caucasians, $p < 0.001$) and knowledge about energy expenditure (6.22 L·week^{-1} in unknowledgeable adolescents vs. 4.26 L·week^{-1} in adolescents who underestimated, 3.73 L·week^{-1} in adolescents who overestimated, and 3.64 L·week^{-1} in adolescents who correctly responded on the energy expenditure required to eliminate an SSB unit, $p = 0.033$). To conclude, community-based health promotion strategies should (1) focus on the physical effort needed to negate SSB consumption rather than the nutritional energy from SSB units and (2) highlight how to achieve sustainable lifestyles and provide tools for greater understanding and positive action.

Keywords: consumption behavior; knowledge; Melanesian; Pacific; physical activity; sugar-sweetened beverage; noncommunicable diseases; weight status; self-weight perception

1. Introduction

Adolescent overweight and obesity are associated with lifestyle factors like low physical activity (PA) and frequent consumption of energy-dense foods high in saturated fats and refined carbohydrates [1]. Sugar-sweetened beverages (SSBs), in particular, are a frequent source of refined carbohydrates in adolescent nutrition [2–4]. According to the 2010 Dietary Guidelines for Americans, SSBs are "liquids that are sweetened with various forms of sugars that add calories. These beverages include, but are not limited to, soda and fruit drinks, and sports and energy drinks" [5]. SSBs are the largest source of added sugars and major energy contributors to diet [6]. Harnack et al. [2] showed that US school children drinking an average of 265 mL or more of soft drinks daily consumed almost 835 kJ more total energy per day than those drinking no soft drinks. Moreover, epidemiological studies have quantified the positive relationships between SSB consumption and long-term weight gain, type 2 diabetes mellitus and cardiovascular diseases [6,7].

SSB consumption is also related to weight status [8], self-weight perception and body dissatisfaction [8], and PA [9,10]. It may also be related to knowledge or opinions about SSB [6,11]. For example, Park et al. [6] found that SSB consumption was higher among adults who disagreed that SSBs contribute to weight gain, whereas knowledge about the energy content of regular soda was not associated with SSB intake. Conversely, other authors found that adolescents or young adults (college students) with the poorest nutrition knowledge had the highest SSB consumption [11].

The Pacific Island Countries and Territories (PICTs) are also facing problems of obesity, overweight and changing nutrition patterns [4]. Kessaram et al. [10] reported the high prevalence of overweight and obesity in adolescents, likely explained by environmental mutations and shifts in nutrition and PA [12]. Traditional diets of root crops, vegetables, fruits and fresh fish and meat have been steadily replaced by imported, processed, energy-dense, low-nutrient foods [13], including SSBs. In six PICTs, 42% of 13- to 15-year-old students declared drinking SSBs daily [10]. Pak et al. [14] assessed soft drink consumption and reported 84 L/person in Palau in 2011.

Obesity and comorbidities are a health concern for young adults in Oceania, especially those in New Caledonia [15]. New Caledonia is a French archipelago in the South Pacific located between 162° E–169° E longitude and 19° S–23° S latitude. Melanesians were the first inhabitants of this archipelago, and consecutive arrivals of different populations since the era of colonization have now provided a multi-ethnic society with several "ethnic communities" that are representative of the Pacific populations. Melanesian (39%), European (or Caucasian) (27%), Polynesian (8%), Asian (2.5%) and other populations live together [16]. In 1989, New Caledonia was divided into three provinces: the Southern Province, the Northern Province and the Loyalty Islands Province. The capital city Noumea (Southern Province) is nevertheless the center for most economic activities. As a consequence, Noumea and its suburbs are the only areas that can be considered urban. The lifestyles of urban and rural areas differ greatly, and cultural and socioeconomic differences are also observed among the main ethnic groups, especially in rural areas. Indeed, New Caledonia's economy is overall on par with that of the Western world, especially in Noumea and other small towns, although half the population lives a traditional Pacific lifestyle. The traditional lifestyle is characterized by daily physical activities oriented toward agriculture, fishing or other activities to meet a family's daily needs. Disparities are seen in all age groups including school-going adolescents. Whereas an "equitable school system" exists—i.e., offering every adolescent the same access to school and a standardized academic curriculum, as well as a health education program [17]—the differences between the ethnic communities may lead to dramatic consequences for health in future generations [18]. Although few studies have focused on 11- to 16-year-old adolescents in New Caledonia [13,19,20], the prevalence of overweight or obesity was found to be three times greater in New Caledonian adolescents than in French adolescents in the same age range [21]. In addition, Frayon et al. [13] showed that in this multi-ethnic society, the risk of being overweight/obese was significantly greater in Polynesian and Melanesian adolescents. Adolescent overweight was also associated with rural lifestyles and low socioeconomic status (SES) for girls and breakfast skipping for boys [22]. Melanesian adolescents were more physically active and had a higher body mass percentage, mainly in rural girls compared with urban girls [20]. PA and food intake, and adolescent knowledge about and consumption of SSBs remain inadequately explored in the New Caledonian population, but research suggests that socio-environmental variables should be taken into account. We therefore hypothesized that SSB consumption would be associated with ethnicity (i.e., being Melanesian), living environment (i.e., rural) and knowledge about SSBs (i.e., sugar contained in SSBs, energy expenditure to eliminate consumed SSBs and association with weight gain).

This study aimed to broaden the vision on health among the 11- to 16-year-old adolescents in New Caledonia by assessing their SSB consumption behaviors and the associations with individual and socio-environmental factors.

2. Materials and Methods

2.1. Data Collection and Participants

Our study was part of a community-based obesity prevention project conducted in five selected representative school sites in the three provinces (Northern Province, Southern Province and Loyalty Islands) of New Caledonia. The schools were selected on the basis of the following criteria: (1) a representative repartition of the schools between rural and urban areas (respectively, 63% and 37% of the population), and (2) sufficient school size ($n > 200$). Eight schools were eligible in the Southern Province (urban), four in the Northern Province (rural) and only one in the Loyalty Islands (rural). Selected schools were then randomly drawn among these eligible schools: two in the Southern Province, two in the Northern Province and one in the Loyalty Islands. The school and participant selection process are further described elsewhere [19].

Data were collected between July 2015 and April 2016 from 696 school-going adolescents (11–16 years old) during class time. In each school, only 95% of the expected participants responded due to absences or parental refusal. Adolescents with missing data (no height, no weight, no PA, inconsistent or no response: $n = 221$) were then excluded from this study, as were adolescents from an ethnic community other than Caucasian or Melanesian (mostly Asian and Polynesian: $n = 28$), as these subsamples were too small. The final total sample was 447 adolescents.

Parents gave informed written consent prior to the children's participation in the study, in line with the legal requirements and the Declaration of Helsinki. The protocol was also approved by the Ethics Committee of the University of New Caledonia.

2.2. Measures

2.2.1. Anthropometric Parameters

All anthropometric data, including body mass index (BMI) and the International Obesity Task Force (IOTF) criteria [23], were collected by trained staff (the senior researcher) in the school nurse's office. Height was measured to the nearest 0.1 cm using a portable stadiometer (Leicester Tanita HR 001, Tanita Corporation, Tokyo, Japan). Weight was determined to the nearest 0.1 kg using a scale (Tanita HA 503, Tanita Corporation, Tokyo, Japan), with adolescents weighed in light clothing. Body mass index (BMI) was calculated by dividing weight in kilograms by height squared in meters.

The BMI standard deviation score (BMI-SDS) and percentile were calculated by the LMS method using the IOTF reference values. Weight status was defined according to the IOTF criteria, which are used to classify BMI values according to age and gender as thin (underweight), normal weight, overweight, or obese, based on adult BMI cutoffs at 18 years [23].

2.2.2. Sociodemographic Characteristics

Ethnicity was self-reported by the adolescents using an anonymous survey tool and categorized as recommended in the report on New Caledonia [24] from the *Institut National de la Santé Et de la Recherche Médicale* (INSERM; National Institute of Health and Medical Research). Three SES categories were generated according to the National Statistics Socio-Economic Classification [25]: managerial and professional occupations (high), intermediate occupations (medium), and routine and manual occupations (low). According to the latest census in New Caledonia [26] and a European standard for the degree of urbanization [27], Noumea and its suburbs were classified as urban and the other areas were classified as rural.

2.2.3. SSB Consumption

SSB consumption was assessed by first asking: "Do you drink SSBs?" Average amounts were then assessed with the question: "How many glasses (250 mL), cans (330 mL), small bottles (500 mL) or big bottles (1500 mL) do you drink per week on average?" The total SSB intake per week, converted to liters, was calculated by adding up the volumes of the total number of glasses, cans and bottles. Adolescents who answered "No" to the first question were considered as consuming 0 L per week.

2.2.4. Self-Weight Perception

Adolescents were asked about their self-weight perception with the following question: "Given your age and height, would you say that you are about the right weight, too big, or too skinny?" [28]

2.2.5. Physical Activity

The self-report International Physical Activity Questionnaire-Short Form (IPAQ-SF) was filled out on the research day with the researchers' assistance. The total number of days and minutes of PA was calculated for each participant [29]. Total PA time was converted to hours per week.

2.2.6. Knowledge and Opinion about SSBs

Three parameters assessed participants' knowledge about SSBs.

First, participants expressed their opinion about the effects of SSBs on weight by responding to this statement: "Drinking regular sodas, fruit drinks, sports or energy drinks, and other sugar-sweetened drinks can cause weight gain." Responses were categorized as: agree (strongly/somewhat agree) or disagree (disagree completely, strongly/somewhat disagree).

Second, participants answered the following question to assess their "knowledge about sugar": "How many sugar lumps does a regular can of, for example, non-diet cola contain?" Responses were categorized as: underestimated (<5 lumps), accurate (5–10 lumps), overestimated (>10 lumps), and don't know.

Last, participants answered the following question to assess their "knowledge about energy expenditure": "How much time do you need to run (at moderate speed) to eliminate the energy intake from drinking a regular can of, for example, non-diet cola?" The four response categories were: underestimated (<30 min), accurate (30–60 min), overestimated (>60 min), and don't know.

2.3. Statistics

All analyses were conducted using R 3.1.0. [30] with a significance level of $p = 0.05$.

First, differences between categories for each explanatory factor were tested one by one. Differences were tested with the χ^2 test or Fisher's exact test (according to implementation conditions) for categorical variables and with means equality tests (Student, Welch or Wilcoxon) for numerical variables with binary factors. One-way ANOVA and the Kruskal-Wallis test were coupled with a post-hoc t-test and Nemenyi's test, respectively, when needed for numerical variables with other factors. The PA-quantity of SSB consumption correlation was determined and tested with Spearman's test because Pearson's test was not applicable.

The adolescents' quantified SSB consumption was globally assessed by multiple regression and multifactorial ANOVA to detect associations, possible interactions and a confounding bias between factors. The significant pairwise interactions were included in the regression and ANOVA.

3. Results

Table 1 shows that socioeconomic factors were not discriminant for the "prevalence" of SSB consumption. Sex, living environment, ethnic community, SES and weight status were not significant factors and generally about 90% of the adolescents declared consuming SSBs. In addition, boys were significantly more physically active than girls (14.31 h·week^{-1} for boys vs. 12.18 h·week^{-1} for girls, $p = 0.01$), Melanesians were significantly more physically active than Caucasians (11.23 h·week^{-1} for Caucasians vs. 14.05 h·week^{-1} for Melanesians, $p < 0.01$), and adolescents were significantly more physically active in rural areas than in urban areas (13.64 h·week^{-1} in rural vs. 10.88 h·week^{-1} in urban, $p < 0.01$).

Table 1. Population: proportions of weight status, weight perception, SSB consumption (yes or no) and physical activity according to sex, living environment, ethnic community, socioeconomic status (SES) and weight status (n = 447).

		Size	Weight Status (%)				Self-Weight Perception (%)				SSB Consumption (%)			Physical Activity (h·week⁻¹)	
			UnN *	Overweight	Obese	p-Value #	Too Skinny	Normal	Too Big	p-Value #	Yes	No	p-Value #	Mean ± SD	p-Value †
Sex	Boys	194	65.5	19.1	15.5	0.453	13.9	67.5	18.6	0.393	90.7	9.3	0.946	14.31 ± 9.31	0.011
	Girls	253	64.0	23.3	12.7		16.6	61.3	22.1		90.9	9.1		12.18 ± 7.81	
Living environment	Rural	361	60.9	23.0	16.1	0.002	15.2	63.7	21.1	0.873	91.7	8.3	0.278	13.64 ± 8.68	0.007
	Urban	86	80.2	15.1	4.7		16.3	65.1	18.6		87.2	12.8		10.88 ± 7.62	
Ethnic community	Caucasian	149	75.8	12.8	11.4	0.001	15.4	67.8	16.8	0.354	87.9	12.1	0.183	11.23 ± 8.67	0.001
	Melanesian	298	59.1	25.8	15.1		15.4	62.1	22.5		92.3	7.7		14.05 ± 8.34	
SES	Low	205	58.1	24.9	17.1	0.041	16.1	62.9	21.0	0.831	89.8	10.2	0.751	12.69 ± 8.03	0.586
	Medium	115	65.2	20.9	13.9		17.4	61.7	20.9		92.2	7.8		13.21 ± 8.94	
	High	127	74.8	16.5	8.7		12.6	67.7	19.7		91.3	8.7		13.68 ± 9.28	
Weight status	UnN *	289					23.5	71.6	4.8	<0.001	92.4	7.6	0.289	13.25 ± 8.62	0.731
	Overweight	96					1.0	56.3	42.7		88.5	11.5		13.18 ± 8.36	
	Obese	62					0.0	40.3	59.7		87.1	12.9		12.32 ± 8.56	

* UnN: underweight and normal. # χ² test or Fisher's exact test. † Binary factors: Student's or Welch's t-test. Other factors: one-way ANOVA.

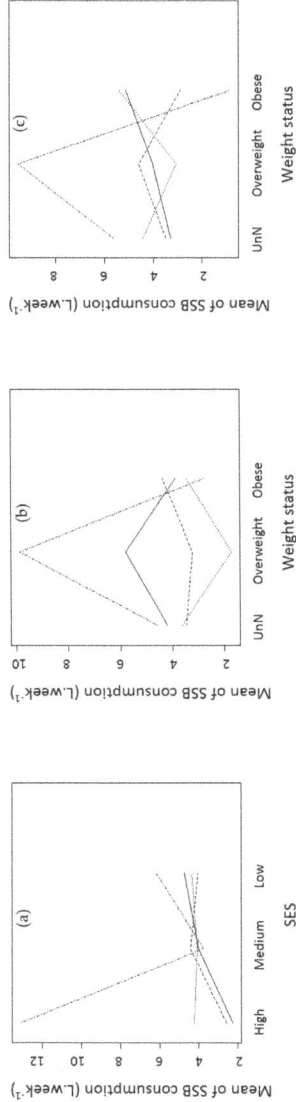

Figure 1. Pairwise factor interaction plots for SSB consumption: (**a**) Socioeconomic status (SES) vs. knowledge about energy expenditure, p = 0.005; (**b**) Weight status vs. knowledge about sugar, p = 0.011; (**c**) Weight status vs. knowledge about energy expenditure, p = 0.002. Type of line corresponds to knowledge. Solid line: adolescents who overestimated; dashed line: adolescents who gave accurate answers; dotted line: adolescents who underestimated; dotted-dashed line: adolescents who did not know.

The analysis of factor interactions revealed significant pairwise interactions between SES and knowledge about energy expenditure ($p < 0.01$), weight status and knowledge about sugar ($p = 0.01$), weight status and knowledge about energy expenditure ($p < 0.01$), and PA and knowledge about energy expenditure ($p = 0.02$). Figure 1 shows the significant pairwise interactions between these categorical factors.

Table 2 shows that sex, SES, weight status, self-weight perception, knowledge about sugar, opinion about SSBs and weight gain, and PA were not significantly associated with quantity of SSB consumption. Conversely, living environment, ethnic community and knowledge about energy expenditure were significantly related to the quantity of SSBs consumed. In this general model, only interactions between SES and knowledge about energy expenditure ($p = 0.01$) and between PA and knowledge about energy expenditure ($p = 0.02$) were significant.

SSB consumption was significantly higher in rural environments than in urban environments, with respective values of 4.49 L·week^{-1} and 1.94 L·week^{-1} ($p < 0.01$, Table 2).

Melanesian adolescents consumed many more SSBs than their Caucasian counterparts, with respective values of 4.77 L·week^{-1} and 2.46 L·week^{-1} ($p < 0.01$, Table 2).

Weight status and self-weight perception were not significant factors of SSB consumption ($p = 0.94$ and 0.59, respectively). However, weight status significantly interacted with knowledge about sugar (Figure 1b, $p = 0.01$) and knowledge about energy expenditure (Figure 1c, $p < 0.01$), but these interactions were not satisfactory factors in the general ANOVA model (Table 2, $p = 0.15$ and $p = 0.37$, respectively).

The correlation between PA and the quantity of SSB consumption was $\rho = 0.026$ and this was not significant ($p = 0.583$). However, PA has to be taken into account to explain SSB consumption (even if $p = 0.11$) because of the significant interactions between PA and knowledge about energy expenditure ($p = 0.02$).

Knowledge about sugar was not a significant factor for SSB consumption ($p = 0.12$, Table 2), but most of the adolescents (192 for "accurate" and 153 for "overestimated", i.e., 77%) reported knowing that there is a lot sugar in an SSB can. Conversely, knowledge about energy expenditure was a significant factor ($p = 0.03$), and the adolescents categorized as "don't know" for energy expenditure knowledge consumed significantly more SSBs (6.22 L·week^{-1}) than the others did (4.26 L·week^{-1} for adolescents who underestimated, 3.64 L·week^{-1} for adolescents who gave an accurate answer, and 3.73 L·week^{-1} for adolescents who overestimated the energy expenditure required to eliminate a SSB unit). The multiple regression in Table 2 shows that the higher the estimated expenditure, the lower the SSB consumption (B = −6.18 for "underestimated", B = −7.75 for "accurate" and B = −8.29 for "overestimated").

Opinion about the SSB consumption−weight gain relationship was not a significant factor for SSB consumption (B = 0.57, $p = 0.20$) and most of the adolescents (349, i.e., 78%) agreed with the statement "consuming SSBs can cause weight gain."

Table 2. SSB consumption: quantity, multifactorial regression and ANOVA (n = 447).

		Size	Quantity (L·week⁻¹)		Multiple Regression [1] (R² = 0.25; R²adj = 0.18)		Multifactorial ANOVA [1]
			Mean ± SD	p-Value *	B ± SE (95% CI)	p-Value	p-Value
Sex	Boys	194	4.25 ± 4.30	0.258	0.50 ± 0.38 (−0.24;1.24)	0.187	0.187
	Girls	253	3.81 ± 4.00				
Living environment	Rural	361	4.49 ± 4.31	<0.001	−1.67 ± 0.51 (−2.67;−0.66)	0.001	0.001
	Urban	86	1.94 ± 2.39				
Ethnic community	Caucasian	149	2.46 ± 3.23	<0.001	1.91 ± 0.43 (1.07;2.75)	<0.001	<0.001
	Melanesian	298	4.77 ± 4.32				
SES [†]	Low	205	4.44 ± 4.17 [a]	0.014	−11.08 ± 3.23 (−17.42;−4.74)	0.001	0.607
	Medium	115	4.20 ± 3.83 [a,b]		−11.06 ± 3.19 (−17.34;−4.79)	0.001	
	High	127	3.11 ± 4.23 [b]				
Weight status	Underweight and normal	289	3.86 ± 3.91	0.392			0.943
	Overweight	96	4.51 ± 4.75		1.86 ± 2.62 (−3.28;7.01)	0.477	
	Obese	62	3.87 ± 4.09		−1.54 ± 3.09 (−7.61;4.53)	0.618	
Weight perception	Too skinny	69	4.31 ± 4.30	0.748			0.590
	Normal	286	3.99 ± 4.09		−0.35 ± 0.53 (−1.39;0.69)	0.511	
	Too big	92	3.81 ± 4.18		−0.75 ± 0.73 (−2.19;0.69)	0.305	
How many sugar lumps in a SSB can?	Do not know	24	5.23 ± 5.72	0.071			0.124
	Underestimate	78	3.25 ± 3.61		−0.52 ± 1.30 (−3.08;2.03)	0.689	
	Accurate	153	3.53 ± 3.59		−0.30 ± 1.26 (−2.77;2.16)	0.808	
	Overestimate	192	4.53 ± 4.42		−0.11 ± 1.23 (−2.53;2.32)	0.932	
How much running is needed to eliminate the sugar contained in a SSB can?	Do not know	27	6.22 ± 6.39	0.174			0.033
	Underestimate	137	4.26 ± 4.23		−6.18 ± 3.09 (−12.26;−0.10)	0.046	
	Accurate	201	3.64 ± 3.75		−7.75 ± 3.03 (−13.71;−1.79)	0.011	
	Overestimate	82	3.73 ± 3.74		−8.29 ± 3.15 (−14.47;−2.10)	0.009	
Consuming SSBs can cause weight gain	Agree	349	3.77 ± 4.06	0.027	0.57 ± 0.45 (−0.31;1.46)	0.204	0.204
	Disagree	98	4.82 ± 4.28				
Physical activity		447			0.29 ± 0.11 (0.08;0.50)	0.006	0.111

[1] Analyses adjusted by the significant pairwise interactions: SES and knowledge about energy expenditure (p = 0.011), weight status and knowledge about sugar (p = 0.147), weight status and knowledge about energy expenditure (p = 0.367), and physical activity and knowledge about energy expenditure (p = 0.017). * Binary factors: Student's, Welch's or Wilcoxon's test. Other factors: one-way ANOVA or Kruskal-Wallis' test. [†] One or several subscripted letters in a cell indicate a post-hoc pairwise t-test result. Similar letters: no significant difference between two groups. Post-hoc pairwise t-test p-values: p = 0.604 for low and medium, p = 0.013 for low and high and p = 0.081 for medium and high.

4. Discussion

The main result of this study was that 90% of the New Caledonian adolescents claimed to regularly drink SSBs. Moreover, the entire population was concerned since they reported regular consumption regardless of sex, living environment, ethnic community, socioeconomic status and weight status. Notably, the quantity of SSBs was strongly correlated with social factors like living environment and ethnic community but weight status and self-weight perception were surprisingly not linked to quantity.

Knowledge about sugar was not significantly linked to quantity of SSB consumption but knowledge about energy expenditure was.

4.1. Sociodemographic Factors

In New Caledonia, the living environment, ethnic community and SES are interconnected factors. For example, most of the people living in rural environments have tribal lifestyles and are Melanesian, and most of the people from other ethnic communities (such as Caucasians) live in the urban environments of Noumea and its suburbs. Moreover, rural inhabitants are usually classified as low SES since they generally live of food crops [4]. Therefore, it is unsurprising that the quantity of consumed SSBs presented in Table 2 was significantly higher in rural environments, Melanesian adolescents, and low-SES adolescents as these factors are very much intertwined. This also may explain why, although the high-SES adolescents consumed significantly fewer SSBs than the low-SES adolescents, this factor was not significant in the general regression model (Table 2).

Adolescents living in rural areas reported significantly higher SSB consumption than those living in urban areas (4.49 L·week^{-1} vs. 1.94 L·week^{-1}, respectively). This has also been observed in other countries. Indeed, Park et al. [6] reported that SSB intake differs significantly among US adults according to geographic region. They found that the proportion of adults who consumed SSBs $\geq$2 times per day, or more than 3.5 L·week^{-1}, was highest among adults living in the East South Central region of the US [6]. Sharkey et al., who studied eating behaviors among rural and urban adults, found that the prevalence and high level of SSB consumption ($\geq$3 cans or glasses of SSB per day, or more than 5 L·week^{-1}) were greater among rural adults (52.4% prevalence and 17.7% high consumption) compared with urban counterparts (43.7% prevalence and 10.5% high consumption) [31]. The differences were partially explained by cultural norms, SSB availability, and/or state and local obesity prevention programs [6,31]. In New Caledonia, SSBs are widely available near all schools before, during and after the school day, and health education programs are delivered to all areas of the archipelago. Media access is nevertheless easier in the urban environments, and the media often provide strong warnings about the sugar in industrial products and its impact on health [10]. Moreover, Hughes and Lawrence [12] pointed out some of the factors that have changed Pacific Islanders' behaviors, notably the acceptance and/or belief that foreign (imported) goods are superior. This may explain why Melanesian adolescents reported consuming significantly more SSBs than their Caucasian counterparts (4.77 L·week^{-1} and 2.46 L·week^{-1}, respectively). In addition, a recent review evaluated the interventions targeting the consumption of high-sugar products by Pacific Island adolescents [10]. The authors reported that school and community-based interventions have had little success in reducing the consumption of these products for the moment [10].

As studies have shown, SSBs may also replace water as the daily beverage [32], and access to potable water might explain our observation in parts of rural New Caledonia [33]. In particularly remote areas, the water comes from desalination plants and/or the treated water may be of poor bacteriological quality [33]. People living in environments where access to drinking water is a problem might become suspicious of this essential natural resource, especially as the taste can be unpleasant. This might explain the preference for SSBs among some rural populations.

Several factors and their mutual interactions may in fact explain the prevalence of SSB consumption in rural environments and should be considered in the future: (1) drinking tap water may be not safe, so it is better to drink something else; (2) drinking SSBs or giving money to children to buy SSBs may be a way to ostensibly show personal earning power (more than buying bottled water); and (3) adolescent eating habits are influenced by media campaigns that communicate health and nutrition warnings, especially in urban environments.

4.2. Weight Status and Self-Weight Perception

A previous study reported that weight status might be linked to SSB intake [10], although another study found no association [34]. Researchers have explained this non-significant finding as underreported intake [35] or reduced intake by overweight and obese adolescents wanting to lose weight [34]. Our study shows that neither weight status ($p = 0.94$) nor self-weight perception ($p = 0.59$) was a significant explanatory factor for the quantity of SSB consumption (Table 2).

Previous studies conducted in New Caledonia have shown that people are aware that obesity can exacerbate noncommunicable diseases but they may not know the actual definition of obesity [36] and thus whether they are concerned. Adolescents have also shown a mismatch between weight perception and reality [19]. It is therefore possible that some of the overweight adolescents in the current study were not aware of their own weight status. In addition, overweight is overall associated with unhealthy lifestyles—not only SSB consumption but also other energy-dense food consumption. The total energy intake was unfortunately not assessed in this study and this might explain why weight status was not a significant explanatory factor for quantity of SSB consumption.

However, weight status related to knowledge may be linked to SSB intake (Figure 1) although, as shown in Table 2, the interactions between weight status and knowledge were not significant in the multiple regression ($p = 0.15$ for interactions between weight status and knowledge about sugar; $p = 0.37$ for interactions between weight status and knowledge about energy expenditure). Jasti et al. [11] found that overweight status modified the effect of SSB knowledge on SSB consumption. In their study, less SSB knowledge was associated with higher SSB consumption (OR = 3.56) only among overweight students, with no association in non-overweight students [11]. Our analysis of pairwise interactions (Figure 1b,c) showed that among the adolescents categorized as "don't know" for sugar knowledge, those who were overweight had higher SSB intake than the others. Their overweight status may have been due in part to their lack of knowledge: they did not know how to behave healthily. On the contrary, the obese adolescents categorized as "don't know" consumed fewer SSBs. This might be explained by medical monitoring: these adolescents had undoubtedly been warned against excessive SSB consumption and thus they refrained from drinking "too much" even if they had little knowledge about SSBs (sugar content and energy expenditure). In addition, the more highly the overweight adolescents estimated the sugar quantity in a can, the higher their SSB intake was. This may be due to fatalistic feelings or enjoyment being prioritized over health, especially when friends also drink SSBs: "There's a lot of sugar in sweetened beverages, it's unhealthy and it may cause weight gain, but sweetened beverages are so good and my friends are drinking a can . . . So, yes! I drink a can too!" [37]. But these observations should be carefully considered because of the small sample sizes in some subcategories.

4.3. Physical Activity

Bibiloni et al. [9] found that even though beverage intake and beverage total energy intake were positively associated with PA in Spanish adolescents, there was no association between PA and SSB intake (fruit drinks, soda or energy/sport beverages). In this study, inactive boys claimed that they drank more than 9 L·week^{-1} of SSBs (370.8 mL fruit drinks, 441.6 mL soda and 495.0 mL energy/sport beverages per day) and active boys claimed drinking more than 8 L·week^{-1} (338.3 mL fruit drinks, 474.0 mL soda and 337.1 mL energy/sport beverages per day). Inactive girls claimed drinking more than 6.5 L·week^{-1} of SSBs (312.6 mL fruit drinks, 400.4 mL soda and 233.3 mL energy/sport beverages per day) and active girls also claimed drinking more than 6.5 L·week^{-1} (269.7 mL fruit drinks, 365.4 mL soda and 330.0 mL energy/sport beverages per day) [9]. Our method differed from that of Bibiloni et al. Indeed, PA was not categorized but was processed as a continuous variable; for this reason, any comparisons must be cautiously made. However, when the active and inactive adolescents in New Caledonia were mixed, they reported drinking fewer SSBs than the Spaniards (4.25 L·week^{-1} in boys and 3.81 L·week^{-1} in girls, Table 2). In contrast to Bibiloni et al.'s study, our findings showed a positive correlation between PA and quantity of SSB consumption (B = 0.29, $p \leq 0.01$). To explain this result, we need to consider that being active at school in a year-round subtropical climate requires high levels of hydration [38] and adolescents may prefer drinking other drinks than tap water in some remote areas (see Section 4.1.). In addition, the adolescents were significantly more active when they were boys (14.31 h·week^{-1} in boys vs. 12.18 h·week^{-1} in girls, p = 0.01), Melanesian (14.05 h·week^{-1} for Melanesians vs. 11.23 h·week^{-1} for Caucasians, p < 0.01), and living in rural areas (13.64 h·week^{-1} for rural adolescents vs. 10.88 h·week^{-1} for urban adolescents, p < 0.01) (Table 1). These results are in accordance with Zongo et al.'s study [20] and they support the observation that the interactions between sociocultural factors and behavioral factors are mutual in New Caledonia.

4.4. Knowledge and Opinion

Interestingly, knowledge about sugar was not a satisfactory explanatory factor (p = 0.12). This finding lines up with Park et al.'s findings [6] but is opposed to those of Jasti et al. [11]. The non-explanatory nature of this factor seems to indicate that thinking SSBs contain a lot of sugar does not affect the New Caledonian adolescents' consumption. Notably, many of them gave an accurate answer or overestimated the quantity of sugar, and consequently they "knew"—or certainly thought they knew – that there was a lot of sugar, but that knowledge was not always totally accurate. In addition, despite this often vague knowledge, they consumed SSBs. However, knowledge about energy expenditure seemed to encourage the young people to consume less [39]. Indeed, the adolescents who were categorized as "don't know" claimed that they drank many more SSBs than the others (6.22 L·week^{-1} for the "don't know" vs. <4.3 L·week^{-1} for the others). Moreover, more than 78% reported agreeing with the statement "consuming SSBs can cause weight gain" and the adolescents who agreed that drinking SSBs can cause weight gain drank less than the others (3.77 L·week^{-1} for "agree" vs. 4.82 L·week^{-1} for "disagree", p = 0.03). Similarly, Park et al. found many more individuals (≥29%) with high SSB consumption (more than 3.5 L·week^{-1}, ≥2 servings per day) among those who did not think that drinking SSBs contributes to weight gain, compared with those who agreed about the SSB-weight gain relationship (18.3% consumed 3.5L·week^{-1}, ≥2 times per day) [6]. Nevertheless, opinion about the SSB consumption–weight gain relationship was not a satisfactory predictive factor (B = 0.57, p = 0.20), i.e., statistically, the B coefficient can be assumed to be zero. This seems to suggest that thinking SSBs can cause weight does not influence the SSB consumption in the adolescents of New Caledonia.

Our findings suggest that the key factor is "the notion of effort" related to SSB intake rather than "accurately knowing." Indeed, the adjusted analyses showed that the "don't know" adolescents consumed many more SSBs than the others, and the adolescents who thought that high energy expenditure was needed to eliminate the content of a SSB unit—that is, the "overestimators"—claimed consuming fewer SSBs than those who "underestimated" or were "accurate" (Table 2). Having an accurate answer seemed to be not that important as long as the notion of the physical effort needed to negate SSB intake had been learned. Moreover, even though most of the New Caledonian adolescents thought consuming SSBs can cause weight gain, they nonetheless drank them. Further studies are now needed to explain this observation.

4.5. Limitations and Strengths of the Study

This cross-sectional study does not provide evidence of causal associations or trends in the long term. However, the data were directly collected in the schools of interest: anthropometric measures were obtained during medical examination, providing more reliable assessments [19], and the survey was filled out on research days in the presence of researchers.

Adolescents were asked about their SSB consumption, PA, and knowledge and opinions about SSBs. The questions seemed to be easily understood and produced straightforward answers [39]. Yet some adolescents still gave aberrant answers probably because of a misunderstanding about the weekly average and the container volumes, and these answers were removed from analysis. The significant results were nevertheless based on robust statistical tests and thus were not impacted. Moreover, some of the adolescents might have taken sips from the drinks of the regular consumers. We assume that they took these small quantities into account in their responses, even though such quantities were probably negligible compared to drinking from one's own container.

This study examined self-reported data, as well: SSB consumption, ethnic community and PA. These measures are subjective, especially PA quantification, but the associated surveys are commonly used to obtain this type of data [29,40]. This limitation might explain the non-significance of PA in explaining the quantity of SSB consumption. Future studies will therefore need to use objective data to assess PA.

As noted, the total energy intake was not assessed in this study even though weight status was introduced as an explanatory factor. It was therefore not possible to adjust the multiple regression with the total energy intake.

This study aimed to determine associations between SSB consumption and sociodemographic characteristics, including ethnic community, in adolescents of New Caledonia. However, for statistical reasons—that is, the sample size—only the two main ethnic communities were retained, i.e., Caucasian and Melanesian. This may have introduced a bias for comparisons with the general population of New Caledonia.

5. Conclusions

This study provides insight into the links between SSB consumption and socioeconomic factors, actual weight status and self-weight perception, PA, and knowledge and opinions about SSBs in New Caledonian adolescents.

First, this study showed that SSB consumption in New Caledonia is strongly associated with ethnic community and living environment. This result should contribute to developing community-based health promotion strategies.

Second, New Caledonian adolescents seem to have an inadequate understanding of the associations between PA, food consumption and health, which raises questions about health communication campaigns from an educational point of view [4,6]. Notably, knowing how much physical effort is needed to negate an SSB seems to have more influence than knowing the sugar quantity in an SSB can. As noted, the "notion of effort" related to SSB intake may best drive adolescents to moderate SSB consumption.

Yet more studies are needed on how New Caledonian youths relate to issues of health, nutrition and physical activity. Longitudinal and qualitative studies should examine why adolescents drink so many SSBs even when they "know"—that "knowledge" often being quite inexact—that there is too much sugar in them and they think SSBs can cause weight gain.

Author Contributions: S.F. and O.G. conceived and designed the study. S.F., S.C., Y.C. and Y.L. collected data. G.W. conducted the statistical analyses and drafted the manuscript. All the authors revised and approved the final submitted version of the manuscript.

Funding: This research received no external funding.

Acknowledgments: We thank the school teaching teams and administrative staff for their help and support in our investigations, especially the Department 'Promotion de la santé en milieu scolaire' of the Vice-Rectorat of New Caledonia.

Conflicts of Interest: The authors declare no conflict of interest.

References

1. Stubbs, C.O.; Lee, A.J. The obesity epidemic: Both energy intake and physical activity contribute. *Med. J. Aust.* **2004**, *181*, 489–491. [PubMed]
2. Harnack, L.; Stang, J.; Story, M. Soft Drink Consumption Among US Children and Adolescents: Nutritional Consequences. *J. Am. Diet. Assoc.* **1999**, *99*, 436–441. [CrossRef]
3. Grimm, G.C.; Harnack, L.; Story, M. Factors associated with soft drink consumption in school-aged children. *J. Am. Diet. Assoc.* **2004**, *104*, 1244–1249. [CrossRef] [PubMed]
4. Aldwell, K.; Caillaud, C.; Galy, O.; Frayon, S.; Allman-Farinelli, M. Tackling the Consumption of High Sugar Products among Children and Adolescents in the Pacific Islands: Implications for Future Research. *Healthcare* **2018**, *6*, 81. [CrossRef] [PubMed]
5. United States Department of Agriculture. *Department of Health and Human Services Nutrition and your health: Dietary Guidelines for Americans, 2010*, 7th ed.; United States Department of Agriculture: Washington, DC, USA, 2010.
6. Park, S.; Onufrak, S.; Sherry, B.; Blanck, H.M. The relationship between health-related knowledge and sugar-sweetened beverage intake among US adults. *J. Acad. Nutr. Diet.* **2014**, *114*, 1059–1066. [CrossRef] [PubMed]
7. Malik, V.S.; Hu, F.B. Sweeteners and Risk of Obesity and Type 2 Diabetes: The Role of Sugar-Sweetened Beverages. *Curr. Diab. Rep.* **2012**, *12*, 195–203. [CrossRef] [PubMed]
8. Mardiyati, N.; Song, W.; Opoku-Acheampong, A.; Miller, C.; Kidd, T.; Wang, W. Effects of Body Weight Perception and Goals on Consumption Behaviour among College Students. *FASEB J.* **2015**, *29*, 900.22.
9. Bibiloni, M.D.; Özen, A.E.; Pons, A.; González-Gross, M.; Tur, J.A. Physical Activity and Beverage Consumption among Adolescents. *Nutrients* **2016**, *8*, 389. [CrossRef]
10. Kessaram, T.; McKenzie, J.; Girin, N.; Merilles, O.E.A.; Pullar, J.; Roth, A.; White, P.; Hoy, D. Overweight, obesity, physical activity and sugar-sweetened beverage consumption in adolescents of Pacific islands: Results from the Global School-Based Student Health Survey and the Youth Risk Behavior Surveillance System. *BMC Obes.* **2015**, *2*, 34. [CrossRef]
11. Jasti, S.; Rubin, R.; Doak, C.M. Sugar-sweetened Beverage Knowledge and Consumption in College Students. *Health Behav. Policy Rev.* **2017**, *4*, 37–45. [CrossRef]
12. Hughes, R.G.; Lawrence, M.A. Globalization, food and health in Pacific Island countries. *Asia Pac. J. Clin. Nutr* **2005**, *14*, 298–306. [PubMed]
13. Frayon, S.; Cherrier, S.; Cavaloc, Y.; Wattelez, G.; Lerrant, Y.; Galy, O. Relationship of body fat and body mass index in young Pacific Islanders: A cross-sectional study in European, Melanesian and Polynesian groups. *Pediatric Obes.* **2018**, *13*, 357–364. [CrossRef] [PubMed]
14. Pak, N.; Mcdonald, A.M.; McKenzie, J.; Tukuitonga, C. Soft drink consumption in Pacific Island countries and territories: A review of trade data. *Pac. Health Dialog* **2014**, *20*, 59–66. [PubMed]
15. Corsenac, P.; Annesi-Maesano, I.; Hoy, D.; Roth, A.; Rouchon, B.; Capart, I.; Taylor, R. Overweight and obesity in New Caledonian adults: Results from measured and adjusted self-reported anthropometric data. *Diabetes Res. Clin. Pract.* **2017**, *133*, 193–203. [CrossRef] [PubMed]
16. ISEE – Communautés. Available online: http://www.isee.nc/population/recensement/communautes (accessed on 16 November 2017).
17. Congrès de la Nouvelle-Calédonie. *Délibération n°106 du 15 janvier 2016 relative à l'avenir de l'école calédonienne*; Congrès de la Nouvelle-Calédonie: Nouméa, Nouvelle-Calédonie, 2016; Available online: https://www.ac-noumea.nc/IMG/pdf/de_libe_ration_no106_du_15.01.16_relative_a_l_avenir_de_l_e_cole_cale_donienne.pdf (accessed on 31 January 2019).
18. Eurisouke, V.; Gambey, C.; Welepa, P.; Bedon, P.; Berthou, L.; Demaneuf, T.; Eyherabide, M.; Poncet, E.; Bazenet, F.; Thomas, O.; et al. *Do Kamo Plan de Santé Calédonien 2018–2028*; Gouvernement de la Nouvelle-Calédonie: Nouméa, Nouvelle-Calédonie, 2018; p. 140. Available online: https://gouv.nc/sites/default/files/atoms/files/brochure_do_kamo_etre_epanoui_0.pdf (accessed on 31 January 2019).
19. Frayon, S.; Cherrier, S.; Cavaloc, Y.; Wattelez, G.; Touitou, A.; Zongo, P.; Yacef, K.; Caillaud, C.; Lerrant, Y.; Galy, O. Misperception of weight status in the pacific: Preliminary findings in rural and urban 11- to 16-year-olds of New Caledonia. *BMC Public Health* **2017**, *17*, 25. [CrossRef]

20. Zongo, P.; Frayon, S.; Antoine-Jonville, S.; Wattelez, G.; Le Roux, P.-Y.; Hue, O.; Galy, O. Anthropometric Characteristics and Physical Fitness in Rural and Urban 11- to 16-Year-Old Melanesian Adolescents: A Cross-sectional Study in New Caledonian Schools. *Asia Pac. J. Public Health* **2017**, *29*, 589–598. [CrossRef] [PubMed]

21. Tassié, J.; Papoz, L.; Barny, S.; Simon, D. Nutritional status in adults in the pluri-ethnic population of New Caledonia. *Int. J. Obes.* **1997**, *21*, 61–66. [CrossRef]

22. Frayon, S.; Cherrier, S.; Touitou, A.; Zongo, P.; Wattelez, G.; Yacef, K.; Caillaud, C.; Galy, O. Nutrition behaviors and sociodemographic factors associated with overweight in the multi-ethnic adolescents of New Caledonia. *Ethn. Health* **2017**, *24*, 194–210. [CrossRef]

23. Cole, T.J.; Lobstein, T. Extended international (IOTF) body mass index cut-offs for thinness, overweight and obesity. *Pediatric Obes.* **2012**, *7*, 284–294. [CrossRef]

24. Institut national de la santé et de la recherche médicale. *687 Situation sociale et comportements de santé des jeunes en Nouvelle-Calédonie. Premiers résultats*; Institut national de la santé et de la recherche médicale: Villejuif, France, 2008; p. 112.

25. Krieger, N.; Rose, D.; Pevalin, D.J. A Researcher's Guide to the National Statistics Socio-Economic Classification. *J. Public Health Policy* **2003**, *24*, 467. [CrossRef]

26. ISEE—Structure de la population et évolutions. Available online: http://www.isee.nc/population/recensement/structure-de-la-population-et-evolutions (accessed on 16 November 2017).

27. The European Union Labour Force Survey—Methods and Definitions—2001 (Eurostat, Guidelines, Labour Statistics, Survey). Available online: https://unstats.un.org/unsd/EconStatKB/KnowledgebaseArticle10230.aspx (accessed on 16 November 2017).

28. Jackson, S.E.; Johnson, F.; Croker, H.; Wardle, J. Weight perceptions in a population sample of English adolescents: Cause for celebration or concern? *Int. J. Obes.* **2015**, *39*, ijo2015126. [CrossRef] [PubMed]

29. *IPAQ Research Committee Guidelines for Data Processing and Analysis of the International Physical Activity Questionnaire (IPAQ)—Short and Long Forms*. The IPAQ group (www.ipaq.ki.se). 2005. Available online: https://docs.google.com/viewer?a=v&pid=sites&srcid=ZGVmYXVsdGRvbWFpbnx0aGVpcGFxfGd4OjE0NDgxMDk3NDU1YWRlZTM (accessed on 31 January 2019).

30. R Core Team. *A Language and Environment for Statistical Computing*; R Foundation for Statistical Computing: Vienna, Austria, 2014.

31. Sharkey, J.; Johnson, C.; Dean, W. Less-healthy eating behaviors have a greater association with a high level of sugar-sweetened beverage consumption among rural adults than among urban adults. *Food Nutr. Res.* **2011**, *55*, 5819. [CrossRef] [PubMed]

32. Lee, H.-S.; Park, S.; Kim, M.-H. Factors associated with low water intake among South Korean adolescents - Korea National Health and Nutrition Examination Survey, 2007–2010. *Nutr. Res. Pract.* **2014**, *8*, 74–80. [CrossRef] [PubMed]

33. Chavroche, J. *Contribution à l'élaboration d'un cadre réglementaire visant la distribution publique de l'eau en Nouvelle-Calédonie: Fondements sanitaires et propositions*; ENGEES, ENSP, DASS-NC: DASS Nouvelle-Calédonie; Ecole Nationale de Génie de l'eau et de l'environnement de Strasbourg: Strasbourg, France, 2005; p. 82. Available online: http://fulltext.bdsp.ehesp.fr/Ensp/Memoires/2005/igs/chavroche.pdf (accessed on 31 January 2019).

34. Park, S.; Sherry, B.; Foti, K.; Blanck, H.M. Self-Reported Academic Grades and Other Correlates of Sugar-Sweetened Soda Intake among US Adolescents. *J. Acad. Nutr. Diet.* **2012**, *112*, 125–131. [CrossRef] [PubMed]

35. Lioret, S.; Touvier, M.; Balin, M.; Huybrechts, I.; Dubuisson, C.; Dufour, A.; Bertin, M.; Maire, B.; Lafay, L. Characteristics of energy under-reporting in children and adolescents. *Br. J. Nutr.* **2011**, *105*, 1671–1680. [CrossRef] [PubMed]

36. ASS NC. *L'équilibre alimentaire: Rapport d'étude omnibus, Novembre 2011*; Agence Sanitaire et Sociale de la Nouvelle-Calédonie: Nouméa, Nouvelle-Calédonie, 2011.

37. Lawrence, H.; Nathan Reynolds, A.; Joseph Venn, B. Perceptions of the Healthfulness of Foods of New Zealand Adults Living with Prediabetes and Type 2 Diabetes: A Pilot Study. *J. Nutr. Educ. Behav.* **2017**, *49*, 339–345. [CrossRef] [PubMed]

38. Galy, O.; Antoine-jonville, S.; Reuillard, E.; Hue, O. Free hydration and well-being during physical education in tropical climate. In *Educ. St. Sociétés*; Editions des archives contemporaines: Paris, France, 2016; Volume 2, pp. 79–92.

39. Francis, J.; Martin, K.; Costa, B.; Christian, H.; Kaur, S.; Harray, A.; Barblett, A.; Oddy, W.H.; Ambrosini, G.; Allen, K.; et al. Informing Intervention Strategies to Reduce Energy Drink Consumption in Young People: Findings From Qualitative Research. *J. Nutr. Educ. Behav.* **2017**, *49*, 724–733. [CrossRef]

40. Lee, P.H.; Macfarlane, D.J.; Lam, T.; Stewart, S.M. Validity of the international physical activity questionnaire short form (IPAQ-SF): A systematic review. *Int. J. Behav. Nutr. Phys. Act.* **2011**, *8*, 115. [CrossRef]

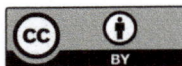

nutrients

MDPI

Article

Socioeconomic Disparities in Diet Vary According to Migration Status among Adolescents in Belgium

Manon Rouche [1,*], Bart de Clercq [2], Thérésa Lebacq [1,3], Maxim Dierckens [2], Nathalie Moreau [1,3], Lucille Desbouys [1], Isabelle Godin [4] and Katia Castetbon [1,3]

[1] Research Center in Epidemiology, Biostatistics and Clinical Research, School of Public Health, Université libre de Bruxelles (ULB), 1040 Brussels, Belgium; theresa.lebacq@ulb.ac.be (T.L.); nathalie.moreau@ulb.ac.be (N.M.); lucille.desbouys@ulb.ac.be (L.D.); katia.castetbon@ulb.ac.be (K.C.)
[2] Department of Public Health and Primary Care, Ghent University (UGent), 9000 Ghent, Belgium; b.declercq@ugent.be (B.d.C.); maxim.dierckens@ugent.be (M.D.)
[3] Service d'Information Promotion Education Santé (SIPES), School of Public Health, Université libre de Bruxelles (ULB), 1040 Brussels, Belgium
[4] Research Centre in Social Approaches to Health, School of Public Health, Université libre de Bruxelles (ULB), 1040 Brussels, Belgium; isabelle.godin@ulb.ac.be
* Correspondence: manon.rouche@ulb.ac.be; Tel.: +32-2-555-40-59

Received: 11 March 2019; Accepted: 6 April 2019; Published: 10 April 2019

Abstract: Little information concerning social disparities in adolescent dietary habits is currently available, especially regarding migration status. The aim of the present study was to estimate socioeconomic disparities in dietary habits of school adolescents from different migration backgrounds. In the 2014 cross-sectional "Health Behavior in School-Aged Children" survey in Belgium, food consumption was estimated using a self-administrated short food frequency questionnaire. In total, 19,172 school adolescents aged 10–19 years were included in analyses. Multilevel multiple binary and multinomial logistic regressions were performed, stratified by migration status (natives, 2nd- and 1st-generation immigrants). Overall, immigrants more frequently consumed both healthy and unhealthy foods. Indeed, 32.4% of 1st-generation immigrants, 26.5% of 2nd-generation immigrants, and 16.7% of natives consumed fish ≥two days a week. Compared to those having a high family affluence scale (FAS), adolescents with a low FAS were more likely to consume chips and fries ≥once a day (vs. <once a day: Natives aRRR = 1.39 (95%CI: 1.12–1.73); NS in immigrants). Immigrants at schools in Flanders were less likely than those in Brussels to consume sugar-sweetened beverages 2–6 days a week (vs. ≤once a week: Natives aRRR = 1.86 (95%CI: 1.32–2.62); 2nd-generation immigrants aRRR = 1.52 (1.11–2.09); NS in 1st-generation immigrants). The migration gradient observed here underlines a process of acculturation. Narrower socioeconomic disparities in immigrant dietary habits compared with natives suggest that such habits are primarily defined by culture of origin. Nutrition interventions should thus include cultural components of dietary habits.

Keywords: migration status; dietary habits; food frequency questionnaire; socioeconomic disparities; adolescents

1. Introduction

High consumption of foods such as chips and fries [1] and sugar-sweetened beverages (SSB) [2] might be associated with increased noncommunicable diseases (NCD); by contrast, adequate consumption of fruits, vegetables [2,3], fish [2], and dairy products [4] might reduce NCD and all-cause mortality. Furthermore, it has been estimated that up to two-thirds of NCD social inequalities may be explained by dietary disparities [5,6].

In addition, evidence indicates that dietary habits during adolescence may continue into adulthood [7–9]. To implement effective prevention of NCD throughout the lifetime, disparities in adolescent eating behavior warrant elucidation. However, information on this topic is scarce in Western countries. Although several studies have pointed out the association between dietary habits and socioeconomic status (SES) among adolescents [10,11], SES may not explain all observed variations.

Among other determinants of dietary habits, migration status may play a role [12,13]; however, published studies are rare, even among adults, and are often oriented towards a specific ethnic group [12,13]. Studies on health related to migration have revealed a mortality advantage in immigrants compared to natives, despite the lower SES of most immigrants [14]. This paradox could be explained by the "healthy-migrant effect", i.e., positive self-selection, and an unhealthy return-migration effect, also known as the "salmon-bias hypothesis" [14]. However, these selection processes are subject to caution; "beneficial cultural and behavioral factors", like dietary habits, may be the most plausible explanation for this paradox [14]. The immigrant health advantage may also tend to wear off with length of stay in the host country, mostly due to an acculturation process [15,16], wherein foreign individuals partially integrate behaviors and cultural aspects of the host population while maintaining their roots [17]. This has been highlighted in some adult dietary studies and suggests gradual adaptation to the natives' eating habits according to years spent in the host country [18]. In adolescents, dietary habits varying according to migration status (including a gradient across migration generations) might also be expected, but such investigations have thus far been limited [19,20].

An effect modification between migration status and socioeconomic characteristics was emphasized in a previous study on adult self-rated health: A gradient was revealed across social classes in natives, which was not the case for immigrants from poor countries [21]. Similarly, in adolescents, a clear gradient throughout family affluence categories was observed for health-related quality of life in natives but not in immigrants [22]. Therefore, a possible effect modification of migration status on socioeconomic characteristics should be considered when evaluating disparities in dietary habits.

The aim of this study was to estimate socioeconomic disparities in dietary habits of school adolescents from different migration backgrounds. We first hypothesized that adolescent immigrants have healthier dietary habits than natives and that food consumption frequencies increase or decrease gradually according to the migration generation, related to an acculturation process. Secondly, we assumed that migration status might modify the association between socioeconomic characteristics and dietary habits in adolescents.

2. Materials and Methods

Research was carried out using data from the "Health Behavior in School-Aged Children" (HBSC) survey conducted in 2014 in Belgium. The cross-national HBSC survey takes place every four years in around 40 countries in Europe and North America under the aegis of the World Health Organization (WHO) Regional Office for Europe. Its goal is to produce comprehensive indicators supporting implementation of health prevention and promotion policies and interventions. Questionnaires are self-administrated in the classroom, and anonymity and data confidentiality are guaranteed [23].

Belgium has a regionalized administration in which wide demographic variations are observed, including those concerning migration. In 2014 in Belgium, this study was carried out separately in French- and Dutch-speaking schools covering the three regions, Wallonia, Flanders, and Brussels, with the latter including both French- and Dutch-speaking schools.

This survey was carried out according to guidelines articulated in the Declaration of Helsinki. For French-speaking schools, the survey was approved by school authorities. This protocol was not submitted to a medical ethics committee in view of the topics and methods used for data collection (Belgian law of May 7, 2004 and Advisory Committee on Bioethics of Belgium, opinion n°40, 12/2/2007). For Dutch-speaking schools, the study was approved by the ethics review committee of the University Hospital of Ghent (project EC/2013/1145). Following advice from school authorities, no written consent was requested for French-speaking schools; for the Dutch-speaking schools, consent was passive. Adolescents were clearly informed about survey content and about their full right to refuse to fill out the questionnaire or answer specific questions. All procedures used during data collection enabled confidentiality and anonymity.

2.1. Sampling

The French- and Dutch-speaking surveys were conducted on a random sample stratified proportionally with the school networks and included public and private schools. In addition, in the French-speaking part, the sample was stratified proportionally with the province ($n = 6$); in the Dutch-speaking part, it was stratified proportionally with the form of education (ordinary, general, technical, vocational, art secondary education, and non-native newcomer classes).

In all regions, schools were first randomly selected based on an official list. Next, classes from fifth grade elementary school (corresponding to adolescents aged $\pm$ 10 years) to the final grade of the secondary school (corresponding to adolescents aged $\pm$ 18 years) were selected in each grade among the schools that agreed to participate in the study. All adolescents from selected classes were invited to participate on a voluntary basis. In French-speaking schools, classes were randomly selected. In Dutch-speaking schools, distributions of gender, grade, and form of education from the previous survey were used as temporary proxies to select classes.

In 2014, 781 schools in the French-speaking schools and 208 schools in the Dutch-speaking schools were invited to participate. Among these schools, 168 in the French- and 98 in the Dutch-speaking areas actually participated, corresponding, respectively, to a participation rate of 21.5% and 47.1%.

In total, 23,552 questionnaires were collected (Figure 1). Since, in Dutch-speaking schools, adolescents aged 20 or over were not questioned, only adolescents 10 to 19 years old were included in the joint database ($n = 23,031$). The basis sample included all participants who responded to all covariates and to the food consumption variable that was most frequently filled in, i.e., fruits. Thus, the maximum number of adolescents included in the analyses was 19,172 (Figure 1). For food consumption other than fruits, the sample size was slightly lower.

2.2. Measures

Food Frequency Questionnaire. Food data were collected using a validated short food frequency questionnaire (FFQ) [24,25] that included a total of 22 food groups (17 in the Dutch part, 18 in the French part, including 13 in common). Seven answer categories were proposed: "more than once a day"; "once a day"; "5–6 days a week"; "2–4 days a week"; "once a week"; "less than once a week"; and "never".

Migration status. Adolescents born abroad and whose parents were not both born in Belgium were considered "1st-generation immigrants". Adolescents born in Belgium and who had at least one parent born abroad were considered "2nd-generation immigrants". Adolescents whose parents were born in Belgium were considered to be "natives".

Geographical area of origin. Based on countries of origin of adolescents for 1st-generation immigrants and of parents for 2nd-generation immigrants, five categories were defined for complementary analyses: (1) Europe; (2) America; (3) Asia; (4) Middle East and North Africa; (5) Sub-Saharan Africa. For 2nd-generation immigrants, in the particular case where the parents were from two different geographical areas, the category was randomly chosen between the mother's and the father's area of origin.

Family affluence. The family affluence scale (FAS) is composed of six items and has been validated in Europe [26]. The FAS score ranged from 0 to 13 and was divided into three categories after ridit analysis transformation—"low", "medium", and "high"—corresponding, in the national sample, to the 20% of adolescents with the lowest FAS scores, the 60% of adolescents with the intermediate score, and the 20% of adolescents with the highest FAS scores, respectively.

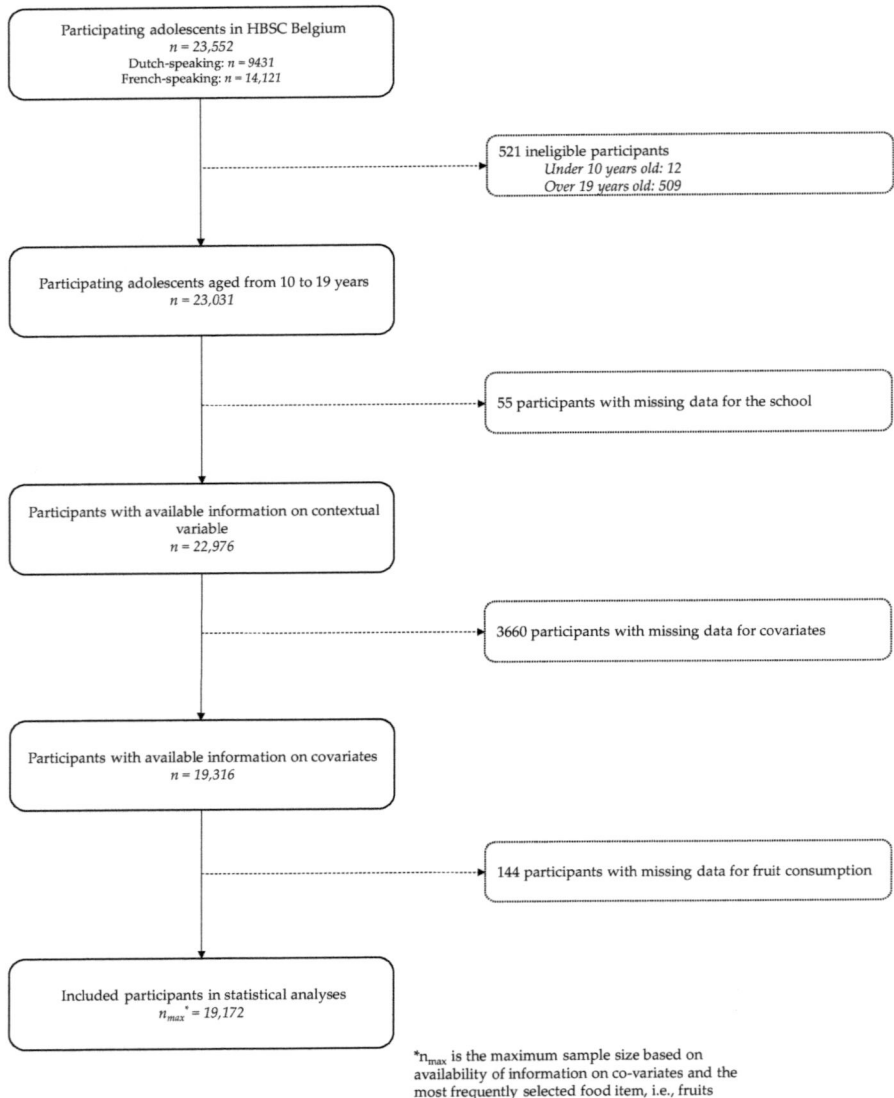

Figure 1. Inclusion diagram of adolescents in Belgium, "Health Behavior in School-Aged Children" (HBSC), 2014.

Parental working status. Based on parental employment and reason for parental unemployment, four categories were defined: (1) Adolescents with both parents working; (2) adolescents with parent(s) not working (those with a parent not working and without a second parent were placed in this category (n = 365)); (3) adolescents with one working parent and the other at home (housewife/husband, pre-retired, disabled or student); (4) adolescents with one working parent and the other "absent" from home (seeking a job, or adolescent not living with the second parent).

In addition, gender, age, family structure, siblings, and school region were taken into account in the analyses.

2.3. Statistical Analyses

2.3.1. Reprocessing Data

For all food items, categorization was defined so as to correspond as closely as possible to Belgian nutritional policies [27] but was also determined by the original answer modalities. Food consumption was first divided into three categories: A category corresponding as closely as possible to the Belgian nutritional policies, a category further removed from Belgian nutritional policies, and an intermediate category. If the intermediate category did not provide additional information, categorization was reduced to two categories. Frequency of *fruit and vegetable consumption* was classified into three categories: ">once a day", "5–7 days a week" (low frequency), and "<5 days a week" (very low frequency). Frequency of *fish consumption* was classified into: "≥two days a week" and "<two days a week" (low frequency). Milk (whole and semi-skimmed/skimmed), cheese, and other dairy product frequencies were transformed into consumption per month of 30 days and added up to obtain frequency of *dairy consumption*; this was then divided into total consumption of 31 days or more, which corresponded to consumption ">once a day", or else to consumption "≤once a day" (low frequency). Consumption of chips and fries and SSB was similarly processed. Frequency of *chips and fries* consumption was classified into: "<once a day", strictly corresponding to consumption under 25 days, and "≥once a day" (high frequency). Frequency of *SSB consumption* was classified into: "≤once a week", corresponding to total consumption under 5 days, "2–6 days a week" (high frequency) and "≥once a day" (very high frequency), corresponding to a total of 25 days or more.

2.3.2. Modeling

Due to a significant effect modification of migration status on several covariates for each food group analyzed, analyses were stratified by migration status. Since individuals were nested within schools, multilevel models were used. In each model for each food group, the school effect was controlled and estimated. The "null" model referred to the estimation of the school effect. Associations between covariates and a given food consumption were then evaluated by univariate regression, corresponding to "model 1". Multilevel binary logistic regression was performed for food groups with consumption frequencies in two categories (odds ratio (OR) and 95% CI); multilevel multinomial logistic regression was used for food groups with consumption frequencies falling into three categories (relative risk ratio (RRR) and 95%CI). The reference category was assumed to be the most favorable category in terms of health. All covariates with a p value < 0.20 were included in the initial multivariable regression model. Manual backward stepwise selection was used to determine the final model: It consisted of iteratively removing the predictor with the highest p value, and higher than 0.05. Following removal, confounding was evaluated with a tolerance threshold for variation of OR and RRR set at 10%. If variation was greater than 10%, the variable was then retained in the model. In order to facilitate comparisons between migration strata, a predictor significantly associated with food consumption in a given migration status group was retained for all other migration status groups. The results of the regressions are graphically presented and available as supplementary tables (Supplementary Tables S1–S6).

In order to estimate the role of the immigrants' geographical area of origin on socioeconomic and sociodemographic disparities, the same modeling was carried out only in immigrant adolescents and adjusted for the geographical area of origin.

Colinearity and fitting of models were verified. Statistical significance of tests was set at 0.05. All analyses were performed using Stata/IC 14® (StataCorp, College Station, TX, USA).

3. Results

The sample of 19,172 school participants included 69.6% natives, 22.0% 2nd-generation immigrants, and 8.4% 1st-generation immigrants. In univariate analyses, differences in sociodemographic and socioeconomic characteristics were observed according to migration status (Table 1).

Table 1. Sociodemographic and socioeconomic characteristics of the sample overall and by migration status—HBSC, Belgium, 2014.

Variables	Sample (n = 19,172) %	Natives (n = 13,353) %	2nd-Generation Immigrants (n = 4214) %	1st-Generation Immigrants (n = 1605) %	p value
Gender					<0.001 [†]
Boys	50.6	51.5	47.5	51.7	
Girls	49.4	48.5	52.5	48.3	
Age					<0.001 [¥]
10–12 years	28.8	29.6	28.7	22.5	
13–16 years	50.2	49.9	50.6	51.4	
17–19 years	21.0	20.5	20.7	26.1	
Family structure [a]					<0.001
Two parents	66.4	66.1	67.9	65.0	
Blended family	14.1	15.8	9.9	12.0	
Single-parent family	19.5	18.1	22.2	23.0	
Family Affluence Scale [a]					<0.001
High	19.4	20.6	17.0	16.4	
Medium	63.7	66.1	59.8	53.6	
Low	16.9	13.3	23.2	30.0	
Parental working status [a]					<0.001
Both parents working	68.4	76.1	51.9	47.0	
One working, the other at home	17.4	13.4	27.8	23.7	
One working, the other not at home	8.1	7.2	8.5	14.0	
None working	6.1	3.3	11.8	15.3	
Siblings					<0.001 [†]
Single child	9.3	9.8	7.5	10.5	
Siblings	90.7	90.2	92.5	89.5	
School Region					<0.001
Brussels-Capital	11.4	3.4	29.2	31.7	
Wallonia	46.6	48.7	43.0	38.2	
Flanders	42.0	47.9	27.8	30.1	
Geographical area of origin					<0.001 *
Europe			43.7	59.8	
America			3.0	6.7	
Asia			7.3	7.7	
Middle East and South Africa			36.0	13.1	
Sub-Saharan Africa			10.0	12.7	

[a] For details, see *Methods* section, [†] Nonsignificant difference between natives and 1st-generation immigrants, [¥] Nonsignificant difference between natives and 2nd-generation immigrants, * Comparison between 1st- and 2nd-generation immigrants.

Irrespective of migration status, one adolescent out of five ate fruits (17.2%) or vegetables (18.8%) >once a day and fish ≥two days a week (20.2%) (data not tabulated). Eight pupils out of ten (79.6%) ate dairy products >once a day. Nearly half of the adolescents (43.7%) drank SSB ≥once a day; fewer than one-eighth (12.2%) ate chips and fries ≥once a day (data not tabulated).

Immigrants significantly more often ate fruits (>once a day and 5–7 days a week), vegetables (>once a day) and fish (≥two days a week) than did natives (Figure 2). In addition, immigrants significantly more often consumed SSB (≥once a day), and chips and fries (≥once a day) than natives. Moreover, the proportion of 2nd-generation immigrants having low or very low intake of vegetables, fish, chips and fries was significantly at an intermediate level, i.e., higher (or lower) than that of natives, and lower (or higher) than that of 1st-generation immigrants. However, a significant difference in dairy product consumption was observed only between 2nd-generation immigrants and natives (Figure 2).

In immigrants only, and compared with immigrants from a European country, statistically significant differences in food consumption frequencies were found in those from the Middle East and North Africa areas, and from sub-Saharan Africa, for vegetable, fish, dairy, chips and fries, and SSB (Supplementary Table S7). Immigrants from America also slightly differed regarding SSB and chips and fries consumption, and those from Asia for chips and fries consumption. Overall, estimates of the SES characteristics were not modified by the addition of origins in the modeling except only for siblings in 1st-generation immigrants for chips and fries consumption (data not shown).

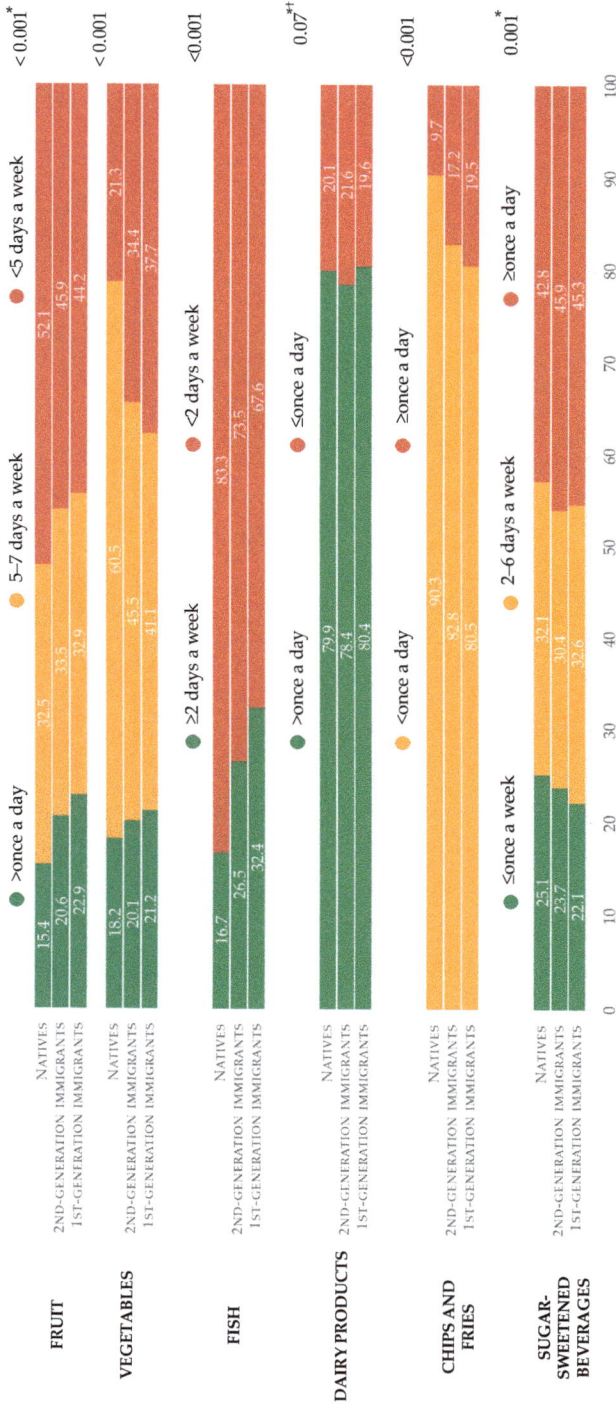

Figure 2. Distribution of food consumption frequencies by migration status in the sample, HBSC, Belgium, 2014. Favorable, moderately favorable, and unfavorable behaviors are represented, respectively, in green, orange, and red. * Nonsignificant difference between 2nd- and 1st-generation immigrants, † nonsignificant difference between natives and 1st-generation immigrants.

3.1. Fruit Consumption (Reference Category: >Once a Day)

In all migration strata, the likelihood of very low fruit consumption frequency (<5 days a week) significantly decreased with the FAS (except in 1st-generation immigrants: NS for medium FAS vs. high FAS) (Figure 3). In addition, natives having a medium FAS were more likely to eat fruits 5–7 days a week (low frequency) than those with a high FAS. Native adolescents in blended families were more likely to declare very low or low fruit consumption compared to adolescents with two parents; native adolescents in single-parent families also had greater odds of very low frequency. There was no significant association with parental working status. In all migration strata, adolescents in Flanders were significantly more likely to declare low or very low fruit consumption than adolescents in Brussels-Capital (Figure 3).

Moreover, age was significantly associated with fruit consumption frequency in all migration strata (Figure 3). This was also the case for gender in natives and 2nd-generation immigrants, whereas the existence of siblings was associated with fruit consumption frequency only in natives. The school effect upon the very low fruit consumption of all migration groups was significant, as was its effect upon the low frequency found in natives (Figure 3).

3.2. Vegetable Consumption (Reference Category: >Once a Day)

In natives and 1st-generation immigrants only, the odds of very low vegetable consumption frequency (<5 days a week) decreased with FAS (Figure 4). The same applied to low frequency (5–7 days a week) in natives. In 2nd-generation immigrants, adolescents having a medium FAS were more likely to declare very low or low vegetable consumption than those with a high FAS; in addition, adolescents having a low FAS were more likely to eat vegetables <5 days a week.

Compared with adolescents with two parents, native adolescents from a single-parent family were at greater odds of consuming vegetables <5 days a week (Figure 4). Native adolescents with two working parents were more likely to declare a low frequency than adolescents with one parent who worked and the other who stayed at home. Moreover, 2nd-generation immigrants with both working parents were less likely to declare a very low frequency. Compared with adolescents in Brussels-Capital, adolescents in Flanders were more likely to eat vegetables 5–7 days a week in all migration strata; in addition, immigrants in Flanders were more likely to declare a very low frequency, whereas 2nd-generation immigrants in Wallonia were less likely to do so (Figure 4).

Gender was significantly associated with vegetable consumption frequency in all migration strata. This was also the case for age in natives and 2nd-generation immigrants, while the existence of siblings was associated only in natives. The school effect was significant only in natives (Figure 4).

3.3. Fish Consumption (Reference Category: ≥Two Days a Week)

In natives and 2nd-generation immigrants, the likelihood of eating fish at low frequency (<two days a week) decreased with FAS. Moreover, low fish consumption was more frequent in adolescents from blended families than in those having two parents (Figure 5). Compared with adolescents with one working parent and the other who stayed at home, 2nd-generation immigrants with no working parents were less likely to eat fish at low frequency. In 1st-generation immigrants, adolescents whose parents both worked were more likely to declare low fish-eating frequency. For all migration strata, compared with Brussels-Capital, adolescents in Flanders and Wallonia were significantly more likely to declare low frequency (Figure 5).

In addition, gender was significantly associated with fish consumption frequency in natives and 2nd-generation immigrants. The school effect was significant in natives and 2nd-generation immigrants.

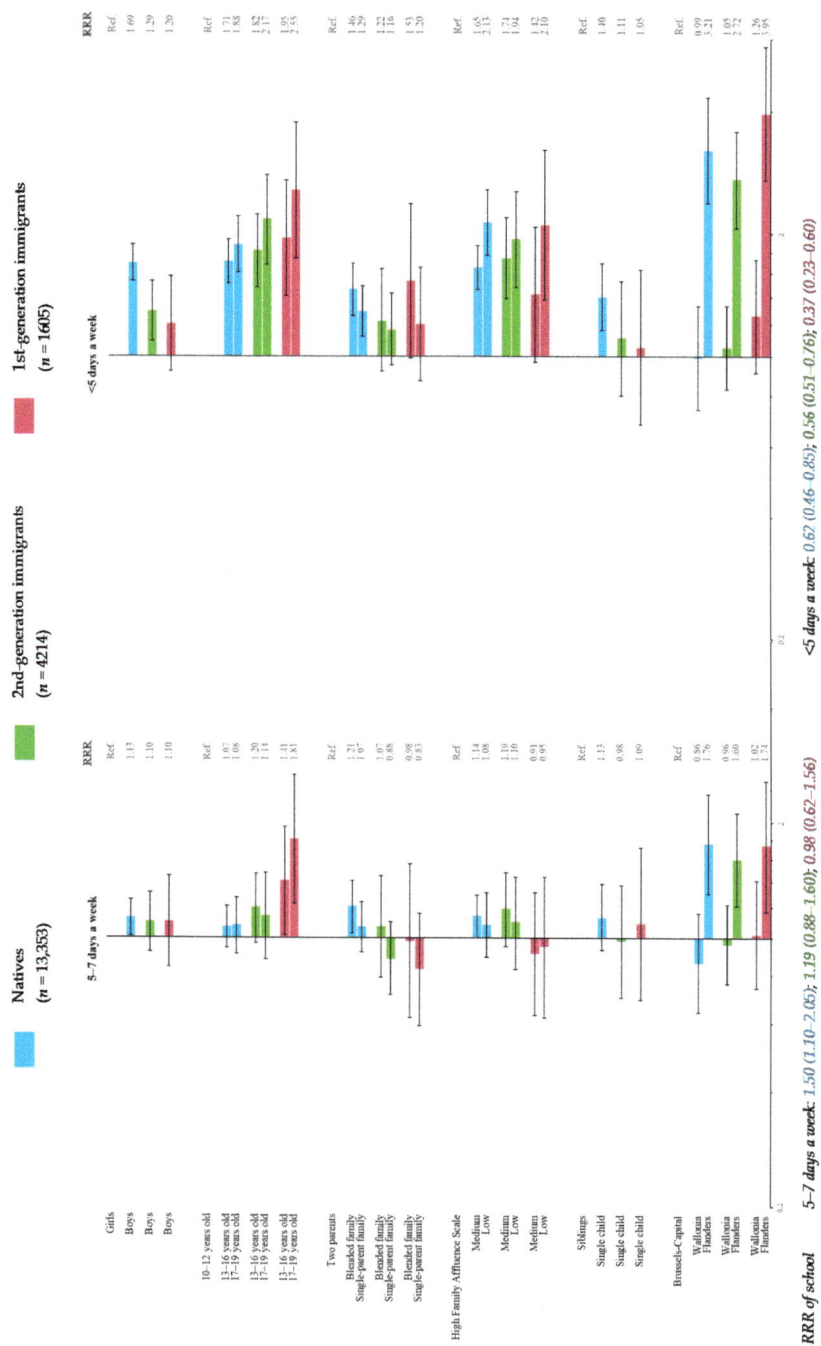

Figure 3. Multiple multilevel multinomial regression* for fruit consumption (reference category: >once a day) stratified by migration status—HBSC, Belgium, 2014 (*n* = 19,172). * RRR < 1: More favorable for health; RRR > 1: Less favorable for health.

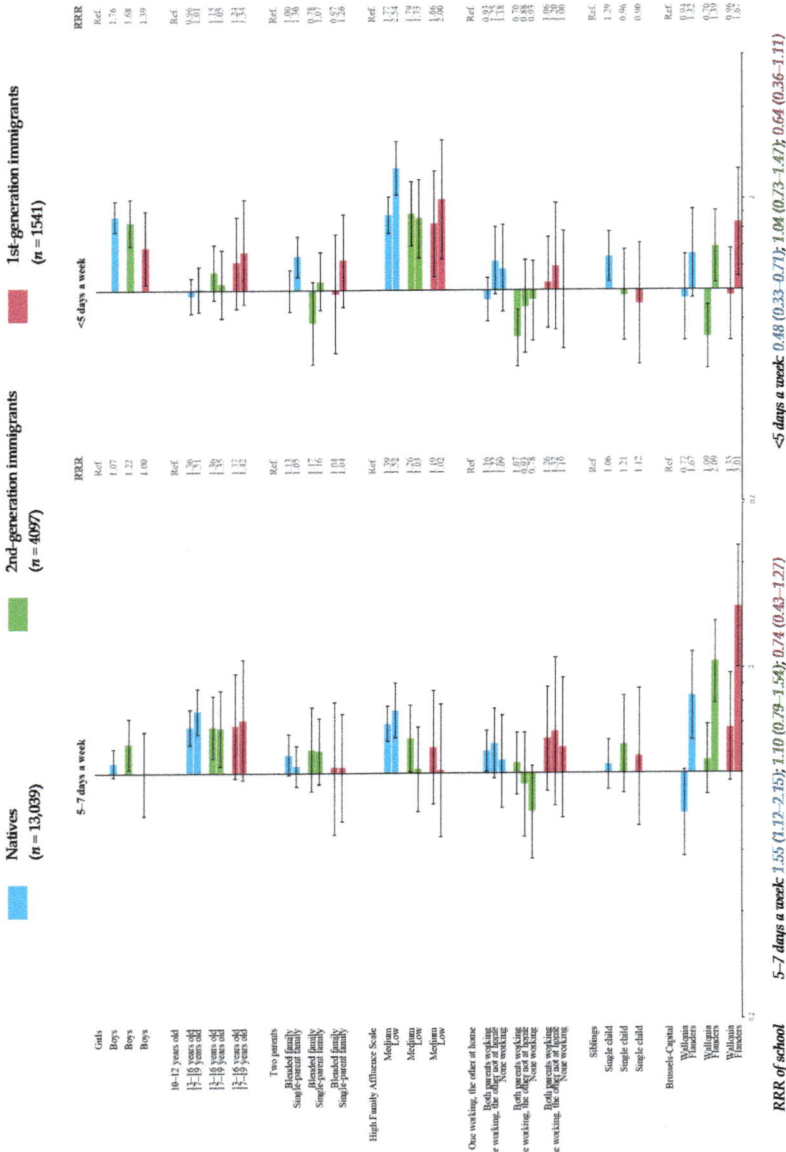

Figure 4. Multiple multilevel multinomial regression* for vegetable consumption (reference category: >once a day) stratified by migration status—HBSC, Belgium, 2014 (*n* = 18,974). * RRR < 1: More favorable for health; RRR > 1: Less favorable for health.

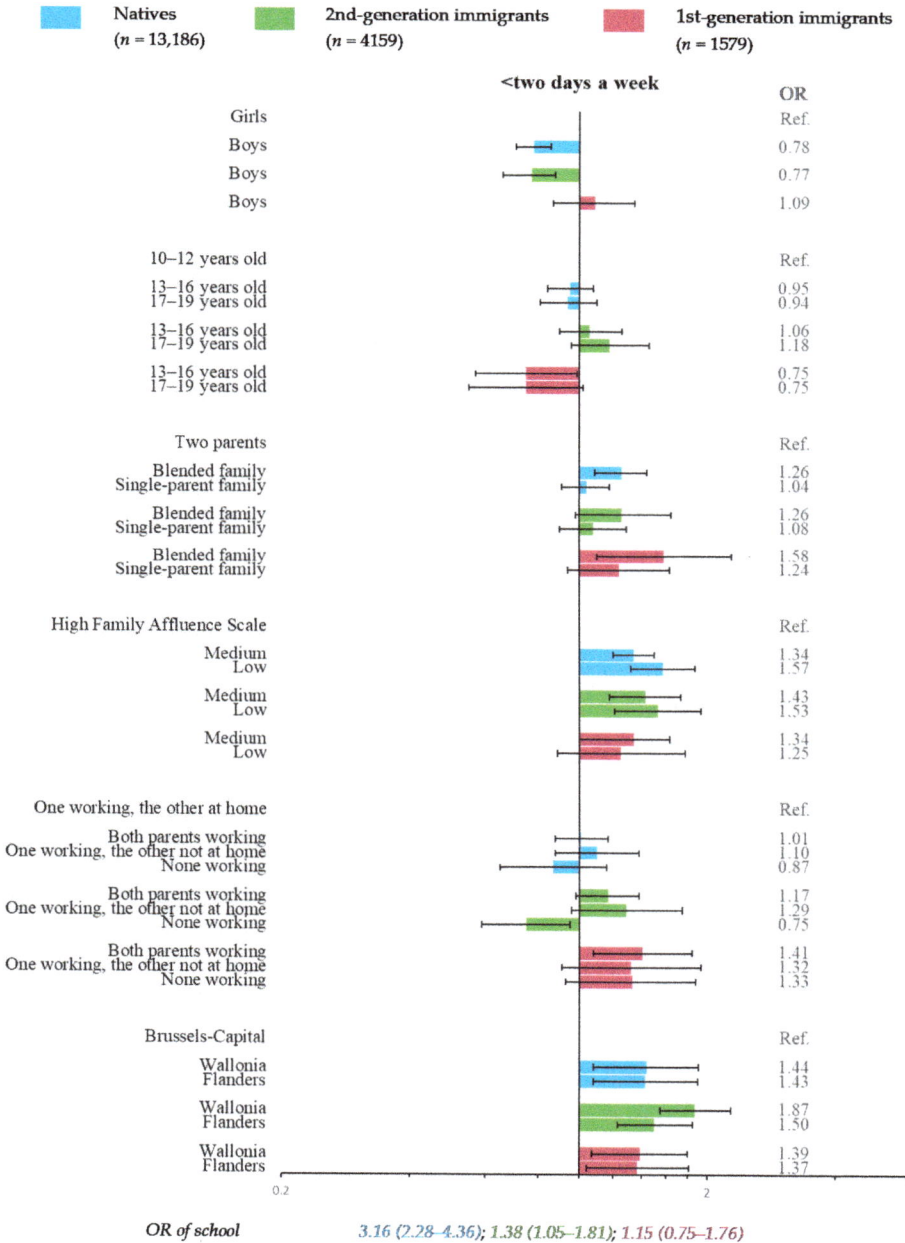

Figure 5. Multiple multilevel logistic regression* for fish consumption (reference category: ≥two days a week) stratified by migration status—HBSC, Belgium, 2014 (*n* = 18,924). * OR < 1: More favorable for health; OR > 1: Less favorable for health.

3.4. Dairy Product Consumption (Reference Category: >Once a Day)

For all migration situations, neither FAS nor family structure nor parental working status was significantly associated with dairy consumption (Figure 6). Compared with Brussels-Capital, natives and 2nd-generation immigrants in Flanders were at significantly lower odds of consuming dairy foods ≤once a day (Figure 6).

In addition, dairy consumption frequency was significantly associated with gender in all migration strata and with age in natives and 2nd-generation immigrants, whereas the presence of siblings was significant only in natives. The school effect was significant in all migration strata (Figure 6).

3.5. Chips and Fries Consumption (Reference Category: <Once a Day)

Compared with those having a high FAS, natives with a low FAS were significantly more likely to declare frequent eating of chips and fries (≥once a day) (Figure 7). High frequency was also more likely in natives from blended or single-parent families than in those with two parents. Compared with adolescents having one working parent and the other who stayed at home, adolescents with two working parents were less likely to consume chips and fries ≥once a day whatever their migration status. In natives and 2nd-generation immigrants with no working parents, high frequency was more likely. In Flanders, compared to Brussels-Capital, adolescents among all migration groups were significantly less likely to declare high consumption of chips and fries; in Wallonia, this was also the case for 2nd- and 1st-generation immigrants (Figure 7).

In addition, frequent eating of chips and fries was significantly associated with gender in all migration strata, and with age in natives and 2nd-generation immigrants. Sibling presence was significantly associated only in 1st-generation immigrants. The school effect was significant in all migration strata (Figure 7).

3.6. Sugar-Sweetened Beverages (Reference Category: ≤Once a Week)

In natives and 2nd-generation immigrants, the odds of declaring very high SSB consumption (≥once a day) decreased with FAS (Figure 8). For all migration strata, adolescents from blended families were significantly more likely to declare very high frequency. In addition, natives from blended families were more likely to consume SSB at high frequency (2–6 days a week). In natives and 2nd-generation immigrants, very high SSB frequency was more often seen in adolescents from single-parent families (vs. two-parent families) and in adolescents with nonworking parents (vs. one working parent and the other at home) and was less likely in adolescents with both parents working. In 2nd-generation immigrants only, very high SSB frequency was also less likely in adolescents with one parent working and the other absent from the home. In Flanders, compared with Brussels-Capital, natives and 2nd-generation immigrants were more likely to consume SSB 2–6 days a week.

In addition, "gender and age" was significantly associated with SSB frequency in all migration strata, whereas "siblings" was significant only in natives. The school effect was significant only in natives (Figure 8).

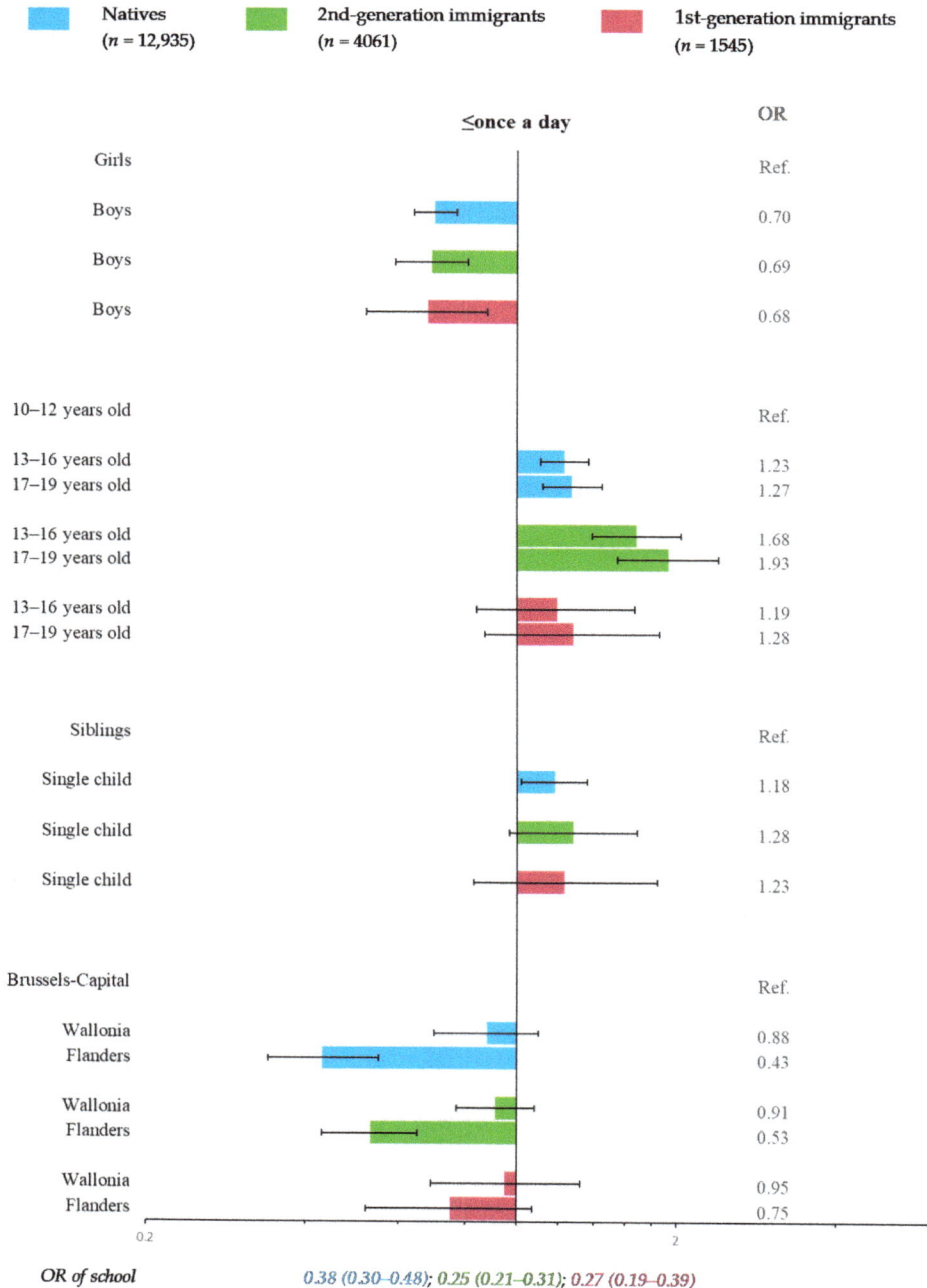

Figure 6. Multiple multilevel logistic regression* for dairy product consumption (reference category: >once a day) stratified by migration status—HBSC, Belgium, 2014 (*n* = 18,541). * OR < 1: More favorable for health; OR > 1: Less favorable for health.

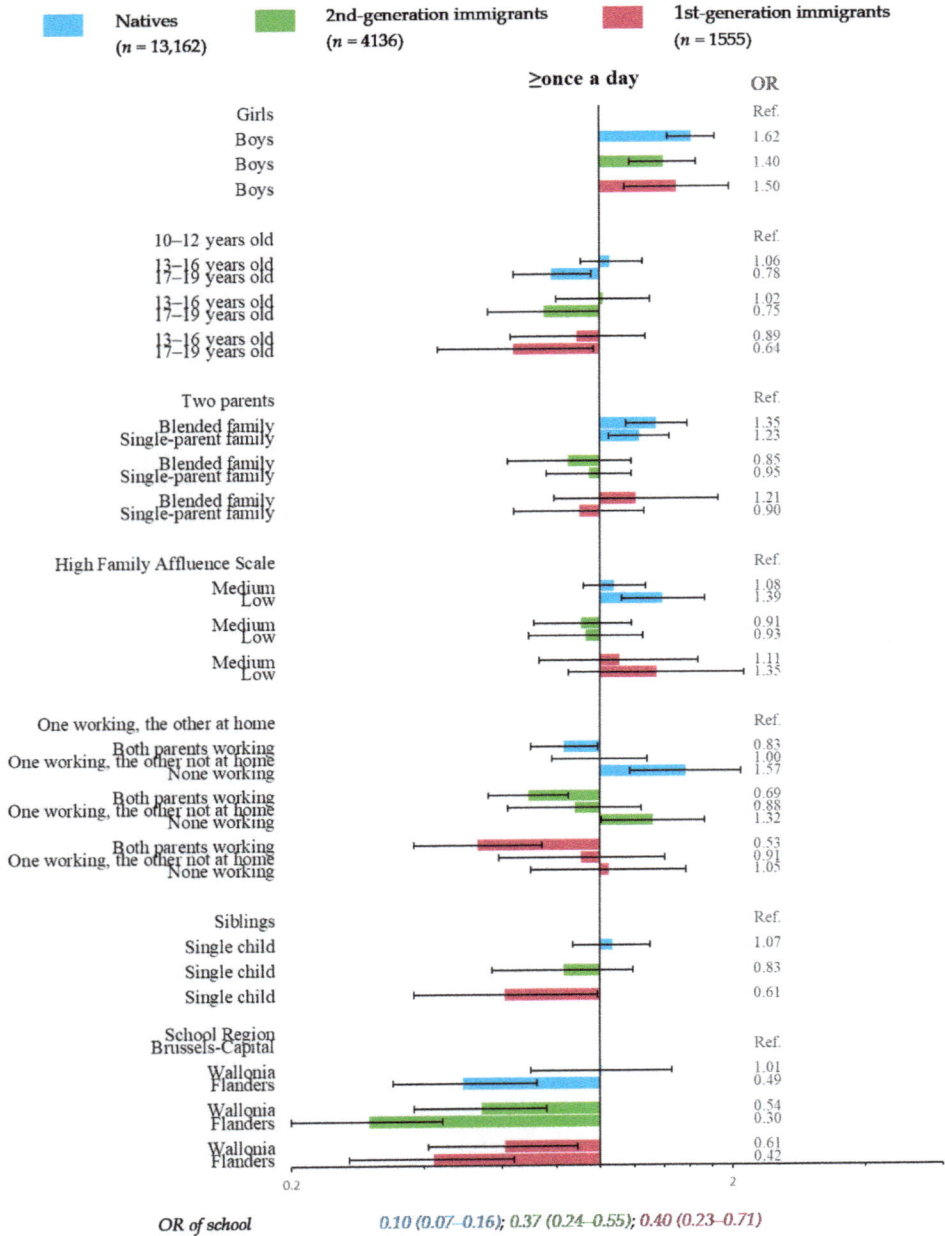

Figure 7. Multiple multilevel logistic regression* for chips and fries consumption (reference category: <once a day) stratified by migration status—HBSC, Belgium, 2014 (*n* = 18,853). * OR < 1: More favorable for health; OR > 1: Less favorable for health.

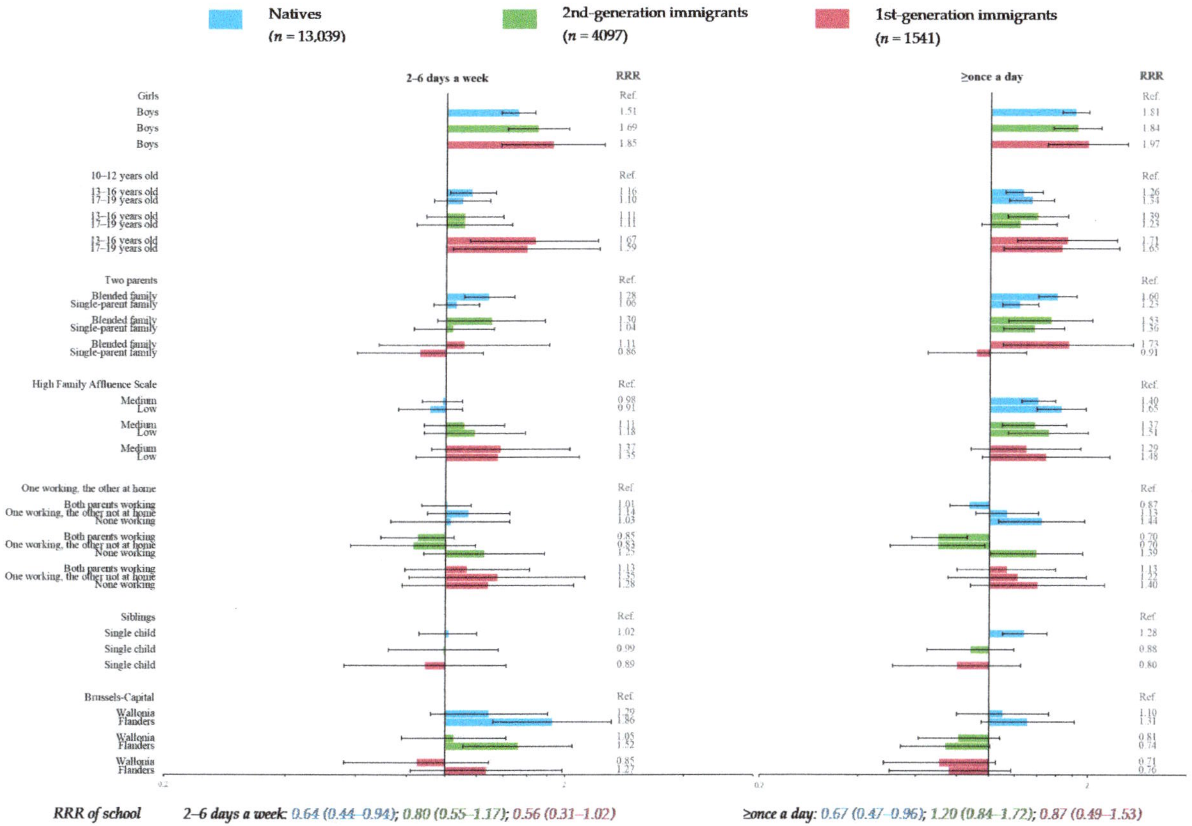

Figure 8. Multiple multilevel multinomial regression* for sugar-sweetened beverages consumption (reference category: ≤once a week) stratified by migration status—HBSC, Belgium, 2014 (*n* = 18,642). * RRR < 1: More favorable for health; RRR > 1: Less favorable for health.

4. Discussion

The aim of the present study was to estimate socioeconomic disparities in dietary habits of school adolescents in Belgium from different migration backgrounds. Our results emphasize that the migration component that was rarely considered in previous studies is fundamental regarding dietary behavior at these ages. Indeed, dietary habits differed according to migration strata. Furthermore, socioeconomic disparities varied amongst the migration groups: For all food groups, disparities were particularly wide in natives and more limited in 1st-generation immigrants. Overall, the sociodemographic and socioeconomic disparities observed in immigrants did not change after adjusting for their geographical area of origin. By food group, the widest socioeconomic and cultural disparities were observed for SSB and vegetables, and the least for dairy foods. Such findings provide interesting and original hypotheses that could further support the development of health promotion interventions in the future.

4.1. Dietary Acculturation

In descriptive analyses, immigrant adolescents, whether of the 1st or 2nd generation, were more likely to frequently consume both healthy (fruits, vegetables, and fish, but not dairy products) and unhealthy foods (chips and fries, SSB). In addition, a migration gradient in food frequencies was underlined for vegetables, fish, and chips and fries: Consumption gradually increased (for healthy food) or decreased (for unhealthy food) from natives to 2nd-generation immigrants, and from 2nd-generation immigrants to 1st-generation immigrants. However, no significant differences were found between 1st- and 2nd-generation immigrants regarding consumption of fruits, dairy products, and SSB.

The situation of 2nd-generation immigrants in terms of food consumption, intermediate between natives and 1st-generation immigrants, suggests ongoing acculturation. The interplay of host behavior and culture with that of immigrants may lead to a mixture of healthy and unhealthy dietary habits. Indeed, at a given age, 2nd-generation immigrants have probably been in Belgium much longer than 1st-generation immigrants and are therefore more likely to be further engaged in the process of integration of culinary habits of the host country and partial substitution of family roots, as reported for adults in different countries [18]. In addition to the migration generation, the region of origin may play differently in the acquisition of European dietary habits for immigrants. Indeed, differences in dietary habits were of lower size between European, American, and Asian, than between European and African and Middle-East immigrants. Nevertheless, the results could not be precisely interpreted due to the cultural heterogeneity remaining in this categorization by the geographical area of origin.

The acculturation process may depend on factors such as accessibility and affordability, acting as an "external push", and on individual factors such as curiosity, acting as an "internal pull" [28], which might encourage the adding of novel foods to the traditional diet, thus offering wider diversity. Such diversity could result in greater intake via gradual adaptation to new food products [29]. This may also explain why immigrants more frequently ate almost each food group studied. Maintaining traditional food habits implies the availability and accessibility of such food; when this is not the case, then people of foreign culture might progressively abandon their diet in favor of the host diet [30]. The acculturation process should also be further studied by considering the age of arrival in Belgium of the 1st-generation immigrants, unavailable in this survey.

4.2. Socioeconomic Disparities in Dietary Habits

Our results emphasize several socioeconomic disparities in dietary habits in adolescents, mainly in natives and 2nd-generation immigrants. Indeed, adolescents with lower FAS less frequently ate healthy foods like fruits and more frequently consumed unhealthy foods like SSB, consistent with previous studies [10,11]. These disparities may be explained by a lower level of familiarity or adoption of dietary recommendations by parents [31], and by the affordability of healthy foods [32].

Some disparities related to family structure were also revealed, mainly in natives and 2nd-generation immigrants. In line with previous studies [33,34], adolescents from blended or single-parent families more frequently ate chips and fries and SSB and less frequently ate fruits, vegetables and fish. Single-parent families often have fewer financial resources, thereby impairing their access to healthy foods [32]. Indeed, in our sample, 30.8% of adolescents belonging to a single-parent family were in a low FAS compared to 14.0% of adolescents from two-parent families and 15.7% of adolescents from blended families (data not shown). In addition, single parents may also have less time for monitoring meals compared to dual-parent families [33,35]. Adolescents from blended families also tended to have less healthy food habits than adolescents from two-parent families. Indeed, stepparents may have fewer opportunities for active involvement in their stepchildren's education and health [33].

Moreover, parental work status disparities were observed, mainly in natives and 2nd-generation immigrants. In our study, parental working status was mainly related to the socioeconomic condition: 10.2% of adolescents with both parents working had a low FAS, while 51.8% of adolescents with no parents working fell into this category ($p < 0.001$; 24.1% in those with one parent working and one at home, 31.5% for one parent working and the other "absent" from home). After adjustment for FAS and other covariates, our results related to parental working status were mixed. Indeed, compared to adolescents with both parents working, those with no working parents were more likely to frequently eat vegetables and fish, but they also more frequently ate chips and fries and SSB (data not shown). These results might appear surprising if we assume that parental working status is related only to socioeconomic conditions. However, they suggest an interplay between free time and work. Indeed, parental working status might also indicate that fully employed parents have less time to cook [36].

For all migration strata, eating habits varied according to the school region. Numerous differences were found in consumption frequencies between adolescents attending schools in Flanders, mainly Dutch-speaking, and those in Brussels and Wallonia, both primarily French-speaking. Another study indicating similar regional linguistic specificities in consumption of vegetables, dairy products, fish, and SSB in Switzerland hypothesized a possible influence of culture and eating habits of neighboring countries [37], which might also apply to Belgium: Culinary customs in Flanders may be strongly influenced by the Netherlands, while those in Brussels, although they do not border, and in Wallonia, may be influenced by France, which shares the same language, i.e., French. Further, several differences were pointed out between Brussels and Wallonia, mainly concerning 1st- and 2nd-generation immigrants. In 2011, nearly half of the inhabitants of the Brussels-Capital Region (42.4%) were born outside of Belgium, compared to 10.2% in Flanders and 14.1% in Wallonia [38]. Since the Brussels-Capital region is multicultural, this vast proportion of immigrants might contribute to slowing down the acculturation process; indeed, immigrants are usually surrounded by other immigrants [17]. By contrast, in Wallonia, such a process may have been accelerated, meaning that food habits in immigrants would differ from those of immigrants in Brussels.

Socioeconomic disparities were measurable in all food groups, except for dairy products, for which disparities were statistically significant only for the school region. The absence of socioeconomic disparities in consumption of dairy foods (milk, cheese, and other) could be explained by the diversity of these products and their overall affordability.

4.3. Sociodemographic Disparities in Dietary Habits

Our results underlined gender disparities in food consumption in almost all migration strata. Compared to boys, girls were more likely to more frequently eat fruits and vegetables, which could be explained by taste preferences [39,40], health beliefs, and greater concern about weight [41].

After adjustment for other covariates, sibling disparities continued to be unfavorable to the single child (except for chips and fries in 1st-generation immigrants). The sibling role in food consumption might be explained by two opposite phenomena: "Modeling" leads to imitation of the model (i.e., of the sibling), whereas "de-identification" leads to differentiation from the sibling [42]. The absence of sibling disparities in immigrants could be explained by the manner in which society views sibling relationships and their respective roles [43]. Thus, immigrants in our study might come from countries that do not promote sibling relationships. However, the sibling role has rarely been examined in dietary studies irrespective of migration status [44], thus preventing interpretation. Certain psychologists have suggested that older siblings may influence health behavior [45]; thus, birth order should be considered when evaluating the association between diet and siblings.

4.4. Strengths and Limitations

Due to the cross-sectional design of the HBSC survey and use of self-administrated questionnaires, a substantial sample size was obtained in each region of Belgium, along with a wide range of topics addressed. Although both Dutch- and French-speaking surveys were conducted separately and in different languages, standardization of the questionnaires according to the international HBSC protocol made it possible to combine data sets [23]. However, the two surveys were not identical. For instance, they were differently stratified in order to reach the representativeness of the linguistic regions. Therefore, the generalization of the results to the school population in Belgium should be interpreted cautiously. A second point related to the independence of studies is the use of reverse order categorization for food frequencies ("never" to ">once a day" for the Dutch-speaking survey versus ">once a day" to "never" for the French-speaking survey) may have contributed to lower frequencies of fruit and vegetable consumption in Flanders compared to Wallonia, since initial responses may have been chosen more frequently. This discrepancy could explain why we obtained results differing from the final national food consumption survey (based on 24-h recall) [46]. The short HBSC FFQ might also lead to inaccuracies due to use of large food group names rather than exact food names, and to the overestimation of consumption frequencies [25]. However, it has been validated in Belgium through a comparison with a seven-day record [24,25]. The conclusion was that it can be considered reliable for "ranking subjects according to consumption of the individual food items" [25]. In addition, we can only conclude about frequencies and the results must be interpreted as such given that a more frequent consumption does not necessarily imply—nor rules out—a higher food amount or a higher energy intake.

A significant strength of the current study was the use of multilevel analyses controlling for the school effect and, therefore, cluster bias. Nevertheless, further interpreting the school effect is difficult given that food-related school characteristics were unavailable in this study. To better understand such effects, further studies should simultaneously consider contextual characteristics of the schools, such as implementation of nutritional actions and canteen use. For some food groups (fruits, vegetables, and SSB), categorization was in three instead of two, as is the case in numerous studies using categorization and FFQ. Although disparities were narrower for the intermediate category and, therefore, little difference from the reference category was observed, intermediate categories provided new information in certain cases. Indeed, in natives and 2nd-generation immigrants, age-related disparities existed for vegetables 5–7 days a week but not for vegetables <5 days a week; in addition, school-region-related disparities existed for SSB consumption 2–6 days a week but not for SSB $\geq$once a day. Although difficult to interpret, the school effect for natives might be a protective factor for fruits 5–7 days a week and a risk factor for fruits <5 days a week.

Another limitation was the rather small sample size of 1st-generation immigrants (n_{max} = 1605), leading to fewer participants in some categories (n_{min} = 159) and resulting in loss of statistical power. However, confidence intervals of OR and RRR (Figures 3–8) suggested that nonsignificant results in 1st-generation immigrants were mainly due to fewer disparities rather than a lack of precision. This rather small sample size was also restrictive for in-depth analysis stratified by countries or continental regions of origin. To get around the small sample, results were subsequently adjusted for geographical areas of origin. Nevertheless, some cultural heterogeneity remained in this categorization and did not help to precisely interpret the findings.

Several biases could also be highlighted. First, adolescents may have overreported consumption of healthy foods and underreported consumption of unhealthy products due to social pressure [47]. Second, we observed differential distribution of fish and SSB consumption and of several covariates (migration status, gender, family structure, FAS, parental working status, and school region) between included participants and eligible participants not included in analyses due to missing data (Supplementary Table S8), leading to selection bias. Interpretation of results should thus be approached with caution, although some differences in percentages were slight, and statistical significance was mainly due to the large sample size. The generalization of the results is limited to the school adolescents, especially for the eldest beyond the legal school age (18 years of age in Belgium). It should also be interpreted cautiously due to the relatively low participation rate of schools.

5. Conclusions

Overall, rather poor adolescent dietary habits indicate that efforts should be made to improve knowledge and further prevent NCD in adulthood. The process of acculturation of dietary habits pointed out here warrants confirmation, taking into consideration the number of years in the host country and the age of arrival in that country. Narrower socioeconomic disparities in dietary habits among 2nd- and 1st-generation immigrants compared to natives suggest the prevailing role of culture in immigrant dietary habits with respect to socioeconomic conditions. Finally, our study reveals that interventions aimed at improving dietary habits in adolescents must take into account the cultural component of dietary habits, especially in immigrant adolescents. However, further research is needed to better understand the role of culture and its interaction with socioeconomic components in dietary habits.

Supplementary Materials: The following are available online at http://www.mdpi.com/2072-6643/11/4/812/s1, Table S1: Multilevel multinomial regressions for fruit consumption (reference category: >once a day) stratified by migration status—HBSC, Belgium, 2014 (n = 19,172), Table S2: Multilevel multinomial regressions for vegetable consumption (reference category: >once a day) stratified by migration status—HBSC, Belgium, 2014 (n = 18,974), Table S3: Multilevel logistic regressions for fish consumption (reference category: $\geq$two days a week) stratified by migration status—HBSC, Belgium, 2014 (n = 18,924), Table S4: Multilevel logistic regressions for dairy product consumption (reference category: >once a day) stratified by migration status—HBSC, Belgium, 2014 (n = 18,541), Table S5: Multilevel logistic regressions for chips and fries consumption (reference category: <once a day) stratified by migration status—HBSC, Belgium, 2014 (n = 18,853), Table S6: Multilevel multinomial regressions for sugar-sweetened beverages consumption (reference category: $\leq$once a week) stratified by migration status—HBSC, Belgium, 2014 (n = 18,642), Table S7: Multilevel logistic regressions* for food consumption stratified by migration status—HBSC, Belgium, 2014, Table S8: Comparisons of food consumptions, cultural, and sociodemographic characteristics between participants included in the analyses and those excluded due to missing data.

Author Contributions: Conceptualization, M.R. and K.C.; methodology, M.R. and K.C.; formal analysis, M.R.; investigation, M.R.; resources, B.d.C., N.M. and I.G.; data curation, B.d.C., N.M. and I.G.; writing—original draft preparation, M.R. and K.C.; writing—review and editing, B.d.C., T.L., M.D., N.M., L.D. and I.G.; visualization, M.R.; supervision, K.C.; project administration, K.C..; funding acquisition, I.G., K.C. and B.d.C.

Funding: The Wallonia-Brussels Federation (FWB), the Birth and Children Office (ONE), the Walloon Region, the Brussels-Capital Region, and the Government of Flanders (Grant No. GEO-1GDD2A-WT) provided financial support for carrying out the 2014 Health Behavior in School-aged Children (HBSC) study. This work was supported by the French Community of Belgium, as part of the "Actions de Recherche Concertée" funding program. Researchers performed the study (study design, data collection, analyses, interpretation and writing) independently of the funding bodies.

Acknowledgments: The authors thank the schools and students for their participation in the French-speaking and Dutch-speaking Belgian HBSC surveys. They also thank the HBSC International Coordination Center (University of St Andrews, United Kingdom) and the HBSC data Management Center (University of Bergen, Norway) for their scientific support, as well as Maud Dujeu, Camille Pedroni and Patrick De Smet (SIPES, Université libre de Bruxelles, Belgium) for their collaboration in data cleaning and management, and Jerry Bram for editing reviewing.

Conflicts of Interest: The authors declare no conflicts of interest.

References

1. Grootveld, M.; Percival, B.C.; Grootveld, K. Chronic Non-Communicable Disease Risks Presented by Lipid Oxidation Products in Fried Foods. *HepatoBiliary Surg. Nutr.* **2018**, *7*, 305–312. [CrossRef] [PubMed]
2. Schwingshackl, L.; Schwedhelm, C.; Hoffmann, G.; Lampousi, A.-M.; Knuppel, S.; Iqbal, K.; Bechthold, A.; Schlesinger, S.; Boeing, H. Food groups and risk of all-cause mortality: A systematic review and meta-analysis of prospective studies. *Am. J. Clin. Nutr.* **2017**, *105*, 1462–1473. [CrossRef] [PubMed]
3. Aune, D.; Giovannucci, E.; Boffetta, P.; Fadnes, L.T.; Keum, N.; Norat, T.; Greenwood, D.C.; Riboli, E.; Vatten, L.J.; Tonstad, S. Fruit and vegetable intake and the risk of cardiovascular disease, total cancer and all-cause mortality—A systematic review and dose-response meta-analysis of prospective studies. *Int. J. Epidemiol.* **2017**, *46*, 1029–1056. [CrossRef]
4. Fardet, A.; Rock, E. In vitro and in vivo antioxidant potential of milks, yoghurts, fermented milks and cheeses: A narrative review of evidence. *Nutr. Res. Rev.* **2018**, *31*, 52–70. [CrossRef] [PubMed]
5. Stringhini, S.; Dugravot, A.; Shipley, M.; Goldberg, M.; Zins, M.; Kivimäki, M.; Marmot, M.; Sabia, S.; Singh-Manoux, A. Health behaviours, socioeconomic status, and mortality: Further analyses of the British Whitehall II and the French GAZEL prospective cohorts. *PLoS Med.* **2011**, *8*, e1000419. [CrossRef]
6. Méjean, C.; Droomers, M.; Van Der Schouw, Y.T.; Sluijs, I.; Czernichow, S.; Grobbee, D.E.; Bueno-de-Mesquita, H.B.; Beulens, J.W.J. The contribution of diet and lifestyle to socioeconomic inequalities in cardiovascular morbidity and mortality. *Int. J. Cardiol.* **2013**, *168*, 5190–5195. [CrossRef]
7. Lien, N.; Jacobs, D.R.; Klepp, K.-I. Exploring predictors of eating behaviour among adolescents by gender and socio-economic status. *Public Health Nutr.* **2002**, *5*, 671–681. [CrossRef] [PubMed]
8. Kelder, S.H.; Perry, C.L.; Klepp, K.I.; Lytle, L.L. Longitudinal tracking of adolescent smoking, physical activity, and food choice behaviors. *Am. J. Public Health* **1994**, *84*, 1121–1126. [CrossRef] [PubMed]
9. Lake, A.A.; Mathers, J.C.; Rugg-Gunn, A.J.; Adamson, A.J. Longitudinal change in food habits between adolescence (11–12 years) and adulthood (32–33 years): The ASH30 Study. *J. Public Health* **2006**, *28*, 10–16. [CrossRef]
10. Drouillet-Pinard, P.; Dubuisson, C.; Bordes, I.; Margaritis, I.; Lioret, S.; Volatier, J.-L. Socio-economic disparities in the diet of French children and adolescents: A multidimensional issue. *Public Health Nutr.* **2017**, *20*, 870–882. [CrossRef]
11. Béghin, L.; Dauchet, L.; de Vriendt, T.; Cuenca-García, M.; Manios, Y.; Toti, E.; Plada, M.; Widhalm, K.; Repasy, J.; Huybrechts, I.; et al. Influence of parental socio-economic status on diet quality of European adolescents: Results from the HELENA study. *Br. J. Nutr.* **2014**, *111*, 1303–1312. [CrossRef]
12. Allen, M.L.; Elliott, M.N.; Morales, L.S.; Diamant, A.L.; Hambarsoomian, K.; Schuster, M.A. Adolescent participation in preventive health behaviors, physical activity, and nutrition: Differences across immigrant generations for Asians and Latinos compared with Whites. *Am. J. Public Health* **2007**, *97*, 337–343. [CrossRef]
13. Brown, A.G.M.; Houser, R.F.; Mattei, J.; Rehm, C.D.; Mozaffarian, D.; Lichtenstein, A.H.; Folta, S.C. Diet quality among US-born and foreign-born non-Hispanic blacks: NHANES 2003-2012 data. *Am. J. Clin. Nutr.* **2018**, *107*, 695–706. [CrossRef]
14. Deboosere, P.; Gadeyne, S. Adult Migrant Mortality Advantage in Belgium: Evidence Using Census and Register Data. *Population* **2005**, 655–698. [CrossRef]
15. Neuman, S. Are immigrants healthier than native residents? *IZA World Labor* **2014**. [CrossRef]
16. Vandenheede, H.; Willaert, D.; de Grande, H.; Simoens, S.; Vanroelen, C. Mortality in adult immigrants in the 2000s in Belgium: A test of the 'healthy-migrant' and the 'migration-as-rapid-health-transition' hypotheses. *Trop. Med. Int. Health* **2015**, *20*, 1832–1845. [CrossRef]
17. Barker, G.G. Choosing the best of both worlds: The acculturation process revisited. *Int. J. Intercult. Relat.* **2015**, *45*, 56–69. [CrossRef]
18. Méjean, C.; Traissac, P.; Eymard-Duvernay, S.; Delpeuch, F.; Maire, B. Influence of acculturation among Tunisian migrants in France and their past/present exposure to the home country on diet and physical activity. *Public Health Nutr.* **2009**, *12*, 832–841. [CrossRef]
19. Llull, R.; Bibiloni, M.; Pons, A.; Tur, J.A. Food consumption patterns of Balearic Islands' adolescents depending on their origin. *J. Immigr. Minor Health* **2015**, *17*, 358–366. [CrossRef]

20. Te Velde, S.J.; Wind, M.; van Lenthe, F.J.; Klepp, K.-I.; Brug, J. Differences in fruit and vegetable intake and determinants of intakes between children of Dutch origin and non-Western ethnic minority children in the Netherlands—A cross sectional study. *Int. J. Behav. Nutr. Phys. Act.* **2006**, *3*, 31. [CrossRef]

21. Malmusi, D.; Borrell, C.; Benach, J. Migration-related health inequalities: Showing the complex interactions between gender, social class and place of origin. *Soc. Sci. Med.* **2010**, *71*, 1610–1619. [CrossRef]

22. Pantzer, K.; Rajmil, L.; Tebé, C.; Codina, F.; Serra-Sutton, V.; Ferrer, M.; Ravens-Sieberer, U.; Simeoni, M.-C.; Alonso, J. Health related quality of life in immigrants and native school aged adolescents in Spain. *J. Epidemiol. Community Health* **2006**, *60*, 694–698. [CrossRef]

23. Currie, C.; Griebler, R.; Inchley, J.; Theunissen, A.; Molcho, M.; Samdal, O.; Dür, W. *Health Behaviour in School-Aged Children (HBSC) Study Protocol: Background, Methodology and Mandatory Items for the 2009/10 Survey*; CAHRU: St Andrews, Hong Kong, China, 2010.

24. Vereecken, C.A.; Maes, L. A Belgian study on the reliability and relative validity of the Health Behaviour in School-Aged Children food-frequency questionnaire. *Public Health Nutr.* **2003**, *6*, 581–588. [CrossRef]

25. Vereecken, C.A.; Rossi, S.; Giacchi, M.V.; Maes, L. Comparison of a short food-frequency questionnaire and derived indices with a seven-day diet record in Belgian and Italian children. *Int. J. Public Health* **2008**, *53*, 297–305. [CrossRef]

26. Torsheim, T.; Cavallo, F.; Levin, K.A.; Schnohr, C.; Mazur, J.; Niclasen, B.; Currie, C. Psychometric Validation of the Revised Family Affluence Scale: A Latent Variable Approach. *Child. Indic. Res.* **2016**, *9*, 771–784. [CrossRef]

27. Conseil Supérieur de la Santé. *Recommandations Nutritionnelles pour la Belgique 2016. Avis n°9285*; Conseil Supérieur de la Santé: Bruxelles, Belgium, 2016.

28. Hartwell, H.J.; Edwards, J.S.A.; Brown, L. Acculturation and food habits: Lessons to be learned. *Br. Food J.* **2011**, *113*, 1393–1405. [CrossRef]

29. Raynor, H.A.; Vadiveloo, M. Understanding the Relationship Between Food Variety, Food Intake, and Energy Balance. *Curr. Obes. Rep.* **2018**, *7*, 68–75. [CrossRef]

30. Papadaki, S.; Mavrikaki, E. Greek adolescents and the Mediterranean diet: Factors affecting quality and adherence. *Nutrition* **2015**, *31*, 345–349. [CrossRef]

31. Skårdal, M.; Western, I.M.; Ask, A.M.S.; Øverby, N.C. Socioeconomic differences in selected dietary habits among Norwegian 13–14 year-olds: A cross-sectional study. *Food Nutr. Res.* **2014**, *58*. [CrossRef]

32. Morris, M.A.; Hulme, C.; Clarke, G.P.; Edwards, K.L.; Cade, J.E. What is the cost of a healthy diet? Using diet data from the UK Women's Cohort Study. *J. Epidemiol. Community Health* **2014**, *68*, 1043–1049. [CrossRef]

33. Stewart, S.D.; Menning, C.L. Family structure, nonresident father involvement, and adolescent eating patterns. *J. Adolesc. Health* **2009**, *45*, 193–201. [CrossRef]

34. Baek, Y.J.; Paik, H.Y.; Shim, J.E. Association between family structure and food group intake in children. *Nutr. Res. Pract.* **2014**, *8*, 463–468. [CrossRef]

35. Reicks, M.; Banna, J.; Cluskey, M.; Gunther, C.; Hongu, N.; Richards, R.; Topham, G.; Wong, S.S. Influence of Parenting Practices on Eating Behaviors of Early Adolescents during Independent Eating Occasions: Implications for Obesity Prevention. *Nutrients* **2015**, *7*, 8783–8801. [CrossRef]

36. Bauer, K.W.; Hearst, M.O.; Escoto, K.; Berge, J.M.; Neumark-Sztainer, D. Parental employment and work-family stress: Associations with family food environments. *Soc. Sci. Med.* **2012**, *75*, 496–504. [CrossRef]

37. Chatelan, A.; Beer-Borst, S.; Randriamiharisoa, A.; Pasquier, J.; Blanco, J.M.; Siegenthaler, S.; Paccaud, F.; Slimani, N.; Nicolas, G.; Camenzind-Frey, E.; et al. Major Differences in Diet across Three Linguistic Regions of Switzerland: Results from the First National Nutrition Survey menuCH. *Nutrients* **2017**, *9*, 1163. [CrossRef]

38. Census/Statbel. Population par Lieu de Résidence (Province), Sexe, Position dans le Ménage (C), État Civil, Situation sur le Marché de L'emploi (A) et Lieu de Naissance (A). Available online: http://census2011.fgov.be/censusselection/selectionFR.html (accessed on 16 July 2018).

39. Bere, E.; Brug, J.; Klepp, K.-I. Why do boys eat less fruit and vegetables than girls? *Public Health Nutr.* **2008**, *11*, 321–325. [CrossRef]

40. Caine-Bish, N.L.; Scheule, B. Gender differences in food preferences of school-aged children and adolescents. *J. Sch. Health* **2009**, *79*, 532–540. [CrossRef]

41. Wardle, J.; Haase, A.M.; Steptoe, A.; Nillapun, M.; Jonwutiwes, K.; Bellisle, F. Gender differences in food choice: The contribution of health beliefs and dieting. *Ann. Behav. Med.* **2004**, *27*, 107–116. [CrossRef]

42. Salvy, S.-J.; Vartanian, L.R.; Coelho, J.S.; Jarrin, D.; Pliner, P.P. The role of familiarity on modeling of eating and food consumption in children. *Appetite* **2008**, *50*, 514–518. [CrossRef]
43. McHale, S.M.; Updegraff, K.A.; Whiteman, S.D. Sibling Relationships and Influences in Childhood and Adolescence. *J. Marriage Fam.* **2012**, *74*, 913–930. [CrossRef]
44. Berge, J.M.; Meyer, C.; Maclehose, R.F.; Crichlow, R.; Neumark-Sztainer, D. All in the Family: Correlations between Parents' and Adolescent Siblings' Weight and Weight-related Behaviors. *Obesity* **2015**, *23*, 833–839. [CrossRef]
45. Senguttuvan, U.; Whiteman, S.D.; Jensen, A.C. Family Relationships and Adolescents' Health Attitudes and Weight: The Understudied Role of Sibling Relationships. *Fam. Relat.* **2014**, *63*, 384–396. [CrossRef]
46. De Ridder, K.; Bel, S.; Brocatus, L.; Cuypers, K.; Lebacq, T.; Moyersoen, I.; Ost, C.; Teppers, E. Enquête de Consommation Alimentaire 2014-2015: Rapport 4: La Consommation Alimentaire. Available online: https://fcs.wiv-isp.be/nl/Gedeelde%20%20documenten/FRANS/Rapport%204/Resume_rapport_4_finaal_finaal.pdf (accessed on 13 August 2018).
47. Moore, G.F.; Tapper, K.; Moore, L.; Murphy, S. Cognitive, behavioral, and social factors are associated with bias in dietary questionnaire self-reports by schoolchildren aged 9 to 11 years. *J. Am. Diet. Assoc.* **2008**, *108*, 1865–1873. [CrossRef]

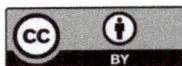

nutrients

MDPI

Article

The Association of Breakfast Frequency and Cardiovascular Disease (CVD) Risk Factors among Adolescents in Malaysia

Norashikin Mustafa [1], Hazreen Abd Majid [2,3], Zoi Toumpakari [1], Harriet Amy Carroll [1], Muhammad Yazid Jalaludin [4], Nabilla Al Sadat [2] and Laura Johnson [1,*]

[1] Centre for Exercise Nutrition and Health Sciences, School for Policy Studies, University of Bristol, Bristol BS8 1TZ, UK; norashikinmus@gmail.com (N.M.); z.toumpakari@bristol.ac.uk (Z.T.); hc12591@my.bristol.ac.uk (H.A.C.)
[2] Centre for Population Health (CePH) and Department of Social & Preventive Medicine, Faculty of Medicine, University of Malaya, 50603 Kuala Lumpur, Malaysia; hazreen@ummc.edu.my (H.A.M.); drnabilla@gmail.com (N.A.S.)
[3] Faculty of Public Health, Universitas Airlangga, Surabaya 60115, Indonesia
[4] Department of Paediatrics, Faculty of Medicine, University of Malaya, 50603 Kuala Lumpur, Malaysia; yazidj@ummc.edu.my
* Correspondence: Laura.Johnson@bristol.ac.uk

Received: 22 February 2019; Accepted: 24 April 2019; Published: 28 April 2019

Abstract: Breakfast frequency is associated with cardiovascular disease (CVD) risk in Western populations, possibly via the types of food eaten or the timing of food consumption, but associations in Malaysian adolescents are unknown. While the timing of breakfast is similar, the type of food consumed at breakfast in Malaysia differs from Western diets, which allows novel insight into the mechanisms underlying breakfast–CVD risk associations. We investigated foods eaten for breakfast and associations between breakfast frequency and CVD risk factors in the Malaysian Health and Adolescents Longitudinal Research Team study (MyHeARTs). Breakfast (frequency of any food/drink reported as breakfast in 7-day diet history interviews) and CVD risk factors (body mass index (BMI), waist circumference, fasting blood glucose, triacylglycerol, total cholesterol, high-density lipoprotein (HDL), low-density lipoprotein (LDL), and systolic and diastolic blood pressure) were cross-sectionally associated using linear regression adjusting for potential confounders ($n = 795$, age 13 years). Twelve percent of adolescents never ate breakfast and 50% ate breakfast daily, containing mean (SD) 400 ($\pm$127) kilocalories. Commonly consumed breakfast foods were cereal-based dishes (primarily rice), confectionery (primarily sugar), hot/powdered drinks (primarily Milo), and high-fat milk (primarily sweetened condensed milk). After adjustment, each extra day of breakfast consumption per week was associated with a lower BMI (-0.34 kg/m^2, 95% confidence interval (CI) -0.02, -0.66), and serum total (-0.07 mmol/L 95% CI -0.02, -0.13) and LDL (-0.07 mmol/L 95% CI -0.02, -0.12) cholesterol concentrations. Eating daily breakfast in Malaysia was associated with slightly lower BMI and total and LDL cholesterol concentrations among adolescents. Longitudinal studies and randomized trials could further establish causality.

Keywords: breakfast; obesity; cardiovascular; health; BMI; waist circumference; cholesterol; blood pressure; MyHeARTs

1. Introduction

Cardiovascular disease (CVD) is the number one cause of death globally [1]. In Malaysia, CVD is the biggest cause of mortality, accounting for 36% of total deaths [2]. Although the incidence of CVD (e.g., myocardial infarction and stroke) does not emerge until adulthood, CVD risk factors often present during adolescence [3]. For example, Malaysian children and adolescents have the highest prevalence of overweight and obesity across the South and Southeast Asian countries, at 22.5% (95% confidence interval (CI) 19.1–26.1) in boys and 19.1% (95% CI 16.1–22.6) in girls [4].

Over 50 cross-sectional studies, primarily in Europe and the United States, have reported consistent inverse associations between breakfast skipping and increased risk of overweight and obesity (odds ratio (OR) 1.55, 95% CI 1.46, 1.65) [5]. Outside of Europe and the United States, a meta-analysis of 19 cross-sectional studies in Asian populations also reported an increased risk of overweight and obesity (OR 1.76, 95% CI 1.48, 2.08) for breakfast skippers versus consumers [6], suggesting that the association is not limited to Western populations. Several causal mechanisms have been hypothesized to explain why eating breakfast may protect against CVD risk (Figure 1). In pathway 1, eating breakfast is hypothesized to reduce subsequent snacking, resulting in lower overall daily energy intake, thus maintaining energy balance and a lower body weight. Although in observational studies, breakfast is typically associated with higher total daily energy intakes [7]. In pathway 2, breakfast is associated with better food choices. For example, the kinds of foods typically eaten at breakfast in the United States and Europe tend to have cardio-protective properties e.g., wholegrain cereals that are high in fiber and micronutrients [8]. However, as foods typically eaten for breakfast vary widely across cultures, consistent associations of breakfast frequency across diverse countries could point to the timing of eating as more important than the type of food eaten. In pathway 3, it is hypothesized that eating in the morning is specifically better suited to circadian rhythms in metabolism, such that food ingested earlier in the day is metabolized more efficiently. The hypothesized circadian pathway is supported by acute randomized crossover experiments in adults, whereby the timing of food intake (but not the type of food consumed) is manipulated such that delaying breakfast is related to poorer appetite control, lower resting energy expenditure, impaired fasting lipid profiles, and reduced postprandial insulin sensitivity [9–12]. However more recent longer-term free-living trials that manipulated the timing of the first meal or randomized participants to receive simple advice to "eat breakfast" or not, have cast doubt on whether observational associations are causal but instead confounded i.e., eating breakfast may simply be an indicator of a generally healthy lifestyle [13–15]. Further research exploring breakfast frequency and the types of food eaten for breakfast in non-western populations is required to further understand existing observed associations.

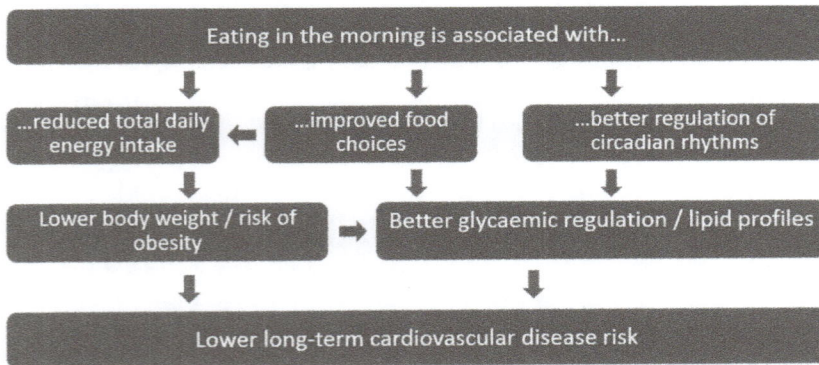

Figure 1. Hypothesized mechanisms for associations of breakfast with cardiovascular disease risk.

Most research on breakfast and health has been conducted in adults, with some work in children, but far less research has been dedicated to adolescents. However, adolescence represents a unique phase of life involving rapid growth, hormonal fluctuations, insulin resistance [16,17], and circadian dysregulation [18]. Considering the insulin resistance and circadian dysregulation can be influenced by breakfast consumption [19], it is important to understand the role of breakfast consumption on health in adolescents. In children aged 9–10 years in the 2011–2013 multi-country ISCOLE study, eating breakfast frequently (6–7 days/week), which varied from 58% in Brazil to 95% in Colombia, was associated with lower body mass index (BMI) z scores in some but not all countries [20]. This observation is supported by a systematic review including 10 longitudinal studies of children and adolescents of which eight provided evidence of inverse associations of more frequent breakfast consumption and adiposity [21]. In Malaysia, four cross-sectional studies have identified breakfast as the most frequently skipped meal among children and adolescents [22–25], with the prevalence of skipping breakfast varying from 17% [25] to 40% [24]. Only one cross-sectional study has examined breakfast consumption in relation to adiposity and obesity among Malaysian 12–19 year old adolescents [26]. Adolescents consuming breakfast five or more days/week had lower body weight, BMI, waist circumference, body fat mass, and percentage of body fat compared to those consuming breakfast less than five days/week. Overall, observational evidence on the association of a higher breakfast frequency with lower adiposity in adolescents is consistent worldwide.

Given that higher adiposity is associated with poorer CVD risk profiles [27], and breakfast frequency is associated with adiposity, one might expect to see similar associations with breakfast frequency and cardiovascular risk. However, evidence for associations of breakfast consumption with other CVD risk factors is less consistent. For example, fasted blood glucose concentrations were lowest among U.K. adolescents [28] and European boys [29] reporting daily breakfast consumption, but there was no evidence of a similar cross-sectional association among U.S. [30], Finnish [31], Taiwanese [32], or Japanese [33] adolescents. Lower systolic blood pressure has been observed among daily breakfast consumers in Taiwan [32] and in a European sample of boys, but no evidence of a similar cross-sectional association was observed among European girls and U.K., Japanese [33], U.S., Finnish, or Iranian [34] samples. Among Australian 9–15 year old children and adolescents followed-up as adults (aged 26–36 years), persistent breakfast skipping (defined as not eating between 0600 h and 0900 h as a child and adult) compared to consuming breakfast consistently was longitudinally associated with a higher waist circumference (mean difference 4.6, 95% CI 1.72, 7.53 cm), fasting serum insulin (mean difference 2.02, 95% CI 0.75, 3.29 mU/L), total cholesterol (mean difference 0.40, 95% CI 0.13, 0.68 mmol/L), and low density lipoprotein (LDL) cholesterol (mean difference 0.40, 95% CI 0.16, 0.64 mmol/L) concentrations [35]. Among Swedish 16 year-olds followed-up to age 43 years, eating breakfast only showed robust evidence of association with hyperglycemia (OR 1.75, 95% CI 1.01, 3.02), but not low high density lipoprotein (HDL) concentrations or hypertension [36]. Differences in sample sizes (ranging from 367 to 13,486 participants), diverse definitions of breakfast habits, and variation in adjustment for confounders may explain the inconsistency in findings to date.

Another possible explanation for inconsistent associations between breakfast consumption and CVD risk in adolescents is a lack of concurrent information on breakfast composition or diet quality. Existing evidence has typically relied on simple self-reported questions on usual breakfast frequency leaving it unclear how regular breakfast consumption relates to the types of food specifically eaten in the morning. Detailed dietary assessment methods like a food diary, 24-h diet recall, or diet history provide data on both the time of consumption and the food and nutrient content of breakfast, enabling both the frequency and composition of breakfast to be characterized and separate possible mechanisms to be explored. Finally, a proposed method for improved causal inference in observational research, by reducing the possibility that associations are confounded, is to explore the consistency of associations across high, middle- or low-income countries where the confounding structure may differ [37]. Therefore, adding to the existing evidence base on associations between breakfast and CVD risk, that is primarily in Western populations, by using Malaysian data may improve our understanding of the importance of breakfast.

No study to date has investigated the association of breakfast and CVD risk in Malaysian adolescents. In addition, few previous studies were able to explore what is eaten for breakfast in addition to breakfast frequency. The purpose of our study was to provide a detailed description of what adolescents ate for breakfast and investigate the association of breakfast frequency with CVD risk factors among adolescents using data from the Malaysian Health and Adolescent Longitudinal Research study

(MyHeARTs), including 7-day diet history enabling adjustment for potential confounders including concurrent diet quality.

2. Methods

2.1. Study Overview and Population

MyHeARTs is a prospective cohort study of 1351 schoolchildren (aged 13 years old at baseline) that attended 15 public secondary schools from central (Kuala Lumpur and Selangor) and northern (Perak) regions of Peninsular Malaysia. A detailed description of the MyHeARTs can be found elsewhere [38]. All procedures in MyHeARTs were approved by the Medical Ethics Committee, University Malaya Medical Centre according to the Declaration of Helsinki. Participation in the study was voluntary and written informed assent and consent was obtained from participants and parents/guardians of participants, respectively.

2.2. Dietary Assessment

Dietary intake was assessed using a seven-day diet history, which has been shown to give the most valid estimates of energy intake in children and adolescents (Burrows et al. 2010). Dietitians conducted open-ended interviews with the students to collect information on foods and drinks consumed during breakfast, mid-morning snack, lunch, afternoon tea, dinner and supper over the previous seven days. Pictures of local food and household measurement items were used to assist participants in estimating portion sizes consumed. Food and drink energy and nutrient intakes were calculated using the Nutritionist Pro™ Diet Analysis (Axxya Systems, Redmond, WA, USA) and Nutrient Composition of Malaysian Foods [39,40].

To compute breakfast consumption, energy intake from all foods or drink reported during the meal-slot identified as breakfast was combined on each day. Frequency of breakfast intake (days/week) was calculated as the number of days where any food or drinks were reported at breakfast. This was categorized for descriptive analyses by grouping into daily, 4–6 days/week, 1–3 days/week, and 0 days/week. The types of food and drink reported were investigated by grouping food items into 44 groups and then analyzing the frequency that each food group was reported across all food items in each breakfast occasions. Under-reporting of energy intake was assessed by comparing reported energy intake to estimated basal metabolic rate and participants defined as under-reporters ($n = 497$) were excluded [41]. Excluded participants were 43% male, 57% urban, 78% Malay, 12% Chinese, 7% Indian, and 2% other ethnicity, with age mean 12.9 ($\pm$0.3) years, BMI mean ($\pm$SD) 22.2 ($\pm$5.6) kg/m^2, and a mean daily energy intake of 1126 ($\pm$278) kcal.

A dietary pattern score for each adolescent was derived using reduced rank regression [42]. The score is a weighted linear combination of the 44 food groups (Supplementary Table S1) which predict the maximum variation in intermediate variables hypothesized to be on the pathway between food group intake and cardiovascular health, i.e., energy density (kJ/gram), fiber density (g/MJ), and percentage of energy intake from fat (%). A high pattern score represents an energy dense, low-fiber diet, which is characterized by high consumption of processed meat, bread products, chocolate, egg dishes and energy-dense Malaysian kuih (Malaysian snacks and desserts), and a low consumption of fruit, vegetables and vegetables dishes, and soups (unpublished results).

2.3. Anthropometric and Clinical Measurements

Height was measured without socks and shoes using a calibrated vertical stadiometer (Seca Portable 217, Seca, Birmingham, UK). Weight was measured with light clothing using a digital electronic weighing scale (Seca 813, Seca, Birmingham, UK). Body mass index was calculated as weight in kilograms divided by the square of height in meters (kg/m^2). Waist circumference was measured to the nearest millimeter using a non-elastic Seca measuring tape (Seca 201, Seca, Birmingham, UK). Systolic and diastolic blood pressure were calculated as the average of three readings using a stethoscope and a mercury sphygmomanometer. Fasting (≥10 h) venous blood samples were obtained from each participant and analyzed for serum total cholesterol, LDL cholesterol, HDL cholesterol, triacylglycerol (TAG), and blood glucose concentrations. More information on the way anthropometric and clinical measures were obtained can be found elsewhere [38].

2.4. Confounders

Physical activity was self-reported using the physical activity questionnaire (in Malay) for older children (PAC-Q). Sex, ethnicity (Malay, Chinese, Indian, other), smoking status (yes/no), and alcohol intake (yes/no) were self-reported in student questionnaires.

2.5. Statistical Analysis

Variables are described using mean (SD) if continuous and normal, or frequency (%) if categorical. Normality was checked via visual inspection of histograms. Analysis of variance (ANOVA) was performed to test the mean difference between breakfast frequency groups and continuous CVD risk factors. Tests for linear trend were performed using a likelihood ratio test comparing a model containing breakfast frequency (days/week) as a continuous variable with a model containing breakfast frequency as a categorical variable (daily, 4–6 days/week, 1–3 days/week, and 0 days/week). The chi-squared test was used to test for associations between breakfast frequency groups and categorical confounders. Multiple linear regression analysis was used to examine the independent relationship between breakfast frequency (days/week) and CVD risk factors. Risk factors analyzed as dependent variables were BMI, waist circumference, fasting serum glucose, TAG, total cholesterol, HDL and LDL concentrations, and systolic and diastolic blood pressure. Model 1 included only breakfast frequency as an independent variable. Model 2 included breakfast frequency, sex, ethnicity, physical activity level, smoking status, and alcohol intake. Model 3 included model 2 variables as well as BMI. Model 4 included model 3 variables together with total energy (kcal/day), total carbohydrate (% daily energy), total protein (% energy), total fat (% energy), total cholesterol (mg/1000 kcal), total saturated fatty acid (% energy), total sodium (mg/1000 kcal), total calcium (mg/1000 kcal), total iron (mg/1000 kcal), total fiber (g/1000 kcal), and total sugar (% energy). Model 5 included model 4 variables together with dietary pattern score. Statistical analyses were performed using SPSS (version 21, IBM), Stata (version 15, StataCorp LLC, College Station, Texas, USA), and SAS (version 9.4, Marlow, Buckinghamshire, UK).

3. Results

Figure 2 shows that 795 participants had complete data based on the variables of interest and were included in the current analysis. The characteristics of participants overall and stratified by breakfast frequency are presented in Table 1. Fifty one percent of the sample were daily breakfast eaters, 25% consumed breakfast 4–6 days/week, 15% consumed breakfast 1–3 days/week, and 10% of the sample never consumed breakfast. Adolescents of Indian ethnicity were more likely to be daily breakfast eaters (71%) compared to the overall sample, while no Chinese adolescents were identified as breakfast skippers. Boys were more likely than girls to consume breakfast daily (58% vs. 47%). Few differences in breakfast frequency were observed for any other individual characteristics.

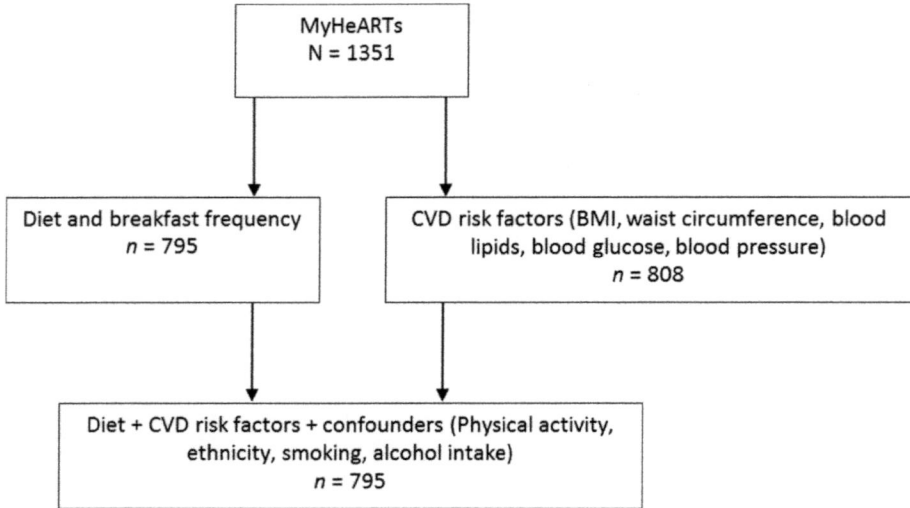

Figure 2. Number of participants with data available based on the variables of interest. CVD: cardiovascular disease; MyHeARTs: Malaysian Health and Adolescents Longitudinal Research Team study.

In terms of diet, adolescents who consumed breakfast but infrequently (1–3 days/week) consumed the least total daily energy, calcium, and sugar compared to both breakfast skippers and daily consumers (Table 1). Daily breakfast consumers had a positive dietary pattern score i.e., a more energy dense and lower fiber density diet, compared to infrequent breakfast eaters and breakfast skippers who, on average, had a negative dietary pattern score. Breakfasts reported in MyHeARTs contained a mean (SD) 400 ± 127 kcal. The most frequent food groups of all food items reported at breakfast were cereal-based mixed meals (19%), chocolate and confectionery (14%), hot and powdered drinks (13%), high fat milk (12%), and bread (6%) (Figure 3). Cereal-based mixed meals, were mainly rice in coconut milk (34% of cereal based mixed meals food items), fried rice (30%), and fried noodles (12%) (Supplementary Material Table S1). Chocolate and confectionery refer to granulated sugar (99% of chocolate and confectionery items reported at breakfast), while hot and powdered drinks, are mostly Milo (a chocolate and malt powder drink) (40%) and malted milk powder (38%). High fat milk and cream was primarily sweetened condensed milk (90% of items in that group) (Supplementary Material Table S1).

Table 1. Characteristics of MyHeARTs participants by breakfast frequency groups.

	Total	Breakfast Frequency				p-Value
		0 days/week	1–3 days/week	4–6 days/week	Daily	
All children, n (%)	795 (100)	76 (10)	115 (15)	196 (25)	408 (51)	-
Age (years), mean (SD)	12.9 (0.3)	12.9 (0.3)	12.9 (0.4)	12.8 (0.3)	12.9 (0.3)	-
Sex						
Boys, n (%)	298 (37)	32 (10)	36 (12)	58 (19)	172 (58)	0.01 [a]
Girls, n (%)	497 (63)	44 (9)	79 (16)	138 (28)	236 (47)	
Urbanicity						
Urban, n (%)	401 (50)	17 (4)	53 (13)	114 (28)	217 (54)	<0.001 [a]
Rural, n (%)	394 (50)	59 (15)	62 (16)	82 (21)	191 (48)	
Ethnicity						
Malay, n (%)	650 (82)	68 (10)	100 (15)	162 (25)	320 (49)	0.03 [a]
Chinese, n (%)	44 (6)	0 (0)	8 (18)	12 (27)	24 (55)	
Indian, n (%)	69 (14)	5 (7)	3 (4)	12 (17)	49 (71)	
Others, n (%)	32 (6)	3 (9)	4 (13)	10 (31)	15 (47)	
Smoking status						
Yes, n (%)	73 (9)	11 (15)	12 (16)	13 (18)	37 (51)	0.23 [a]
No, n (%)	722 (91)	65 (9)	103 (14)	183 (25)	371 (51)	
Alcohol intake						
Yes, n (%)	23 (3)	3 (13)	5 (22)	4 (17)	11 (48)	0.55 [a]
No, n (%)	772 (97)	73 (9)	110 (14)	192 (25)	397 (51)	
Physical activity (in last 7 days)						

Table 1. *Cont.*

| | Total | Breakfast Frequency | | | | *p*-Value |
		0 days/week	1–3 days/week	4–6 days/week	Daily	
Never n (%)	237 (30)	27 (11)	35 (15)	55 (23)	120 (51)	0.35 [a]
1–2 times last week n (%)	361 (45)	32 (8)	58 (16)	89 (25)	182 (50)	
3–4 times last week n (%)	113 (14)	8 (7)	13 (12)	31 (27)	61 (54)	
5–6 times last week n (%)	34 (4)	2 (6)	8 (24)	8 (24)	16 (47)	
7+ times last week n (%)	50 (6)	7 (14)	1 (2)	13 (26)	29 (58)	
Total daily intake						
Energy (kcal/day)	1673 (332)	1744 (433)	1573 (276)	1594 (267)	1726 (339)	<0.001 [b]
Protein (% of total energy)	15 (2)	15 (2)	15 (2)	15 (2)	15 (2)	0.63 [b]
Fat (% of total energy)	29.930 (5)	30 (5)	30 (4)	30 (5)	30 (4)	0.87 [b]
Carbohydrate (% of total energy)	55 (5)	55 (5)	56 (5)	55 (5)	55 (6)	0.62 [b]
Cholesterol (mg/1000 kcal)	133 (52)	137 (58)	139 (50)	131(47)	132 (54)	0.53 [b]
SFA (% of total energy)	6 (2)	6 (2)	5 (2)	6 (3)	6 (2)	0.14 [b]
Sodium (mg/1000 kcal)	1387 (345)	1328 (380)	1363 (352)	1400 (329)	1399 (344)	0.32 [b]
Calcium (mg/1000 kcal)	226 (91)	229 (116)	195 (827)	222 (81)	236 (92)	<0.001 [b]
Iron (mg/1000 kcal)	9 (3)	9 (3)	8 (6)	8 (2)	9 (2)	0.42 [b]
Crude fiber (g/1000 kcal)	2 (1)	2 (1)	2 (1)	2 (11)	2 (1)	0.51 [b]
Sugar (% of total energy)	8 (4)	8 (4)	7 (3)	9 (4)	8 (4)	0.04 [b]
Dietary pattern score (SD units)	0.01 (1.10)	−0.06 (1.18)	−0.09 (1.02)	−0.12 (1.081)	0.12 (1.10)	0.05 [b]

[a] Pearson's chi-squared; [b] ANOVA. Abbreviations—ANOVA: analysis of variance; SD: standard deviation; SFA: saturated fatty acid.

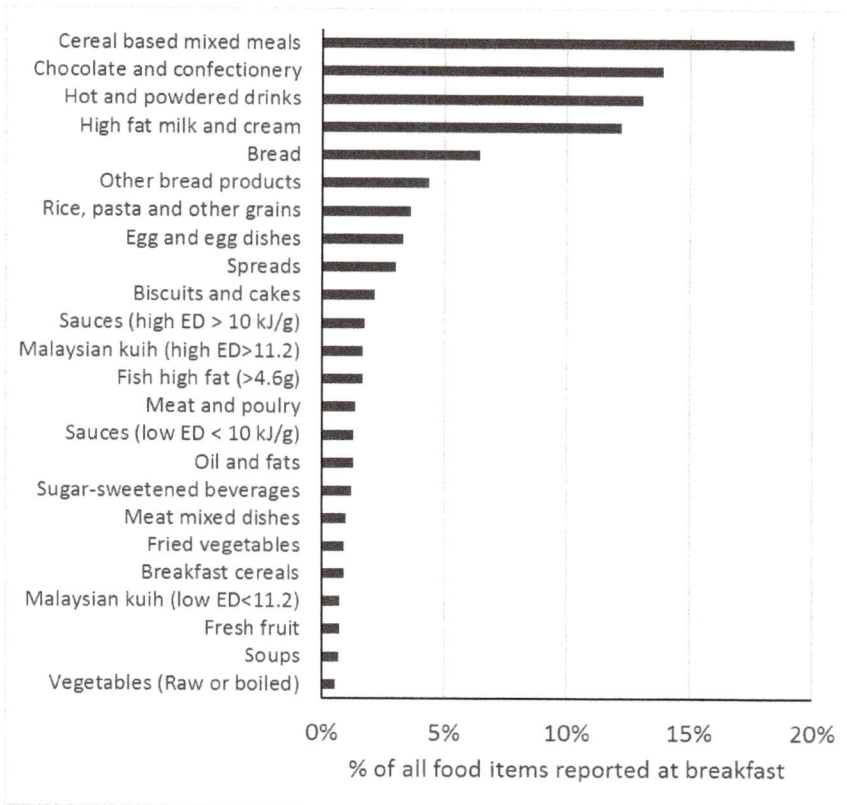

Figure 3. Food groups eaten for breakfast. Bars represent percentage of each food group from all food items reported in breakfast occasions ($n = 15{,}507$ food items reported at breakfast). Only food groups contributing 1% or more to all food items are displayed. Energy density (ED).

3.1. Mean of Cardiovascular Disease Risk Factors

A description of CVD risk factors by breakfast frequency is presented in Table 2. Compared to daily breakfast consumers, those who never ate breakfast had slightly higher serum total cholesterol concentrations (4.6 vs. 4.8 mmol/L, $p = 0.01$), driven by higher LDL cholesterol (2.7 vs. 2.9 mmol/L, $p = 0.01$) (Figure 4). These associations were linear across the breakfast categories. Unlike the other CVD risk variables, there was weak evidence ($p_{trend} = 0.06$) that the relationship between breakfast consumption and BMI may be non-linear. Those consuming breakfast daily had the lowest BMI (19.2 kg/m^2), but participants who consumed breakfast infrequently (1–3 days/week), rather than never, had the highest BMI (20.9 kg/m^2; Table 2 and Figure 4). There was no evidence of other CVD risk factors, i.e., fasting serum glucose, TAG, or HDL concentration and blood pressure, varying by breakfast frequency, though there was some weak evidence suggesting that waist circumference was 2 cm smaller in daily vs. never breakfast consumers ($p = 0.06$).

Table 2. Description of cardiovascular disease (CVD) risk factors by breakfast frequency (*n* = 795).

	Breakfast Frequency				*p*-Value (ANOVA)	*p*trend
	0 days/week (*n* = 76)	1–3 days/week (*n* = 115)	4–6 days/week (*n* = 196)	Daily (*n* = 408)		
	Mean (SD)	Mean (SD)	Mean (SD)	Mean (SD)		
BMI (kg/m^2)	19.9 (5.7)	20.9 (5.3)	20.0 (4.4)	19.2 (4.7)	0.003	0.06
WC (cm)	70.1 (12.9)	71.0 (13.4)	69.0 (10.6)	67.9 (11.6)	0.06	0.91
FBG (mmol/L)	4.9 (0.4)	4.9 (0.4)	4.9 (0.4)	4.9 (0.8)	0.79	0.61
TC (mmol/L)	4.8 (1.0)	4.6 (0.9)	4.7 (0.8)	4.6 (0.8)	0.01	0.32
HDL(mmol/L)	1.5 (0.3)	1.5 (0.3)	1.4 (0.3)	1.5 (0.3)	0.56	0.38
LDL (mmol/L)	2.9 (0.9)	2.8 (0.8)	2.8 (0.7)	2.7 (0.7)	0.01	0.41
SBP (mmHg)	109 (13)	111 (11)	109 (11)	109 (11)	0.32	0.31
DBP (mmHg)	67 (13)	68 (10)	67 (10)	68 (10)	0.45	0.34
TAG (mmol/L)	0.98 (0.60)	0.92 (0.45)	0.99 (0.47)	0.91 (0.46)	0.24	0.23

Abbreviations—ANOVA: analysis of variance; BMI: body mass index; DBP: diastolic blood pressure; FBG: fasting plasma glucose; HDL: high-density lipoprotein; LDL: low-density lipoprotein; TC: total cholesterol; SBP: systolic blood pressure; SD: standard deviation; TAG: triacylglycerol; WC: waist circumference.

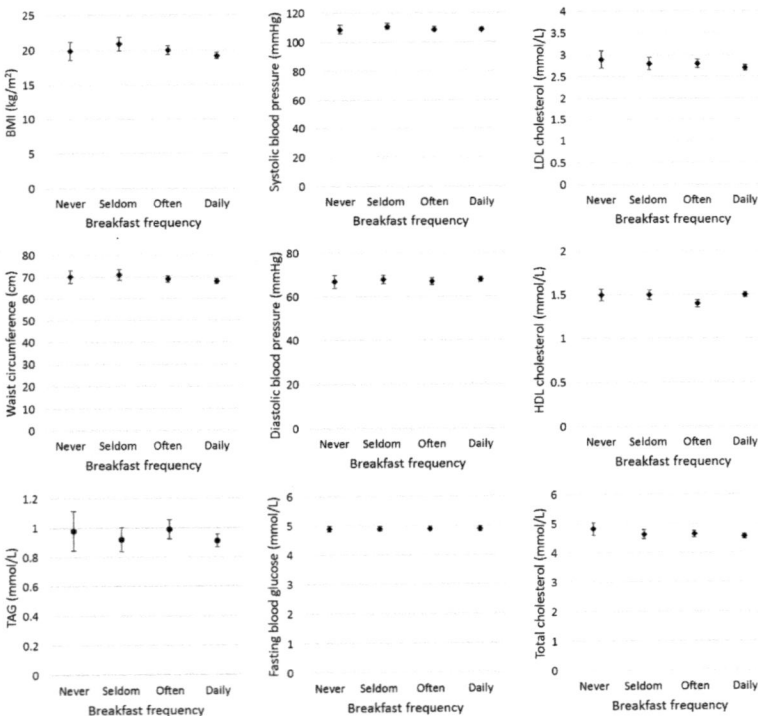

Figure 4. Baseline associations between breakfast frequency and cardiovascular disease (CVD) risk factors in MyHeARTs. Never = 0 days a week, *n* = 76; Seldom = 1–3 days a week, *n* = 115; Often = 4–6 days a week, *n* = 196; Daily = 7 days a week, *n* = 408. Abbreviations—BMI: body mass index; HDL: high-density lipoprotein; LDL: low-density lipoprotein; TAG: triacylglycerol.

3.2. Association of Breakfast Consumption and cardiovascular disease (CVD) Risk Factors

Table 3 shows associations between breakfast frequency and CVD risk factors, before and after adjusting for potential confounders. In the fully adjusted models, each extra day of breakfast was associated with a lower BMI by 0.2 kg/m^2 (95% CI −0.4, −0.1) and lower total cholesterol concentration of −0.03 mmol/L (95% CI −0.06, −0.01). The lower total cholesterol concentration was driven by LDL cholesterol, which was lower by the same order of magnitude for each extra day of breakfast (β −0.03, 95% CI −0.06, −0.01). Waist circumference was 0.5 cm (95% CI −0.84, −0.16 cm) lower per extra day of eating breakfast per week in model 2, but the association was reduced to 0.06 cm/breakfast/week after adjustment for BMI (model 3, Table 3). No evidence of association was observed for fasting serum glucose or TAG concentration, serum HDL cholesterol concentration, and blood pressure.

Table 3. Multiple linear regression analysis of association of breakfast frequency and risk factors of cardiovascular disease independent of potential confounding among participants (*n* = 795).

	β (95% CI)	*p*-Value
Body mass index (kg/m^2)		
Model 1 [a]	−0.21 (−0.35, −0.07)	0.004
Model 2 [b]	−0.20 (−0.34, −0.06)	0.01
Model 4 [d]	−0.20 (−0.34, −0.05)	0.01
Model 5 [f]	−0.18 (−0.33, −0.04)	0.01
Waist circumference (cm)		
Model 1 [a]	−0.44 (−0.78, −0.10)	0.01
Model 2 [b]	−0.50 (−0.84, −0.16)	0.004
Model 3 [c]	−0.06 (−0.21, 0.09)	0.40
Model 4 [e]	−0.07 (−0.22, 0.08)	0.36
Model 5 [g]	−0.06 (−0.21, 0.09)	0.43
Fasting glucose concentration (mmol/L)		
Model 1 [a]	0.00 (−0.02, 0.02)	0.80
Model 2 [b]	0.00 (−0.02, 0.02)	0.88
Model 3 [c]	0.00 (−0.02. 0.02)	0.79
Model 4 [e]	0.00 (−0.02, 0.02)	086
Model 5 [g]	0.00 (−0.02, 0.02)	0.82
Total cholesterol concentration (mmol/L)		
Model 1 [a]	−0.04 (−0.06, −0.01)	0.004
Model 2 [b]	−0.04 (−0.06, −0.01)	0.003
Model 3 [c]	−0.04 (−0.06, −0.01)	0.01
Model 4 [e]	−0.03 (−0.06, −0.01)	0.01
Model 5 [g]	−0.03 (−0.06, −0.01)	0.01
High-density lipoprotein cholesterol concentration (mmol/L)		
Model 1 [a]	0.00 (−0.01, 0.01)	0.68
Model 2 [b]	0.00 (−0.01, 0.01)	0.66
Model 3 [c]	0.00 (−0.01, 0.01)	0.57
Model 4 [e]	0.00 (−0.01, 0.01)	0.80
Model 5 [g]	0.00 (−0.01, 0.01)	0.82

Table 3. *Cont.*

	β (95% CI)	*p*-Value
Low-density lipoprotein cholesterol concentration (mmol/L)		
Model 1 [a]	−0.03 (−0.06, −0.01)	0.002
Model 2 [b]	−0.04 (−0.06, −0.01)	0.001
Model 3 [c]	−0.03 (−0.05, −0.01)	0.03
Model 4 [e]	−0.03 (−0.05, −0.01)	0.01
Model 5 [g]	−0.03 (−0.05, −0.01)	0.01
Systolic blood pressure (mmHg)		
Model 1 [a]	−0.18 (−0.51, 0.15)	0.28
Model 2 [b]	−0.14 (−0.46, 0.18)	0.389
Model 3 [c]	0.04 (−0.25, 0.34)	0.78
Model 4 [e]	0.07 (−0.23, 0.37)	0.65
Model 5 [g]	0.07 (−0.23, 0.37)	0.65
Diastolic blood pressure (mmHg)		
Model 1 [a]	0.11 (−0.19, 0.41)	0.48
Model 2 [b]	0.12 (−0.18, 0.42)	0.44
Model 3 [c]	0.26 (−0.03, 0.55)	0.08
Model 4 [e]	0.27 (−0.03, 0.56)	0.08
Model 5 [g]	0.27 (−0.02, 0.57)	0.07
Triacylglycerol concentration (mmol/L)		
Model 1 [a]	−0.01 (−0.02, 0.01)	0.26
Model 2 [b]	−0.01 (−0.02, 0.01)	0.34
Model 3 [c]	0.00 (−0.01, 0.01)	0.92
Model 4 [e]	0.00 (−0.02, 0.01)	0.82
Model 5 [g]	0.00 (−0.01, 0.01)	0.90

Abbreviations—CI: confidence interval. [a] Model 1 includes only breakfast frequency. [b] Model 2 includes breakfast frequency, physical activity, smoking status, alcohol intake, ethnicity, and sex. [c] Model 3 includes variables in model 2 plus BMI. [d] Model 4 includes variables from model 2 plus total daily energy (kcal), total daily carbohydrate (%), total daily protein (%), total daily fat (%), total daily cholesterol (mg/1000 kcal), total daily saturated fatty acid (%), total daily sodium (mg/1000 kcal), total daily calcium (mg/1000 kcal), total daily iron (mg/1000 kcal), total daily fiber (g/1000 kcal), and total daily sugar (%). [e] Model 4 includes variables from model 3 plus total daily energy (kcal), total daily carbohydrate (%), total daily protein (%), total daily fat (%), total daily cholesterol (mg/1000 kcal), total daily saturated fatty acid (%), total daily sodium (mg/1000 kcal), total daily calcium (mg/1000 kcal), total daily iron (mg/1000 kcal), total daily fiber (g/1000 kcal), and total daily sugar (%). [f] Model 5 includes variables from model 4 [d] plus dietary pattern score. [g] Model 5 includes variables from model 4 [e] plus dietary pattern score.

4. Discussion

In this cross-sectional analysis of a large sample of Malaysian adolescents with detailed dietary data and a broad range of CVD risk factors, we found evidence that breakfast frequency was inversely associated with BMI and fasting total and LDL cholesterol concentrations, but not waist circumference, fasting glucose, HDL or TAG concentrations, or blood pressure.

Among Malaysian adolescents in our study, 10% were breakfast skippers and 51% were daily breakfast consumers, which is similar to a previously reported prevalence in a different Malaysian sample of 12–19 year-olds [26]. A higher prevalence of breakfast skipping has been observed among U.S. and Finnish adolescents (i.e., 13–16% and 16–24% respectively [31,43]) as well as higher prevalence of daily breakfast consumption in other populations (i.e., 94% among U.K. primary school children and 89% among Taiwanese primary school children [28,32]). Differences in daily breakfast consumption could partly be explained by a lack of a consistent definition of breakfast in the literature [44]. For example, some studies defined breakfast based on the time of the day food was consumed, e.g., between 0600 h and 0900 h [35], while others based their definitions on the frequency of breakfast (self-identified by the participant) during the week [29,32,34] or only during weekdays [31]. In addition, adolescents with the same breakfast frequency may be in different groups across studies, e.g., breakfast skippers in the current study are those who never consumed breakfast, while in other studies those who never consumed breakfast are combined with irregular consumers [29].

4.1. Breakfast Associations with Cardiovascular Disease Risk Factors

Our findings agree with previous observational studies across the world showing consistent inverse associations between frequency of breakfast consumption and BMI [5,6]. Only one study previously investigated Malaysian adolescents (*n* = 236) [26], finding breakfast consumption to be associated with lower BMI, concordant with our analysis. Interestingly, we did not find strong evidence for a linear relationship potentially suggesting that never eating breakfast is not problematic per se, but rather irregular consumption of breakfast on some days but not others makes energy balance more difficult to regulate. Nurul-Fadhilah et al. [26] further found an inverse relationship between breakfast consumption and waist circumference, which our analysis supports, but the association was not robust to adjustment for BMI. Similar waist circumferences were found between the two studies for infrequent breakfast consumers (~70 cm) but the waist circumference observed in frequent breakfast consumers differed, where Nurul-Fadhilah et al. [26] found lower waist circumferences (~64 cm) compared with MyHeARTs (~68 cm). The differences in these findings may be explained by the comparatively homogenous sample (mostly Malay from Kelantan) with a smaller sample size compared to the larger and more diverse MyHeARTs sample.

Our study found frequent breakfast consumption was associated with lower total cholesterol driven by lower LDL cholesterol concentrations compared to infrequent breakfast consumption. These findings are in agreement with some [29,35], but not all [28–30,33] previous studies. However the effect sizes in our analyses were small and likely not clinically meaningful (~0.03 mmol/L difference in plasma total and LDL cholesterol concentrations for each extra day of breakfast), as ≥ 1.0 mmol/L reduction in LDL concentration is needed to reduce the risk of all-cause mortality by 10% in adults [45].

Previous research has reported inconsistent associations between breakfast consumption and HDL cholesterol concentrations [30–33]. Our analyses however provided no evidence of association in accordance with several studies [30,31,33,35]. Whilst others found statistically significant associations [32,46], the differences in HDL cholesterol concentrations observed elsewhere were small and unlikely to be clinically meaningful at reducing CVD risk (difference of <2 mg/dL). Importantly, all categories of breakfast consumption in this study were associated with plasma HDL cholesterol concentrations within the range associated with lowest CVD and mortality risk in adults [47]. Such findings may suggest that there is limited power in detecting associations between CVD risk markers such as HDL concentrations in an overall healthy sample. Despite the inconsistencies in statistical significance between studies, taken together there appears to be no meaningful association between HDL cholesterol concentrations and breakfast consumption in adolescents, in line with our results.

We did not observe evidence of association between breakfast consumption and blood pressure, which may partially be explained by the similar sodium intakes between breakfast consumption categories. As with HDL cholesterol concentrations, previous research has provided mixed results regarding the relationship between breakfast consumption and blood pressure in adolescents. Ahadi et al. [34] found breakfast consumption to be associated with lower blood pressure, supporting previous research showing a reduced risk of hypertension [31]. The latter study however only showed lower hypertension risk in girls who were semi-regular breakfast consumers. Our findings do however support other research demonstrating no association between breakfast consumption and diastolic [28,30,36,46] and systolic [30,36,46] blood pressure.

Our analysis did not find an association between breakfast consumption frequency and plasma TAG concentrations, supporting most other studies [28–30,48]. Smith et al. [35] found breakfast skipping to be longitudinally associated with increased serum TAG concentrations compared to regular breakfast consumption, potentially suggesting changes to TAG concentrations occur over a longer period. Such a time effect may be physiologically plausible; blood TAG concentrations are typically due to greater adiposity, but such an effect is not necessarily immediate. Since breakfast skipping has consistently been associated with greater adiposity [5], it may be that the associations with TAG are chronic adaptations to higher fat mass.

Lower fasting glucose concentrations have previously been associated with regular breakfast consumption in adolescents in some [28,29,36] but not all [30,32] studies, with others finding mixed results [31,35]. Our analyses provide no evidence for an association. However, we were unable to investigate markers of insulin resistance (e.g., Homeostatic model assessment HOMA) due to lack of insulin data; such a measure provides useful data due to the insulin resistance exhibited during adolescence [16,17]. This may explain the more consistent finding (compared to fasting plasma glucose concentrations alone) of regular breakfast consumption being associated with lower insulin resistance in adolescents [28–30,35].

There is a lack of causal data in adolescents pertaining to glycemic regulation and breakfast consumption. In adults, short-term experimental manipulations to meal regularity (including breakfast omission) have detrimental effects on acute postprandial glycemic and insulinemic responses [9,49], although longer-term breakfast consumption versus omission does not appear to negatively influence glycemic regulation [13]. Equally, in schoolchildren, fasted plasma glucose concentrations were unaffected by participation (compared to non-participation) in a nine-month school breakfast program [50], supporting our analysis. Such findings suggest chronic adaptations to blood glucose possibly occur mitigating the acute-effects of breakfast omission.

4.2. Comparisons of Breakfast Definitions

The differences in the way breakfast is defined and how frequencies are combined in each study make it hard to directly compare associations with health and may be responsible for the disparate findings [51]. For example Nurul-Fadhilah et al. [26] used two broad categories of breakfast, i.e., <5 days/week versus ≥5 days/week, which could explain the evidence for association observed for waist circumference, in comparison to the weaker evidence observed in our study, which included a greater number of breakfast categories. Furthermore, our study adjusted for aspects of adiposity and diet quality, which was not the case in previous studies showing associations for fasting glucose concentrations and blood pressure [28,32]. Different ranges of CVD risk factors could also explain the diverse findings; for example, mean diastolic blood pressure was higher among U.K. primary children [28] compared to our sample. Additional explanations could be the inclusion of younger and smaller sample sizes [28,30] and the inclusion of healthier adolescents compared to the average population [33].

4.3. Breakfast Composition and Meal Timing

Overall, our findings show some, albeit limited, evidence for a protective association between breakfast consumption and some CVD risk factors, such as BMI, and total and LDL cholesterol concentrations. One reason for which breakfast might be protective is the consumption of particular foods during breakfast. The fiber contained in cereal and the high protein content of eggs have been shown to increase satiety and improve appetite control [44,52,53]. This may explain the protective effect of breakfast in some populations. For example, European children and adolescents typically consume micronutrient-dense breakfast cereal (with milk) and bread [54], while in our sample the most commonly consumed breakfast foods were cooked rice dishes, sugar, malt drinks, and sweetened condensed milk. Considering the differences in the types of foods consumed at breakfast between populations, it is more likely that, if causal, breakfast relates to health because of the timing of food intake in relation to circadian metabolic rhythms rather than the type of food consumed.

The timing of eating has been associated with improved gluco-regulatory responses in adults (e.g., Farshchi et al. [9]). Improved postprandial metabolic responses may be of particular importance in adolescents because of the increased insulin resistance in this population compared to childhood and adulthood [16,17], as well as the circadian dysregulation, which often skews adolescents towards evening chronotypes [18] typically associated with poorer general health [55]. In adults, such circadian misalignment is causally implicated in poorer cardiometabolic health (e.g., Scheer et al. [56]), with observational research suggesting similar health outcomes in adolescents [57]. Compared to the evening, morning ingestion of nutrients results in lower postprandial glycemia and insulinemia, conducive to lower CVD risk [58], making breakfast a particularly important meal. Breakfast consumption may therefore act to improve cardiometabolic health via both circadian entrainment [59], and via exploiting the favorable postprandial response found when ingesting nutrients in the morning compared to the evening [60], though causal research specifically in adolescents is lacking and should be a priority for future studies.

4.4. Strengths and Limitations

One of the main strengths of our study is that the MyHeARTs is the largest study in Malaysia, involving adolescents from three main ethnicities, three regions, and the inclusion of rural and urban participants, providing superior representativeness than previous studies (e.g., Nurul-Fadhilah et al. [26]). The ethnic diversity in our analyses is a particular strength, demonstrating higher breakfast eating prevalence among Indian participants, and no cases of skipping breakfast every day in Chinese participants. Dietary intake was measured using a seven-day diet history, which is a valid method for estimating the energy and nutrient intake among adolescents (Burrows et al. 2010). A broad range of demographic data, with student lifestyle and information on parents enabled us to model the independent association of breakfast frequency with CVD risk factors, including multiple biomarkers.

Whilst the strengths of this study mean we have provided novel data on breakfast and cardiometabolic health in Malaysian adolescents, several limitations also need to be acknowledged. Breakfast is notoriously difficult to define, particularly in epidemiological studies due to limitations in data availability (e.g., wake time not being recorded). In our study, breakfast was self-defined by the participant. Recent research has aimed to define breakfast and has proposed a wake-time-dependent definition of within two or three hours of waking [44]. In data collection for MyHeARTs, dietitians asked participants when their breakfast time was, and if this was after 1030 h, the meal was not recorded as 'breakfast' but as a morning snack instead. Owing to early school start times in Malaysia (~0730 h), our definition of breakfast on week days is likely to have classified some breakfasts outside of 2–3 h of waking, thus capturing a slightly extended morning fast.

Future studies should further explore different types of breakfast which may help provide novel insights into the role of breakfast on cardiometabolic health. For example, in our sample, adolescents typically consumed foods such as rice and noodles for breakfast which, despite being high carbohydrates, differ in nutritional composition to typical breakfast foods in Europe, such as cereal, which is a vehicle for milk consumption in European children [54]. Differences in breakfast composition may help explain some of the aforementioned disparities compared to previous research. Future studies could explore this using meal coding, as has been done previously, to understand meal-based dietary patterns in adults [61,62]. Additionally, understanding breakfast composition may help elucidate whether the consistent associations with BMI are driven by breakfast food composition or timing of nutrient intake. In the case of the latter, this would explain why we observed a protective association with breakfast despite daily breakfast consumers having a more energy-dense, lower fiber overall dietary pattern score, which is associated with greater adiposity in the United Kingdom [63]. This may additionally suggest further cultural differences, as typically breakfast consumption in Western populations is associated with less obesogenic diets [64].

Physical activity and diet were both self-reported. Although validated methods were used to obtain these data minimizing risk of bias, there is known error within these measures, such as energy intake underreporting bias. As such, we aimed to control for dietary misreporting by excluding under-reporters. Finally, the cross-sectional and observational nature of the study prevents causal inference for the associations observed owing to the possibility of reverse causation and residual confounding. Thus, both longitudinal and randomized controlled studies are required in order to establish the causality of the relationship between breakfast consumption and lower CVD risk factors in this population. Longitudinal studies are particularly valuable in adolescents as some research has suggested breakfast skipping is cross-sectionally, but not longitudinally associated with higher BMI in adolescents with overweight, and vice versa in those in the normal BMI range [65]. Our study has provided valuable information for hypothesis generation to aid in developing such studies.

5. Conclusion

In conclusion, the present study suggests that adolescents in Malaysia who eat breakfast more frequently have a lower BMI, and lower plasma total and LDL cholesterol concentrations independent of a range of confounders. Our study results specifically highlight that the benefits of breakfast (if causal) are not limited to the types of foods typically eaten in Western populations such as breakfast cereals, milk, or bread, but may be independent of the type of food consumed and instead related to the timing of food intake. Furthermore, our data suggested that irregular habits may be more detrimental to CVD risk than uniform breakfast eating vs. skipping. Previous longitudinal studies or long-term randomized trials have not explored the potential impact of consistent versus irregular breakfast habits or been able to differentiate changes in the timing of eating from the type of food eaten. Future research should aim to examine whether the content, timing, or regularity of breakfast intake is associated with lower CVD risk both longitudinally and causally within trials in adolescents.

Supplementary Materials: The following are available online at http://www.mdpi.com/2072-6643/11/5/973/s1, Table S1: Food groups and their contents (% reported is the proportion of specific food items out of all items reported consumed for breakfast in that group).

Author Contributions: N.M. and L.J. formulated the research question and designed the analysis; H.A.M., N.A.S., and M.Y.J. conceived the idea of the overall MyHeART study, obtained funding, and were involved with data collection; H.A.M. coordinated all main data entry; N.M. analyzed the data and wrote the first draft of the article. Z.T. and H.A.C. analyzed data. L.J. supervised the analyses. L.J., Z.T., and H.A.C. revised the article including comments from H.A.M. and M.Y.J. All authors approved the final manuscript.

Acknowledgments: We are grateful for the support and guidance provided by MyHeART study group members (Nik Rubiah Nik Abdul Rashid and Zarihah Mohd Zain (Ministry of Health, Malaysia), Maizurah Omar (USM), Mohamad Haniki Nik Mohamed (UIA), Khadijah Shamsuddin (UKM), Rosnah Sutan (UKM), and Sim Pei Ying, Ms Liyana Ramli, Tin Tin Su, Nahar Azmi, and Maznah Dahlui (University of Malaya).

Conflicts of Interest: Laura Johnson received research funding from Kellogg Europe for a project on breakfast in European adults from 2015 to 2016.

Financial Support: The MyHeARTs study is funded by the University of Malaya Research Grant (H.A.M.: UMRP022A-14HTM, M.Y.J.: UMRP022C-14HTM) and Vice-Chancellor Research Grant (NAS: UMQUB3D-2011). Z.T., L.J., H.A.C., and H.A.M. are supported by Medical Research Council grant MR/P013821/1.

References

1. Mendis, S.; Puska, P.; Norrving, B. *Global Atlas on Cardiovascular Disease Prevention and Control*; World Health Organization: Geneva, Switzerland.

2. Noncommunicable Diseases Country Profiles 2014. Available online: https://www.who.int/nmh/publications/ncd-profiles-2014/en/ (accessed on 30 June 2017).

3. Raitakari, O.T.; Juonala, M.; Kahonen, M.; Taittonen, L.; Laitinen, T.; Maki-Torkko, N.; Jarvisalo, M.J.; Uhari, M.; Jokinen, E.; Ronnemaa, T.; et al. Cardiovascular risk factors in childhood and carotid artery intima-media thickness in adulthood: the Cardiovascular Risk in Young Finns Study. *JAMA* **2003**, *290*, 2277–2283. [CrossRef]

4. Ng, M.; Fleming, T.; Robinson, M.; Thomson, B.; Graetz, N.; Margono, C.; Mullany, E.C.; Biryukov, S.; Abbafati, C.; Abera, S.F.; et al. Global, regional, and national prevalence of overweight and obesity in children and adults during 1980–2013: A systematic analysis for the Global Burden of Disease Study 2013. *Lancet* **2013**, *384*, 766–781. [CrossRef]

5. Brown, A.W.; Bohan Brown, M.M.; Allison, D.B. Belief beyond the evidence: using the proposed effect of breakfast on obesity to show 2 practices that distort scientific evidence. *Am. J. Clin. Nutr.* **2013**. [CrossRef] [PubMed]

6. Horikawa, C.; Kodama, S.; Yachi, Y.; Heianza, Y.; Hirasawa, R.; Ibe, Y.; Saito, K.; Shimano, H.; Yamada, N.; Sone, H. Skipping breakfast and prevalence of overweight and obesity in Asian and Pacific regions: A meta-analysis. *Prev. Med.* **2011**, *53*, 260–267. [CrossRef]

7. Purslow, L.R.; Sandhu, M.S.; Forouhi, N.; Young, E.H.; Luben, R.N.; Welch, A.A.; Khaw, K.T.; Bingham, S.A.; Wareham, N.J. Energy Intake at Breakfast and Weight Change: Prospective Study of 6,764 Middle-aged Men and Women. *Am. J. Epidemiol.* **2008**, *167*, 188–192. [CrossRef]

8. Mente, A.; de Koning, L.; Shannon, H.S.; Anand, S.S. A systematic review of the evidence supporting a causal link between dietary factors and coronary heart disease. *Arch. Intern. Med.* **2009**, *169*, 659–669. [CrossRef] [PubMed]

9. Farshchi, H.R.; Taylor, M.A.; Macdonald, I.A. Deleterious effects of omitting breakfast on insulin sensitivity and fasting lipid profiles in healthy lean women. *Am. J. Clin. Nutr.* **2005**, *81*, 388–396. [CrossRef] [PubMed]

10. Clayton, D.J.; Stensel, D.J.; James, L.J. Effect of breakfast omission on subjective appetite, metabolism, acylated ghrelin and GLP-17-36 during rest and exercise. *Nutrition* **2016**, *32*, 179–185. [CrossRef] [PubMed]

11. Bo, S.; Fadda, M.; Castiglione, A.; Ciccone, G.; De Francesco, A.; Fedele, D.; Guggino, A.; Parasiliti Caprino, M.; Ferrara, S.; Vezio Boggio, M.; et al. Is the timing of caloric intake associated with variation in diet-induced thermogenesis and in the metabolic pattern? A randomized cross-over study. *Int. J. Obes. (Lond)* **2015**, *39*, 1689–1695. [CrossRef] [PubMed]

12. Bandin, C.; Scheer, F.A.; Luque, A.J.; Avila-Gandia, V.; Zamora, S.; Madrid, J.A.; Gomez-Abellan, P.; Garaulet, M. Meal timing affects glucose tolerance, substrate oxidation and circadian-related variables: A randomized, crossover trial. *Int. J. Obes. (Lond)* **2015**, *39*, 828–833. [CrossRef]

13. Betts, J.A.; Richardson, J.D.; Chowdhury, E.A.; Holman, G.D.; Tsintzas, K.; Thompson, D. The causal role of breakfast in energy balance and health: a randomized controlled trial in lean adults. *Am. J. Clin. Nutr.* **2014**, *100*, 539–547. [CrossRef]

14. Chowdhury, E.A.; Richardson, J.D.; Holman, G.D.; Tsintzas, K.; Thompson, D.; Betts, J.A. The causal role of breakfast in energy balance and health: A randomized controlled trial in obese adults. *Am. J. Clin. Nutr.* **2016**, *103*, 747–756. [CrossRef]

15. Dhurandhar, E.J.; Dawson, J.; Alcorn, A.; Larsen, L.H.; Thomas, E.A.; Cardel, M.; Bourland, A.C.; Astrup, A.; St-Onge, M.P.; Hill, J.O.; et al. The effectiveness of breakfast recommendations on weight loss: a randomized controlled trial. *Am. J. Clin. Nutr.* **2014**, *100*, 507–513. [CrossRef]

16. Amiel, S.A.; Sherwin, R.S.; Simonson, D.C.; Lauritano, A.A.; Tamborlane, W.V. Impaired insulin action in puberty. A contributing factor to poor glycemic control in adolescents with diabetes. *N. Engl. J. Med.* **1986**, *315*, 215–219. [CrossRef]

17. Hannon, T.S.; Janosky, J.; Arslanian, S.A. Longitudinal study of physiologic insulin resistance and metabolic changes of puberty. *Pediatr. Res.* **2006**, *60*, 759–763. [CrossRef]

18. Crowley, S.J.; Acebo, C.; Carskadon, M.A. Sleep, circadian rhythms, and delayed phase in adolescence. *Sleep Med.* **2007**, *8*, 602–612. [CrossRef]

19. Jakubowicz, D.; Wainstein, J.; Landau, Z.; Raz, I.; Ahren, B.; Chapnik, N.; Ganz, T.; Menaged, M.; Barnea, M.; Bar-Dayan, Y. Influences of Breakfast on Clock Gene Expression and Postprandial Glycemia in Healthy Individuals and Individuals With Diabetes: A Randomized Clinical Trial. *Diabetes. Care* **2017**, *40*, 1573–1579. [CrossRef]

20. Zakrzewski, J.K.; Gillison, F.B.; Cumming, S.; Church, T.S.; Katzmarzyk, P.T.; Broyles, S.T.; Champagne, C.M.; Chaput, J.P.; Denstel, K.D.; Fogelholm, M.; et al. Associations between breakfast frequency and adiposity indicators in children from 12 countries. *Int. J. Obes. Suppl.* **2015**, *5*, S80–S88. [CrossRef] [PubMed]

21. Blondin, S.A.; Anzman-Frasca, S.; Djang, H.C.; Economos, C.D. Breakfast consumption and adiposity among children and adolescents: An updated review of the literature. *Pediatr. Obes.* **2016**. [CrossRef] [PubMed]

22. Chin, Y.S.; Mohd Nasir, M.T. Eating Behaviors among Female Adolescents in Kuantan District, Pahang, Malaysia. *Pak. J. Nutr.* **2009**, *8*, 425–432. [CrossRef]

23. Koo, H.-C.; Abdul Jalil, S.N.; Ruzita, A.T. Breakfast Eating Pattern and Ready-to-Eat Cereals Consumption among Schoolchildren in Kuala Lumpur. *Malays. J. Med. Sci.* **2015**, *22*, 32–39.

24. Law, L.S.; Mohd-Nasir, M.T.; Hazizi, A.S. Factors associated with breakfast skipping among school going adolescents in Sarawak, Malaysia. *Malays. J. Nutr.* **2013**, *19*, 401–407.

25. Ming, F.M.; Ying, G.C.; Kassim, S.Z.M. Eating patterns of school children and adolescent in Kuala Lumpur. *Malays. J. Nutr.* **2006**, *12*, 1–10.

26. Nurul-Fadhilah, A.; Teo, P.S.; Huybrechts, I.; Foo, L.H. Infrequent breakfast consumption is associated with higher body adiposity and abdominal obesity in Malaysian school-aged adolescents. *PLoS ONE* **2013**, *8*, e59297. [CrossRef]

27. Abdelaal, M.; le Roux, C.W.; Docherty, N.G. Morbidity and mortality associated with obesity. *Ann. Transl. Med.* **2017**, *5*, 161. [CrossRef] [PubMed]

28. Donin, A.S.; Nightingale, C.M.; Owen, C.G.; Rudnicka, A.R.; Perkin, M.R.; Jebb, S.A.; Stephen, A.M.; Sattar, N.; Cook, D.G.; Whincup, P.H. Regular Breakfast Consumption and Type 2 Diabetes Risk Markers in 9- to 10-Year-Old Children in the Child Heart and Health Study in England (CHASE): A Cross-Sectional Analysis. *PLoS Med.* **2014**, *11*, e1001703. [CrossRef] [PubMed]

29. Hallström, L.; Labayen, I.; Ruiz, J.R.; Patterson, E.; Vereecken, C.A.; Breidenassel, C.; Gottrand, F.; Huybrechts, I.; Manios, Y.; Mistura, L.; et al. Breakfast consumption and CVD risk factors in European adolescents: the HELENA (Healthy Lifestyle in Europe by Nutrition in Adolescence) Study. *Publi. Health Nutr.* **2013**, 1296–1305. [CrossRef]

30. Marlatt, K.L.; Farbakhsh, K.; Dengel, D.R.; Lytle, L.A. Breakfast and fast food consumption are associated with selected biomarkers in adolescents. *Prev. Med. Rep.* **2016**, *3*, 49–52. [CrossRef]

31. Jaaskelainen, A.; Schwab, U.; Kolehmainen, M.; Pirkola, J.; Jarvelin, M.R.; Laitinen, J. Associations of meal frequency and breakfast with obesity and metabolic syndrome traits in adolescents of Northern Finland Birth Cohort 1986. *Nutr. Metab. Cardiovasc. Dis.* **2013**, *23*, 1002–1009. [CrossRef]

32. Ho, C.-Y.; Huang, Y.-C.; Lo, Y.-T.C.; Wahlqvist, M.L.; Lee, M.-S. Breakfast is associated with the metabolic syndrome and school performance among Taiwanese children. *Res. Dev. Dis.* **2015**, *43*, 179–188. [CrossRef]

33. Yoshinaga, M.; Hatake, S.; Tachikawa, T.; Shinomiya, M.; Miyazaki, A.; Takahashi, H. Impact of Lifestyles of Adolescents and Their Parents on Cardiovascular Risk Factors in Adolescents. *J. Atheroscler. Thromb.* **2011**, *18*, 981–990. [CrossRef] [PubMed]

34. Ahadi, Z.; Qorbani, M.; Kelishadi, R.; Ardalan, G.; Motlagh, M.E.; Asayesh, H.; Zeynali, M.; Chinian, M.; Larijani, B.; Shafiee, G.; et al. Association between breakfast intake with anthropometric measurements, blood pressure and food consumption behaviors among Iranian children and adolescents: The CASPIAN-IV study. *Publ. Health* **2015**, *129*, 740–747. [CrossRef] [PubMed]

35. Smith, K.J.; Gall, S.L.; McNaughton, S.A.; Blizzard, L.; Dwyer, T.; Venn, A.J. Skipping breakfast: longitudinal associations with cardiometabolic risk factors in the Childhood Determinants of Adult Health Study. *Am. J. Clin. Nutr.* **2010**, *92*, 1316–1325. [CrossRef]

36. Wennberg, M.; Gustafsson, P.E.; Wennberg, P.; Hammarstrom, A. Poor breakfast habits in adolescence predict the metabolic syndrome in adulthood. *Publ. Health Nutr.* **2015**, *18*, 122–129. [CrossRef]

37. Brion, M.J.; Lawlor, D.A.; Matijasevich, A.; Horta, B.; Anselmi, L.; Araujo, C.L.; Menezes, A.M.; Victora, C.G.; Smith, G.D. What are the causal effects of breastfeeding on IQ, obesity and blood pressure? Evidence from comparing high-income with middle-income cohorts. *Int. J. Epidemiol.* **2011**, *40*, 670–680. [CrossRef]

38. Hazreen, M.A.; Su, T.T.; Jalaludin, M.Y.; Dahlui, M.; Chinna, K.; Ismail, M.; Murray, L.; Cantwell, M.; Al Sadat, N.; MyHe, A.R.T.S.G. An exploratory study on risk factors for chronic non-communicable diseases among adolescents in Malaysia: overview of the Malaysian Health and Adolescents Longitudinal Research Team study (The MyHeART study). *BMC Publ. Health.* **2014**, *14*, S6. [CrossRef]

39. Nutritient Composition of Malaysian Foods. Available online: http://www.nutriscene.org.my/books/Tee%20et%20al%201997%20-%20Nutr%20Comp%20of%20Malaysian%20Foods.pdf (accessed on 26 April 2019).

40. Mohd Yusoff, N.A.; Safii, N.A.; Ghazali, R.; Ahmed, R.; Shahar, S. *Atlas of Food Exchanges and Portion Sizes*, 2nd ed.; MDC Publisher Sdn Bhd: Kuala Lumpur, Malaysia, 2009.

41. Abdul Majid, H.; Ramli, L.; Ying, S.P.; Su, T.T.; Jalaludin, M.Y.; Abdul Mohsein, N.A. Dietary Intake among Adolescents in a Middle-Income Country: An Outcome from the Malaysian Health and Adolescents Longitudinal Research Team Study (the MyHeARTs Study). *PLoS ONE* **2016**, *11*, e0155447. [CrossRef]

42. Johnson, L.; Toumpakari, Z.; Papadaki, A. Social Gradients and Physical Activity Trends in an Obesogenic Dietary Pattern: Cross-Sectional Analysis of the UK National Diet and Nutrition Survey 2008–2014. **2018**, *10*, 388. [CrossRef]

43. Timlin, M.T.; Pereira, M.A.; Story, M.; Neumark-Sztainer, D. Breakfast Eating and Weight Change in a 5-Year Prospective Analysis of Adolescents: Project EAT (Eating Among Teens). *Pediatrics* **2008**, *121*, e638–e645. [CrossRef]

44. O'Neil, C.E.; Byrd-Bredbenner, C.; Hayes, D.; Jana, L.; Klinger, S.E.; Stephenson-Martin, S. The Role of Breakfast in Health: Definition and Criteria for a Quality Breakfast. *J. Acad. Nutr. Diet.* **2014**, *114*, S8–S26. [CrossRef]

45. Soran, H.; Dent, R.; Durrington, P. Evidence-based goals in LDL-C reduction. *Clin. Res. Cardiol.* **2017**, *106*, 237–248. [CrossRef]

46. Shafiee, G.; Kelishadi, R.; Qorbani, M.; Motlagh, M.E.; Taheri, M.; Ardalan, G.; Taslimi, M.; Poursafa, P.; Heshmat, R.; Larijani, B. Association of breakfast intake with cardiometabolic risk factors. *J. Pediatr. (Rio. J.)* **2013**, *89*, 575–582. [CrossRef]

47. Marz, W.; Kleber, M.E.; Scharnagl, H.; Speer, T.; Zewinger, S.; Ritsch, A.; Parhofer, K.G.; von Eckardstein, A.; Landmesser, U.; Laufs, U. HDL cholesterol: reappraisal of its clinical relevance. *Clin. Res. Cardiol.* **2017**, *106*, 663–675. [CrossRef] [PubMed]

48. Silva, F.A.; Padez, C.; Sartorelli, D.S.; Oliveira, R.M.S.; Netto, M.P.; Mendes, L.L.; Candido, A.P.C. Cross-sectional study showed that breakfast consumption was associated with demographic, clinical and biochemical factors in children and adolescents. *Acta. Paediatr.* **2018**. [CrossRef] [PubMed]

49. Farshchi, H.R.; Taylor, M.A.; Macdonald, I.A. Regular meal frequency creates more appropriate insulin sensitivity and lipid profiles compared with irregular meal frequency in healthy lean women. *Eur. J. Clin. Nutr.* **2004**, *58*, 1071–1077. [CrossRef] [PubMed]

50. Ramirez-Lopez, E.; Grijalva-Haro, M.I.; Valencia, M.E.; Antonio Ponce, J.; Artalejo, E. Effect of a School Breakfast Program on the prevalence of obesity and cardiovascular risk factors in children. *Salud Publica Mex* **2005**, *47*, 126–133.

51. Dialektakou, K.D.; Vranas, P.B. Breakfast skipping and body mass index among adolescents in Greece: Whether an association exists depends on how breakfast skipping is defined. *J. Am. Diet. Assoc.* **2008**, *108*, 1517–1525. [CrossRef]

52. Bayham, B.E.; Greenway, F.L.; Johnson, W.D.; Dhurandhar, N.V. A randomized trial to manipulate the quality instead of quantity of dietary proteins to influence the markers of satiety. *J. Diabetes Complic.* **2014**, *28*, 547–552. [CrossRef]

53. Rebello, C.J.; Johnson, W.D.; Martin, C.K.; Xie, W.; O'Shea, M.; Kurilich, A.; Bordenave, N.; Andler, S.; Klinken, B.J.W.v.; Chu, Y.-F.; et al. Acute Effect of Oatmeal on Subjective Measures of Appetite and Satiety Compared to a Ready-to-Eat Breakfast Cereal: A Randomized Crossover Trial. *J. Am. Coll. Nutr.* **2013**, *32*, 272–279. [CrossRef] [PubMed]

54. Alexy, U.; Wicher, M.; Kersting, M. Breakfast trends in children and adolescents: frequency and quality. *Publ. Health Nutr.* **2010**, *13*, 1795–1802. [CrossRef] [PubMed]

55. Randler, C. Association between morningness-eveningness and mental and physical health in adolescents. *Psychol. Health Med.* **2011**, *16*, 29–38. [CrossRef]

56. Scheer, F.A.; Hilton, M.F.; Mantzoros, C.S.; Shea, S.A. Adverse metabolic and cardiovascular consequences of circadian misalignment. *Proc. Natl. Acad. Sci. USA* **2009**, *106*, 4453–4458. [CrossRef]

57. Kong, A.P.; Wing, Y.K.; Choi, K.C.; Li, A.M.; Ko, G.T.; Ma, R.C.; Tong, P.C.; Ho, C.S.; Chan, M.H.; Ng, M.H.; et al. Associations of sleep duration with obesity and serum lipid profile in children and adolescents. *Sleep Med.* **2011**, *12*, 659–665. [CrossRef] [PubMed]

58. Van Cauter, E.; Polonsky, K.S.; Scheen, A.J. Roles of circadian rhythmicity and sleep in human glucose regulation. *Endocr. Rev.* **1997**, *18*, 716–738. [CrossRef] [PubMed]

59. Mendoza, J. Circadian clocks: Setting time by food. *J. Neuroendocrinol.* **2007**, *19*, 127–137. [CrossRef] [PubMed]

60. Qian, J.; Scheer, F. Circadian System and Glucose Metabolism: Implications for Physiology and Disease. *Trends. Endocrinol. Metab.* **2016**, *27*, 282–293. [CrossRef] [PubMed]
61. Woolhead, C.; Gibney, M.J.; Walsh, M.C.; Brennan, L.; Gibney, E.R. A generic coding approach for the examination of meal patterns. *Am. J. Clin. Nutr.* **2015**, *102*, 316–323. [CrossRef]
62. Murakami, K.; Livingstone, M.B.E.; Sasaki, S. Establishment of a Meal Coding System for the Characterization of Meal-Based Dietary Patterns in Japan. *J. Nutr.* **2017**, *147*, 2093–2101. [CrossRef] [PubMed]
63. Johnson, L.; Mander, A.P.; Jones, L.R.; Emmett, P.M.; Jebb, S.A. Energy-dense, low-fiber, high-fat dietary pattern is associated with increased fatness in childhood. *Am. J. Clin. Nutr.* **2008**, *87*, 846–854. [CrossRef] [PubMed]
64. Matthys, C.; De Henauw, S.; Bellemans, M.; De Maeyer, M.; De Backer, G. Breakfast habits affect overall nutrient profiles in adolescents. *Publ. Health Nutr.* **2007**, *10*, 413–421. [CrossRef] [PubMed]
65. Berkey, C.S.; Rockett, H.R.; Gillman, M.W.; Field, A.E.; Colditz, G.A. Longitudinal study of skipping breakfast and weight change in adolescents. *Int. J. Obes. Relat. Metab. Disord.* **2003**, *27*, 1258–1266. [CrossRef] [PubMed]

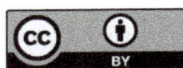

nutrients

MDPI

Article

Melanocortin-4 Receptor and Lipocalin 2 Gene Variants in Spanish Children with Abdominal Obesity: Effects on BMI-SDS after a Lifestyle Intervention

Lydia Morell-Azanza [1,2], **Ana Ojeda-Rodríguez** [1,2], **Johanna Giuranna** [3], **Mª Cristina Azcona-SanJulián** [2,4], **Johannes Hebebrand** [3], **Amelia Marti** [1,2,5,*] **and Anke Hinney** [3]

[1] Department of Nutrition, Food Sciences and Physiology, University of Navarra, c/Irunlarrea, 1. 31008 Pamplona, Spain; lmorell.1@alumni.unav.es (L.M.-A.); aojeda.5@alumni.unav.es (A.O.-R.)

[2] IdiSNA, Instituto de Investigación Sanitaria de Navarra, c/Irunlarrea, 3. 31008 Pamplona, Spain; cazcona@unav.es

[3] Department of Child and Adolescent Psychiatry, Psychosomatics and Psychotherapy, University Hospital Essen, University of Duisburg-Essen, Virchowstr. 174, D-45147 Essen, Germany; johanna.giuranna@uni-due.de (J.G.); johannes.hebebrand@uni-duisburg-essen.de (J.H.); anke.hinney@uni-due.de (A.H.)

[4] Department of Paediatrics, Clínica Universidad de Navarra, Paediatric Endocrinology Unit, c/Piío XII, 36. 31008 Pamplona, Spain

[5] Biomedical Research Centre Network on Obesity and Nutrition (CIBERobn), Physiopathology of Obesity and Nutrition, Institute of Health Carlos III, Av. Monforte de Lemos, 3-5. 28029 Madrid, Spain

* Correspondence: amarti@unav.es; Tel.: +34-948-425600 (ext. 806244)

Received: 11 March 2019; Accepted: 24 April 2019; Published: 26 April 2019

Abstract: Mutations leading to a reduced function of the melanocortin-4 receptor (MC4R) exert a major gene effect on extreme obesity. Recently it was shown that the bone derived hormone lipocalin 2 (LCN2) binds to the MC4R and activates a MC4R dependent anorexigenic pathway. We identified mutations in both genes and screened the effects of *MC4R* and *LCN2* mutations on eating behavior and weight change after a lifestyle intervention. One hundred and twelve children (11.24 ± 2.6 years, BMI-SDS 2.91 ± 1.07) with abdominal obesity participated in a lifestyle intervention. *MC4R* and *LCN2* coding regions were screened by Sanger sequencing. Eating behavior was assessed at baseline with the Children Eating Behavior Questionnaire (CEBQ). We detected three previously described non-synonymous *MC4R* variants (Glu42Lys, Thr150Ile, and Arg305Gln) and one non-synonymous polymorphism (Ile251Leu). Regarding *LCN2*, one known non-synonymous variant (Thr124Met) was detected. Eating behavior was described in carriers of the *MC4R* and *LCN2* mutation and in non-carriers. *MC4R* and *LCN2* mutations were detected in 2.42% and 0.84%, respectively, of Spanish children with abdominal obesity. A number of subjects with functional mutation variants in *MC4R* and *LCN2* were able to achieve a reduction in BMI-SDS after a lifestyle intervention.

Keywords: childhood obesity; CEBQ; eating behavior and Ile251Leu

1. Introduction

Obesity has been defined by the World Health Organization (WHO) as an abnormal or excessive body fat accumulation that may impair health [1]. Both environmental and genetic factors have an influence on weight gain [2]. The impact of genetics on obesity is heterogeneous. For a small number of subjects obesity is caused by mutations in single genes, for the majority of the population obesity has a polygenic nature [2,3].

One of the most common single genes harboring variants associated with obesity is the melanocortin-4 receptor gene (*MC4R*) [4,5]. It is known as a regulator of energy homeostasis due to its effect on food intake and energy expenditure via neuronal melanocortinergic pathways [6]. More than 369 mutations including non-synonymous, nonsense, and frameshift mutations have been identified mainly in obese individuals [7,8]. Most of the non-synonymous mutations lead to partial or complete loss of function of the *MC4R* [9]. The polymorphism Ile251Leu leads to an increased function of MC4R and is associated with a reduced BMI [7].

The protein lipocalin 2 has been associated with obesity [10,11] and was thought to be secreted from adipose tissue as an adipokine [12]. However recent studies discovered a ten-fold higher expression in osteoblasts than in adipose tissue. In this line, recent studies have shown that lipocalin 2 (LCN2) binds to the MC4R to activate MC4R-dependent anorexigenic pathways [13]. It has also been observed that obese participants heterozygous for *MC4R* mutations leading to impaired function have higher levels of plasma LCN2 than BMI-matched MC4R wild-type controls [13].

Our aim was to screen for mutations in the *MC4R* and *LCN2* genes in a Spanish pediatric population with abdominal obesity. Moreover, we investigated the effects on eating behavior and weight change after participating in a one-year lifestyle intervention for carriers versus non-carriers of *MC4R* and *LCN2* variants.

2. Materials and Methods

2.1. Subjects

For this study, a total of 112 children between 7 to 16 years of age and with abdominal obesity defined as a waist circumference higher than the 90th percentile [14] participate in a lifestyle intervention. The IGENOI study is a 2-year lifestyle intervention program for children with abdominal obesity carried out by GENOI group (*"Grupo de Estudio Navarro de la Obesidad infantil"*). This study is a randomized control trial (NCT03147261) conducted in Pamplona, Spain. Children were recruited from the Pediatric Endocrinology at "Clinica Universidad de Navarra" and "Complejo hospitalario de Navarra", and from health care centers around Pamplona and its neighborhoods.

Participants with previous diabetes, presence of other diseases beside obesity, major psychiatric illness including bulimia nervosa, pharmacological treatment, food intolerance, or treatment with special diets, or frequent alcohol or drug consumption were excluded. Children and their parents signed a written informed consent in the screening visit. The study protocol was performed in accordance with the ethical standards of the Declaration of Helsinki (Fortaleza, Brasil, October 2013), and was approved by the ethics committee of the University of Navarra (Reference number 044/2014).

2.2. Experimental Design

The lifestyle intervention comprises an 8-week intensive phase ($N = 104$ subjects) and a follow-up period of 10 months ($N = 85$ subjects, 1 year). The dropout rate was 7% at week 8 and 24% at 1 year of follow up.

A multidisciplinary team conformed by dietitians, pediatricians, nurses, physical activity experts, and laboratory technicians were involved in the development of the study protocol. Participants were randomly assigned into two different groups: intensive care and usual care group, following a 3:1 ratio. The first one was given a moderate hypocaloric Mediterranean diet, as previously described [15], while the usual care group received usual pediatric advice with healthy diet recommendations [16]. Specifically, intensive care participants were prescribed with a moderate hypocaloric diet based on a fixed full-day meal plan. The restriction, not to interfere with growth, was calculated depending on the degree of obesity (from −10% to −40% of total energy intake). A Mediterranean-style diet based consists of high consumption of fruit, vegetables, whole grains, legumes, nuts, seeds, and olive oil, minimally processed foods; moderate consumption of dairy products, fish, and poultry; and low consumption of red meat [15]. Both groups were encouraged to increase their physical activity to at least 200 minutes per week as recommended by The American College of Sports Medicine to prevent weight gain [17].

The intervention group participants had 30-minute individual sessions with the dietitian every two weeks during the 8-week treatment phase. In these sessions a follow-up about the accomplishment of the diet and anthropometric measurements was performed. In addition, the parents or legal guardians had one parallel group session where they received education about their role in the study and obesity related problems, while intensive care participants were encouraged to make healthy lifestyle decisions about food choices, eating behavior, sedentary activities, and physical activity. On the other hand, usual care participants and their parents received one 30-min individual session with the dietitian and five monitoring visits to assess anthropometric parameters.

During the follow-up period, participants had monitoring visits at 3, 4,5,6,9, and 12 months from the baseline visit.

2.3. Anthropometric, Clinical and Biochemical Measurements

All anthropometric measurements were performed at baseline, after 8 weeks, and at 1 year of follow up according to standard procedures and calibrated tools in the paediatric population [18]. Measurements were performed by trained personnel in a wide space, while the participants were asked to stand barefoot and wore light clothing, without hair ornaments or jewels.

Body weight and body fat were determined using a digital scale BC-418 Segmental Body Composition Analyzer according to manufacturer instructions (Tanita, Tokyo, Japan). To measure height, participants were asked to stand on stadiometer with the feet placed parallel and slightly apart, and heels, buttocks, scapula, and occipital head area touching the vertical board at the same time. A non-stretchable measuring tape (type SECA 200) was used for measuring waist circumference (WC) and hip circumference (HC) by standard procedures (Type SECA 200). The waist-to-hip and waist-to-height ratios were also calculated.

Body mass index was calculated as weight divided by squared height (Kg/m^2). BMI-standard deviation (BMI-SDS) is BMI values converted into standard deviation using age and specific cut-points according to Spanish reference growth charts [19]. Pubertal status was determined using Tanner stage and was evaluated by a paediatrician. The presence of *Acanthosis Nigricans* was diagnosed by pediatricians of the team at baseline. Blood pressure was measured following standard procedures, as described elsewhere [20].

Venous blood samples were obtained by specialized trained nurses at the Hospital after an overnight fast. Glucose, insulin leptin, and lipid profiles were determined by standard autoanalyzer techniques at baseline. Insulin resistance was calculated from the homeostasis model assessment of insulin resistance (HOMA-IR).

2.4. Physical Activity

Moderate-to-vigorous physical activity was assessed at baseline using triaxial accelerometry (Actigraph wGT3X-BT, Actigraph LLC, Penascola, FL, USA). Briefly, participants wore the accelerometer around the non-dominant waist for four days, including, at least, two weekend days, as described elsewhere [21]. Accelerometry data were analysed using ActiLife 6.0 software (Actigraph LLC, Penascola, FL, USA) as describe elsewhere [22].

2.5. Children Eating Behavior Questionnaire (CEBQ)

The Children Eating Behaviour Questionnaire (CEBQ) is a multidimensional parent-reported questionnaire about their children's eating behaviour [23]. It includes 35 items regarding eating styles that are clustered into eight subscales. The eight subscales are classified into two dimensions: food approach or food avoidance. The food approach dimension comprises the following subscales: "Emotional overeating", "Enjoyment of food", "Desire for drink", and "Food responsiveness". Food avoidance is represented by the following: "Slowness in eating", "Satiety responsiveness", "and Emotional undereating", and "Food fussiness". It was fulfilled by parents or legal guardians at baseline.

For each behaviour subscale parents report their children's behaviour on a five-point Likert Scale, that ranges from never, rarely, sometimes, often, or always (1 to 5). A ratio was calculated between the sums of the food approach vs. the sum of the food avoidance subscales.

2.6. DNA Extraction

Venous blood samples were obtained on ethylendiaminetetraacetic acid (EDTA) tubes, which were centrifuged 30 minutes after the extraction at 3500 rpm for 15 minutes at 4 °C. DNA was extracted from the buffy coat fraction using a commercial kit MasterPure DNA purification kit for Blood Version II (Epicenter Biotechnologies, Madison, WI, USA). Its quality and quantity were determined with a Nanodrop spectrometer ND-1000 (Nanodrop Technologies, Wilmington, Delware, USA) and it was stored at −80 °C until processing.

2.7. Mutation Screen

MC4R and *LCN2* genes were screened for mutations. All subjects were heterozygous for the mutations. *MC4R* was analyzed with one PCR fragment, while *LCN2* was divided into four PCR fragments. Methodological details can be obtained from the authors.

All samples were commercially Sanger sequenced by LGC Genomics (Berlin, Germany). Analyses of the sequences were performed by two experienced individuals in Essen (Germany). Samples with discrepancies were re-sequenced by Seqlab laboratories (Göttingen, Germany).

2.8. Statistical Analysis

Statistical analyses were performed using STATA version 12 (StataCorp, College Station, TX, USA). Normality was assessed by Shapiro-Wilk. All the tests were two-sided and the significance level was set at $\alpha = 0.05$. We did not correct for multiple testing.

We used Wilcoxon rank-sum test for the comparison between subjects with Ile 251Leu MC4R mutation and without MC4R mutation for the variables studied at baseline.

Paired t-test was applied for assessing changes in BMI-SDS between baseline vs. week 8, and baseline vs. 1 year. Furthermore, we performed a comparison between subjects with Ile 251Leu MC4R mutation and without MC4R mutation for changes in BMI-SDS (week 8 and one year, Wilcoxon rank-sum test).

3. Results

One hundred and twelve children with abdominal obesity (mean age 11.24 years, males 38%, BMI-SDS 2.93) participated in the study.

3.1. Description of Identified Variants

Mutation screen of the coding region of MC4R identified a total of four variants, three known nonsynonymous variants, rs776051881 (Glu42Lys), rs766665118 (Thr150Ile), and rs775382722 (Arg305Gln), and one nonsynonymous polymorphism rs52820871 (Ile251Leu) (Table 1). First, we classified variants as leading to reduced receptor function or similar to the wild type MC4R function. Three previously reported variants (Glu42Lys, Thr150Ileu, and Arg305Gln) lead to a reduced MC4R function as classified by in-silico predictors [24] that claim them to be disease causing. Furthermore, some in-vitro analyses had described reduced function for the mutations Thr150Ileu and Arg305Gln [9,25,26]. Our study shows a frequency of 2.52% of MC4R mutations leading to a reduced function in our sample of Spanish of children with abdominal obesity.

Table 1. MC4R and LCN2 genetic variants in Spanish children with abdominal obesity.

Gene Subject	N° of Subjects	Aminoacid Exchange	rs Number	In-silico Prediction*	Function	Reference of Functional Analysis
MC4R Mutations						
Glu42Lys	1	p.Glu42Lys	rs776051881	Disease causing	Not known	-
Thr150Ile	1	p.Thr150Ile	rs766665118	Disease causing	Reduced	[9,25]
Arg305Gln	1	p.Arg305Gln	rs775382722	Disease causing	Reduced	[26]
Polymorphisms						
Ile251Leu	5	p.Ile251Leu	rs52820871	Disease causing	Like wild type	[27–31]
LCN2 Mutations						
Thr124Met	1	p.Thr124Met	rs79993583	Probably harmless	-	-

Abdominal obesity was defined as waist circumference (WC) above the sex and age-specific 90th percentile. * In-silico prediction was performed by mutation taster www.mutationtaster.org.

The mutation screen of the coding region of LCN2 identified a total of twelve variants, eleven are located in intronic regions (rs2232632, rs202024127, rs11794980, rs2232629, rs2232625, rs2232626, rs116745581, rs2232628, rs568419305, rs2232631, rs2232632) and one is a known nonsynonymous variant: rs79993583 (Thr124Met). The analysis of all detected variants by in-silico predictors show that three of them could be disease causing (Supplementary Table S1).

3.2. Phenotypic Description of Mutation Carriers

In Table 2 phenotypic characteristics of participants with mutations at MC4R and LCN2 genes at baseline are described in detail. We also provide data from obese participants of IGENOI study without mutations in the coding regions of these genes.

For 103 children (37.8% males) with a mean age of 11.32 years no mutations in MC4R and LCN2 genes were found, they are wild type carriers. Mutated subjects are compared with them in the subsequent analyses. All wild type carriers were also obese (BMI-SDS: 2.92 ± 1.10) and 41.7% showed clinical evidence for insulin resistance in the presence of Acanthosis Nigricans that was accompanied by a HOMA-IR of 4.03 ± 3.17.

A 14 year-old girl was heterozygous for the Glu42Lys mutation at the MC4R gene. She suffers from severe-obesity (BMI-SDS:4.04) reflected in a fat mass of 40.8%. The main clinical features of this participant were leptin levels higher than expected for the BMI [32], and the presence of insulin resistance observed as hyperinsulinemia, increased HOMA-IR (4.23), and Acanthosis Nigricans.

Mutation Thr150Ileu at the MC4R gene was observed in an eight year-old boy with a BMI-SDS of +3.5. Biochemical parameters were normal and the participant was physically active (50.65 min/day). One participant carries two variants at the MC4R gene: Arg305Gln and the polymorphism Ile251Leu. She is a 12 year-old girl with a BMI-SDS of 2.91, and a fat mass of 43.2% (measured by bioimpedance). Five independent children also carried the polymorphism Ile251Leu. They had a mean age of nine years and a mean BMI-SDS of 2.69. In comparison with the participants with the wild type receptor, none of the participants carrying this polymorphism showed Acanthosis Nigricans.

The polymorphism Ile251Leu of MC4R was observed in five participants with a mean age of nine years old. We found increased levels of total cholesterol and LDL-cholesterol in comparison to participants without MC4R mutation ($p = 0.004$ and $p = 0.013$; Wilcoxon rank-sum test). These differences persist when subjects with the Ile251Leu MC4R mutation were compared to age and sex matched subjects without MC4R mutation (Supplementary Table S2).

One male 15 year-old heterozygously carried the mutation Thr124Met at the LCN2 gene. Clinical characteristics of this participant included severe obesity (BMI-SDS = +4.01) accompanied by an elevated percentage of fat mass (38.7%). Also, a remarkable difference of higher levels of MVPA was detected in comparison with the wild type population. The carrier of this mutation was much more active than the wild-type controls (120.92 min/day vs. 44.82 min/day, $p = 0.088$). We also evaluated the siblings (three girls) of the index patient, all of them were obese. Two of them were also carriers of Thr124Met (BMI-SDS: 3.47 and BMI-SDS: 3.76). The MAF for this variant in the LCN2 gene in the study population is 0.44%.

Table 2. Baseline characteristics of heterozygous MC4R and LCN2 variant carriers and wild type Spanish children with abdominal obesity.

		MC4R Mutations				LCN2 Mutation
	Wt Population	Glu42Lys	Thr150Ile	Arg305Gln+Ile251Leu	Ile251Leu	Thr124Met
N	103	1	1	1	5	1
Age (years)	11.32 (2.46)	14	8	12	9 (1)	15
Sex (Male/Female)	39/64	Female	Male	Female	2/3	Male
Tanner (I/II/III/IV/V)	31/17/18/6/24	V	I	II	4/-/1/-/-	V
Height (cm)	151.23 (12.72)	168	137.8	151	137.3 (13.86)	175.9
Weight (Kg)	66.71 (18.77)	97	49.1	67.2	49.94 (17.87)	112.9
BMI (Kg/m^2)	28.55 (4.51)	34.4	25.85	29.5	25.64 (3.53)	36.5
BMI-SDS	2.92 (1.10)	4.04	3.5	2.91	2.69 (1.05)	4.01
WHR	0.88 (0.06)	0.90	0.89	0.93	0.86 (0.04)	0.82
% fat mass	37.22 (6.33)	40.8	32.1	43.2	33.98 (9.28)	38.7
Acantosis nigricans (+/-)	43/52	+	-	-	0/5	+
Glucose (mg/dL)	89.04 (6.58)	85	88	78	88.25 (6.84)	87
Insulin (μu/mL)	17.92 (13.29)	20.2	7	13.5	11.87 (6.43)	11.4
HOMA-IR	4.03 (3.17)	4.23	1.52	2.6	2.66 (1.68)	2.44
Total Colesterol (mg/dL)	162.65 (24.97)	116	162	157	198.75 (14.88)*	160
HDL-colesterol (mg/dL)	46.70 (9.96)	42	53	46	56.75 (12.25)	41
LDL-colesterol (mg/dL)	97.67 (21.15)	64	96	97	125.75 (16.82)*	99
Triglycerides (mg/dL)	94.48 (44.73)	49	64	68	81.25 (41.65)	98
Leptin (ng/mL)	36.41 (18.60)	90.8	14	NA	33.52 (13.11)	8.1
MVPA (min/day)	44.88 (23.69)	37.5	50.65	30.93	44.55 (18.37)	120.92
CEBQ ratio	1.22 (0.42)	0.82	1.25	NA	1.01 (0.12)	0.85

Data are expressed as mean (SD), * $p < 0.05$ for the comparison between Ile 251Leu MC4R mutation subjects and subjects without MC4R mutation, Wilcoxon rank-sum test was applied Abdominal obesity was defined as WC above the sex and age-specific 90th percentile. BMI-SDS, standard deviation score for body mass index; CEBQ, Children Eating Behavior Questionnaire Ratio; MVPA, moderate to vigorous physical activity; WHR: waist to height ratio.

3.3. Children Eating Behavior

The eating behavior scores with four dimension charts of children with abdominal obesity at baseline is described in Figure 1. Wild type subjects (no mutations in MC4R and LCN2 genes) had a score of 1.19. Carriers of the MC4R Thr150Ileu and LCN2 Thr124Met variants had nominally higher scores than wild type subjects, while participants with Ile251Leu polymorphism have lower score.

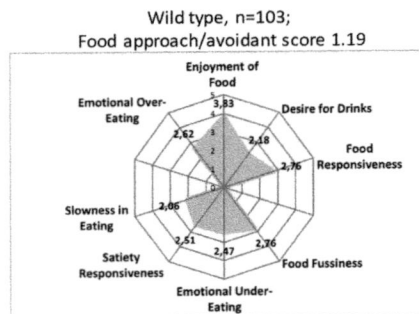

Figure 1. *Cont.*

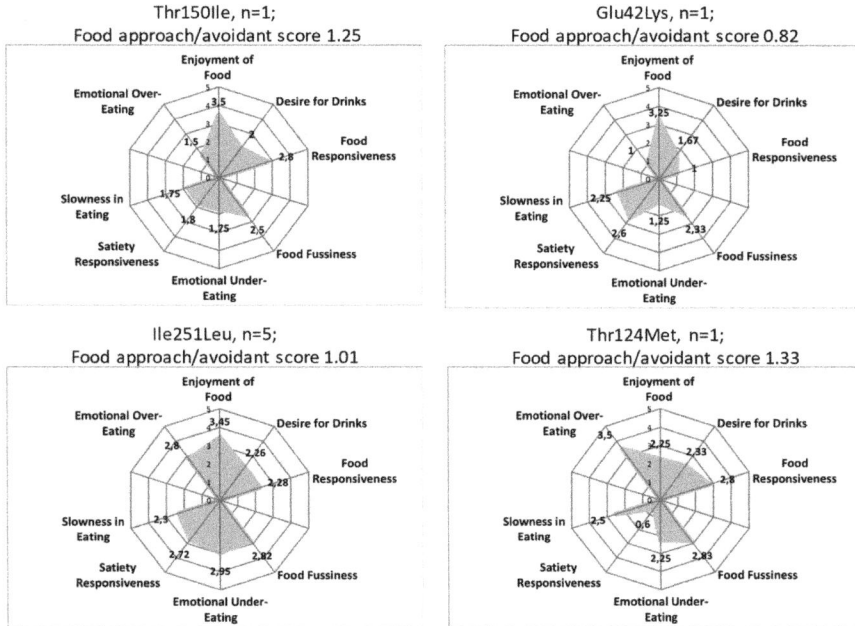

Figure 1. Childhood Eating Behavior Score (CEBQ) in Spanish children with abdominal obesity. The Food approach/avoidant score refers to the quotient between the sums of scores of the "food approach" subscales divided by the sum of the scores of the "food avoidant" subscales. Subjects with mutations in MC4R (Thr124Met, Thr150Ileu) and LCN2 (Thr124Met) genes were evaluated.

3.4. *Change in BMI-SDS and Mutations in MC4R and LCN2 After 8-Week and 1-Year of Follow Up*

Carriers of mutations that lead to a reduced function in MC4R and LCN2 genes showed a disparity of responses to the lifestyle intervention (Table 3). Changes in BMI-SDS of the five subject carriers of the Ile251Leu polymorphism are quite variable with two of them not showing any improvement at 1 year. Moreover, no significant differences in BMI-SDS changes were found after eight weeks or one-year of follow up in mutated carriers vs. non carriers subjects in analysis conducted in matched age and sex subjects with and without a functional mutation in MC4R (Supplementary Table S3).

Table 3. Changes in BMI-SDS according to MC4R and LCN2 variants after an 8-week and 1-year lifestyle intervention.

		ΔBMI-SDS			
		8 Week		1 Year	
		Mutation Carriers	Non Carriers	Mutation Carriers	Non Carriers
Usual Care Group			$n = 27$ −0.44 (0.66)***		$n = 22$ −0.47 (0.52)***
MC4R: Glu42Lys		−0.51		Drop out	
MC4R: Thr150Ile		−0.67		−0.90	
Intensive Care group			$n = 68$ −0.51 (0.38)***		$n = 56$ −0.60 (0.72)***
MC4R: Arg305Gln + Ile251Leu		−0.13		−0.81	
MC4R: Ile251Leu	Mean ($n = 5$)	−0.74 (0.41)**		−1.02 (1.21)	
	Carrier 1	−0.95		−1.47	
	Carrier 2	−0.10		0.07	
	Carrier 3	−0.56		0.38	
	Carrier 4	−1.14		−1.56	
	Carrier 5	−0.97		−2.53	
LCN2: Thr124Met		−0.59		Drop out	

Data are expressed as mean (SD). Paired t-test for changes between baseline vs. 8 week, and baseline vs. 1 year was applied (** < 0.010, *** < 0.001).

4. Discussion

To our knowledge, this is the first study evaluating *MC4R* and *LCN2* gene variants, in a population of children and adolescents with abdominal obesity. In addition, we measured the eating behavior in all participants with the CEBQ. Finally, we reported changes in BMI-SDS achieved after eight weeks and 1 year of follow-up according to the two different strategies (usual care or intensive care) and the presence of *MC4R* and *LCN2* gene variants.

The rate of participants carrying a *MC4R* mutation leading to a reduced function was 2.67 %. This frequency is in accordance with the reported values in Czech children with obesity being 2.4% [33]. Previously, a wide variability (ranging from 0.5 to 5.8%) in the frequency of *MC4R* mutations had been described in children and adolescents with obesity in different populations [33–36].

In our population, we found one extremely obese participant (BMI-SDS +4.04) carrying the *MC4R* mutation Glu42Lys. This mutation was previously reported in 5.6% of Turkish children with obesity [37]. In our case, the minor allele frequency (MAF) for this mutation was 0.89%.

Moreover, an eight year-old boy with a BMI-SDS of +3.5 was a heterozygous carrier of the *MC4R* Thr150Ileu variation. This mutation had previously been described in an obese Chilean child with a BMI-SDS of +2.79 [38]. In the Chilean population the MAF for this variant was 0.45% similar to the observed value in our Spanish population (0.84%).

Mutation Arg305Gln of the *MC4R* gene was characterized in functional studies as a variation that causes a decrease in MC4R constituently activity and in the response to the agonist [9]. We found this mutation in a 12 year-old girl with obesity (43.2% body fat mass and BMI-SDS +2.91). This participant also carries the Ile251Leu polymorphism. There is also a German obese boy harboring this Arg305Gln variation (BMI-SDS +2.5) [39]. The frequency of this variation in our population is 0.84% while in the German population was 0.19%.

Two polymorphisms in the *MC4R* (Val103Ileu and Ile251Leu) had been demonstrated to reduce the risk of obesity [40–42]. Val103Ileu was described in white Europeans with frequencies between 1–4% [2]. In our study, we did not observe carriers of this variation. In other independent studies in Spanish children the frequencies of this polymorphism were lower than in other European countries [43–45]. The frequency of the Ile251Leu variation in our studied sample was 5.04% (6 children with abdominal obesity), which is higher than the observed values in other Spanish and Polish pediatric populations [28,43,44]. Heterozygous subjects for the Ile251Leu SNP showed higher levels of total cholesterol and LDL-cholesterol. There are studies on the association between *MC4R* variants and other lipid markers in several populations [31,46].

To our knowledge this is the first study evaluating non-common variants in the *LCN2* gene in children with abdominal obesity. We found one heterozygous carrier of the Thr124Met variant that was severely obese (BMI-SDS: + 4.01) despite being physically active (more than 2 hours per day on moderate-to-vigorous physical activity).

It has been demonstrated that LCN2 suppresses appetite by signaling trough MC4R [13]. For this reason we evaluated eating behavior in our population with the children eating behavior questionnaire (CEBQ), for which solid reproducibility and high internal consistency had been reported [47]. In particular we represent graphically the multidimensionality of participants carrying *MC4R* and *LCN2* mutations. We observed that carriers of the Thr150Ile (*MC4R*) and Thr124Met (*LCN2*) variants showed slightly higher eating behavior scores than obese individuals without *MC4R* variants. This tentatively suggests an effect of these mutations on eating behavior, as mutation carriers showed lower scores on food avoidance subscales. However, as the number of mutation carriers is very low, meaningful statistical analyses are not possible.

Regarding the mutation Thr150Ile of the *MC4R* gene, an association between this variant and eating behavior in three Chilean obese carriers was reported. These participants had a cognitive restraint measured by the TFEQ-R18 questionnaire [48].

The participant carrying the *LCN2* Thr124Met allele showed lower satiety responsiveness (0.6 out of 5). This could be explained by a potential effect of LCN2 on appetite-suppressing activities [13]. Participants carrying the Ile251Leu polymorphism of the *MC4R* had lower scores in satiety responsiveness than the wild type population (1.01 vs. 1.19). Nevertheless, carrying the infrequent allele at *MC4R* Ile251Leu seems not to have an influence on eating behavior compared to children with obesity and variations in the *MC4R* gene. A previous study had described association between *MC4R* polymorphism rs17782313 (in the 3′ region of the gene) and childhood eating behavior. Satiety responsiveness dimension was decreased and enjoyment of food was increased in carriers of the CC allele [38]. However, the lack of significance in our results should be seen under the limited statistical power as we analyzed rare variants in a relatively small study group.

In our population, participants carrying mutations in *MC4R* and *LCN2* that lead to a reduced function were able to achieve similar or greater reduction in BMI-SDS than children without mutation in these genes after a lifestyle intervention. These results are in concordance with previous weight loss *MC4R* studies [4,39]. It had been demonstrated that children with mutations in *MC4R* had a significantly greater beneficial effect from the short lifestyle interventions than wild type carriers [49]. However, in our study one carrier of Arg305Gln only achieved a successful reduction in BMI-SDS after one year of intervention. When the polymorphism Ile251Leu of the *MC4R* gene was analyzed, some participants showed a reduction in BMI-SDS similar to that of wild type subjects after the intervention. Limitations of our study comprise of a relatively small sample size, the lack of a normal-weight study group, that no functional in vitro tests were performed, and also that we cannot exclude the presence of mutations in other genes involved in monogenic obesity.

5. Conclusions

In summary, *MC4R* and *LCN2* mutations were detected in 2.42% and 0.84%, respectively, of Spanish children with abdominal obesity. Our data suggests a putative association between profiles of eating behavior and functional mutations in *MC4R* gene. Specifically, *MC4R* and *LCN2* mutation carriers having abdominal obesity were able to reduce BMI-SDS after a lifestyle intervention.

Supplementary Materials: The following are available online at http://www.mdpi.com/2072-6643/11/5/960/s1, Table S1: *LCN2* genetic variants in Spanish children with abdominal obesity. Table S2: Baseline characteristics from a subpopulation of matched age and sex subjects with the Ile251Leu MC4R mutations and without the mutation. Table S3: Changes in anthropometric and biochemical from a subpopulation of matched age and sex subjects with the Ile251Leu MC4R mutations and without the mutation.

Author Contributions: Conceptualization, M.C.A.-S., A.H. and A.M.; methodology, L.M.-A., A.O.-R. and J.G.; formal analysis, L.M.-A., J.G., A.O.-R. and A.H.; resources, M.C.A.-S., J.H., A.H., and A.M.; data curation, L.M.-A. and A.H.; writing—original draft preparation, L.M.-A.; writing—review and editing, A.O.-R., J.G., M.C.A.-S., J.H., A.H. and A.M.; supervision, A.H.; project administration, M.C.A.-S. and A.M.; funding acquisition, M.C.A.-S., J.H., A.H. and A.M.

Funding: The IGENOI study was supported by a MERCK foundation grant and Laboratories ORDESA (Sant Boi de Llobregat; Barcelona, España)-FEI-AEP grant. A.H. and J.H. were supported by the Deutsche Forschungsgemeinschaft (DFG; HI 865/2-1) and the BMBF (01GS0820). A.H. and J.G. were supported by the 'Landesprogramm für Geschlechtergerechte Hochschulen-Programmstrang Förderung von Denominationen in der Genderforschung.

Acknowledgments: We thank all the children and families in the trial for their enthusiastic and maintained collaboration, and other investigators of the IGENOI group for their participation in the recruitment process and the acquisition of the data. We are indebted to S. Düerkop and J. Andrä for technical support. L.M.-A. and A.O.-R. acknowledge their fellowships from the "la Caixa" Banking Foundation.

Conflicts of Interest: The authors declare no conflict of interest.

References

1. World Health Organization. Obesity and Overweight. Available online: https://www.who.int/news-room/fact-sheets/detail/obesity-and-overweight (accessed on 1 June 2018).
2. Loos, R.J.F. The genetic epidemiology of melanocortin 4 receptor variants. *Eur. J. Pharmacol.* **2011**, *660*, 156–164. [CrossRef] [PubMed]

3. Razquin, C.; Marti, A.; Martinez, J.A. Evidences on three relevant obesogenes: MC4R, FTO and PPARγ. Approaches for personalized nutrition. *Mol. Nutr. Food Res.* **2011**, *55*, 136–149. [CrossRef]

4. Koochakpoor, G.; Hosseini-Esfahani, F.; Daneshpour, M.S.; Hosseini, S.A.; Mirmiran, P. Effect of interactions of polymorphisms in the Melanocortin-4 receptor gene with dietary factors on the risk of obesity and Type 2 diabetes: A systematic review. *Diabet. Med.* **2016**, *33*, 1026–1034. [CrossRef] [PubMed]

5. Saeed, S.; Bonnefond, A.; Manzoor, J.; Shabir, F.; Ayesha, H.; Philippe, J.; Durand, E.; Crouch, H.; Sand, O.; Ali, M.; et al. Genetic variants in *LEP*, *LEPR*, and *MC4R* explain 30% of severe obesity in children from a consanguineous population. *Obesity* **2015**, *23*, 1687–1695. [CrossRef] [PubMed]

6. Zlatohlavek, L.; Hubacek, J.A.; Vrablik, M.; Pejsova, H.; Lanska, V.; Ceska, R. The Impact of Physical Activity and Dietary Measures on the Biochemical and Anthropometric Parameters in Obese Children. Is There Any Genetic Predisposition? *Cent. Eur. J. Public Health* **2015**, *23*. [CrossRef]

7. Hinney, A.; Volckmar, A.-L.; Knoll, N. Chapter Five - Melanocortin-4 Receptor in Energy Homeostasis and Obesity Pathogenesis. In *G Protein-Coupled Receptors in Energy Homeostasis and Obesity Pathogenesis*, 1st ed.; Elsevier Inc.: New York, NY, USA, 2013; Volume 114, pp. 147–191.

8. Collet, T.H.; Dubern, B.; Mokrosinski, J.; Connors, H.; Keogh, J.M.; Mendes de Oliveira, E.; Henning, E.; Poitou-Bernert, C.; Oppert, J.-M.; Tounian, P.; et al. Evaluation of a melanocortin-4 receptor (MC4R) agonist (Setmelanotide) in MC4R deficiency. *Mol. Metab.* **2017**, *6*, 1321–1329. [CrossRef]

9. Lubrano-Berthelier, C.; Dubern, B.; Lacorte, J.M.; Picard, F.; Shapiro, A.; Zhang, S.; Bertrais, S.; Hercberg, S.; Basdevant, A.; Clément, K.; et al. Melanocortin 4 receptor mutations in a large cohort of severely obese adults: Prevalence, functional classification, genotype-phenotype relationship, and lack of association with binge eating. *J. Clin. Endocrinol. Metab.* **2006**, *91*, 1811–1818. [CrossRef]

10. Catalán, V.; Gómez-Ambrosi, J.; Rodríguez, A.; Ramírez, B.; Valentí, V.; Moncada, R.; Silva, C.; Salvador, J.; Frühbeck, G. Peripheral mononuclear blood cells contribute to the obesity-associated inflammatory state independently of glycemic status: involvement of the novel proinflammatory adipokines chemerin, chitinase-3-like protein 1, lipocalin-2 and osteopontin. *Genes Nutr.* **2015**, *10*. [CrossRef]

11. Elkhidir, A.E.; Eltaher, H.B.; Mohamed, A.O. Association of lipocalin-2 level, glycemic status and obesity in type 2 diabetes mellitus. *BMC Res. Notes* **2017**, *10*, 1–6. [CrossRef] [PubMed]

12. Zhang, Y.; Foncea, R.; Deis, J.A.; Guo, H.; Bernlohr, D.A.; Chen, X. Lipocalin 2 expression and secretion is highly regulated by metabolic stress, cytokines, and nutrients in adipocytes. *PLoS ONE* **2014**, *9*, 1–9. [CrossRef] [PubMed]

13. Mosialou, I.; Shikhel, S.; Liu, J.M.; Maurizi, A.; Luo, N.; He, Z.; Huang, Y.R.; Zong, H.H.; Friedman, R.A.; Barasch, J. MC4R-dependent suppression of appetite by bone-derived lipocalin 2. *Nature* **2017**, *543*, 385–390. [CrossRef] [PubMed]

14. Serra Majem, L.; Aranceta Bartrina, J.; Ribas Barba, L.; Pérez Rodrigo, C.; García Closas, R. *Estudio enKid: objetivos y metodología. Crecimiento y desarrollo. Estudio enKid*; Masson S.A.: Barcelona, Spain, 2000; Volume 4.

15. Ojeda-Rodríguez, A.; Zazpe, I.; Morell-Azanza, L.; Chueca, M.J.; Azcona-Sanjulian, M.C.; Marti, A. Improved diet quality and nutrient adequacy in children and adolescents with abdominal obesity after a lifestyle intervention. *Nutrients* **2018**, *10*, 1500. [CrossRef]

16. Aranceta Batrina, J.; Arija Val, V.; Maíz Aldalur, E.; de Victoria Muñoz, E.M.; Ortega Anta, R.M.; Pérez Rodrigo, C.; Quiles Izquierdo, J.; Rodríguez Martín, A.; Román Viñas, B.; Salvador i Castell, G.; et al. Guías alimentarias para la población española (SENC, diciembre 2016); la nueva pirámide de la alimentación saludable. *Nutr. Hosp.* **2015**, *31*, 1–145. [CrossRef]

17. Donnelly, J.E.; Blair, S.N.; Jakicic, J.M.; Manore, M.M.; Rankin, J.W.; Smith, B.K. Appropriate physical activity intervention strategies for weight loss and prevention of weight regain for adults. *Med. Sci. Sports Exerc.* **2009**, *41*, 459–471. [CrossRef]

18. Morell-Azanza, L.; García-Calzón, S.; Rendo-Urteaga, T.; Martin-Calvo, N.; Chueca, M.; Martínez, J.A.; Azcona-Sanjulián, M.C.; Marti, A. Serum oxidized low-density lipoprotein levels are related to cardiometabolic risk and decreased after a weight loss treatment in obese children and adolescents. *Pediatr. Diabetes* **2017**, *18*, 18. [CrossRef]

19. Sobradillo, B.; Aguirre, A.; Uresti, U.; Bilbao, A.; Fernández-Ramos, C.; Lizarraga, A.; Lorenzo, H.; Madariag, L.; Rica, I.; Ruiz, I.; et al. Curvas y tablas de Crecimiento. Estudios Longitudinal y Transversal. Bilbao: Fundación Faustino Orbegozo Eizaguirre. 2004. Available online: https://www.fundacionorbegozo.com/wp-content/uploads/pdf/estudios_2004.pdf (accessed on 20 January 2015).

20. Pickering, T.G.; Hall, J.E.; Appel, L.J.; Falkner, B.E.; Graves, J.; Hill, M.N.; Jones, D.W.; Kurtz, T.; Sheps, S.G.; Roccella, E.J. Recommendations for blood pressure measurement in humans and experimental animals: Part 1: Blood pressure measurement in humans—A statement for professionals from the Subcommittee of Professional and Public Education of the American Heart Association Council on High Blood Pressure Research. *Circulation* **2005**, *111*, 697–716. [CrossRef]

21. Morell-Azanza, L.; Ojeda-Rodríguez, A.; Ochotorena-Elicegui, A.; Martín-Calvo, N.; Chueca, M.; Marti, A.; Azcona-San Julian, C. Changes in objectively measured physical activity after a multidisciplinary lifestyle intervention in children with abdominal obesity: A randomized control trial. *BMC Pediatr.* **2019**, 6–13. [CrossRef]

22. Konstabel, K.; Veidebaum, T.; Verbestel, V.; Moreno, L.A.; Bammann, K.; Tornaritis, M.; Eiben, G.; Molnár, D.; Siani, A.; Sprengeler, O.; et al. Objectively measured physical activity in European children: The IDEFICS study. *Int. J. Obes.* **2014**, *38*, S135–S143. [CrossRef]

23. González, A.; Martínez, J.L.S.; Santos-Martínez, J.L. Adaptación y aplicación del cuestionario de conducta de alimentación infantil CEBQ. Fundam Nutr y Dietética Bases Metod y Apl. 2011, pp. 339–344. Available online: https://dialnet.unirioja.es/servlet/articulo?codigo=6364656 (accessed on 2 March 2017).

24. MutationTaster. Available online: www.mutationtaster.org (accessed on 5 April 2017).

25. Xiang, Z.; Pogozheva, I.D.; Sorenson, N.B.; Wilczynski, A.M.; Holder, J.R.; Litherland, S.A.; Millard, W.J.; Mosberg, H.I.; Haskell-Luevano, C. Peptide and small molecules rescue the functional activity and agonist potency of dysfunctional human melanocortin-4 receptor polymorphisms. *Biochemistry* **2007**, *46*, 8273–8287. [CrossRef] [PubMed]

26. Calton, M.A.; Ersoy, B.A.; Zhang, S.; Kane, J.P.; Malloy, M.J.; Pullinger, C.R.; Bromberg, Y.; Pennacchio, L.A.; Dent, R.; McPherson, R.; et al. Association of functionally significant Melanocortin-4 but not Melanocortin-3 receptor mutations with severe adult obesity in a large North American case-control study. *Hum. Mol. Genet.* **2009**, *18*, 1140–1147. [CrossRef]

27. Thearle, M.S.; Muller, Y.L.; Hanson, R.L.; Mullins, M.; AbdusSamad, M.; Tran, J.; Knowler, W.C.; Bogardus, C.; Krakoff, J.; Baier, L.J. Greater impact of melanocortin-4 receptor deficiency on rates of growth and risk of type 2 diabetes during childhood compared with adulthood in Pima Indians. *Diabetes* **2012**, *61*, 250–257. [CrossRef] [PubMed]

28. Nowacka-Woszuk, J.; Cieslak, J.; Skowronska, B.; Majewska, K.A.; Stankiewicz, W.; Fichna, P.; Switonski, M. Missense mutations and polymorphisms of the MC4R gene in Polish obese children and adolescents in relation to the relative body mass index. *J. Appl. Genet.* **2011**, *52*, 319–323. [CrossRef] [PubMed]

29. Bonnefond, A.; Keller, R.; Meyre, D.; Stutzmann, F.; Thuillier, D.; Stefanov, D.G.; Froguel, P.; Horber, F.F.; Kral, J.G. Eating Behavior, Low-Frequency Functional Mutations in the Melanocortin-4 Receptor (MC4R) Gene, and Outcomes of Bariatric Operations: A 6-Year Prospective Study. *Diabetes Care* **2016**, *39*, 1384–1392. [CrossRef] [PubMed]

30. Rovite, V.; Petrovska, R.; Vaivade, I.; Kalnina, I.; Fridmanis, D.; Zaharenko, L.; Peculis, R.; Pirags, V.; Schioth, H.B.; Klovins, J. The role of common and rare MC4R variants and FTO polymorphisms in extreme form of obesity. *Mol. Biol. Rep.* **2014**, *41*, 1491–1500. [CrossRef]

31. Melchior, C.; Schulz, A.; Windholz, J.; Kiess, W.; Schneberg, T.; Krner, A. Clinical and functional relevance of melanocortin-4 receptor variants in obese german children. *Horm. Res. Paediatr.* **2012**, *78*, 237–246. [CrossRef] [PubMed]

32. Koester-Weber, T.; Valtuena, J.; Breidenassel, C.; Beghin, L.; Plada, M.; Moreno, S.; Huybrechts, I.; Palacios, G.; Gomez-Martinez, S.; Albers, U.; et al. Valores de referencia para leptina, Cortisol, Insulina y glucosa entre los adolescentes europeos y su asociaciÓn con adiposidad: Estudio helena. *Nutr. Hosp.* **2014**, *30*, 1181–1190. [CrossRef] [PubMed]

33. Hainerova, I.; Larsen, L.H.; Holst, B.; Finkova, M. Melanocortin 4 Receptor Mutations in Obese Czech Children: Studies of Prevalence, Phenotype Development, Weight Reduction Response, and Functional Analysis. *J. Clin. Endocrinol. Metab.* **2007**, *92*, 3689–3696. [CrossRef]

34. Hinney, A.; Bettecken, T.; Tarnow, P.; Brumm, H.; Reichwald, K.; Lichtner, P.; Scherag, A.; Nguyen, T.T.; Schlumberger, P.; Rief, W.; et al. Prevalence, spectrum, and functional characterization of melanocortin-4 receptor gene mutations in a representative population-based sample and obese adults from Germany. *J. Clin. Endocrinol. Metab.* **2006**, *91*, 1761–1769. [CrossRef] [PubMed]

35. Miraglia del Giudice, E.; Cirillo, G.; Nigro, V.; Santoro, N.; D'Urso, L.; Raimondo, P.; Cozzolino, D.; Scafato, D.; Perrone, L. Low frequency of melanocortin-4 receptor (MC4R) mutations in a Mediterranean population with early-onset obesity. *Int. J. Obes.* **2002**, *26*, 647–651. [CrossRef]

36. Stutzmann, F.; Tan, K.; Vatin, V.; Dina, C.; Jouret, B.; Tichet, J.; Balkau, B.; Potoczna, N.; Horber, F.; O'Rahilly, S.; et al. Prevalence of melanocortin-4 receptor deficiency in europeans and their age-dependent penetrance in multigenerational pedigrees. *Diabetes* **2008**, *57*, 2511–2518. [CrossRef]

37. Demiralp, D.O.; Berberoğlu, M.; Akar, N. Melanocortin-4 receptor polymorphisms in Turkish pediatric obese patients. *Clin. Appl. Thromb.* **2011**, *17*, 70–74. [CrossRef] [PubMed]

38. Valladares, M.; Domínguez-Vásquez, P.; Obregón, A.M.; Weisstaub, G.; Burrows, R.; Maiz, A.; Santos, J.L. Melanocortin-4 receptor gene variants in Chilean families: Association with childhood obesity and eating behavior. *Nutr. Neurosci.* **2010**, *13*, 71–78. [CrossRef]

39. Reinehr, T.; Hebebrand, J.; Friedel, S.; Toschke, A.M.; Brumm, H.; Biebermann, H.; Hinney, A. Lifestyle Intervention in Obese Children With Variations in the Melanocortin 4 Receptor Gene. *Obesity* **2009**, *17*, 382–389. [CrossRef] [PubMed]

40. Young, E.H.; Wareham, N.J.; Farooqi, S.; Hinney, A.; Hebebrand, J.; Scherag, A.; O'rahilly, S.; Barroso, I.; Sandhu, M.S. The V103I polymorphism of the MC4R gene and obesity: Population based studies and meta-analysis of 29 563 individuals. *Int. J. Obes.* **2007**, *31*, 1437–1441. [CrossRef] [PubMed]

41. Stutzmann, F.; Vatin, V.; Cauchi, S.; Morandi, A.; Jouret, B.; Landt, O.; Tounian, P.; Levy-Marchal, C.; Buzzetti, R.; Pinelli, L.; et al. Non-synonymous polymorphisms in melanocortin-4 receptor protect against obesity: The two facets of a Janus obesity gene. *Hum. Mol. Genet.* **2007**, *16*, 1837–1844. [CrossRef] [PubMed]

42. Wang, D.; Ma, J.; Zhang, S.; Hinney, A.; Hebebrand, J.; Wang, Y.; Wang, H.J. Association of the MC4R V103I polymorphism with obesity: A chinese case-control study and meta-analysis in 55,195 individuals. *Obesity* **2010**, *18*, 573–579. [CrossRef]

43. Ochoa, M.C.; Razquin, C.; Azcona, C.; García-Fuentes, M.; Martínez, J.A. Val103Ile and Ile251Leu polymorphisms in MC4R gene in Spanish children and adolescents. *Rev. Española Obes.* **2005**, *3*, 250–272.

44. Ochoa, M.C.; Azcona, C.; Biebermann, H.; Brumm, H.; Razquin, C.; Wermter, A.K.; Martínez, J.A.; Hebebrand, J.; Hinney, A.; Moreno-Aliaga, M.J.; et al. A novel mutation Thr162Arg of the melanocortin 4 receptor gene in a Spanish children and adolescent population. *Clin. Endocrinol. (Oxf).* **2007**, *66*, 652–658. [CrossRef]

45. Marti, A.; Corbala, M.S.; Forga, L.; Martinez, J.A.; Hinney, A.; Hebebrand, J. A novel nonsense mutation in the melanocortin-4 receptor associated with obesity in a Spanish population. *Int. J. Obes.* **2003**, *27*, 385–388. [CrossRef] [PubMed]

46. Fernandes, A.E.; de Melo, M.E.; Fujiwara, C.T.H.; Pioltine, M.B.; Matioli, S.R.; Santos, A.; Cercato, C.; Halpern, A.; Mancini, M.C. Associations between a common variant near the MC4R gene and serum triglyceride levels in an obese pediatric cohort. *Endocrine* **2015**, *49*, 653–658. [CrossRef]

47. Ashcroft, J.; Semmler, C.; Carnell, S.; van Jaarsveld, C.H.M.; Wardle, J. Continuity and stability of eating behaviour traits in children. *Eur. J. Clin. Nutr.* **2008**, *62*, 985–990. [CrossRef] [PubMed]

48. Santos, J.L.; Amador, P.; Valladares, M.; Albala, C.; Martinez, J.A.; Marti, A. Obesity and eating behaviour in a three-generation Chilean family with carriers of the Thr150Ile mutation in the melanocortin-4 receptor gene. *J. Physiol. Biochem.* **2008**, *64*, 205–210. [CrossRef] [PubMed]

49. Zlatohlavek, L.; Vrablik, M.; Motykova, E.; Ceska, R.; Vasickova, L.; Dlouha, D.; Hubacek, J.A. FTO and MC4R gene variants determine BMI changes in children after intensive lifestyle intervention. *Clin. Biochem.* **2013**, *46*, 313–316. [CrossRef] [PubMed]

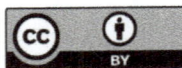

nutrients

MDPI

Review

International Study of Childhood Obesity, Lifestyle and the Environment (ISCOLE): Contributions to Understanding the Global Obesity Epidemic

Peter T. Katzmarzyk [1,*], Jean-Philippe Chaput [2], Mikael Fogelholm [3], Gang Hu [1], Carol Maher [4], Jose Maia [5], Timothy Olds [4], Olga L. Sarmiento [6], Martyn Standage [7], Mark S. Tremblay [2] and Catrine Tudor-Locke [8]

[1] Pennington Biomedical Research Center, 6400 Perkins Road, Baton Rouge, LA 70808, USA; gang.hu@pbrc.edu
[2] Children's Hospital of Eastern Ontario Research Institute, Ottawa, ON K1H 8L1, Canada; jpchaput@cheo.on.ca (J.-P.C.); mtremblay@cheo.on.ca (M.S.T.)
[3] Department of Food and Environmental Sciences, University of Helsinki, 00014 Helsinki, Finland; mikael.fogelholm@helsinki.fi
[4] School of Health Sciences, Sansom Institute, University of South Australia, Adelaide, SA 5001, Australia; Carol.Maher@unisa.edu.au (C.M.); timothy.olds@unisa.edu.au (T.O.)
[5] Faculdade de Desporto, University of Porto, Rua Dr. Plácido Costa, 91, 4200-450 Porto, Portugal; jmaia@fade.up.pt
[6] School of Medicine, Universidad de los Andes, Bogota 11001000, Colombia; osarmien@uniandes.edu.co
[7] Department for Health, University of Bath, Bath BA2 7AY, UK; m.standage@bath.ac.uk
[8] Department of Kinesiology, University of Massachusetts, Amherst, MA 01003, USA; ctudorlocke@umass.edu
* Correspondence: peter.katzmarzyk@pbrc.edu; Tel.: +1-225-763-2536

Received: 22 February 2019; Accepted: 10 April 2019; Published: 15 April 2019

Abstract: The purpose of this review is to summarize the scientific contributions of the International Study of Childhood Obesity, Lifestyle and the Environment (ISCOLE) in extending our understanding about obesity in children from around the world. ISCOLE was a multi-national study of 9 to 11 year-old children from sites in 12 countries from all inhabited continents. The primary purpose was to investigate relationships between lifestyle behaviors and obesity, and the influence of higher-order characteristics such as behavioral settings, and physical, social and policy environments. ISCOLE has made several advances in scientific methodology related to the assessment of physical activity, dietary behavior, sleep and the neighborhood and school environments. Furthermore, ISCOLE has provided important evidence on (1) epidemiological transitions in obesity and related behaviors, (2) correlates of obesity and lifestyle behaviors at the individual, neighborhood and school levels, and (3) 24-h movement behaviors in relation to novel analytical techniques. A key feature of ISCOLE was the development of a platform for international training, data entry, and data quality for multi-country studies. Finally, ISCOLE represents a transparent model for future public-private research partnerships across low, middle and high-income countries.

Keywords: pediatric; overweight; epidemiological transition; collaboration

1. Introduction

The prevalence of childhood obesity has increased significantly in recent years and remains high in many countries [1]. Given the global nature of the problem, a greater understanding of context-specific correlates of obesity is required in order to develop effective interventions that can be translated from one setting to another. To date, there have been only limited attempts to understand the correlates of adiposity or obesity in specific world regions using standardized methods. Large multi-country studies of childhood obesity and/or related behavioral risk factors (physical activity, diet, etc.) have been largely limited to the European region [2–6]. Therefore, the primary aim of the International Study of Childhood Obesity, Lifestyle and the Environment (ISCOLE) was to investigate relationships between lifestyle behaviors and obesity, and the influence of higher-order characteristics such as behavioral settings, and the physical, social and policy environments, on the observed relationships within and between countries that vary widely in levels of human development [7]. ISCOLE was a multi-national study of 9–11 year-old children from research sites in 12 countries from all inhabited continents ranging widely in environmental and socio-cultural contexts.

The purpose of this paper is to summarize the scientific contributions of ISCOLE in extending our understanding about obesity in children from around the world. The focus is primarily on the results from analyses that utilized the 12-country dataset; nevertheless, a large number of papers have also been generated using country-specific datasets or data from small clusters of countries. A complete list of scientific peer-reviewed papers to date from ISCOLE can be found in the online Supplementary Materials (Supplementary File S1).

2. Study Design

A detailed description of the ISCOLE design and methods has been published elsewhere [7]. Briefly, ISCOLE was a multi-national, cross-sectional study conducted in 12 countries (Australia, Brazil, Canada, China, Colombia, Finland, India, Kenya, Portugal, South Africa, United Kingdom, United States) from all inhabited continents. A total of 7372 9–11 year old children participated in ISCOLE [8]. In addition to including sites from countries across a wide range of human development, children were sampled across a range of family socio-economic status within each country. By design, the ISCOLE samples are not representative of the populations from which the participants were drawn. However, an analysis of ISCOLE data compared to other available studies across many world regions suggests that there is no evidence that the ISCOLE samples are systematically biased [9]. These results suggest that ISCOLE data could be used cautiously to inform the development of country-level interventions when other data are lacking.

Table 1 provides descriptive characteristics of the sample by study site, ranked according to the prevalence of obesity. The Human Development Index (HDI) of the study sites ranged from 0.509 in Kenya to 0.929 in Australia. The average age of the sample was 10.4 years, and the prevalence of obesity ranged from 5.4% in Finland to 23.7% in China. Level of parental education also varied among the study sites; with the proportion of the sample with parents having at least a bachelor's degree ranging from 12.9% in South Africa to 73.4% in India.

All ISCOLE data were collected under a standardized research protocol using the same instrumentation at all study sites. Data included objectively measured indicators of adiposity and obesity (body mass index (BMI), waist circumference, body fat), lifestyle behaviors related to obesity (diet, physical activity, sleep, etc.), demographics and family health history, the home and neighborhood environment, and the school environment. All information was entered remotely (anthropometry, questionnaires, etc.) or uploaded (accelerometry) on a secure web-based data entry platform. ISCOLE employed a rigorous quality assurance and quality control program. This program included comprehensive in-person training and certification of all investigators and staff, random remote source data verification, in-person site monitoring visits, and data cleaning and final source data verification [7].

Table 1. Descriptive characteristics of the study sample from the International Study of Childhood Obesity, Lifestyle and the Environment (ISCOLE).

Study Site	HDI *	Boys (n)	Girls (n)	Age (year) **	NW (%)	OV (%)	OB (%)	Parent Education (%)		
								1	2	3
China (Tianjin)	**0.687**	**293**	**259**	**9.9 (0.4)**	**58.9**	**17.4**	23.7	33.0	44.4	22.6
Brazil (Sao Paulo)	0.718	287	297	10.5 (0.5)	56.3	22.8	20.9	24.3	52.8	22.9
United States (Baton Rouge)	0.910	281	370	10.0 (0.6)	58.8	22.4	18.7	8.9	44.6	46.6
Portugal (Porto)	0.809	358	419	10.4 (0.3)	52.8	29.7	17.5	46.7	32.8	20.5
Canada (Ottawa)	0.908	239	328	10.5 (0.4)	69.3	18.9	11.8	2.0	27.7	70.4
South Africa (Cape Town)	0.619	223	327	10.3 (0.7)	73.6	15.6	10.7	48.0	39.0	12.9
Australia (Adelaide)	0.929	243	285	10.7 (0.4)	62.1	27.5	10.4	11.4	47.7	40.9
India (Bangalore)	0.547	292	328	10.4 (0.5)	66.3	23.4	10.3	4.8	21.7	73.4
United Kingdom (Bath)	0.863	237	288	10.9 (0.5)	69.7	20.6	9.7	3.0	51.6	45.4
Kenya (Nairobi)	0.509	262	301	10.2 (0.7)	78.9	14.6	6.6	13.9	45.7	40.4
Colombia (Bogota)	0.710	454	465	10.5 (0.6)	77.2	17.1	5.8	31.8	50.7	17.5
Finland (Helsinki)	0.882	253	283	10.5 (0.4)	76.3	18.3	5.4	2.8	55.1	42.1

* Human Development Index [10]; ** Mean (SD); NW: normal weight; OV: overweight; OB: obese. Parent education levels are 1 <high school and some high school, 2 completed high school and some post-secondary (e.g., vocational diploma or certificate); 3 bachelor degree and post-graduate.

3. Advances in Scientific Methodology Related to the Assessment of Physical Activity, Sleep, Dietary Behavior, and the Neighborhood, Home and School Environments

Mounting a multi-national study of the scale of ISCOLE required the development of novel methods and the adaptation of existing tools that could be applied in sites that ranged considerably in level of human development. This section summarizes some of the methodological advances that were developed during the planning and implementation of ISCOLE. As described above, we have made all of our protocols and algorithms publicly available, and we have summarized our contributions to the use of accelerometry in large studies in detail elsewhere [11,12].

3.1. Physical Activity

A major strength of ISCOLE was the objective assessment of physical activity and sedentary behavior using a waist-mounted accelerometer protocol that was deployed in all study sites [7,11]. Awake-time wear protocols typically require the participants to remove their accelerometer before going to bed and then to reapply it in the morning upon waking. Concerns about wear time compliance have led some investigators to adopt a wrist-mounted rather than a waist-mounted protocol [13]. For example, the U.S. National Health and Nutrition Examination Survey (NHANES) switched from a waist-mounted to a wrist-mounted protocol between the 2005–2006 and 2011–2012 cycles of the survey [13]. In ISCOLE, we chose to attempt to improve wear time compliance by using a waist-mounted 24-h protocol rather than moving to a wrist-mounted protocol [7,14].

The 24-h protocol employed in ISCOLE resulted in impressive increases in wear time in comparison to previous studies. The average wear time in ISCOLE was 22.8 h per day [8]. Given that NHANES used a wake-only protocol, no direct comparisons can be made for total wear time. However, we conducted a study comparing the US ISCOLE site with the 2003–2006 NHANES (that used the waist mounted protocol), and the awake wear time in ISCOLE was 14.7 h per day compared to 13.7 h per day in NHANES, which represents a one hour per day improvement when using the 24-h protocol [14].

Using a 7-day protocol allowed us to estimate the reliability of accelerometer-determined physical activity and sedentary behavior [15]. The estimated minimum number of days needed to achieve a reliability of $G \geq 0.8$ ranged from 5 to 9 for boys and 3 to 11 for girls for light physical activity; 5 to 9 and 3 to 10 for moderate-to-vigorous intensity physical activity; 5 to 10 and 4 to 10 for total activity counts; and 7 to 11 and 6 to 11 for sedentary time, respectively [15]. The results demonstrate that, in most cases, close to seven days of monitored time is required to achieve adequate reliability; and future studies should take this into account when designing their protocols.

3.2. Sleep

The availability of seven days of 24-h accelerometry data in ISCOLE provided an opportunity to develop algorithms to objectively identify the sleep period [16,17]. Over several months, we developed a fully automated algorithm for identifying the nocturnal total sleep episode time in two stages. The first step was to develop and validate an initial algorithm against expert visual inspection of the data [16]. The initial algorithm combined aspects of the Sadeh algorithm [18] for sleep–wake scoring, made use of the inclinometer function in the accelerometer, and built upon the framework of the publicly available non-wear algorithm developed by the National Cancer Institute [19]. The initial algorithm identified sleep onset (i.e., 'bedtime') and sleep offset (i.e., 'waking') times. The second step was to refine the algorithm by adding the ability to identify disrupted nocturnal sleep episodes (and exclude episodes of nighttime non-wear/wakefulness) and avoid misclassification of daytime non-wear or sedentary behavior as sleep [17]. Compared with sleep logs, we achieved acceptable levels of accuracy (<10% mean absolute percent difference) [17]. The Pennington Biomedical Research Center (PBRC) hosts public web-based access to both the original [20] and refined [21] algorithms. As a companion to the sleep algorithms, we have published a full catalog of nocturnal sleep-related variables in ISCOLE [22].

3.3. Dietary Behavior

The primary dietary information used in ISCOLE was collected using a Food Frequency Questionnaire (FFQ) adapted from the Health Behavior in School-aged Children Survey [23]. The ISCOLE FFQ asks about the consumption of 23 food items, and was adapted for use in each of the 12 study sites [7]. We conducted a reliability and validity study in three culturally different study sites (Finland, US, and Colombia) [24]. Reliability correlation coefficients from two surveys completed ~5 weeks apart ranged from 0.37 to 0.78 and gross misclassification for all food groups was <5%. Validity correlation coefficients were below 0.5 for 22/23 food groups and gross misclassification was <5% for 22/23 food groups. Over- or underestimation did not appear for 19/23 food groups [24].

To identify dietary patterns, principal components analyses (PCA) were carried out using weekly portions as input variables [25]. Both site-specific and pooled data showed that dietary behaviors in ISCOLE to be well defined by two component solutions. We labelled the first component as the "unhealthy diet pattern", which included sugar-sweetened sodas, fast foods, ice cream, fried food, French fries, potato chips, and cakes. The second component we characterized as the "healthy diet pattern", which included dark-green vegetables, orange vegetables, fish, cheese, whole grains and fruits. Figure 1 presents the loadings for the two principal components.

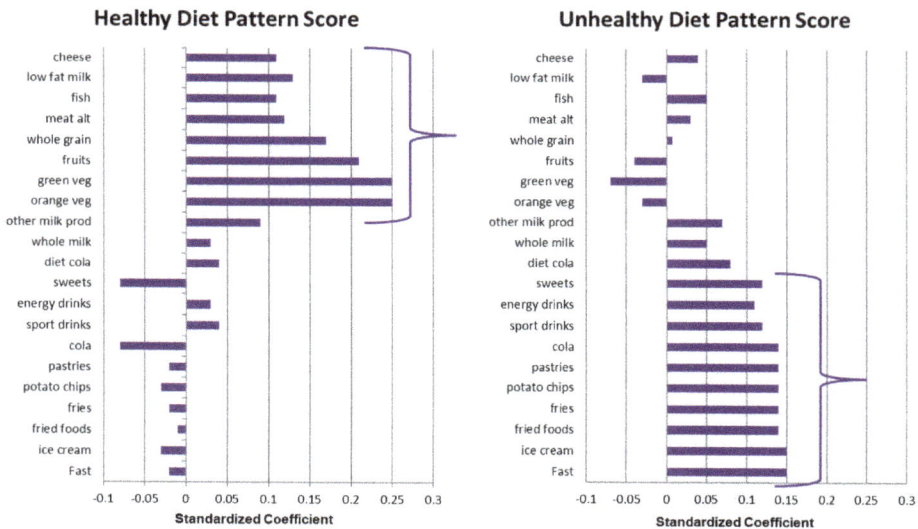

Figure 1. Principal component loadings for the healthy and unhealthy diet pattern scores in the International Study of Childhood Obesity, Lifestyle and the Environment (ISCOLE) (all sites combined), from Mikkila et al. [25].

3.4. Neighborhood, Home and School Environments

Information on several aspects of the neighborhood, home and school environments were collected in ISCOLE using a variety of approaches. A neighborhood and home environment questionnaire, which was based on the Neighborhood Impact on Kids (NIK) survey [26], was completed by parents/guardians. The school environment was assessed using two approaches. First, a school administrator questionnaire, which covered school facilities, healthy eating and physical activity policies, extracurricular activities, frequency of physical education and breaks (recess), and availability of healthy and unhealthy food, was completed by a school official [7]. Second, a school audit of the physical environment was performed at each participating school by one of the study staff. Each site completed a reliability audit (simultaneous audits by two independent, certified data collectors) for a minimum of two schools or at least 5% of their school sample [27]. For the assessed environmental features, inter-rater reliability (kappa) ranged from 0.37 to 0.96; 18 items (42%) were assessed with almost perfect reliability (K = 0.80–0.96), and a further 24 items (56%) were assessed with substantial reliability (K = 0.61–0.79) [27]. These results suggest that the ISCOLE school audit can be used to conduct reliable objective audits of the school environment across diverse, international school settings. However, the administration of the school audit tool can be challenging in some contexts, such as in countries where snow may cover or change aspects of the school environment. Furthermore, research is required to validate these tools under different environmental conditions.

4. Epidemiological Transitions in Obesity and Related Behaviors

The theory of epidemiologic transition characterizes long-term changes in patterns of morbidity and mortality away from causes related to undernutrition and infectious diseases towards chronic 'man-made' diseases as countries become more developed [28]. Related to the concept of epidemiological transition, theories about parallel nutritional and physical activity transitions have been described [29,30]. The nutrition transition is characterized by a shift away from traditional diets that were based on staple grains, local legumes, and fruits and vegetables, towards a diet comprised of more animal-based food products and processed food high in saturated fats and sugar [29]. The physical activity transition is characterized by long-term shifts in physical activity patterns away from necessity (acquiring food, water and shelter, escaping predation, procreation or transport in settings with low motor vehicle availability) towards a largely inactive lifestyle in high-income countries where physical activity has been successfully engineered out of our everyday lives. In high-income countries, humans no longer need to be physically active out of necessity but instead act out of choice to be physically active because of enjoyment, maintenance of body weight, employment, and the prevention of chronic diseases [30]. Whereas in lower-middle income countries where car availability remains relatively low in comparison to high income countries, physical activity could be more reflective of purposeful transport rather than leisure pursuits. These parallel transitions in nutrition and physical activity may contribute to the increased chronic disease burden associated with the epidemiological transition, such as higher rates of obesity, type 2 diabetes, cardiovascular disease, and many cancers.

A review of studies from Western developed countries published between 1990 and 2005 concluded that there was a significant inverse association between socio-economic status and obesity and that positive associations had all but disappeared [31]. However, little is known about how indicators of childhood obesity vary across levels of socio-economic status among countries at different levels of the human development index (HDI). ISCOLE was uniquely positioned to answer this question. Our results demonstrated that BMI and percent body fat were positively associated with family income in countries with low HDI, negatively associated in countries at high HDI, with no association in countries with an HDI in the midrange [32]. Similar patterns were observed for the association between HDI and the prevalence of obesity (Figure 2), reflecting variability in the stages of nutrition and physical activity transitions among countries.

In addition to obesity, we tested for socio-economic gradients in physical activity, dietary patterns and sleep duration in ISCOLE [33–35]. In girls, time spent in moderate-to-vigorous physical activity was negatively associated with family income at the 10th and 50th percentiles HDI (all $p < 0.012$); and positively related with family income at the 90th percentile ($p = 0.044$) [35]. In boys, time spent in moderate-to-vigorous physical activity was also negatively associated with family income at the 10th and 50th percentiles of HDI (both $p < 0.001$) [35]. These results are consistent with the existence of a physical activity transition. A parallel analysis of dietary patterns demonstrated that lower family income was associated with a higher "unhealthy" dietary pattern score and a lower "healthy" dietary pattern score in many countries; however, the pattern was not reflective of a nutrition transition in dietary patterns in these counties [34]. Finally, we also explored the association between sleep duration and family income [33]. No significant associations were observed in any site, and the summary odds ratio was also not significant (OR = 0.94; 95% Confidence Interval (CI) = 0.60 – 1.47) [33].

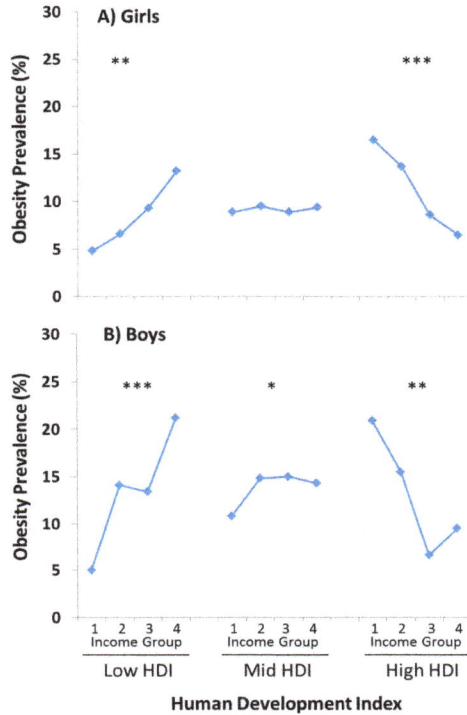

Figure 2. Income gradients in obesity prevalence across levels of HDI in (**A**) girls and (**B**) boys from ISCOLE. Low, middle and high human development index (HDI) correspond to the 10th, 50th and 90th percentiles of the ISCOLE sample (HDI = 0.52, 0.72 and 0.91, respectively). Tests for linear trend are indicated: * $p < 0.05$; ** $p < 0.001$; *** $p < 0.0001$. Figure is adapted from Broyles et al. [32].

In summary, in ISCOLE, we found evidence of epidemiological transitions in obesity and physical activity, but not for dietary patterns and sleep duration. Furthermore, research is required to better characterize country-level changes in these behaviors using temporal surveillance data in countries undergoing rapid economic and social development.

5. Correlates of Obesity and Lifestyle Behaviors at Multiple Levels

5.1. The Socio-Ecological Model

The socio-ecological model is a variant of the root Ecological Systems Theory firstly developed by Bronfenbrenner [36]. Socio-ecological models have been proposed as frameworks to think about the influences of factors at several levels (individual, social, physical and policy environments) on obesity, physical activity and dietary intake [37–39]. ISCOLE was designed to help answer some questions about the contributions of factors at multiple levels of the socio-ecological model to childhood obesity and related behaviors. Our study was a nested design, with individuals (Level 1) nested within schools (Level 2), which were in turn nested within study sites (Level 3). This design necessitated the use of multi-level mixed models for data analysis. This approach also allowed us to partition the percentage of the variance in several variables that is explained by factors at all three levels. The multilevel model is highly elegant in its statistical formulation [40], as well as its versatility [41] which made it a valid model to use with the hierarchical system of information gathered from different levels as in ISCOLE—individuals nested within schools which are nested within research sites. Furthermore, within-level as well as cross-level interactions were considered as per the ISCOLE framework, and these were modeled and statistically tested to verify their substantive tenability.

We undertook an analysis that estimated the proportion of the variance in several key variables at the study site, school and individual levels [42]. The proportion of the variance in BMI and waist circumference explained at the individual level is greater than 90%; the proportion of the variance explained in dietary patterns, sleep, physical activity and sedentary time at the individual level ranges between 66% and 88%, while the proportion of the variance in in-school physical activity and in-school sedentary behavior explained at the site and school levels is between 46% and 75%, with less of a contribution from individual-level factors [42]. These results suggest that interventions that target policy and environmental changes for increasing school-based physical activity and reducing in-school sedentary behavior may enhance obesity intervention efforts.

5.2. Obesity

Several analyses have been undertaken to identify the correlates of obesity in ISCOLE. Our first investigation involved determining the associations between several lifestyle traits (healthy diet patterns, unhealthy diet patterns, moderate-to-vigorous physical activity, TV viewing time, and sleep duration) and the presence of obesity [8]. The odds ratios for obesity (per standard deviation of the predictor variable) were 0.51 (95% CI: 0.45–0.57) for moderate-to-vigorous physical activity, 0.79 (95% CI: 0.72–0.86) for sleep duration, and 1.11 (95% CI: 1.04–1.19) for TV viewing time, while the diet pattern scores were not related to obesity [8]. The results were consistent in boys and girls. These findings led to an in-depth examination of the associations among obesity and accelerometer-derived measures of physical activity and sedentary behavior [43]. In the overall sample, the odds ratios for obesity (per standard deviation of each predictor variable) were significant for sedentary time (1.19; 1.08–1.30), moderate-to-vigorous physical activity (0.49; 95% CI, 0.44–0.55), and vigorous physical activity (0.41; 0.37–0.46). Furthermore, the associations of moderate-to-vigorous physical activity and vigorous physical activity with obesity were significant in all 12 sites, whereas the association between sedentary time and obesity was significant in five of the 12 sites [43].

Active school transport is one potential opportunity for children to accumulate physical activity during the day. Thus, we examined the association between active school transport and indicators of adiposity in ISCOLE [44]. After adjusting for several covariates, children who reported active school transport were less likely to be obese (odds ratio = 0.72, 95% CI: 0.60–0.87) and had a lower BMI z-score, percent body fat and waist circumference (all $p < 0.05$) compared with those who reported motorized travel [44]. Furthermore, the associations between active school transport and obesity did not differ by country or by sex.

Although we found that dietary patterns were not related to obesity in ISCOLE [8], we further explored the association between specific dietary behaviors and obesity. For example, frequent breakfast consumption was associated with lower BMI z-scores compared with occasional ($p < 0.0001$) and rare ($p < 0.0001$) consumption, as well as lower percentage body fat compared with occasional ($p < 0.0001$) and rare ($p < 0.0001$) consumption [45]. These associations differed significantly across study sites, and further research is required to understand these differences. We also explored the association between soft drink consumption and obesity [46]. There was a significant linear trend for increasing BMI z-scores across increasing consumption of regular soft drinks in boys ($p = 0.049$), but not in girls. On the other hand, there was no significant linear trend across categories of diet soft drink consumption in boys, but there was a graded, positive association in girls for BMI z-score ($p = 0.0002$) [46].

Evidence from high-income countries has identified associations between gestational diabetes and birth weight with subsequent childhood obesity. We explored these associations in the multi-national sample from ISCOLE. Compared to children with mothers who did not experience gestational diabetes, children with mothers who experienced gestational diabetes had an odds ratio of 1.53 (95% CI: 1.03–2.27) for obesity, 1.73 (95% CI: 1.14–2.62) for central obesity, and 1.42 (95% CI: 0.90–2.26) for high percentage body fat [47]. Furthermore, the odds ratios for obesity were 1.45 (95% CI: 1.10–1.92) for those with birthweight of 3500–3999 g and 2.08 (95% CI: 1.47–2.93) for those with birthweight ≥4000 g, compared with those with birthweight of 2500–2999 g [48]. The positive association between birth weight and obesity was linear in girls, whereas it was U-shaped in boys. We further explored the association between birthweight and obesity by examining interactions with physical activity and sedentary behavior. Interestingly, the positive association between birthweight and obesity was significant among children with either low moderate-to-vigorous physical activity or high sedentary time, but not among children with either high moderate-to-vigorous physical activity or low sedentary time [49].

Building upon the evidence supporting the inter-generational transmission of obesity, we found that parental overweight was associated with childhood overweight in the overall ISCOLE sample [50]. Furthermore, parental education was differentially associated with childhood overweight across the ISCOLE study sites, and more research is required to understand the context-specific associations between parental education and childhood overweight and obesity.

5.3. Physical Activity and Sedentary Behavior

Current public health recommendations call for children and youth to accumulate at least 60 min of moderate-to-vigorous physical activity every day [51]. In ISCOLE, 4.8% of children achieved ≥60 min of moderate-to-vigorous physical activity for all seven days of the week, while 25.5% attained the recommendation ≥5 days [52]. Furthermore, a total of 18.8% of the sample did not accumulate ≥60 min of moderate-to-vigorous on any of the monitored days [52]. There was variability in compliance to the guidelines across sites: the mean number of days of compliance ranged from 1.8 days per week in the United States to 3.5 days per week in Colombia [52]. Given the availability of 24-h, time-stamped accelerometry data and detailed information about the start and stop times for each student's school in ISCOLE, we were able to differentiate between before-school, during-school and after-school physical activity and sedentary behavior.

Physical education classes are an important opportunity for physical activity in children and youth. In ISCOLE, approximately 25% of participants reported attending physical education classes on three or more days per week [53]. After adjusting for several covariates, children who took physical education classes were more likely to have higher levels of physical activity and shorter time in spent in sedentary behavior both in and out of school during the school week [53].

We also found that children who used active school transportation had significantly higher weekday moderate-to-vigorous physical activity and significantly lower light physical activity before school compared with children who used motorized transport to school [54]. On average, children who used active transportation accumulated 6.0 (95% CI: 4.7–7.3) min more moderate-to-vigorous physical activity per day than children who used motorized transportation. There was wide variability in the prevalence of active school transportation across study sites, which varied from 5.2% in India to 79.4% in Finland [55]. We found wide variability in the correlates that were associated with active school transport across study sites. Longer trip duration (≥16 min vs. ≤15 min) was associated with lower odds of active school transportation in eight sites; whereas individual and neighborhood factors were associated with active school transportation in three sites or less [55].

In ISCOLE, we also investigated home and neighborhood correlates of physical activity. Across sites, children with at least one piece of electronic media in their bedroom had lower levels of moderate-to-vigorous physical activity than those who did not ($p < 0.001$) [56]. More frequent physical activity in the home and yard, ownership of more frequently used play equipment, and higher social support for physical activity were also associated with higher moderate-to-vigorous physical activity ($p < 0.0001$). However, association between play equipment ownership and moderate-to-vigorous physical activity varied across study sites ($p_{interaction} < 0.01$), suggesting that cultural differences should be studied further when developing interventions or making recommendations [56].

Aspects of the neighborhood social environment (collective efficacy and perceived crime) were also studied in ISCOLE as potential correlates of moderate-to-vigorous physical activity [57]. Collective efficacy was inversely associated with moderate-to-vigorous physical activity among children in low/lower-middle-income countries ($\beta = -1.96$; 95% CI: -3.72, -0.19) while it was positively associated with moderate-to-vigorous physical activity among children in high-income countries ($\beta = 1.86$; 95% CI: 0.76, 2.96) [57]. Perceived crime was significantly associated with lower moderate-to-vigorous physical activity ($\beta = -2.12$; 95% CI: -3.18, -1.06) among children in high-income countries but was not significantly associated with moderate-to-vigorous physical activity among children from low/lower-middle-income countries or upper-middle-income countries [57]. These results demonstrate heterogeneity in associations between aspects of the neighborhood environment and physical activity that need to be taken into account when developing strategies that target these correlates in different settings.

In addition to physical activity, we also investigated associations of 21 potential correlates with accelerometer-determined sedentary time and self-reported TV viewing time [58]. Boys reported greater TV viewing time than girls, while in 9 of 12 sites, girls engaged in more objectively-measured sedentary time than boys. Common correlates of sedentary time and TV viewing time included excess weight status, not meeting physical activity recommendations, and having a TV in the bedroom [58].

The associations between sleep and movement behaviors are currently of great interest [59]. In ISCOLE, sleep duration was negatively associated with moderate-to-vigorous physical activity and sedentary time, while sleep efficiency was negatively related to moderate-to-vigorous physical activity and positively associated with sedentary time [60]. The availability of time-stamped accelerometry data allowed us to examine temporal associations between sleep, physical activity and sedentary time [61]. Results showed that the relationships between sleep and physical activity and sedentary time are bi-directional. For example, for each one standard deviation (SD) unit increase in sleep duration, sedentary behavior was 0.04 SD units lower the following day, while light physical activity and moderate-to-vigorous physical activity were 0.04 and 0.02 SD units higher, respectively. Sleep duration was 0.02 SD units lower and 0.04 SD units higher for each one SD unit increase in sedentary time and moderate-to-vigorous physical activity, respectively [61]. While these results highlight the interactions between sleep and movement behaviors, the small effect sizes suggest that the clinical implications may be modest.

5.4. Dietary Patterns

As previously described, "healthy" and "unhealthy" dietary pattern scores were derived from FFQ data in ISCOLE [25]. Figure 3 presents the mean dietary scores across study sites. The results demonstrate variability in dietary pattern scores across countries, with the highest healthy dietary pattern score found in Canada, while the lowest is found in Colombia. Finland had the lowest unhealthy dietary pattern score while South Africa had the highest.

We explored the potential home and school environments as correlates of dietary patterns [62]. Here, we found that more meals eaten outside home and school were associated with higher unhealthy diet pattern scores. Furthermore, low availability of empty-calorie foods at home was found to be more important than high availability of wholesome foods at keeping unhealthy diet pattern scores low. The availability of wholesome foods at home was positively associated with the healthy diet pattern scores, while food availability at school was not associated with the dietary patterns [62]. In the ISCOLE sample, the home food environment was more significant than the school food environment in predicting the child's dietary patterns.

Given the availability of objective measures of sleep in ISCOLE, coupled with the FFQ data, we were able to study the association between sleep and dietary variables [60,63]. Both sleep duration and sleep efficiency were negatively associated with the unhealthy diet pattern score [60]. Interestingly, shorter sleep duration was associated with higher intake of regular soft drinks, while earlier bedtimes were associated with lower intake of regular soft drinks and higher intake of energy drinks and sports drinks [63]. More research is required to better understand the underlying mechanisms that might link beverage consumption to sleep patterns.

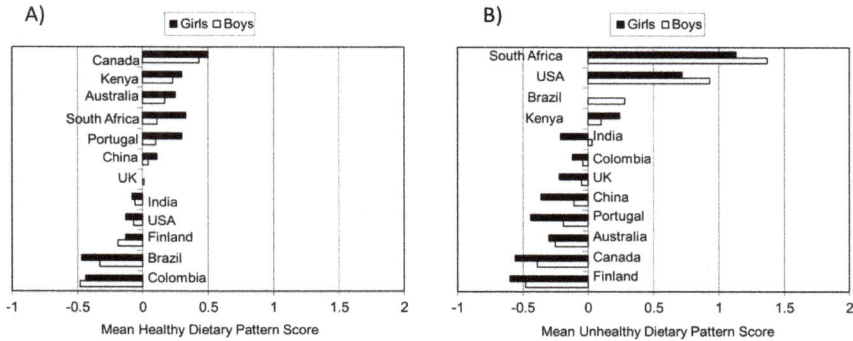

Figure 3. Mean dietary pattern scores across ISCOLE study sites. (**A**) presents the mean scores for the "healthy dietary pattern" and (**B**) presents the mean scores for the "unhealthy dietary pattern". Data were obtained from Mikkila et al. [25].

5.5. Higher-Order Correlates

Given that ISCOLE data were collected across multiple seasons in several geographical regions of the world, we were able to explore associations with other potential "higher-order" correlates of obesity and lifestyle behaviors. For example, we explored the association between moon phase, sleep and physical activity using data from 33,710 24-h accelerometer recordings of sleep and activity [64]. While differences in moderate-to-vigorous physical activity, light physical activity, and sedentary time between moon phases were negligible and non-significant (<2 min/day), sleep duration was significantly shorter (~5 min/night) during the full moon phase compared to the new moon phase [64]. Despite the statistical significance of the association between moon phase and sleep duration, the magnitude of the difference is unlikely to be clinically important.

The associations of weather with physical activity and sedentary time were explored using data from the Australian and Canadian ISCOLE sites [65]. Daily maximal temperature was significantly associated with physical activity and sedentary time in both Australia and Canada, and daily rainfall was negatively associated with physical activity in Australia and positively associated with sedentary time in Canada [65]. The results from both countries indicated that the best levels of physical activity and sedentary time occurred in a range between 20° and 25° Celsius. These results highlight the importance of taking weather into account in the development of intervention and surveillance strategies related to physical activity and sedentary behavior.

The associations of outdoor time with BMI, physical activity, sedentary time and dietary patterns were also explored in ISCOLE [66,67]. Time spent outside and dietary patterns were assessed by questionnaire, while time spent in physical activity and sedentary behavior were determined by accelerometry [7]. Time spent outside was not associated with BMI z-scores; however, each additional hour per day spent outdoors was associated with higher moderate-to-vigorous and light physical activity, and lower sedentary time [67]. Effect sizes were generally weaker in lower-middle-income countries. However, the evaluation of the Ciclovia in Colombia to promote physical activity outside on the streets was associated with higher moderate-to-vigorous and light physical activity, and lower sedentary time on Sundays [68]. Furthermore, time spent outdoors was positively associated with higher healthy dietary pattern scores, but there was no association with the unhealthy dietary pattern scores [66]. Similar patterns were observed in boys and girls, and across study sites. Research using longitudinal study designs is required to elucidate the mechanisms behind these observed associations.

6. The 24-h Movement Behavior Cycle in Relation to Integrated Guidelines and Novel Analytical Techniques

The focus of physical activity guidelines in public health has typically been on the promotion of moderate-to-vigorous physical activity. However, there has been increasing interest in understanding the health impacts associated with multiple movement behaviors (i.e., sedentary behavior, light activity, moderate-to-vigorous activity, and sleep) [59]. Canada has recently released *24-h Movement Guidelines for Children and Youth*, which attempts to integrate these movement behaviors [69]. For example, the guidelines recommend that 10 year-old children should accumulate at least 60 min of moderate-to-vigorous physical activity per day, sleep between 9 and 11 h per night, engage in no more than two hours of recreational screen time per day, spend several hours per day in light physical activity, while minimizing the time they spend sitting [69].

Figure 4 presents estimates of the mean proportions (%) of the day spent in sleep, sedentary behavior, and total physical activity (light, moderate and vigorous) in children across the 12 ISCOLE sites [70]. The mean proportions of the day spent in the different behaviors is remarkably similar across countries given the expanded axes of the ternary plot, as one would predict from the proportion of the variance in these variables that is explained at the site level [42]. The mean time spent in the movement behaviors ranges from 508 min in Portugal to 579 in the United Kingdom for sleep, from 486 min in Australia to 573 min in China for sedentary time, and from 336 min in China to 406 min in Kenya for total physical activity [70]. In addition to these three variables that constitute a 24-h day, mean levels of moderate-to-vigorous physical activity ranges from 43 min in China to 69 min in Finland [70].

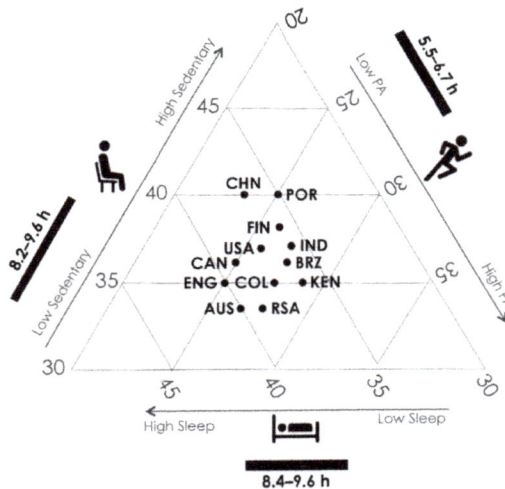

Figure 4. Ternary plot of the average proportions of the 24-h day spent in sleep (bottom axis), sedentary behaviour (left axis) and total physical activity (right axis) in the 12 ISCOLE countries. The black bars represent the range of time (h/day) spent in the various movement behaviours. For sedentary behavior, follow the direct horizontal line to the left axis; for physical activity, follow the lines sloping upwards from left to right to the right axis; for sleep, follow the lines sloping downwards from left to right to the bottom axis. Chinese (CHN) children, for example, spend on average 37% of the day sleeping, 40% of the day sedentary and 23% in physical activity. Compositional means are from Dumuid et al. [70]. AUS = Australia; BRZ = Brazil; CAN = Canada; CHN = China; COL = Colombia; ENG = England; FIN = Finland; IND = India; KEN = Kenya; POR = Portugal; RSA = Republic of South Africa; USA = United States.

Associations between meeting combinations of the 24-h guidelines and obesity [71], health-related quality of life [72], and dietary patterns [73] have been explored in ISCOLE. Overall, the proportion of the sample meeting the overall recommendations (all three behaviors: moderate-to-vigorous physical activity, recreational screen time, and sleep duration) was 7%; individually, 44% of the sample met the physical activity recommendation, 39% met the screen time recommendation, and 42% met the sleep duration recommendation [71]. Meeting all three of the recommendations was associated with much lower odds of obesity (odds ratio = 0.28; 95% CI: 0.18–0.45) [71], higher health-related quality of life scores (51.2 vs. 50.0; $p < 0.05$) [72], higher healthy dietary pattern scores (0.18 vs. −0.01; $p < 0.001$), and lower unhealthy dietary pattern scores (−0.31 vs. −0.02; $p < 0.001$) [73].

A day is constrained by the 24-h period, which presents some challenges for the analysis of multiple movement behaviors together in relation to other health parameters such as obesity [74,75]. Traditional analyses that use Euclidian operations such as linear regression fail to account for the Aitchison geometry of the constrained space [75], and therefore compositional analysis approaches have been proposed as an alternative [76]. Noting the lack of suitable analytical techniques available to handle the analysis of 24-h movements behaviors, Dumuid et al. [77] developed a novel method for predicting change in a continuous outcome based on relative changes within a composition, and for calculating associated confidence intervals to allow for statistical inference. Using data from ISCOLE, we demonstrated the application of compositional multiple linear regression to estimate adiposity from children's 24-h movement behaviors [77]. Furthermore, ISCOLE presented a unique opportunity to compare the results of traditional vs. compositional isotemporal substitution analyses in the associations between 24-h movement behaviors and obesity. The results of this investigation demonstrated that both compositional and traditional models estimated an unfavorable association with percentage body fat when time was reallocated from moderate-to-vigorous physical activity to any other behavior (sleep, sedentary behavior, light physical activity). However, unlike traditional models, compositional models found the differences in adiposity were (A) not necessarily symmetrical when an activity was being displaced, or displacing another movement behavior; (B) not linearly related to the durations of time reallocated; and (C) varied depending on the starting composition [75].

In an attempt to better understand the associations between lifestyle variables and obesity, Dumuid et al. [78] undertook a compositional cluster analysis in which the input variables including sedentary time, light, moderate and vigorous physical activity, sleep duration, TV viewing time, and healthy and unhealthy diet pattern scores were subjected to cluster analysis. Four clusters emerged and were labelled as: (A) Junk Food Screenies; (B) Actives; (C) Sitters; and (D) All-Rounders. Measures of adiposity varied across the clusters, and were highest in the Sitters and lowest in the Actives [78].

In addition to obesity, we have applied compositional data analysis to study the association between 24-h movement behaviors and health-related quality of life [70]. Relative to the other movement behaviors, the association was strongest with moderate-to-vigorous physical activity. Furthermore, this association was moderated by country-level HDI; the association between the moderate-to-vigorous physical activity and health-related quality of life was stronger among countries with a high HDI compared to countries with a lower HDI [70].

7. Other Novel Contributions of ISCOLE

In addition to the work described above, ISCOLE has made several other significant contributions to the literature.

7.1. Body Composition

The majority of the research conducted to date on associations between anthropometry and body fat in children has been in high-income countries, and there is a lack of data on associations in children from low- and middle-income countries. We explored the association between BMI and body fat (from bioelectric impedance) in ISCOLE [79]. Correlations between BMI and total body fat (kg) were >0.90 in all study sites, while correlations between BMI and percentage body fat (%) ranged from 0.76 to 0.96.

Boys from India had higher percentage body fat than boys from several other countries at all levels of BMI, whereas Kenyan girls had lower levels of percentage body fat than girls from several other countries at all levels of BMI. Boys and girls from Colombia had higher values of percentage body fat at low levels of BMI, while Colombian boys at moderate and high levels of BMI also had higher values of percentage body fat than boys in other countries [79].

Given the difficulty in measuring height and weight in some field situations, we explored the utility of using mid-upper-arm circumference as an index of adiposity in ISCOLE [80]. Correlations between mid-upper-arm circumference and percentage body fat were 0.86 in girls ($p < 0.001$) and 0.88 in boys ($p < 0.001$) [80]. Furthermore, results from receiver operating characteristic (ROC) curves demonstrated areas under the curve (AUCs) for the prediction of obesity $\geq$0.97 in both boys and girls, suggesting that mid-upper-arm circumference may be a good screening tool for obesity and excess adiposity in resource-limited settings.

7.2. Identification of Physical Activity Thresholds

We used ROC analyses to estimate the optimal thresholds of moderate-to-vigorous physical activity that were related to the identification of obesity in ISCOLE [43]. The results indicated that the optimal thresholds were 55 (95% CI: 50–64) minutes per day in the total sample, 65 (95% CI: 55–75) minutes per day in boys, and 49 (95% CI: 43–62) minutes per day in girls [43]. These thresholds are comparable to the global physical activity recommendation, which call for children to accumulate at least 60 min per day of moderate-to-vigorous physical activity [51].

Given the recent interest in the health effects associated with sedentary behavior, and the possible interaction between sedentary behavior and physical activity on health outcomes [81], we attempted to identify the optimal thresholds of moderate-to-vigorous physical activity at different levels of sedentary behavior [82]. The results showed that the optimal thresholds of moderate-to-vigorous physical activity to predict obesity ranged from 37.9 to 75.9 min per day in boys and from 32.5 to 62.7 min per day in girls across levels of sedentary behavior [82]. The incorporation of sedentary behavior did not alter or improve the prediction of obesity in this sample, suggesting that the current physical activity guidelines may apply broadly to all children, regardless of their level of sedentary behavior.

7.3. Inequality in Lifestyle and Obesity

Most studies examining associations between obesity and movement behaviors such as physical activity, sedentary behavior, and sleep duration have focused on average values, despite important within and between country variability in these behaviors. Using data from the accelerometers in smartphones in a sample of adults distributed across 111 countries, Althoff et al. [83] found that country-level inequality in physical activity (quantified using the Gini coefficient applied to the accelerometer steps/day data) was a better correlate of obesity prevalence than average physical activity volume (mean steps/day). We explored this issue in ISCOLE, and expanded the focus to include sedentary behavior and sleep as potential correlates of obesity [84].

Our results showed that average moderate-to-vigorous physical activity (hours/day) was a better correlate of obesity than moderate-to-vigorous physical activity inequality (r = −0.77 vs. r = 0.00, $p = 0.03$) [84] (see Figure 5). Along the same lines, average sedentary time (hours/day) was also a better correlate of obesity than sedentary time inequality (r = 0.52 vs. r = 0.32, $p = 0.05$). The differences in associations for mean vs. inequality measures for screen time and sleep period time were not statistically significant [84]. Although there is promise in further exploring associations between inequality in lifestyle behaviors and health outcomes, our results suggest that mean estimates of behavior are still important correlates of obesity in children.

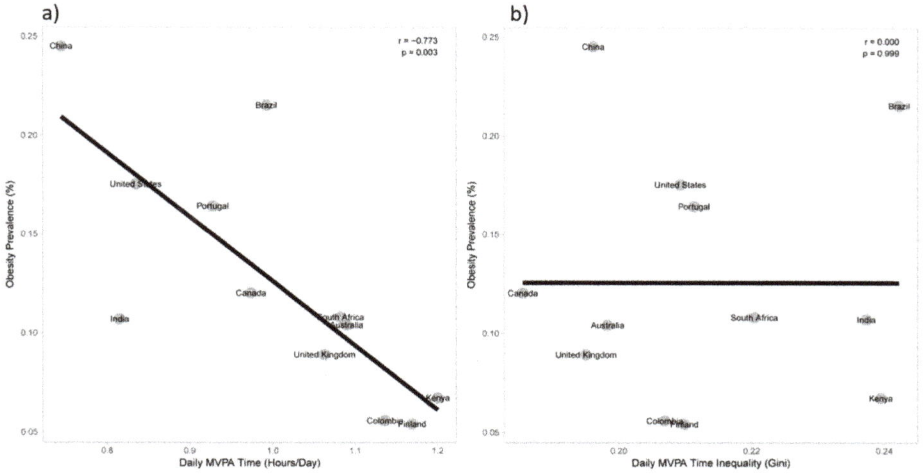

Figure 5. Association between moderate-to-vigorous physical activity (MVPA) and obesity. (**a**) shows the correlation between average MVPA and obesity, while (**b**) shows the correlation between MVPA inequality (Gini coefficient) and obesity. Boys and girls are combined for analysis. Correlation coefficients were compared using a Steiger's Z-test ($p = 0.029$), adapted from Chaput et al. [84].

8. Summary of Research Contributions

As described above, ISCOLE has made many significant research contributions related to understanding global patterns of obesity across countries at different levels of human development and identifying correlates of obesity, physical activity, sedentary behavior, and dietary intake. Furthermore, ISCOLE generated several important methodological advances to the field over the course of the study. Table 2 provides a summary of the major research contributions made by ISCOLE related to the global childhood obesity epidemic. The results from ISCOLE can help inform the development of interventions targeting promising correlates of obesity in different settings. Some findings were robust across all study sites; while other findings were limited to either higher or lower income countries. A careful examination of the patterns of results across countries will be required to deploy the most effective intervention in a given setting.

Table 2. Major research contributions of the International Study of Childhood Obesity, Lifestyle and the Environment (ISCOLE) to understanding the global obesity epidemic.

Research Area	Major Contribution
Global Patterns of Obesity and Related Behaviors	• There is evidence for global epidemiological transitions in obesity and physical activity across countries at different levels of human development; however, there is less evidence for epidemiological transitions in dietary behaviors and sleep duration • Inequality in lifestyle behaviors is not a better correlate of obesity than mean levels of lifestyle behaviors in countries at different levels of human development
Correlates of Obesity	• The proportion of the variance in BMI and waist circumference explained at the individual level is greater than 90%, with the remainder being explained at the school and site levels • Moderate-to-vigorous physical activity is a robust correlate of obesity across all study sites; active school transportation was also related to a lower odds of obesity • Sedentary behavior and TV viewing are both related to a higher odds of obesity • General dietary patterns (healthy/unhealthy) are not related to obesity; however, regular breakfast consumption was related to a lower odds of obesity; regular soft drink consumption was related to a higher odds of obesity in boys and diet soft drink consumption was related to a higher odds of obesity in girls • Parental overweight, gestational diabetes and high birth weight are related to a higher odds of obesity; high moderate-to-vigorous activity and low sedentary time seem to negate the effects of birthweight on childhood obesity • Meeting all three 24-h movement guidelines (moderate-to-vigorous physical activity, TV viewing, sleep) was associated with much lower odds of obesity
Correlates of Physical Activity & Sedentary Behavior	• Participation in physical education classes is associated with higher levels of moderate-to-vigorous physical activity and less sedentary behavior • Active transportation to school is associated with higher weekday moderate-to-vigorous physical activity and lower light physical activity before school • There is wide variability in the correlates of active school transport across study sites. Longer trip duration was associated with lower odds of active school transportation in eight sites; whereas individual and neighborhood factors were associated with active school transportation in three sites or less • Children with at least one piece of electronic media in their bedroom had lower levels of moderate-to-vigorous physical activity • More frequent physical activity in the home and yard, ownership of more frequently used play equipment, and higher social support for physical activity were associated with higher moderate-to-vigorous physical activity; the association between play equipment ownership and moderate-to-vigorous physical activity varied across sites • Collective efficacy was inversely associated with moderate-to-vigorous physical activity among children in low/lower-middle-income countries, while it was positively associated with moderate-to-vigorous physical activity among children in high-income countries. • Perceived crime was significantly associated with lower moderate-to-vigorous physical activity in high-income countries but not in low/lower-middle-income countries or upper-middle-income countries • Common correlates of sedentary time and TV viewing time were excess weight status, not meeting physical activity recommendations, and having a TV in the bedroom • Greater time spent outdoors was associated with higher moderate-to-vigorous and light physical activity, and lower sedentary time
Correlates of Dietary Intake	• More meals eaten outside home and school was associated with higher unhealthy diet pattern scores • Low availability of empty-calorie foods at home was more important than high availability of wholesome foods for a lower unhealthy diet pattern • Availability of wholesome foods at home was positively associated with a healthy diet pattern; food availability at school was not associated with the dietary patterns • Sleep duration and sleep efficiency were negatively associated with an unhealthy diet • Shorter sleep duration was associated with higher intake of regular soft drinks, while earlier bedtimes were associated with lower intake of regular soft drinks and higher intake of energy drinks and sports drinks • Meeting all three 24-h movement guidelines (moderate-to-vigorous physical activity, TV viewing, sleep) was associated with higher healthy dietary pattern scores and lower unhealthy dietary pattern scores
Methodological Advances	• Creation and validation of an automated algorithm to determine sleep parameters from 24-h waist-worn accelerometry • Development and application of a novel compositional data analysis approach to be used with 24-h movement behavior data • Adaptation and reliability assessment of a school environmental audit tool • Adaptation and validation of a food frequency questionnaire for use in different cultural settings

9. A Platform for International Training, Data Entry, and Data Quality for Multi-Country Research Studies

In addition to its scientific contributions, ISCOLE provided a platform for research capacity development around the world. The study was governed by a standardized protocol implemented using strict quality control procedures, including in-person and online study personnel training, site visits, and remote source data verification. All investigators shared responsibility for quality control. A major component of study management was a shared website, which allowed access to all study documents, training materials, remote data entry, accelerometer data uploads, and real-time data validation. This system, based on a common data model, facilitated timely communication and data transfers between the sites and coordinating center. The enrollment target for ISCOLE was 6000 children; however, the final sample size was 7372. We believe the successful recruitment and high data quality are the result of well trained and prepared research staff and co-ownership and investigator investment in the study. Over 240 people have worked on ISCOLE, including senior and junior faculty, post-doctoral fellows, students, and research staff. To date, 25 students (12 doctoral, 10 masters and 3 undergraduate) from 10 countries have used ISCOLE as the foundation for their thesis. ISCOLE has had a tremendous impact on developing research capacity in countries spanning a wide range of HDI.

10. Strengths and Limitations

There are several strengths and limitations associated with the design and implementation of ISCOLE. Marked strengths of the study include the implementation of a standardized research protocol using the same instruments (adapted to the local context as required) and equipment at all study sites, and the inclusion of research sites and investigators from countries that varied widely in human development [7]. Furthermore, the deployment of a web-based data collection and staff training infrastructure that allowed for real-time data entry and verification increased the assurance of quality data. The publication of the study questionnaires, protocols and data algorithms in peer-reviewed journals, which allows for transparency and reproducibility of the results, is another strength of the study. Such resources are also immensely beneficial to other researchers interested in similar or related research. The timely and thorough publication and presentation of ISCOLE findings helped maximize the dissemination and impact of the research, including, but not limited to the notable scientific and methodological advances discussed in this paper. ISCOLE also contributed markedly to capacity building via the personal skill development of research trainees.

There are several limitations of ISCOLE that warrant discussion. First, the fundamental design of ISCOLE is a cross-sectional study, which limits inferences about cause-and-effect relationships. Second, the ISCOLE study sites represent urban and semi-urban populations, and the samples do not include children from rural areas. The decision to exclude rural samples was based on logistical limitations related to data collection; further research is required to better understand urban-rural differences in the correlates of obesity and related behaviors in multi-national studies. This is of particular importance in low- and middle-income countries where the majority of people live in rural environments. We deployed a rigorous research protocol; however, the assessment of dietary intake in free-living children remains a challenge. We used a validated and widely used FFQ to assess dietary intake patterns; however, the FFQ was short and we were unable to precisely quantify dietary intake (kcals, macronutrients, etc.). Furthermore, research is required to develop better methods of dietary assessment in children.

11. A Transparent Model for Public-Private Research Partnerships

ISCOLE was funded by the Coca-Cola Company through a research contract with PBRC. PBRC, in turn, executed sub-contracts with each of the study site institutions. With the exception of requiring that the study be global in nature, the funder had no role in the design and conduct of the study; collection, management, analysis and interpretation of the data, preparation of manuscripts, and the decision whether to publish the results or not. The overall study design, protocol, and all study procedures were developed solely by the principal investigators, co-investigators and research staff. During the period of the research contract (2011–2014), the research team provided regular updates to the funder about the study progress on a quarterly basis. These reports focused on the achievement of operational milestones such as completion of protocols, staff training, field site implementation, achieving recruitment targets, remote site monitoring, and progress on data management.

Given the increased scrutiny associated with industry-sponsored research, we took several precautions to ensure the integrity of the study methods and results. First, we established an External Advisory Board that was charged with assessing the overall progress, rigor and objectivity of ISCOLE, as well as providing an unbiased assessment of the science and the role of the sponsor. Second, we published the design and methods of ISCOLE in an open-access journal, and included the questionnaires and survey instruments in an online appendix [7]. Third, we have made our accelerometer manual of procedures and algorithms freely available online so that they can be tested, replicated and utilized by other scientists [14,16,17]. Fourth, wherever possible, we have published the results from ISCOLE in open-access, peer-reviewed journals so that they can be freely available to a wide audience. Furthermore, all scientific presentations and publications have clearly acknowledged the funding source and the role of the funder. To date, we have published more than 100 scientific papers that have all undergone peer-review and have been found worthy to make significant contributions to the extant literature. Moreover, the large number of students and young researchers who were engaged in ISCOLE highlights the research capacity building that occurred across low-, middle- and high-income countries. Finally, we have declared our data available upon reasonable request for researchers who wish to replicate or challenge our research findings.

Despite our concerted efforts to ensure transparency and rigor in the design and conduct of ISCOLE, we experienced skepticism about the role of the sponsor. We have received several Freedom of Information requests for access to emails from the study investigators and the sponsor. To date, we have provided emails to several media organizations and the US Right to Know organization. This correspondence was the subject of a manuscript that attempted to understand the relationship between "an industry sponsor and public health academics" [85]. The primary conclusion of the study in the first line of the conclusions section is that "Overall, apart from influencing the total number of study sites, we found no evidence of Coca-Cola exerting 'hard power' over the Pennington PIs, where the funder directly changes core methodological principles or points in the research" [85]. The authors tried to make the case that the funder was involved in the study design since they negotiated the number of study sites with the principal investigators as we developed the budget. However, we maintain that the overall study design was not impacted by the number of study sites, i.e., whether the study included 12, 13 or 14 countries; rather, this was purely a budgetary issue, where the budget largely drove the number of study sites that could be recruited [86]. The selection of study sites was at the discretion of the principal investigators. While the funder made suggestions about potential sites to include in order to ensure global representation, the final slate of study sites was selected solely by the principal investigators, and did not include specific sites recommended by the funder.

In summary, the ISCOLE investigators acted in good faith while developing and executing the ISCOLE protocol. Despite a high level of scrutiny (and review of thousands of our emails) from the media and other organizations, we have conducted ISCOLE with transparency and integrity and we are immensely proud of it. We hope that such scrutiny of our work will not dissuade other researchers from developing appropriately managed and transparent public-private partnerships to tackle important public health issues. We feel that ISCOLE represents a successful and transparent model for future public-private partnerships with academics.

12. Conclusions

ISCOLE was a collaboration of scientists, students and staff from 12 countries ranging widely in levels of human and economic development. Using a model of shared ownership, ISCOLE surpassed all recruitment and quality control goals. To date, more than 100 peer-reviewed papers have been published from ISCOLE. In addition to being an engine of research capacity development, ISCOLE has made many significant contributions to our understanding of the global childhood obesity epidemic in a short period of time. The findings of ISCOLE could, in turn, inform global efforts, such as the World Health Organization Global Action Plan on Physical Activity 2018–2030 [87], and the achievement of the United Nation's Sustainable Development Goals [88]. Furthermore, the results from ISCOLE can inform the development of culturally tailored interventions that can be deployed and tested across a range of settings, and we encourage future collaborations that will build upon ISCOLE to improve the health of children across the world.

Supplementary Materials: The following are available online at http://www.mdpi.com/2072-6643/11/4/848/s1, File S1: ISCOLE Publications List.

Author Contributions: P.T.K. wrote the initial draft of the manuscript. All authors edited the manuscript, provided critical input, and approved the manuscript for publication.

Funding: This research was funded by the Coca-Cola Company.

Acknowledgments: We wish to thank the ISCOLE External Advisory Board and the ISCOLE participants and their families who made this study possible. The ISCOLE Research Group includes: Coordinating Center, Pennington Biomedical Research Center: Peter T. Katzmarzyk, PhD (Co-PI), Timothy S. Church, MD, PhD (Co-PI), Denise G. Lambert, RN (Project Manager), Tiago Barreira, PhD, Stephanie Broyles, PhD, Ben Butitta, BS, Catherine Champagne, PhD, RD, Shannon Cocreham, MBA, Kara Dentro, MPH, Katy Drazba, MPH, Deirdre Harrington, PhD, William Johnson, PhD, Dione Milauskas, BS, Emily Mire, MS, Allison Tohme, MPH, Ruben Rodarte MS, MBA; Data Management Center, Wake Forest University: Bobby Amoroso, BS, John Luopa, BS, Rebecca Neiberg, MS, Scott Rushing, BS; Australia, University of South Australia: Timothy Olds, PhD (Site Co-PI), Carol Maher, PhD (Site Co-PI), Lucy Lewis, PhD, Katia Ferrar, B Physio (Hon), Effie Georgiadis, BPsych, Rebecca Stanley, BAppSc (OT) Hon; Brazil, Centro de Estudos do Laboratório de Aptidão Física de São Caetano do Sul (CELAFISCS): Victor Keihan Rodrigues Matsudo, MD, PhD (Site PI), Sandra Matsudo, MD, PhD, Timoteo Araujo, MSc, Luis Carlos de Oliveira, MSc, Leandro Rezende, BSc, Luis Fabiano, BSc, Diogo Bezerra, BSc, Gerson Ferrari, MSc; Canada, Children's Hospital of Eastern Ontario Research Institute: Mark S. Tremblay, PhD (Site Co-PI), Jean-Philippe Chaput, PhD (Site Co-PI), Priscilla Bélanger, BSc, Mike Borghese, MSc, Charles Boyer, MA, Allana LeBlanc, MSc, Claire Francis, B.Sc.,Geneviève Leduc, PhD; China, Tianjin Women's and Children's Health Center: Pei Zhao, MD (Site Co-PI), Gang Hu, MD, PhD (Site Co-PI), Chengming Diao, MD, Wei Li, MD, Weiqin Li, MSc, Enqing Liu, MD, Gongshu Liu, MD, Hongyan Liu, MSc, Jian Ma, MD, Yijuan Qiao, MSc, Huiguang Tian, PhD, Yue Wang, MD, Tao Zhang, MSc, Fuxia Zhang, MD; Colombia, Universidad de los Andes: Olga Sarmiento, MD, PhD (Site PI), Julio Acosta, Yalta Alvira, BS, Maria Paula Diaz, Rocio Gamez, BS, Maria Paula Garcia, Luis Guillermo Gómez, Lisseth Gonzalez, Silvia Gonzalez, RD, Carlos Grijalba, MD, Leidys Gutierrez, David Leal, Nicolas Lemus, Etelvina Mahecha, BS, Maria Paula Mahecha, Rosalba Mahecha, BS, Andrea Ramirez, MD, Paola Rios, MD, Andres Suarez, Camilo Triana; Finland, University of Helsinki: Mikael Fogelholm, ScD (Site-PI), Elli Hovi, BS, Jemina Kivelä, Sari Räsänen, BS, Sanna Roito, BS, Taru Saloheimo, MS, Leena Valta; India, St. Johns Research Institute: Anura Kurpad, MD, PhD (Site Co-PI), Rebecca Kuriyan, PhD (Site Co-PI), Deepa P. Lokesh, BSc, Michelle Stephanie D'Almeida, BSc, Annie Mattilda R, MSc, Lygia Correa, BSc, Vijay D, BSc; Kenya, Kenyatta University: Vincent Onywera, PhD (Site Co-PI), Mark S. Tremblay, PhD (Site Co-PI), Lucy-Joy Wachira, PhD, Stella Muthuri, PhD; Portugal, University of Porto: Jose Maia, PhD (Site PI), Alessandra da Silva Borges, BA, Sofia Oliveira Sá Cachada, Msc, Raquel Nichele de Chaves, MSc, Thayse Natacha Queiroz Ferreira Gomes, MSc, Sara Isabel Sampaio Pereira, BA, Daniel Monteiro de Vilhena e Santos, PhD, Fernanda Karina dos Santos, MSc, Pedro Gil Rodrigues da Silva, BA, Michele Caroline de Souza, MSc; South Africa, University of Cape Town: Vicki Lambert, PhD (Site PI), Matthew April, BSc (Hons), Monika Uys, BSc (Hons), Nirmala Naidoo, MSc, Nandi Synyanya, Madelaine Carstens, BSc(Hons); United Kingdom, University of Bath: Martyn Standage, PhD (Site PI), Sean Cumming, PhD, Clemens Drenowatz, PhD, Lydia Emm, MSc, Fiona Gillison, PhD, Julia Zakrzewski, PhD; United States, Pennington Biomedical Research Center: Catrine Tudor-Locke, PhD (Site-PI), Ashley Braud, Sheletta Donatto, MS, LDN, RD, Corbin Lemon, BS, Ana Jackson, BA, Ashunti Pearson, MS, Gina Pennington, BS, LDN, RD, Daniel Ragus, BS, Ryan Roubion, John Schuna, Jr., PhD; Derek Wiltz. The ISCOLE External Advisory Board includes Alan Batterham, PhD, Teesside University, Jacqueline Kerr, PhD, University of California, San Diego; Michael Pratt, MD, Centers for Disease Control and Prevention, Angelo Pietrobelli, MD, Verona University Medical School.

Conflicts of Interest: The authors declare no conflicts of interest. With the exception of requiring that the study was global in nature, the funder had no role in the design of the study; in the collection, analyses, or interpretation of data; in the writing of the manuscript, or in the decision to publish the results.

References

1. NCD Risk Factor Collaboration (NCD-RisC). Worldwide trends in body-mass index, underweight, overweight, and obesity from 1975 to 2016: A pooled analysis of 2416 population-based measurement studies in 128.9 million children, adolescents, and adults. *Lancet* **2017**, *390*, 2627–2642. [CrossRef]
2. Riddoch, C.; Edwards, D.; Page, A.S.; Froberg, K.; Anderssen, S.A.; Wedderkopp, N.; Brage, S.; Cooper, A.R.; Sardinha, L.B.; Harro, M.; et al. The European youth heart study—Cardiovascular disease risk factors in children: Rationale, aims, study design, and validation of methods. *J. Phys. Act. Health* **2005**, *2*, 115–129. [CrossRef]
3. Moreno, L.A.; De Henauw, S.; Gonzalez-Gross, M.; Kersting, M.; Molnar, D.; Gottrand, F.; Barrios, L.; Sjostrom, M.; Manios, Y.; Gilbert, C.C.; et al. Design and implementation of the healthy lifestyle in Europe by nutrition in adolescence cross-sectional study. *Int. J. Obes.* **2008**, *32* (Suppl. 5), S4–S11. [CrossRef]
4. Ahrens, W.; Bammann, K.; Siani, A.; Buchecker, K.; De Henauw, S.; Iacoviello, L.; Hebestreit, A.; Krogh, V.; Lissner, L.; Marild, S.; et al. The IDEFICS cohort: Design, characteristics and participation in the baseline survey. *Int. J. Obes.* **2011**, *35* (Suppl. 1), S3–S15. [CrossRef] [PubMed]
5. Van Stralen, M.M.; te Velde, S.J.; Singh, A.S.; De Bourdeaudhuij, I.; Martens, M.K.; van der Sluis, M.; Manios, Y.; Grammatikaki, E.; Chinapaw, M.J.; Maes, L.; et al. EuropeaN energy balance research to prevent excessive weight gain among youth (ENERGY) project: Design and methodology of the energy cross-sectional survey. *BMC Public Health* **2011**, *11*, 65. [CrossRef]
6. Janssen, I.; Katzmarzyk, P.T.; Boyce, W.F.; Vereeken, C.; Mulvihill, C.; Roberts, C.; Currie, C.; Pickett, W. Comparison of overweight and obesity prevalence in school-aged youth from 34 countries and their relationships with physical activity and dietary patterns. *Obes. Rev.* **2005**, *6*, 123–132. [CrossRef]
7. Katzmarzyk, P.T.; Barreira, T.V.; Broyles, S.T.; Champagne, C.M.; Chaput, J.P.; Fogelholm, M.; Hu, G.; Johnson, W.D.; Kuriyan, R.; Kurpad, A.; et al. The International study of childhood obesity, Lifestyle and the environment (ISCOLE): Design and methods. *BMC Public Health* **2013**, *13*, 900. [CrossRef]
8. Katzmarzyk, P.T.; Barreira, T.V.; Broyles, S.T.; Champagne, C.M.; Chaput, J.P.; Fogelholm, M.; Hu, G.; Johnson, W.D.; Kuriyan, R.; Kurpad, A.; et al. Relationship between lifestyle behaviors and obesity in children ages 9–11: Results from a 12-country study. *Obesity* **2015**, *23*, 1696–1702. [CrossRef]
9. LeBlanc, A.G.; Katzmarzyk, P.T.; Barreira, T.V.; Broyles, S.T.; Chaput, J.P.; Church, T.S.; Fogelholm, M.; Harrington, D.M.; Hu, G.; Kuriyan, R.; et al. Are participant characteristics from ISCOLE study sites comparable to the rest of their country? *Int. J. Obes. Suppl.* **2015**, *5*, S9–S16. [CrossRef]
10. United Nations Development Programme. *Sustainability and Equity: A Better Future for All*; Human Development Report 2011; Palgrave Macmillan: New York, NY, USA, 2011.
11. Tudor-Locke, C.; Barreira, T.V.; Schuna, J.M.; Katzmarzyk, P.T. Unique contributions of ISCOLE to the advancement of accelerometry in large studies. *Int. J. Obes. Suppl.* **2015**, *5*, S53–S58. [CrossRef]
12. Tudor-Locke, C.; Mire, E.F.; Dentro, K.N.; Barreira, T.V.; Schuna, J.M., Jr.; Zhao, P.; Tremblay, M.S.; Standage, M.; Sarmiento, O.L.; Onywera, V.; et al. A model for presenting accelerometer paradata in large studies: ISCOLE. *Int. J. Behav. Nutr. Phys. Act.* **2015**, *12*, 52. [CrossRef]
13. Troiano, R.P.; McClain, J.J.; Brychta, R.J.; Chen, K.Y. Evolution of accelerometer methods for physical activity research. *Br. J. Sports Med.* **2014**, *48*, 1019–1023. [CrossRef]
14. Tudor-Locke, C.; Barreira, T.V.; Schuna, J.M., Jr.; Mire, E.F.; Chaput, J.P.; Fogelholm, M.; Hu, G.; Kuriyan, R.; Kurpad, A.; Lambert, E.V.; et al. Improving wear time compliance with a 24 h waist-worn accelerometer protocol in the international study of childhood obesity, lifestyle and the environment (ISCOLE). *Int. J. Behav. Nutr. Phys. Act.* **2015**, *12*, 172. [CrossRef]
15. Barreira, T.V.; Schuna, J.M.; Tudor-Locke, C.; Chaput, J.-P.; Church, T.S.; Fogelholm, M.; Hu, G.; Kuriyan, R.; Kurpad, A.; Lambert, E.V.; et al. Reliability of accelerometer-determined physical activity and sedentary behavior in school-aged children: A 12 country study. *Int. J. Obes. Suppl.* **2015**, *5*, S29–S35. [CrossRef]
16. Tudor-Locke, C.; Barreira, T.V.; Schuna, J.M., Jr.; Mire, E.F.; Katzmarzyk, P.T. Fully automated waist-worn accelerometer algorithm for detecting children's sleep-period time separate from 24 h physical activity or sedentary behaviors. *Appl. Physiol. Nutr. Metab.* **2014**, *39*, 53–57. [CrossRef]
17. Barreira, T.V.; Schuna, J.M., Jr.; Mire, E.F.; Katzmarzyk, P.T.; Chaput, J.P.; Leduc, G.; Tudor-Locke, C. Identifying children's nocturnal sleep using 24 h waist accelerometry. *Med. Sci. Sports Exerc.* **2015**, *47*, 937–943. [CrossRef]

18. Sadeh, A.; Sharkey, K.M.; Carskadon, M.A. Activity-based sleep-wake identification: An empical test of methodological issues. *Sleep* **1994**, *17*, 201–207. [CrossRef]

19. SAS Programs for Analyzing NHANES 2003-2004 Accelerometer Data. Available online: http://riskfactor. cancer.gov/tools/nhanes_pam/ (accessed on 15 April 2019).

20. Fully Automated Waist-worn Accelerometer Algorithm for Children's Sleep Period Time Separate From 24-h Physical Activity or Sedentary Behaviors. Available online: www.pbrc.edu/SleepPeriodTimeMacro (accessed on 15 April 2019).

21. Identifying Children's Nocturnal Sleep Using 24-h Waist Accelerometry. Available online: http://www.pbrc. edu/pdf/PBRCSleepEpisodeTimeMacroCode.pdf (accessed on 15 April 2019).

22. Tudor-Locke, C.; Mire, E.F.; Barreira, T.V.; Schuna, J.M.; Chaput, J.P.; Fogelholm, M.; Hu, G.; Kurpad, A.; Kuriyan, R.; Lambert, E.V.; et al. Nocturnal sleep-related variables from 24 h free-living waist-worn accelerometry: International Study of Childhood Obesity, Lifestyle and the Environment. *Int. J. Obes. Suppl.* **2015**, *5*, S47–S52. [CrossRef]

23. Currie, C.; Zanotti, C.; Morgan, A.; Currie, D.; de Looze, M.; Roberts, C.; Samdal, O.; Smith, O.R.F.; Barnekow, V. *Social Determinants of Health and Well-Being among Young People*; Health Behaviour in School-Aged Children (HBSC) Study: International Report from the 2009/2010 Survey; Health Policy for Children and Adolescents WHO Regional Office for Europe: Copenhagen, Denmark, 2012.

24. Saloheimo, T.; Gonzalez, S.A.; Erkkola, M.; Milauskas, D.M.; Meisel, J.D.; Champagne, C.M.; Tudor-Locke, C.; Sarmiento, O.; Katzmarzyk, P.T.; Fogelholm, M. The reliability and validity of a short food frequency questionnaire among 9–11 year olds: A multinational study on three middle-income and high-income countries. *Int. J. Obes. Suppl.* **2015**, *5*, S22–S28. [CrossRef]

25. Mikkila, V.; Vepsalainen, H.; Saloheimo, T.; Gonzalez, S.A.; Meisel, J.D.; Hu, G.; Champagne, C.M.; Chaput, J.P.; Church, T.S.; Katzmarzyk, P.T.; et al. An international comparison of dietary patterns in 9–11 year old children. *Int. J. Obes. Suppl.* **2015**, *5*, S17–S21. [CrossRef]

26. Saelens, B.E.; Sallis, J.F.; Frank, L.D.; Couch, S.C.; Zhou, C.; Colburn, T.; Cain, K.L.; Chapman, J.; Glanz, K. Obesogenic neighborhood environments, child and parent obesity: The neighborhood impact on kids study. *Am. J. Prev. Med.* **2012**, *42*, e57–e64. [CrossRef] [PubMed]

27. Broyles, S.T.; Drazba, K.T.; Church, T.S.; Chaput, J.P.; Fogelholm, M.; Hu, G.; Kuriyan, R.; Kurpad, A.; Lambert, E.V.; Maher, C.; et al. Development and reliability of an audit tool to assess the school physical activity environment across 12 countries. *Int. J. Obes. Suppl.* **2015**, *5*, S36–S42. [CrossRef] [PubMed]

28. Omran, A.R. The epidemiologic transition. A theory of the epidemiology of population change. *Milbank Mem. Fund Q.* **1971**, *49*, 509–538. [CrossRef] [PubMed]

29. Popkin, B.M. Nutritional patterns and transitions. *Pop. Dev. Rev.* **1993**, *19*, 138–157. [CrossRef]

30. Katzmarzyk, P.T.; Mason, C. The physical activity transition. *J. Phys. Act. Health* **2009**, *6*, 269–280. [CrossRef] [PubMed]

31. Shrewsbury, V.; Wardle, J. Socioeconomic status and adiposity in childhood: A systematic review of cross-sectional studies 1990–2005. *Obesity* **2008**, *16*, 275–284. [CrossRef]

32. Broyles, S.T.; Denstel, K.D.; Church, T.S.; Chaput, J.-P.; Fogelholm, M.; Hu, G.; Kuriyan, R.; Kurpad, A.; Lambert, E.V.; Maher, C.; et al. The epidemiological transition and the global childhood obesity epidemic. *Int. J. Obes. Suppl.* **2015**, *5*, S3–S8. [CrossRef]

33. Manyanga, T.; Barnes, J.D.; Tremblay, M.S.; Katzmarzyk, P.T.; Broyles, S.T.; Barreira, T.V.; Fogelholm, M.; Hu, G.; Maher, C.; Maia, J.; et al. No evidence for an epidemiological transition in sleep patterns among children: A 12-country study. *Sleep Health* **2018**, *4*, 87–95. [CrossRef]

34. Manyanga, T.; Tremblay, M.S.; Chaput, J.P.; Katzmarzyk, P.T.; Fogelholm, M.; Hu, G.; Kuriyan, R.; Kurpad, A.; Lambert, E.V.; Maher, C.; et al. Socioeconomic status and dietary patterns in children from around the world: Different associations by levels of country human development? *BMC Public Health* **2017**, *17*, 457. [CrossRef]

35. Barreira, T.V.; Broyles, S.T.; Tudor-Locke, C.; Chaput, J.-P.; Fogelholm, M.; Hu, G.; Kuriyan, R.; Kurpad, A.; Lambert, E.V.; Maher, C.; et al. Epidemiological transition in physical activity and sedentary time in children. *J. Phys. Act. Health* **2019**, in press.

36. Bronfenbrenner, U. *The Ecology of Human Development*; Harvard University Press: Cambridge, MA, USA, 1979.

37. Sallis, J.F.; Cervero, R.B.; Ascher, W.; Henderson, K.A.; Kraft, M.K.; Kerr, J. An ecological approach to creating active living communities. *Annu. Rev. Public Health* **2006**, *27*, 297–322. [CrossRef] [PubMed]

38. Story, M.; Kaphingst, K.M.; Robinson-O'Brien, R.; Glanz, K. Creating healthy food and eating environments: Policy and environmental approaches. *Annu. Rev. Public Health* **2008**, *29*, 253–272. [CrossRef]

39. Davison, K.K.; Birch, L.L. Childhood overweight: A contextual model and recommendations for future research. *Obes. Rev.* **2001**, *2*, 159–171. [CrossRef]

40. Goldstein, H. *Multilevel Statistical Models*, 3rd ed.; Oxford University Press: New York, NY, USA, 2003.

41. Corgeau, D. *Methodology and Epistemology of Multilevel Analysis: Approaches from Different Social Sciences*; Kluwer Academic Publishers: Dordrecht, The Netherlands, 2003.

42. Katzmarzyk, P.T.; Broyles, S.T.; Chaput, J.P.; Fogelholm, M.; Hu, G.; Lambert, E.V.; Maher, C.; Maia, J.; Olds, T.; Onywera, V.; et al. Sources of variability in childhood obesity indicators and related behaviors. *Int. J. Obes.* **2018**, *42*, 108–110. [CrossRef]

43. Katzmarzyk, P.T.; Barreira, T.V.; Broyles, S.T.; Champagne, C.M.; Chaput, J.-P.; Fogelholm, M.; Hu, G.; Johnson, W.D.; Kuriyan, R.; Kurpad, A.; et al. Physical activity, sedentary time and obesity in an international sample of children. *Med. Sci. Sports Exerc.* **2015**, *47*, 2062–2069. [CrossRef]

44. Sarmiento, O.L.; Lemoine, P.; Gonzalez, S.A.; Broyles, S.T.; Denstel, K.D.; Larouche, R.; Onywera, V.; Barreira, T.V.; Chaput, J.-P.; Fogelholm, M.; et al. Relationships between active school transport and adiposity indicators in school age children from low-, middle-and high-income countries. *Int. J. Obes. Suppl.* **2015**, *5*, S107–S114. [CrossRef]

45. Zakrzewski, J.K.; Gillison, F.B.; Cumming, S.; Church, T.S.; Katzmarzyk, P.T.; Broyles, S.T.; Champagne, C.M.; Chaput, J.P.; Denstel, K.D.; Fogelholm, M.; et al. Associations between breakfast frequency and adiposity indicators in children from 12 countries. *Int. J. Obes. Suppl.* **2015**, *5*, S80–S88. [CrossRef] [PubMed]

46. Katzmarzyk, P.T.; Broyles, S.T.; Champagne, C.M.; Chaput, J.P.; Fogelholm, M.; Hu, G.; Kuriyan, R.; Kurpad, A.; Lambert, E.V.; Maia, J.; et al. Relationship between soft drink consumption and obesity in 9–11 year old children in a multi-national study. *Nutrients* **2016**, *8*, 770. [CrossRef] [PubMed]

47. Zhao, P.; Liu, E.; Qiao, Y.; Katzmarzyk, P.T.; Chaput, J.P.; Fogelholm, M.; Johnson, W.D.; Kuriyan, R.; Kurpad, A.; Lambert, E.V.; et al. Maternal gestational diabetes and childhood obesity at age 9–11: Results of a multinational study. *Diabetologia* **2016**, *59*, 2339–2348. [CrossRef] [PubMed]

48. Qiao, Y.; Ma, J.; Wang, Y.; Li, W.; Katzmarzyk, P.T.; Chaput, J.P.; Fogelholm, M.; Johnson, W.D.; Kuriyan, R.; Kurpad, A.; et al. Birth weight and childhood obesity: A 12-country study. *Int. J. Obes. Suppl.* **2015**, *5*, S74–S79. [CrossRef]

49. Qiao, Y.; Zhang, T.; Liu, H.; Katzmarzyk, P.T.; Chaput, J.P.; Fogelholm, M.; Johnson, W.D.; Kuriyan, R.; Kurpad, A.; Lambert, E.V.; et al. Joint association of birth weight and physical activity/sedentary behavior with obesity in children ages 9–11 years from 12 countries. *Obesity* **2017**, *25*, 1091–1097. [CrossRef] [PubMed]

50. Muthuri, S.K.; Onywera, V.O.; Tremblay, M.S.; Broyles, S.T.; Chaput, J.P.; Fogelholm, M.; Hu, G.; Kuriyan, R.; Kurpad, A.; Lambert, E.V.; et al. Relationships between parental education and overweight with childhood overweight and physical activity in 9–11 year old children: Results from a 12-country study. *PLoS ONE* **2016**, *11*, e0147746. [CrossRef]

51. World Health Organization. *Global Recommendations on Physical Activity for Health*; World Health Organization: Geneva, Switzerland, 2010.

52. Gomes, T.N.; Katzmarzyk, P.T.; Hedeker, D.; Fogelholm, M.; Standage, M.; Onywera, V.; Lambert, E.V.; Tremblay, M.S.; Chaput, J.P.; Tudor-Locke, C.; et al. Correlates of compliance with recommended levels of physical activity in children. *Sci. Rep.* **2017**, *7*, 16507. [CrossRef]

53. Silva, D.A.S.; Chaput, J.P.; Katzmarzyk, P.T.; Fogelholm, M.; Hu, G.; Maher, C.; Olds, T.; Onywera, V.; Sarmiento, O.L.; Standage, M.; et al. Physical education classes, physical activity, and sedentary behavior in children. *Med. Sci. Sports Exerc.* **2018**, *50*, 995–1004. [CrossRef]

54. Denstel, K.D.; Broyles, S.T.; Larouche, R.; Sarmiento, O.L.; Barreira, T.V.; Chaput, J.-P.; Church, T.S.; Fogelholm, M.; Hu, G.; Kuriyan, R.; et al. Active school transport and weekday physical activity in 9–11 year old children from 12 countries. *Int. J. Obes. Suppl.* **2015**, *5*, S100–S106. [CrossRef] [PubMed]

55. Larouche, R.; Sarmiento, O.L.; Broyles, S.T.; Denstel, K.D.; Church, T.S.; Barreira, T.V.; Chaput, J.P.; Fogelholm, M.; Hu, G.; Kuriyan, R.; et al. Are the correlates of active school transport context-specific? *Int. J. Obes. Suppl.* **2015**, *5*, S89–S99. [CrossRef]

56. Harrington, D.M.; Gillison, F.; Broyles, S.T.; Chaput, J.P.; Fogelholm, M.; Hu, G.; Kuriyan, R.; Kurpad, A.; LeBlanc, A.G.; Maher, C.; et al. Household-level correlates of children's physical activity levels in and across 12 countries. *Obesity* **2016**, *24*, 2150–2157. [CrossRef]

57. Sullivan, S.M.; Broyles, S.T.; Barreira, T.V.; Chaput, J.P.; Fogelholm, M.; Hu, G.; Kuriyan, R.; Kurpad, A.; Lambert, E.V.; Maher, C.; et al. Associations of neighborhood social environment attributes and physical activity among 9-11 year old children from 12 countries. *Health Place* **2017**, *46*, 183–191. [CrossRef]

58. LeBlanc, A.G.; Katzmarzyk, P.T.; Barreira, T.V.; Broyles, S.T.; Chaput, J.P.; Church, T.S.; Fogelholm, M.; Harrington, D.M.; Hu, G.; Kuriyan, R.; et al. Correlates of total sedentary time and screen time in 9-11-year-old children around the world: The international study of childhood obesity, lifestyle and the environment. *PLoS ONE* **2015**, *10*, e0129622. [CrossRef]

59. Chaput, J.P.; Carson, V.; Gray, C.E.; Tremblay, M.S. Importance of all movement behaviors in a 24 hour period for overall health. *Int. J. Environ. Res. Public Health* **2014**, *11*, 12575–12581. [CrossRef]

60. Chaput, J.P.; Katzmarzyk, P.T.; LeBlanc, A.G.; Tremblay, M.S.; Barreira, T.V.; Broyles, S.T.; Fogelholm, M.; Hu, G.; Kuriyan, R.; Kurpad, A.; et al. Associations between sleep patterns and lifestyle behaviors in children: An international comparison. *Int. J. Obes. Suppl.* **2015**, *5*, S59–S65. [CrossRef]

61. Lin, Y.; Tremblay, M.S.; Katzmarzyk, P.T.; Fogelholm, M.; Hu, G.; Lambert, E.V.; Maher, C.; Maia, J.; Olds, T.; Sarmiento, O.L.; et al. Temporal and bi-directional associations between sleep duration and physical activity/sedentary time in children: An international comparison. *Prev. Med.* **2018**, *111*, 436–441. [CrossRef]

62. Vepsalainen, H.; Mikkila, V.; Erkkola, M.; Broyles, S.T.; Chaput, J.P.; Hu, G.; Kuriyan, R.; Kurpad, A.; Lambert, E.V.; Maher, C.; et al. Association between home and school food environments and dietary patterns among 9–11-year-old children in 12 countries. *Int. J. Obes. Suppl.* **2015**, *5*, S66–S73. [CrossRef]

63. Chaput, J.P.; Tremblay, M.S.; Katzmarzyk, P.T.; Fogelholm, M.; Hu, G.; Maher, C.; Maia, J.; Olds, T.; Onywera, V.; Sarmiento, O.L.; et al. Sleep patterns and sugar-sweetened beverage consumption among children from around the world. *Public Health Nutr.* **2018**, *21*, 2385–2393. [CrossRef]

64. Chaput, J.P.; Weippert, M.; LeBlanc, A.G.; Hjorth, M.F.; Michaelsen, K.F.; Katzmarzyk, P.T.; Tremblay, M.S.; Barreira, T.V.; Broyles, S.T.; Fogelholm, M.; et al. Are children like werewolves? Full moon and its association with sleep and activity behaviors in an international sample of children. *Front. Pediatr.* **2016**, *4*, 24. [CrossRef] [PubMed]

65. Lewis, L.K.; Maher, C.; Belanger, K.; Tremblay, M.; Chaput, J.P.; Olds, T. At the mercy of the gods: Associations between weather, physical activity, and sedentary time in children. *Pediatr. Exerc. Sci.* **2016**, *28*, 152–163. [CrossRef]

66. Chaput, J.P.; Tremblay, M.S.; Katzmarzyk, P.T.; Fogelholm, M.; Mikkila, V.; Hu, G.; Lambert, E.V.; Maher, C.; Maia, J.; Olds, T.; et al. Outdoor time and dietary patterns in children around the world. *J. Public Health (Oxf)* **2018**, *40*, e493–e501. [CrossRef]

67. Larouche, R.; Mire, E.F.; Belanger, K.; Barreira, T.V.; Chaput, J.P.; Fogelholm, M.; Hu, G.; Lambert, E.V.; Maher, C.; Maia, J.; et al. Relationships between outdoor time, physical activity, sedentary time, and body mass index in children: A 12-country study. *Pediatr. Exerc. Sci.* **2018**, *31*, 118–129. [CrossRef]

68. Triana Reyes, C.A.; Bravo-Balado, A.; Gonzalez, S.A.; Bolivar, M.A.; Lemoine, P.; Meisel, J.D.; Grijalba, C. Active streets for children: The case of the ciclovia of Bogota. *PLoS ONE* **2019**, in press.

69. Tremblay, M.S.; Carson, V.; Chaput, J.P.; Connor Gorber, S.; Dinh, T.; Duggan, M.; Faulkner, G.; Gray, C.E.; Gruber, R.; Janson, K.; et al. Canadian 24 h movement Guidelines for children and youth: An integration of physical activity, sedentary behaviour, and sleep. *Appl. Physiol. Nutr. Metab.* **2016**, *41*, S311–S327. [CrossRef] [PubMed]

70. Dumuid, D.; Maher, C.; Lewis, L.K.; Stanford, T.E.; Martin Fernandez, J.A.; Ratcliffe, J.; Katzmarzyk, P.T.; Barreira, T.V.; Chaput, J.P.; Fogelholm, M.; et al. Human development index, children's health-related quality of life and movement behaviors: A compositional data analysis. *Qual. Life Res.* **2018**, *27*, 1473–1482. [CrossRef] [PubMed]

71. Roman-Vinas, B.; Chaput, J.P.; Katzmarzyk, P.T.; Fogelholm, M.; Lambert, E.V.; Maher, C.; Maia, J.; Olds, T.; Onywera, V.; Sarmiento, O.L.; et al. Proportion of children meeting recommendations for 24 h movement guidelines and associations with adiposity in a 12-country study. *Int. J. Behav. Nutr. Phys. Act.* **2016**, *13*, 123. [CrossRef] [PubMed]

72. Sampasa-Kanyinga, H.; Standage, M.; Tremblay, M.S.; Katzmarzyk, P.T.; Hu, G.; Kuriyan, R.; Maher, C.; Maia, J.; Olds, T.; Sarmiento, O.L.; et al. Associations between meeting combinations of 24 h movement guidelines and health-related quality of life in children from 12-countries. *Public Health* **2017**, *153*, 16–24. [CrossRef] [PubMed]

73. Thivel, D.; Tremblay, M.S.; Katzmarzyk, P.T.; Fogelholm, M.; Hu, G.; Maher, C.; Maia, J.; Olds, T.; Sarmiento, O.L.; Standage, M.; et al. Associations between meeting combinations of 24-hour movement recommendations and dietary patterns of children: A 12-country study. *Prev. Med.* **2018**, *118*, 159–165. [CrossRef] [PubMed]

74. Chastin, S.F.; Palarea-Albaladejo, J.; Dontje, M.L.; Skelton, D.A. Combined effects of time spent in physical activity, sedentary behaviors and sleep on obesity and cardio-metabolic health markers: A novel compositional data analysis approach. *PLoS ONE* **2015**, *10*, e0139984. [CrossRef] [PubMed]

75. Dumuid, D.; Stanford, T.E.; Pedisic, Z.; Maher, C.; Lewis, L.K.; Martin-Fernandez, J.A.; Katzmarzyk, P.T.; Chaput, J.P.; Fogelholm, M.; Standage, M.; et al. Adiposity and the isotemporal substitution of physical activity, sedentary time and sleep among school-aged children: A compositional data analysis approach. *BMC Public Health* **2018**, *18*, 311. [CrossRef] [PubMed]

76. Pedisic, Z. Measurement issues and poor adjustments for physical activity and sleep undermine sedentary behaviour research—The focus should shift to the balance between sleep, sedentary behaviour, standing and activity. *Kinesiology* **2014**, *46*, 135–146.

77. Dumuid, D.; Stanford, T.E.; Martin-Fernandez, J.A.; Pedisic, Z.; Maher, C.A.; Lewis, L.K.; Hron, K.; Katzmarzyk, P.T.; Chaput, J.P.; Fogelholm, M.; et al. Compositional data analysis for physical activity, sedentary time and sleep research. *Stat. Methods Med. Res.* **2017**, *27*. [CrossRef] [PubMed]

78. Dumuid, D.; Olds, T.; Lewis, L.K.; Martin-Fernandez, J.A.; Barreira, T.; Broyles, S.; Chaput, J.P.; Fogelholm, M.; Hu, G.; Kuriyan, R.; et al. The adiposity of children is associated with their lifestyle behaviours: A cluster analysis of school-aged children from 12 nations. *Pediat.r Obes.* **2018**, *13*, 111–119. [CrossRef]

79. Katzmarzyk, P.T.; Barreira, T.V.; Broyles, S.T.; Chaput, J.P.; Fogelholm, M.; Hu, G.; Kuriyan, R.; Kurpad, A.; Lambert, E.V.; Maher, C.; et al. Association between body mass index and body fat in 9–11-year-old children from countries spanning a range of human development. *Int. J. Obes. Suppl.* **2015**, *5*, S43–S46. [CrossRef] [PubMed]

80. Chaput, J.-P.; Katzmarzyk, P.T.; Barnes, J.D.; Fogelholm, M.; Hu, G.; Kuriyan, R.; Kurpad, A.; Lambert, E.V.; Maher, C.; Maia, J.; et al. Mid-upper arm circumference as a screening tool for identifying children with obesity: A 12-country study. *Pediatric. Obes.* **2017**, *12*, 439–445. [CrossRef]

81. Ekelund, U.; Steene-Johannessen, J.; Brown, W.J.; Fagerland, M.W.; Owen, N.; Powell, K.E.; Bauman, A.; Lee, I.M. Does physical activity attenuate, or even eliminate, the detrimental association of sitting time with mortality? A harmonised meta-analysis of data from more than 1 million men and women. *Lancet* **2016**, *388*, 1302–1310. [CrossRef]

82. Chaput, J.-P.; Barnes, J.D.; Tremblay, M.S.; Fogelholm, M.; Hu, G.; Lambert, E.V.; Maher, C.; Maia, J.; Olds, T.; Onywera, V.; et al. Thresholds of physical activity associated with obesity by level of sedentary behaviour in children. *Pediatr. Obes.* **2018**, *13*, 450–457. [CrossRef]

83. Althoff, T.; Sosic, R.; Hicks, J.L.; King, A.C.; Delp, S.L.; Leskovec, J. Large-scale physical activity data reveal worldwide activity inequality. *Nature* **2017**, *547*, 336–339. [CrossRef]

84. Chaput, J.P.; Barnes, J.D.; Tremblay, M.S.; Fogelholm, M.; Hu, G.; Lambert, E.V.; Maher, C.; Maia, J.; Olds, T.; Onywera, V.; et al. Inequality in physical activity, sedentary behaviour, sleep duration and risk of obesity in children: A 12-country study. *Obes. Sci. Pract.* **2018**, *4*, 229–237. [CrossRef] [PubMed]

85. Stuckler, D.; Ruskin, G.; McKee, M. Complexity and conflicts of interest statements: A case-study of emails exchanged between Coca-Cola and the principal investigators of the International Study of Childhood Obesity, Lifestyle and the Environment (ISCOLE). *J. Public Health Pol.* **2018**, *39*, 49–56. [CrossRef] [PubMed]

86. Katzmarzyk, P.T.; Church, T.S. Letter to the editors. *J. Public Health Pol.* **2018**, *39*, 254–257. [CrossRef] [PubMed]

87. World Health Organization. *Global Action Plan on Physical Activity 2018–2030: More Active People for a Healthier World*; World Health Organization: Geneva, Switzerland, 2018.

88. United Nations. *Transforming Our World: The 2030 Agenda for Sustainable Development*; United Nations: New York, NY, USA, 2015.

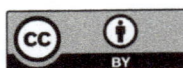

nutrients

MDPI

Review

Interventions Aimed at Increasing Dairy and/or Calcium Consumption of Preschool-Aged Children: A Systematic Literature Review

Victoria Srbely [1], Imtisal Janjua [2], Andrea C. Buchholz [3] and Genevieve Newton [1,*

[1]   Department of Human Health & Nutritional Science, University of Guelph, Guelph, ON N1G2W1, Canada; vsrbely@uoguelph.ca
[2]   Department of Biomedical Sciences, University of Guelph, Guelph, ON N1G2W1, Canada; ijanjua@uoguelph.ca
[3]   Department of Family Relations and Applied Nutrition, University of Guelph, Guelph, ON N1G2W1, Canada; abuchhol@uoguelph.ca
*   Correspondence: newton@uoguelph.ca; Tel.: +1-519-824-4120 (ext. 56822)

Received: 18 February 2019; Accepted: 22 March 2019; Published: 27 March 2019

Abstract: Dairy product consumption is important during childhood, as dairy products provide nutrients to support growth and development. However, a high proportion of children globally are not meeting recommended daily intakes, which may have long-term health implications. Accumulating evidence suggests that interventions aimed at instilling healthy lifestyle habits are most effective when initiated during the preschool years. Therefore, the purpose of the review was to identify the characteristics of effective dairy and/or calcium interventions targeting preschool-aged children. A systematic literature review identified 14 intervention studies published between 1998–2018 addressing dairy/calcium intakes in the preschool population (1.5 to 5 years). Intervention reporting was assessed using intervention intensity, behavior change techniques and Workgroup for Intervention Development and Evaluation Research (WIDER), with the quality of studies evaluated using risk of bias and Grades of Recommendation, Assessment, Development and Evaluation (GRADE). Five of the 14 studies included in the review reported significant improvements in children's dairy (4/5) or calcium (1/5) intake. Characteristics that may enable intervention effectiveness include the delivery of interventions in one setting (preschool facility), using specific behavior change techniques (environmental restructuring and teach to use prompts/cues), and targeting both parent and child. Overall, the interventions assessed demonstrated variable success and highlighted the need for developing effective interventions designed to increase dairy and/or calcium intakes in preschool-aged children.

Keywords: intervention; nutrition; preschool; child; parent; dairy; calcium

1. Introduction

Consumption of dairy products is an important determinant of childhood health and development [1]. Dairy products such as milk, yogurt, and cheese have a rich nutrient profile which includes both macronutrients and micro-nutrients (calcium, vitamin D) that support the optimization and maintenance of good health [2]. Despite the importance of dairy consumption, studies have demonstrated that a significant number of North American children are not meeting recommended intakes, as based on the 2018 Canadian Food Guide [3]. In Canada, 37% of children aged four to nine years do not consume the recommended number of servings of milk and alternatives [3]. Furthermore, between 1977–2001, the proportion of children aged two to 18 years in the United States (U.S.) consuming milk decreased from 94% to 84%, the number of servings consumed decreased from 3.5 to

2.8/day, and the portion size of each serving decreased from 460 to 410 mL [4]. Similar findings have been reported in Europe. For example, the Individuelle Nationale sur les Consommations Alimentaires study conducted in France between 1999–2007 reported a decrease in milk and cheese consumption of 10% and 12%, respectively, in children aged 3 to 10 years old [5]. The Dortmund Nutritional and Anthropometric Longitudinally Designed Study (1986–2001) comprised of German children between the ages of 1–13 years old further demonstrated the global decline in dairy consumption by also reporting a negative trend in milk consumption (−6.5 g/day/study year for children aged 1 to 3; −2.8 to −7.4 g/day/study year for children aged 4 to 13) [5]. A decline in dairy intake from early childhood may have important implications on bone health [6], as well as on the risk of developing a number of costly chronic health conditions such as obesity [7,8], type 2 diabetes [9,10], hypertension [9], and colorectal cancer [11].

Accumulating evidence strongly suggests that interventions aiming to instill healthy lifestyle habits and prevent chronic diseases are most effective when initiated during preschool (≤5 y), as compared to school-age (>5 y) years [12]. For example, Skinner et al. found that the consumption of fruits among school-aged children was predicted by exposure to and consumption of a variety of fruits during preschool years [13]. Marshall et al. (2005) similarly reported that the intake of carbonated beverages, juice drinks, and sugar-sweetened beverages was inversely associated with milk intake in a study of 645 children aged 1 to 5, suggesting the displacement of milk by other beverages [14]. This displacement has potentially significant health consequences, as reported by Dubois et al. (2007), who found that 15.4% of preschoolers in the Québec Longitudinal Study of Child Development who were regular consumers of sugar-sweetened beverages were overweight at 4.5 years of age, as compared to only 6.9% of non-consumers [15]. Furthermore, U.S. data suggest that for each 30-mL reduction in milk consumption by children aged five to 18 years, sugar-sweetened beverage consumption increases by 126 mL, resulting in a net increase of 31 kcal and a loss of 34 mg of calcium for each 30 mL of milk displaced [16]. Collectively, these findings reinforce the need to investigate factors influencing children's dairy intakes during preschool years. Previously published systematic literature reviews have investigated the effects of dietary interventions aiming to increase dairy consumption; however, they targeted children aged 5 to 12 [17] and adolescents aged ≥12 to ≤18 [18], so there is a gap in knowledge regarding dairy intakes in the preschool population.

Enhancing dairy and calcium intake in preschool children is potentially an important step in optimizing children's bone health [6] and mitigating other long-term health consequences associated with insufficient intake. Therefore, the objective of this systematic literature review was to identify the characteristics that constitute effective dairy and/or calcium interventions targeting preschool-aged children. The results of this review will inform the development of future dairy/calcium intervention studies and public health education efforts.

2. Materials and Methods

2.1. Search Method

A list of search terms and keywords were adopted from recent and relevant reviews [17,18], and modified with assistance from an open education resources librarian. The search terms were comprehensive and inclusive, highlighting dairy and/or calcium consumption in preschool-aged children. The search terms were categorized under four headings:

1. Interventions (e.g., intervention, clinical trial, experimental studies)
2. Nutrition (e.g., diet, food, beverage)
3. Population (e.g., preschool, toddler and parent, family)
4. Dairy/Calcium (e.g., yogurt, dairy, milk).

The databases searched included ProQuest, Web of Science, Cochrane Database, Cumulative Index to Nursing and Allied Health Literature, CAB Direct, and PsycINFO. Varying combinations of search terms and keywords were applied to each of the six databases searched (see Supplementary Materials). This allowed for Medical Subject Headings (MeSH) terms to be used along with keywords, where permitted. The final literature search was conducted on 14 June 2018. It included all papers published between 1998–2018, and was restricted to English publications. Grey literature and reference lists of review papers were searched for additional intervention studies focused on dairy consumption. All of the study protocols were registered on 17 July 2018 in PROSPERO (international database of prospectively registered systematic reviews) under the study identification code CRD42018099909.

2.2. Inclusion Criteria

Inclusion criteria limited the selection of studies to: (i) intervention studies with or without control groups, (ii) intervention studies modifying dietary intakes (specifically including dairy and/or calcium intake as a measurement), (iii) the primary or secondary aim of the study being an increase in dairy and/or calcium consumption in preschool-aged children (1.5 to 5 years), including any studies that targeted families (parents and/or children), schools, and/or early education centers, and (iv) intervention studies reporting changes in dairy and/or calcium intakes at either the individual and/or group level.

2.3. Exclusion Criteria

Exclusion criteria included: (i) studies targeting clinical populations (i.e., obese or lactose intolerant groups), (ii) case studies, (iii) studies focused on breast-feeding, allergies, or calcium supplementation, (iv) studies aimed at changing the type of dairy consumption (i.e., regular-fat dairy to low-fat dairy, but not total dairy), (v) publications older than 20 years (i.e., published prior to 1998), and (vi) non-English publications.

2.4. Data Extraction and Synthesis

The Preferred Reporting Items for Systematic Reviews and Meta-Analyses (PRISMA) diagram summarizing the search outcomes is presented in Figure 1. A total of 7178 records were screened (7176 records identified through database searching, two records [19,20] identified through grey literature searching), with 138 articles assessed in full-text based on the specified inclusion and exclusion criteria. A total of 124 articles were excluded based on a lack of access to full-text English publication ($n = 18$), incorrect age range ($n = 38$), not aiming to increase the consumption of dairy and/or calcium ($n = 23$), aiming to change the type of dairy consumption ($n = 16$), focusing on dairy and/or calcium supplementation ($n = 6$), being a case study ($n = 1$), or no intervention ($n = 22$). A total of 14 intervention studies were included in the final analysis.

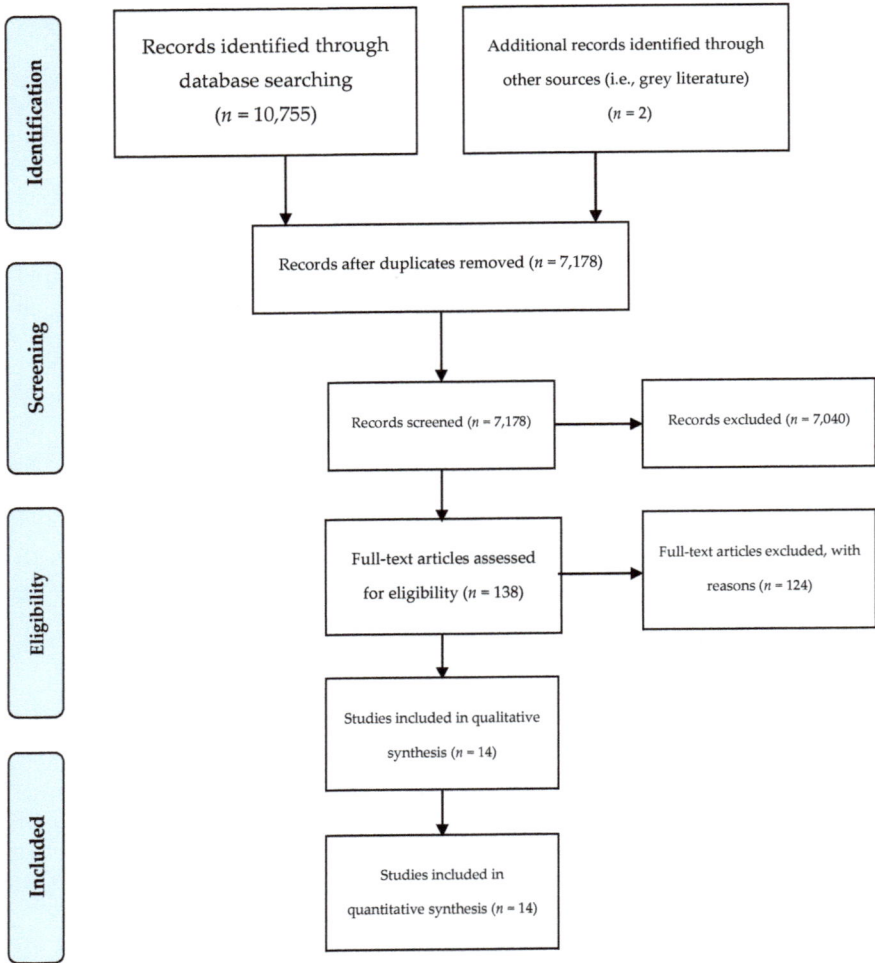

Figure 1. Preferred Reporting Items for Systematic Reviews and Meta-Analyses (PRISMA) four-phase flow diagram of the literature search results. From: Moher, D.; Liberati, A.; Tetzlaff, J.; Altman, D.G.; The PRISMA Group. Preferred reporting items for systematic reviews and meta-analyses: The PRISMA statement. *PLoS Med.* **2009**, *6*, e1000097, doi:10.1371/journal.pmed1000097 [21]. For more information, visit www.prisma-statement.org.

Two independent reviewers (VS, IJ) extracted data from the studies, including the author name and date, population characteristics, description of the intervention, relevant outcome measures, effect size, and effectiveness of the intervention (Table 1). Five assessment tools, including (1) Intervention Intensity Analysis, (2) Coventry, Aberdeen, and London—Refined Taxonomy of Behavior Change Techniques, (3) Workgroup for Intervention Development and Evaluation Research Recommendations, (4) Cochrane Collaboration Risk of Bias Tool, and (5) Grades of Recommendation, Assessment, Development and Evaluation were used to evaluate all of the intervention studies included in the analysis. The five assessment tools are described below.

Table 1. Dairy and calcium intervention studies targeting preschool-aged children: study data extraction table with effect size (*d*) and intervention effectiveness.

Study	Population	Description of Intervention (I = Intervention, C = Control)	Outcome Measure (s)	Intervention Outcome Measurement (s)	Effect Size (*d*)	Effective (Y/N) [1]
Akil (2013) [22]	Parents or caregivers of children aged 3 to 5 (*n* = 140)	I: Parents/caregivers and child followed ordinary HeadStart nutrition curriculum and participated in a nutrition education program (i.e., cooking classes, weekly nutrition newsletters)	Daily number of servings of food groups (i.e., dairy, fruits, and vegetables)	N/A. Study does not report pre/post-intervention consumption.	ND [2]	N
		C: Parents/caregivers and children followed ordinary HeadStart nutrition curriculum				
Bender et al. (2013) [23]	Low income Hispanic mothers (18–35 years old) with children aged 3 to 5 (*n* = 33)	I: Two-phase intervention program; phase I included four biweekly interactive nutrition group lessons, and phase II included six monthly group community activities to reinforce target health behaviors (i.e., nutrition cooking classes)	Beverage (i.e., fruit juice, milk) serving size(s) and number of servings/day	Children's baseline milk consumption in ounces per day (mean (SD)): 14.3 (0.96) Post-intervention milk consumption in ounces per day (mean (SD)): 16.8 (2.1)	ND	N
Cason (2001) [19]	Children aged 3 to 5 (male = 2990, female = 3112)	I: Children participated in a multiple intelligences theory-based nutrition education curriculum (i.e., nutrition education lessons, food tasting)	Daily number of food group servings (i.e., meat, dairy, fruit)	Reported difference in daily servings of dairy in children as mean (SD). Pre-intervention was 0.99 (1.32) and post-intervention was 2.36 (1.54).	ND	Y
Harvey (2008) [24]	Low-income African-American and Hispanic parents (*n* = 25)	I: Parents participated in a weekly nutrition education intervention; they received weekly nutrition newsletters and tracked child daily dietary servings using a kid calendar	Weekly servings for dietary components (i.e., dairy, fruits, vegetables)	Reported changes in weekly servings of low-fat dairy as mean (SD). Baseline measure was 12.44 (7.10) and week 4 post-intervention was 18.04 (7.55).	ND	Y
	Children aged 3 to 5 (female = 13, male = 12)					
Kopetsky (2017) [25]	Parent/caregiver (female = 7)	I: Parent and child attended five, 45-min nutrition education sessions on behavioral strategies (self-monitoring, parental modeling), attended education sessions on MyPlate food groups, and received weekly recipes in the mail	Dietary quality as measured by the Healthy Eating Index (HEI), 2010	HEI 2010 scores quality of dairy in the diet out of 10 points. Baseline and week 5 for dairy consumption (mean (SD)): Baseline: 8.2 (2.5) Week 5: 8.9 (2.0)	0.04	N
	Children aged 3 to 5 (male = 3, female = 3)	C: Parent and child received weekly recipes in the mail				

Table 1. *Cont.*

Study	Population	Description of Intervention (I = Intervention, C = Control)	Outcome Measure (s)	Intervention Outcome Measurement (s)	Effect Size (*d*)	Effective (Y/N) [1]
Korwanich et al. (2008) [26]	Parents (*n* = 219)	I: Nursery schools had implemented a newly developed healthy eating policy (i.e., advising on snack and beverage consumption at school, children engaged in nutrition education activities)	Frequency of dietary intakes per day (i.e., non-sugar milk, fresh fruit)	Frequency of non-sugar milk consumption within groups (mean (SD)). Baseline in intervention group was 0.94 (0.2) and post-intervention was 0.97 (0.2).	0.17	N
	Children aged 4 to 5 years (male = 111, female = 108)	C: No action provided in control schools				
Marquis et al. (2014) [27]	Parent/caregiver (*n* = 201)	I: Parents/caregivers attended weekly meetings for loan payments, entrepreneurship training, and nutrition education on child feeding practices	Frequency of dietary intakes per week (i.e., milk and milk products)	N/A. Study does not report pre/post-intervention consumption.	ND	Y
		C: Parents/caregivers received health education talks				
Munday et al. (2017) [28]	Parents/caregivers (*n* = 16)	I: Children participated in nutrition education sessions, food tasting sessions, sticker reward charts, kindergarten vegetable plots; parents/caregivers participated in cooking classes	Nutrient intake per day (i.e., calcium)	Reported calcium intakes as mean (SD). Baseline intake was 526 (198.4) and post-intervention was 608 (196.2).	ND	Y
	Children aged 3 to 5 (male = 13, female = 4)					
O'Sullivan et al. (2016) [29]	Mothers of children aged 3 to 5 (*n* = 149)	I: Mothers received a community-based home visiting program (i.e., provided information and instruction on parenting practice, emotional support, and access to community services), participated in the Triple P Positive Parenting Program, received child developmental materials and book packs, and were encouraged to attend healthy eating workshops	Proportion of participants meeting daily recommendations (i.e., dairy)	Intakes reported as proportion of participants in the intervention group meeting daily dairy recommendations (mean (SD)). Proportions at each of 18, 24, and 36 months were 0.74 (±0.44), 0.64 (±0.48), and 0.66 (±0.48), respectively.	1.16 to 1.94	N
	Children aged 3 to 5 (*n* = 149)	C: Mothers received child developmental materials and book packs, and were encouraged to attend healthy eating workshops				

Table 1. *Cont.*

Study	Population	Description of Intervention (I = Intervention, C = Control)	Outcome Measure (s)	Intervention Outcome Measurement (s)	Effect Size (*d*)	Effective (Y/N) [1]
Roberts-Gray et al. (2016) [30]	Parent–child dyads (*n* = 608)	I: Parents received nutrition newsletters and participated in parent–child activity stations; children participated in parent–child activity stations and teacher–child classroom activities; nutrition workshops implemented at the organizational level C: No action provided in control schools	Number of dairy servings per day	Number of dairy servings per day (mean (SD)): pre-intervention 0.73 (0.7) and post-intervention 0.79 (0.07).	0.86	N
Salehi et al. (2004) [31]	Parents or caregivers of children <5 years of age	I: Parents/caregivers were exposed to an educational program (i.e., educated on concepts of "food pyramid", taught daily requirements for milk and yogurt intakes)	Quantity of milk consumed (grams)	Reported quantity (g) of milk consumption at beginning of program compared to end. Beginning milk quantity (g) reported as mean (SD) was 50 (13.2), and end was 60 (9.5).	ND	N/A
	Children aged 3 to 5 (*n* = 811)	C: No action provided in control sub-tribes				
Schwartz et al. (2015) [32]	Children aged 3 to 5 (male = 40, female = 45)	I: Children were exposed to one of two feeding practices: (1) fruits, vegetables, and milk were served before the main meal (first course), and (2) fruits, vegetables, and milk were served before the main meal, and meats and grains were removed from the table after the first serving (combination)	Number of Child and Adult Care Food Program (CACFP) servings consumed per meal per day (i.e., milk)	N/A. Not reported as overall pre/post-test consumption.	−0.09 to 0.64	Y
Seward et al. (2018) [20]	Long day childcare services (*n* = 44)	I: Services were provided to staff, including training, receiving a resource pack to support the implementation of nutrition guidelines, having a dietitian complete an audit of the two-week menus, and being allocated an implementation support officer to provide advice and assistance	Number of dietary servings per day (i.e., dairy)	Reported as mean number of daily dairy servings consumed by children as mean (SD). Baseline was 0.55 (0.23) and post-intervention was 1.03 (0.57).	0.03	N
	Children aged 3 to 5 (*n* = 243)	C: Services posted a hard copy of the Caring for Children resource and received regular care from the local health district health promotion staff				

Table 1. *Cont.*

Study	Population	Description of Intervention (I = Intervention, C = Control)	Outcome Measure (s)	Intervention Outcome Measurement (s)	Effect Size (*d*)	Effective (Y/N) [1]
Vereecken et al. (2009) [33]	Parents (mother = 189, father = 11)	I: Children participated in guided and self-guided nutrition activities, were given feedback and reinforcement from teachers, and had access to cooking equipment and healthy foods; parents received nutrition newsletters, engaged in nutrition activities with children, and attended school activities with other parents	Average daily consumption of milk products (mL)	Reported changes in milk intakes in mL. Pre-intervention was 176 mL, and post-intervention was 153 mL. No SD reported.	−2.17	N
	Children aged 3 to 5 (male = 239, female = 237)	C: No action provided in control schools				

[1] Intervention effectiveness is defined as a statistically significant increase (*p* < 0.05) in a dairy or calcium outcome. [2] Abbreviation: ND, no data or not enough data available to calculate effect size.

2.5. Intervention Reporting

2.5.1. Intervention Intensity

Intervention intensity scales have been employed in scientific literature to enhance comparisons of interventions between studies [17]. An intervention intensity scale is a point-scale assessment tool that evaluates the characteristics and degree of an intervention [17]. The intensity score ranks the qualities of each individual intervention as high, medium, or low intensity, facilitating straightforward comparisons of different study designs and/or intervention settings [17].

The intervention intensity scale used was adapted from a recent review [18], assessing four characteristics of interventions on a 5-point ranking scale (1 = low, 2 = low-medium, 3 = medium, 4 = medium–high, and 5 = high), with the exception of "reach of the intervention strategies" [34]. The four characteristics are detailed below:

(1) *Duration of the intervention.* This category ranked the length of the intervention using the following scale: 1 = ≤6 weeks, 2 = 6 to 11 weeks, 3 = 12 weeks to 5 months, 4 = 6 to 12 months, and 5 = ≥12 months.

(2) *Frequency of contact with the intervention.* This characteristic assessed the frequency of contact between participants and the intervention. If the intervention employed multiple points of contact, an average contact score was computed. If the frequency of contact was not clearly stated by authors, the points of contact were divided by the overall duration of the intervention to determine an average frequency of contact. The ranking score that was used for frequency of contact with the intervention was 1 = annually, 2 = bimonthly to quarterly, 3 = monthly, 3.5 = twice a month, 4 = weekly, 4.5 = multiple times per week, and 5 = daily.

(3) *Level of personalization.* This characteristic describes the type and/or level of contact with the intervention. The ranking score used for the level of personalization included: 1 = environmental, 2 = group (parent or child), 2.5 = group (parent and child), 3 = environmental and group (parent or child), 3.5 = environmental and group (parent and child), 4 = group with an individual component (parent or child), 4.5 = group with an individual component (parent and child), and 5 = individual (parent and/or child) or individual, environmental, and group (parent and/or child). If the parent and child experienced different levels of personalization, they were scored independently, and the scores were averaged for a total personalization score out of 5. The more personalized the contact of the intervention, the higher the intensity score.

(4) *Reach of the intervention strategies.* This characteristic assessed the number of different settings (i.e., home, school) used by the researchers to reach their target audience, and used a scale where 1 = one setting, 3 = two settings, and 5 = three or more settings. The greater number of settings used with the intervention, the higher the intensity of the intervention.

The two reviewers (VS, IJ) scored the characteristics and provided an overall intervention intensity score for each intervention included in the analysis. The overall intensity score was the sum of the scores of the four characteristics, giving a total score out of 20. An overall intervention intensity score of greater than or equal to 13.5 was considered a high-intensity intervention, between 10.51–13.49 was rated as medium intensity, and a score of 10.5 or less indicated a low-intensity intervention.

2.5.2. Behavior Change Techniques

Michie et al. (2011) published the Coventry, Aberdeen, and London-Refined (CALO-RE) Taxonomy of Behavior Change Techniques to be used in assessment of interventions targeting healthy eating and physical activity [35]. The refined taxonomy published by Michie et al. (2011) was adopted from the taxonomy of theory-linked behavior change techniques developed by Abraham and Michie (2008) [36], which identified specific behavior change techniques in interventions that enabled effectiveness. The twofold rationale for the use of the CALO-RE Taxonomy is based on determining whether the differences in behavior change techniques observed across studies impacted the effectiveness of each intervention, and secondly, identifying which techniques affected the most significant behavioral change [36].

The CALO-RE Taxonomy provides a behavior change taxonomy of 40 items, which are defined in Supplementary Materials Table S1. Two independent reviewers (VS, IJ) evaluated the behavior change techniques applied in the intervention studies and resolved any discrepancies through discussion. Behavior change techniques three, six, 11, 12, 14, 17, 18, 31, 32, 33, 34, 37, and 40 were excluded from analysis, as these techniques were not employed in any of the interventions assessed.

2.5.3. WIDER Recommendations

The Workgroup for Intervention Development and Evaluation Research (WIDER) [37] developed a framework to assess and report the components of behavior change intervention studies, recommending a set of four criteria by which to evaluate techniques employed in behavior change interventions. The WIDER recommendations were developed to compare behavior change interventions across heterogeneous studies, with the goal of ensuring clarity in reporting of the components of behavior change techniques to ultimately improve the reproducibility of current intervention methods. The description of the four criteria of the WIDER recommendations are outlined in Supplementary Materials Table S2 and detailed below:

(1) The first recommendation addresses the description of the intervention(s) and the level of detail reported by authors. There are eight supplementary recommendations required for discussion throughout the intervention study, including the characteristics of those delivering the intervention, characteristics of the recipients, setting, mode of intervention delivery, intensity, duration, adherence to delivery protocols, and a detailed description of the intervention content for each study group.

(2) The second recommendation addresses the change process employed in the intervention and the design of the intervention. This recommendation requires a description of how the intervention was developed, the behavior change techniques used in the intervention, and the behavioral processes being targeted by the change techniques.

(3) The third recommendation addresses the extent to which the intervention protocols and/or manuals are accessible, as authors must provide easy access to the protocols/manuals for the interventions as supplementary materials (i.e., online).

(4) The fourth recommendation assesses the control group and the control conditions. Authors must describe the characteristics of the interveners delivering the control, characteristics of the control participants, setting, mode of delivery, intensity, duration, compliance to the delivery protocols, and a detailed description of the control content.

Two reviewers (VS, IJ) independently assessed all of the intervention studies using the four WIDER recommendations, and reported whether each intervention satisfied all of the subcomponents of the recommendations [38].

2.6. Quality Criteria

2.6.1. Risk of Bias

The Cochrane Risk of Bias Tool [39] was used to evaluate six types of bias in the individual studies, including selection bias, performance bias, attrition bias, reporting bias, detection bias, and other bias. Within the six types of bias, seven domains exist that aid in assessing the risk of each type of bias:

(1) *Selection bias*: assessed two domains: sequence generation and allocation concealment

(2) *Performance bias*: assessed the blinding procedures implemented in the study

(3) *Detection bias*: assessed the adequacy of the blinding of outcome assessors

(4) *Attrition bias*: assessed all the participant withdrawal from the study that lead to incomplete outcome data

(5) *Reporting bias*: identified the selective reporting of results
(6) *Other bias*: identified any other sources of bias that may be present in the literature, owing to a variety of circumstances or events.

The two reviewers (VS, IJ) evaluated the level of bias within each category for each individual study by assigning a material risk of bias score (high, low, or unclear) for each of the above criteria, including supporting rationale for this score. Material bias is defined as bias significant enough to affect the results and/or conclusions of the study. Examples of criteria used to assess material bias are included in Supplementary Materials Table S3.

The support for the bias judgment is derived from the study and is highlighted by verbatim quotes from the publication, where possible. In this section, review authors may include personal comments and any relevant information supporting the rationale for their judgments. The ambiguity of information within the study can be addressed by indicating 'probably done' or 'probably not done' in addition to an explanation for why they believe so. Lastly, if the primary authors did not provide sufficient information to enable review authors to make clearly defined judgments, this should be clearly indicated.

2.6.2. GRADE

The Grades of Recommendation, Assessment, Development, and Evaluation (GRADE) [40] is a systematic approach that is used to assess the quality of evidence across studies and evaluate the strength of clinical recommendations. Prior to their assessment of the quality of evidence, review authors identify the clinical outcomes on which they will be focusing. If applicable, three items must be clearly defined for each outcome, including the number of studies addressing the specific outcome of interest, the treatment comparison, and the number of participants in each comparison. Then, the quality of evidence addressing the outcomes is evaluated based on the type of evidence provided, quality points, consistency, directness, and effect size.

Two independent reviewers (VS, IJ) used the GRADE criteria to evaluate the quality of evidence across studies. The five GRADE criteria outlined by the British Medical Journal (BMJ) (2012) [40] are detailed in Supplementary Materials Table S4 and summarized below:

(1) *Type of evidence*. Scientific evidence derived from randomized control trials begins at a rating of four points; in contrast, evidence from observational studies is assigned a rating of two.
(2) *Quality points*. A total of three points can be deducted under this category based on inadequacies in follow-up procedures, sparse data, blinding, allocation concealment, and attrition.
(3) *Consistency*. Heterogeneous studies are evaluated under this category, as long as they all address the same outcomes and interventions. A quality point is deducted under this category for inconsistent results between studies while, in contrast, a quality point is added if a dose-response effect is observed or if adjustment of confounders increased the effect size.
(4) *Directness*. A maximum of two points can be deducted for issues affecting the generalizability of the results to the population of interest. Examples of issues affecting directness include co-interventions that are being tested alongside the intervention of interest, as well as the use of samples that are either too broad or too restricted.
(5) *Effect Size*. The GRADE criteria add a quality point for an odds ratio (OR) or relative risk (RR) ≥ 2 and adds two quality points for an OR or RR ≥ 5. One quality point is added for effect sizes >2 (or <0.5), while two quality points are added for effect sizes that are >5 (or <0.2) and are all statistically significant. No quality points are added for effect sizes <2 or statistically insignificant results.

When calculating the final GRADE score for each outcome, a score of at least four points indicates a high quality of evidence, three points suggests a moderate quality of evidence, two points reflects a low quality of evidence, and a score of one or less represents a very low quality of evidence. GRADE scores for independent outcomes are presented in table format, where explanations for the scores and judgments about the quality of evidence are provided. The overall interpretation of the GRADE score does not reflect the methodological quality of a single piece of literature, but rather is a measure of the quality rating of the overall evidence across studies addressing a specific outcome within the target population.

3. Results

3.1. Intervention Studies

3.1.1. Study Description

The present review identified 14 intervention studies published between 1998–2018 that aimed to increase dairy and/or calcium consumption. Of the 14 intervention studies identified, seven (50%) targeted total dairy intake, six (43%) targeted total milk intake, and one (7%) targeted calcium intake; all did so as part of a larger dietary intervention. All of the intervention studies targeted children between the ages of 1.5–5 years, their parents, and/or teachers, as it was acknowledged that interventions may engage the child's caregiver(s), but not be applied to the preschool-aged child(ren). The search methods were exhaustive and retrieved studies conducted globally, allowing for a comprehensive analysis of interventions for populations with differing baselines and habitual dairy and/or calcium intake.

3.1.2. Effectiveness

Intervention effectiveness was determined as a statistically significant ($p < 0.05$) increase in dairy and/or calcium intake. Of the 14 interventions included in the review, five were effective, eight were ineffective, and one did not provide any information on the effectiveness of the intervention (Table 1). Of the five effective interventions, one targeted both parent and child, two targeted only the parent, and two targeted the child alone; importantly, both interventions targeting the child demonstrated effectiveness. The overall intervention effectiveness results reported in this review were lower than those of previously published systematic literature reviews [17,18].

One intervention [30] did not report a statistically significant change in dairy consumption from baseline to six-week post-intervention follow-up, but reported a statistically significant increase in dairy consumption using a treatment-by-time interaction model at 28 weeks post-intervention booster follow-up. (A booster in this context is a reintroduction of the intervention some time after the initial intervention has concluded; it is used to determine whether the behavior changes that were taught/implemented in the initial intervention were maintained over time).

3.1.3. Sample Size, Control Groups, Effect Size

The sample size of intervention studies ranged from very small groups of parents ($n = 7$) and children ($n = 6$) as presented in the study of Kopetsky (2017) [25], to large groups of children ($n = 3112$) enrolled in the Food and Nutrition Services Food Stamp Nutrition Education Program as studied by Cason (2001) [19]. In addition, four (29%) interventions did not have a control group, while only seven (50%) interventions included in the review provided adequate information to calculate effect size. The other 50% had insufficient data (i.e., did not have a control group), or did not provide the data in the correct format to enable effect size calculation.

3.2. Intervention Intensity

The summary of the intervention intensity rating categories associated with effectiveness and overall intervention intensity results are presented in Tables 2 and 3, respectively. In this review, three (23%) interventions were of low intensity, five (~38%) interventions were of medium intensity, and five (~38%) interventions were of high intensity. More than half (60%) of the medium-intensity interventions and 66.7% of the low-intensity interventions reported statistically significant ($p < 0.05$) increases in dairy and/or calcium intakes, whereas none of the high-intensity interventions were effective at increasing dairy and/or calcium consumption.

Table 2. Intervention characteristics and intensity rating categories associated with intervention effectiveness ($n = 13$).

	Effective Interventions	Ineffective Interventions	Total [3]	% Effective [1]
Target of Intervention				
Mixed	5	8	13	38.5
Intervention Intensity				
Low	2	1	3	66.7
Medium	3	2	5	60.0
High	0	5	5	0.0
Duration				
<6 weeks	2	2	4	50.0
6 to 11 weeks	1	0	1	100.0
12 weeks to 5 months	-	-	-	-
6 to 12 months	1	5	6	16.7
>12 months	1	1	2	50.0
Frequency of Contact [2]				
Annually	-	-	-	-
Bimonthly to quarterly	-	-	-	-
Monthly	0	2	2	0.0
Biweekly	1	2	3	33.3
Weekly	2	5	7	28.6
Multiple times per week	2	0	2	100.0
Daily	-	-	-	-
Level of Personalization [2]				
Environmental	1	1	2	50.0
Group (Parent or Child)	3	3	6	50.0
Group (Parent and Child)	-	-	-	-
Environmental + Group (Parent or Child)	1	1	2	50.0
Environmental + Group (Parent and Child)	0	2	2	0.0
Group + Individual (Parent or Child)	1	1	2	50.0
Group + Individual (Parent and Child)	0	1	1	0.0
Individual or Individual + Environmental + Group	0	2	2	0.0
Reach				
1 setting	5	1	6	83.3
2 settings	0	5	5	0.0
3+ settings	0	2	2	0.0

[1] Intervention effectiveness is defined as a statistically significant increase ($p < 0.05$) in a dairy and/or calcium related outcome. [2] Total number of studies in Frequency of Contact and Level of Personalization will not sum to $n = 13$, because some studies used multiple frequencies of contact and multiple levels of personalization throughout the intervention. [3] Salehi et al. (2004) was excluded from the chart and analysis, as the authors did not provide the effectiveness of the intervention.

Table 3. Summary of overall intervention intensity results.

Study (n = 14)	Duration[4]	Frequency[4]	Personalization[4]	Reach[4]	Overall Intensity Score	Overall Intensity Rating[2]	Effective[3]	Group Score
Parent and Child								
Akil (2013) [22]	4	4	3	5	16	High	N	
Bender et al. (2013) [23]	4	3.25	2.5	5	14.75	High	N	
Kopetsky (2017) [25]	1	4	4.5	3	12.5	Medium	N	
Korwanich et al. (2008) [26]	4	4[1]	3.5	3	14.5	High	N	13.5
Munday et al. (2017) [28]	2	4.5	3	1	10.5	Medium	Y	
Roberts-Gray et al. (2016) [30]	1	4	3.5	3	11.5	Medium	N	
Vereecken et al. (2009) [33]	4	4[1]	3.5	3	14.5	High	N	
Parent								
Harvey (2008) [24]	1	4	2	1	8	Low	Y	
Marquis et al. (2014) [27]	5	4	2	1	12	Medium	Y	12.2
Salehi et al. (2004) [31]	4	N/A	Unclear	1	N/A	N/A	N/A	
O'Sullivan et al. (2016) [29]	5	3.5	5	3	16.5	High	N	
Child								
Cason (2001) [19]	4	3.5	3	1	11.5	Medium	Y	9.5
Schwartz et al. (2015) [32]	1	4.5	1	1	7.5	Low	Y	
Childcare Services								
Seward et al. (2018) [20]	4	3	1	1	9	Low	N	9

[1] Frequency of contact with intervention was estimated by review authors; points of contact were divided by the overall duration of the intervention to determine an average frequency of contact. [2] Overall intensity rating score breakdown: low intensity (≤10.5); medium intensity (10.51 to 13.49); high intensity (≥13.5). [3] Intervention effectiveness is defined as a statistically significant increase ($p < 0.05$) in a dairy and/or calcium-related outcome. [4] Intensity ranking scale: *Duration*: 1 = ≤6 weeks; 2 = 6 to 11 weeks; 3 = 12 weeks to 5 months; 4 = 6 to 12 months; 5 = ≥12 months; *Frequency*: 1 = annually; 2 = bimonthly to quarterly; 3 = monthly; 3.5 = twice a month; 4 = weekly; 4.5 = multiple times per week; 5 = daily; *Personalization*: 1 = environmental; 2 = group (parent or child); 2.5 = group (parent and child); 3.5 = environmental + group (parent and child); 4 = group with an individual component (parent and child); 4.5 = group with an individual component (parent and child); 5 = individual (parent and/or child) or individual + environmental + group (parent and/or child); *Reach*: 1 = one setting; 3 = two settings; 5 = three or more settings.

When evaluating the individual intensity rating categories, no relationships appear to exist between duration, frequency of contact or level of personalization, and intervention effectiveness (Table 2). Only one intervention had a duration of 6 to 11 weeks and demonstrated effectiveness. Additionally, the two interventions [28,32] involving contact with participants multiple times per week were effective. None of the levels of personalization were consistently linked with effectiveness, as all were used in both effective and ineffective interventions. Consistent with a previously published systematic literature review [18], all of the studies in which the intervention was conducted and applied in only one setting/environment were effective. Of the six studies using a reach of one setting, five (83.3%) demonstrated significant increases in dairy and/or calcium consumption.

To further assess intervention intensity, the interventions were divided into four groups based on the target population(s): parent and child; parent; child; or childcare services (Table 3). Child-focused interventions had a group score of 9.5 (*n* = 2), indicating a low overall intervention intensity score; however, the interventions in both studies resulted in statistically significant increases in dairy consumption. Interventions that targeted both parent and child had the highest overall group intensity score of 13.5, although only one (14.3%) of the seven interventions resulted in significantly increased calcium consumption. Overall, there was heterogeneity in terms of effectiveness across different categories of intensity and with overall intensity.

3.3. Behavior Change Techniques

The interventions employed a variety of behavior change techniques (BCT). Table 4 outlines the frequency of BCT associated with intervention effectiveness. Salehi et al. (2004) [31] was not included in the BCT analysis, as information about intervention effectiveness was not provided.

Table 4. Behavior change techniques associated with intervention effectiveness.

Behavior Change Technique [1]	Effective (N = 5)	Ineffective (N = 8)	Total (N = 13) [2]	% Effective [3]
1. Provide information on consequences of behavior in general	3	5	8	37.5
2. Provide information on consequences of behavior to the individual	3	6	9	33.3
4. Provide normative information about others' behavior	1	0	1	100.0
5. Goal setting (behavior)	4	8	12	33.3
7. Action planning	5	8	13	38.5
8. Problem solving/barrier identification	2	3	5	40.0
9. Set graded tasks	0	1	1	0.0
10. Review of behavioral goals	1	4	5	20.0
13. Rewards contingent on successful behaviors	2	2	4	50.0
15. Generalization of target behavior	4	7	11	36.4
16. Self-monitoring of behavior	1	3	4	25.0
19. Provide feedback on performance	1	6	7	14.3
20. Provide information on when and where to perform the behavior	4	8	12	33.3
21. Provide instruction on how to perform the behavior	4	8	12	33.3
22. Model/demonstrate the behavior	3	7	10	30.0
23. Teach to use prompts/cues	4	3	7	57.1

Table 4. *Cont.*

Behavior Change Technique [1]	Effective (*N* = 5)	Ineffective (*N* = 8)	Total (*N* = 13) [2]	% Effective [3]
24. Environmental restructuring	5	3	8	62.5
25. Agree on behavioral contract	0	1	1	0.0
26. Prompt practice	4	8	12	33.3
27. Use of follow-up prompts	0	2	2	0.0
28. Facilitate social comparison	0	2	2	0.0
29. Plan social support/social change	2	8	10	20.0
30. Identification as a role model	2	7	9	22.2
35. Relapse prevention/coping planning	0	1	1	0.0
36. Stress management/emotional control training	0	1	1	0.0
38. Time management	0	1	1	0.0
39. General communication skills training	1	2	3	33.3

[1] Behavior change technique numbers three, six, 11, 12, 14, 17, 18, 31, 32, 33, 34, 37, and 40 were removed from the chart and analysis as no studies employed these techniques. [2] Salehi et al. (2004) was excluded from the chart and analysis, as the authors did not provide the effectiveness of the intervention. [3] Intervention effectiveness is defined as a statistically significant increase ($p < 0.05$) in a dairy or calcium outcome.

The most commonly used BCT, which was used in all 13 interventions, was action planning. Other commonly used BCTs were goal setting (behavior) (*n* = 12), providing information on when and where to perform the behavior (*n* = 12), providing instruction on how to perform the behavior (*n* = 12), and prompting practice (*n* = 12). There was one BCT that was used exclusively in the effective intervention by Marquis et al. (2014) [27], which was providing normative information about others' behavior (i.e., providing information about others' behaviors and whether they are common or uncommon in the population). Action planning and environmental restructuring were similarly used in all five effective studies, although both were also used in several ineffective studies. Action planning demonstrated 38.5% efficacy, and environmental restructuring demonstrated 62.5% efficacy. Goal setting (behavior) [19,24,27,28], generalization of the target behavior [19,24,27,28], providing information on when and where to perform the behavior [19,24,27,28], providing instruction on how to perform the behavior [19,24,27,28], teaching how to use prompts/cues [19,24,28,32], and prompt practice [19,24,27,28] were techniques used in four of the five effective interventions. Goal setting (behavior) demonstrated 33.3% efficacy, the generalization of target behavior demonstrated 36.4% efficacy, providing information on when and where to perform the behavior demonstrated 33.3% efficacy, providing instruction on how to perform the behavior had 33.3% efficacy, teaching to use prompts/cues demonstrated 57.1% efficacy, and prompting practice had 33.3% efficacy. The results demonstrate that intervention effectiveness is independent of BCT.

3.4. WIDER

Table 5 provides a summary of WIDER recommendations for each intervention study. Only seven of the 14 studies provided adequate descriptions of their intervention. Similarly, 57% of the studies adequately classified their change processes and design principles. Only three (21%) interventions provided access to intervention protocols, which made it difficult to further evaluate the risk of reporting bias. Four studies (29%) did not have a control group, which classified them under unclear risk of bias for random sequence generation and high risk of bias for allocation concealment. Of the 10 studies that had a control group, only three (30%) had an active control, with two of them providing adequate descriptions of the control.

Table 5. Summary of the Workgroup for Intervention Development and Evaluation Research (WIDER) recommendations.

Study (n = 14)	Description of Intervention	Classification of Change Process and Design Principles	Access to Intervention Manuals and/or Protocols	Description of Active Control Conditions
Akil (2013) [22]	N	N	N	N
Bender et al. (2013) [23]	Y	Y	N	No Control Group
Cason (2001) [19]	N	Y	N	No Control Group
Harvey (2008) [24]	N	N	N	No Control Group
Kopetsky (2017) [25]	Y	Y	N	Y
Korwanich et al. (2008) [26]	N	N	N	No Active Control
Marquis et al. (2014) [27]	Y	N	Y	No Active Control
Munday et al. (2017) [28]	Y	N	N	No Control Group
O'Sullivan et al. (2016) [29]	Y	Y	Y	No Active Control
Roberts-Gray et al. (2016) [30]	Y	Y	N	No Active Control
Salehi et al. (2004) [31]	N	Y	N	No Active Control
Schwartz et al. (2015) [32]	N	N	N	No Active Control
Seward et al. (2018) [20]	Y	Y	Y	Y
Vereecken et al. (2009) [33]	N	Y	N	No Active Control

3.5. Risk of Bias

All 14 intervention studies [19,20,22–33] included in the review were assessed for risk of bias. Figure 2 provides a summary of the authors' (VS, IJ) judgments regarding each risk of bias item for the included intervention studies. The study with the lowest overall risk of bias was O'Sullivan et al. (2016) [29], and the study with the highest overall risk of bias was Munday et al. (2017) [28]. Three studies, two of which were dissertations, had all categories classified as either high or unclear risk of bias [22–24]. Overall, most of the studies had a high or unclear risk of bias in a majority of the categories.

Figure 3 presents the percentages of each risk of bias item across the 14 intervention studies. There was a high percentage (71%) of studies with an unclear risk of bias for random sequence generation. Additionally, six studies inadequately described allocation concealment. All of the studies either had a high or unclear risk of bias in the blinding of participants and personnel. Similarly, only two studies had a low risk of bias in the blinding of outcome assessment. Compared to other categories, there was a high percentage (36%) of studies that had a low risk of bias in incomplete outcome data. For the selective reporting domain, 11 studies had an unclear risk of bias, as they failed to provide protocols, and thus reviewers were unable to make clear judgments about bias risk. Half of the studies (n = 7) had a high risk of other bias due to self-reporting, convenience sampling, crossover bias, and underreporting. A high risk of bias was reported in 50% of the studies across the categories 'other bias' and 'attrition bias', resulting in these two categories having the highest percentage of a high risk of bias. Similarly, the highest percentage (50%) of a low risk of bias was observed in the 'other bias' category. Overall, in four of the seven domains, the percentage of studies with an unclear risk of bias was 50% or greater.

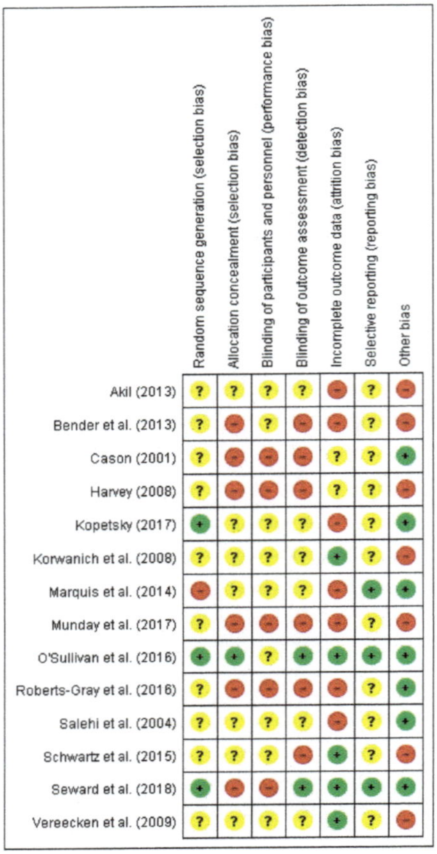

Figure 2. Risk of bias summary: review authors' judgments about each risk of bias item for each included intervention study. Red, yellow, and green circles represent high, unclear, and low risk of bias, respectively.

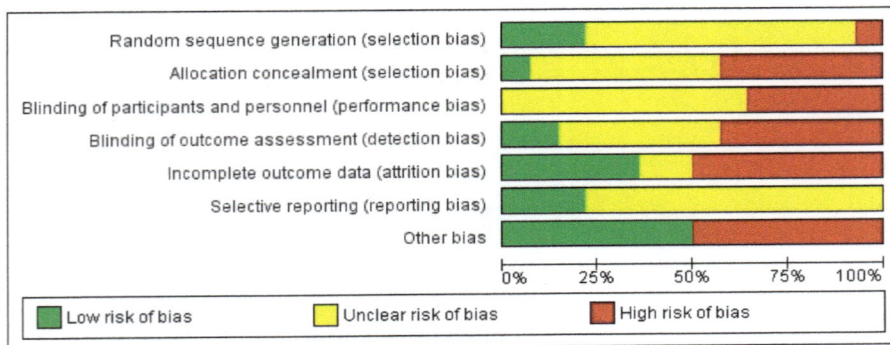

Figure 3. Risk of bias graph: review authors' judgments about each risk of bias item, which are presented as percentages across all of the included intervention studies (*n* = 14).

3.6. GRADE

Thirteen studies were included in the GRADE analysis. One study could not be included, as it was the only intervention assessing calcium intake as an outcome [28]. Table 6 provides a summary of GRADE results for the studies (*n* = 7) that had total dairy intake as an outcome. The overall quality of evidence across these studies was very low, as it received an overall score of zero. Table 7 provides a summary of GRADE results for the studies (*n* = 6) that had total milk intake as an outcome. Similar to total dairy intake, the overall quality of evidence across these studies was also very low, receiving an overall score of one.

Table 6. Summary of Grades of Recommendation, Assessment, Development and Evaluation (GRADE) results for total dairy intake outcome (*n* = 7). Intervention studies evaluated: Akil 2013 [22]; Cason 2001 [19]; Harvey 2008 [24]; Kopetsky 2017 [25]; O'Sullivan et al., 2016 [29]; Roberts-Gray et al., 2016 [30]; and Seward et al., 2018 [20].

GRADE Criteria	Rating	Support for Judgment	Overall Quality of Evidence
Type of Evidence	+4	All of the studies included were intervention studies.	High
Quality Points	−3	Multiple studies had <200 participants. The majority of studies had a high or unclear risk of bias for the blinding and allocation process, as well as attrition.	Low
Consistency	0	Most of the studies reported the ineffectiveness (*n* = 5) versus effectiveness (*n* = 2) of dairy intervention. Dairy outcomes assessed are relatively similar, as the majority of studies reported some variation of the number of servings of dairy consumed.	Moderate
Directness	−1	Generalizability of population was a limitation in several studies.	Moderate
Effect Size	0	*n* = 3 studies did not provide enough information to allow for the calculation of effect size. All of the other studies (*n* = 4) allowed for the calculation of effect size; not all of the effect sizes were >2 or <0.5 and significant.	Low
Overall Score: 0			**Overall Quality of Evidence: Very Low**

Table 7. Summary of GRADE results for total milk intake outcome (*n* = 6). Intervention studies evaluated: Bender et al., 2013 [23]; Korwanich et al., 2008 [26]; Marquis et al., 2014 [27]; Salehi et al., 2004 [31]; Schwartz et al., 2015 [32]; and Vereecken et al., 2009 [33].

GRADE Criteria	Rating	Support for Judgment	Overall Quality of Evidence
Type of Evidence	+4	All of the studies included were intervention studies.	High
Quality Points	−1	All of the studies had a high or unclear risk of bias for blinding and allocation. Three studies had a low risk of attrition bias, with the other three studies having either a high or unclear risk of attrition bias. Generally, sparse data does not appear to be of concern, as the majority of studies had >200 participants.	Moderate
Consistency	−1	Most studies reported ineffectiveness (*n* = 3) versus effectiveness (*n* = 2) of dairy intervention, with one study not reporting effectiveness. Variability in reporting of milk outcomes; studies reported volumes of milk consumed, times consumed per day, or quantity of milk consumed in grams.	Low

Table 7. Cont.

GRADE Criteria	Rating	Support for Judgment	Overall Quality of Evidence
Directness	−1	Generalizability of population was a limitation in multiple studies.	Moderate
Effect Size	0	*n* = 3 studies did not provide enough information to allow for the calculation of effect size. All of the other studies (*n* = 3) allowed for the calculation of effect size; not all of the effect sizes were >2 or <0.5 and significant.	Low
Overall Score: 1			**Overall Quality of Evidence:** Very Low

The type of evidence across both outcomes received a score of +4, as all of the studies that were included in the review were intervention studies. Total dairy intake received the lowest score (−3) for quality points, as a majority of the studies had <200 participants and had a relatively high risk of bias. Conversely, total milk intake had the lowest score (−1) for consistency, as there was variability in the reporting of milk outcomes. Both outcomes received the same scores for directness (−1) and effect size (0). Overall, these results demonstrate heterogeneity between intervention studies.

4. Discussion

The objective of this review was to identify the characteristics of effective interventions aimed at increasing dairy and/or calcium consumption in preschool-aged children. Intervention reporting was evaluated using intervention intensity analysis, behavior change technique taxonomy, and WIDER, with risk of bias and GRADE used to assess the quality of the intervention studies. Only five (35.7%) interventions included in the review reported significant increases in dairy and/or calcium consumption post-intervention, which was lower than the ~70% reported in previously published reviews in other populations [17,18]. Characteristics associated with effectiveness included those interventions delivered in one setting (i.e., preschools, early education centers and/or daycares) versus those delivered in multiple settings, those that included the selected behavior change techniques of environmental restructuring and teach to use prompts/cues, and those that targeted both the parent and child.

The most notable finding was the lack of effectiveness reported by intervention studies aiming to increase dairy and/or calcium intakes in preschool-aged children. The ineffectiveness of most interventions may be attributed to the lack of focus on dairy or calcium intake as the targeted message. All of the interventions in the final analysis included dairy and/or calcium intakes as part of a larger dietary intervention designed to encourage healthy eating and positive dietary habits in preschool-aged children. Hendrie et al. (2012) [17] concluded that interventions specifically targeting dairy or calcium intake independent of other dietary changes were more likely to be effective than those considering dairy/calcium intake in the context of a broader message, such as general healthy eating. These findings suggest that mixed dietary interventions may dilute the impact or preclude adequate communication and/or the adaption of more targeted health and dietary messages. A possible explanation could be that less time and/or effort are allocated to dairy-specific messaging when presented as part of a mixed dietary intervention. Resource availability may also be limited when engaging in broader dietary interventions, directly impacting dairy or calcium messaging and the extent of education and communication about dairy and calcium consumption. The effectiveness of increasing dairy and calcium consumption as part of a larger dietary intervention may be influenced by the behavior change techniques implemented. For example, behavior change techniques that are effective at increasing fruit and vegetable consumption may not be similarly effective at increasing dairy and calcium intake, and therefore may impact the communication of dairy and calcium health messages.

The ineffectiveness of dairy interventions may also be attributed to the heterogeneity of the interventions. The heterogeneity observed between populations may have introduced variability in the communication of dietary messages on the basis of cultural and/or societal norms. For example, Salehi et al. (2004) [31] conducted their interventions on Qashqa'i tribe families in Iran, while Marquis et al. (2014) [27] studied a cohort of rural Ghanaian children. Salehi et al. (2004) [31] aimed to change/improve the customs and cultural practices of the Qashqa'i tribe families through educational program topics such as sanitary waste disposal, water supply, and general dietary consumption guidelines. In contrast, Marquis et al. (2014) [27] focused on improving entrepreneurial training and nutrition education to increase household access to animal food products in rural Ghana. These examples highlight the differences in the availability of resources and/or food sources between cultures, and how this could impact the extent of the dietary health and messaging provided. Secondly, heterogeneity was also observed across participants, with variability in the targets of the interventions (i.e., parent and child, parent, child, or childcare services). The variability observed across intervention targets may significantly influence dietary messaging given that interventions targeting preschool children focus more on simply increasing dairy consumption, whereas those targeting adults are more likely to emphasize the importance or relevance of doing so. Thirdly, heterogeneity existed between the approaches used to communicate dietary messaging, including mass communication, targeted communication, or tailored communication [41]. Mass communication is more generic and most likely used in environmental or group interventions, as this type of communication enables general messages to be delivered to many individuals; in contrast, tailored communication is used when the health messages are specifically designed to individual need. The ineffectiveness and heterogeneity observed across interventions make it difficult to draw reliable conclusions, highlighting the need for future intervention designs to specifically and solely target dairy and/or calcium intake in preschoolers.

The characteristics of effective interventions were determined using intervention intensity analysis. No associations were observed between intervention intensity group scores and intervention effectiveness. Moreover, interventions targeting the parent and child demonstrated the highest intervention intensity scores, but only one of the seven studies demonstrated effectiveness. Both interventions targeting the child alone, by comparison, exhibited low intervention intensity scores, but were effective at increasing dairy intakes. These observations suggest that targeting the child alone may enhance the effectiveness of interventions; although, based on the young age of the preschool children, it is unreasonable to assume that these children would be able to change their intakes without the guidance from their parents and/or caregivers. Targeting both the parent and child may demonstrate higher efficacy in increasing dairy and/or calcium intakes in preschool children, as evidence suggests that parents play an important role in developing preschoolers' eating habits through a variety of mechanisms, including modeling of dietary behaviors [42,43], parental feeding behaviors [44,45], and the availability/accessibility of food products in the home environment [46,47]. Recent evidence from the Guelph Family Health Study, Canada, extended these findings: both mothers' and fathers' involvement of children in meal preparation was associated with lower child nutrition risk (mother beta = -3.45, $p = 0.02$; father beta = -1.74, $p = 0.01$) and healthy home environment scores (mother beta = -8.36, $p < 0.001$; father beta = -2.69, $p = 0.04$) [43]. These results demonstrate the strong parental influence on preschoolers' dietary intakes, supporting the need to target parents as well as children in interventions aiming to increase dairy and/or calcium intakes. Furthermore, when considered as independent categories, no associations were evident between intervention duration, frequency of contact or level of personalization, and overall intervention effectiveness. In contrast, intervention setting did appear to be associated with overall effectiveness, as it was observed that the majority of effective interventions used a reach of only one setting. This is consistent with Marquez et al. (2015) [18], who also reported an 81.8% intervention effectiveness using a reach of one setting, suggesting that a targeted and focused intervention delivered in a single setting may be preferable to interventions delivered across multiple settings. Based on the results of this study, interventions targeting dairy and/or calcium intake should focus on delivery in preschools, early education centers, and/or daycares. Nonetheless, despite the inclusion of 14 interventions in this analysis, the validity of our conclusions regarding the relationship between intervention intensity and effectiveness is limited by the small number of studies in any given category.

Analysis of behavior change techniques was used to investigate the relationship between the use of specific techniques and intervention effectiveness. Overall, the main finding from this analysis indicates some associations between the use of specific behavior techniques and intervention effectiveness. Specifically, environmental restructuring and teaching to use prompts/cues appear to be associated with overall intervention effectiveness. These two techniques are also related, because environmental restructuring prompts the participant to alter their environment to support the target behavior (i.e., put up posters/images) and teaching to use prompt/cues teaches the individual to identify environmental cues to prompt the target behavior. Given that these behavior change techniques are strongly associated with intervention effectiveness, altering the environment to support and encourage dairy/calcium consumption may be effective in the preschool population. As further support, Marquez et al. (2015) [18] reported 66.7% intervention effectiveness with the use of environmental restructuring, which is a result that is comparable to our review. Furthermore, no significant relationships were observed between the target population (i.e., parent and child, parent alone, child alone, or childcare services), the effectiveness of the intervention, and the use of behavior change techniques. These results are consistent with those of Marquez et al. (2015) [18], who concluded that parental involvement and support was not a significant predictor of intervention effectiveness. These findings are in contrast to those published by Hendrie et al. (2012) [17], who reported that effective studies implementing behavior change techniques specifically targeted the parents and/or family, while ineffective studies targeted only the child. Overall, intervention effectiveness appears to be independent of the majority of behavior change techniques, although environmental restructuring and teaching to use prompts/cues may encourage positive behavioral change in the preschool population.

Two assessment tools, risk of bias and GRADE, were used to evaluate the overall quality of the intervention studies included in the analysis. The majority of interventions demonstrated a high or unclear risk of bias in most or all of the risk of bias categories, with the quality appraisal of total dairy and total milk intake outcomes being very low based on the GRADE criteria. This demonstrates an overall lack of reliability and validity of intervention results and conclusions, suggesting a need to further develop standards and consistency in intervention design and the reporting of outcomes related to dairy/calcium intakes. Improving the reporting of outcomes will (i) enable the identification of the outcomes that are most meaningful and relevant in the preschool population, (ii) enable the development of a consensus in this field of research regarding definitions and measures of dairy/calcium outcomes (i.e., servings per day versus amount consumed), and (iii) identify those outcomes that are most likely to promote increases in the effectiveness of dairy/calcium interventions [48]. Finally, consistency in the reporting of outcomes and clarity in intervention design would enable a comparison of study designs, sample sizes, and target populations for the purpose of determining the factors promoting the effectiveness of dairy/calcium consumption in the preschool population. Improving clarity and transparency in outcome reporting and intervention design will in turn increase the reliability and the validity of conclusions about dairy/calcium intakes in preschoolers, and inform initiatives targeting positive health behaviors.

The results of the review should be interpreted considering the limitations. One limitation was a lack of disclosure in the methodology across interventions. This made it difficult to compare the different categories of intervention intensity and determine which behavior change techniques were implemented in interventions. Studies were restricted to those published in English, which may have limited the interventions selected for final analysis. As the primary focus of this review was on interventions aiming to increase dairy and/or calcium consumption, studies that were considered ineffective in this review may have demonstrated effectiveness in changing other dietary and/or physical activity targets in the intervention. Moreover, intervention effectiveness must also be considered in context of study design, as interventions specifically designed to increase dairy and/or calcium consumption may demonstrate increased effectiveness when compared to mixed interventions. Many studies did not report the actual quantities of participants' dairy/calcium intakes, making it difficult to report the degree of intervention efficacy. Lastly, gender bias may also be considered as a limitation, given that some studies included only one parent in the intervention, which was typically the mother. Despite these limitations, the use of several tools to both quantitatively and qualitatively review the included interventions provides a comprehensive critique of this body of literature and yields valuable insight into the characteristics of studies in this research domain.

5. Conclusions

Dietary interventions aiming to increase dairy and/or calcium consumption in preschool-aged children demonstrate variable success. The evidence presented in this review has identified characteristics that may enable the intervention effectiveness of increasing dairy and/or calcium intakes in preschoolers. This includes the delivery of interventions in one setting versus multiple settings, using specific behavior change techniques (such as environmental restructuring and teaching to use prompts/cues), and targeting both the parent and child. Future studies should modify interventions to exclusively target dairy and/or calcium intakes, reduce heterogeneity and/or bias, and improve transparency in the reporting of interventions. Further investigating the relationship and effect of target populations, specifically both parent and child, is another consideration, as it may be necessary and important to work with the parents and/or caregivers of these preschool children to ensure sustainable changes in dairy and/or calcium intakes. A potential avenue for future research includes exploring the use and effectiveness of booster periods for sustaining positive behavioral change over time in the preschool population. In the meantime, public health initiatives should aim to improve the dairy and calcium intake of preschool-aged children for the purpose of instilling healthy dietary habits at a young age, and mitigate the health consequences associated with insufficient intakes. Overall, the findings of this review demonstrate the need for developing effective interventions designed to increase dairy and/or calcium intakes in preschool-aged children.

Supplementary Materials: The following are available at http://www.mdpi.com/2072-6643/11/4/714/s1, Search Method and Inclusion/Exclusion Criteria; Table S1: Description of the 40 behavior change techniques used in the CALO-RE Taxonomy for assessment of interventions; Table S2: Description of the four criteria of the WIDER recommendations; Table S3: Description of the Risk of Bias assessment tool; Table S4: The GRADE scoring system used to evaluate the quality of scientific evidence.

Author Contributions: V.S.: literature searching, screening of articles, data extraction and analysis, manuscript writing, and editing; I.J.: literature searching, screening of articles, data extraction and analysis, writing of results, and manuscript editing; A.C.B.: study design, manuscript editing, supervised overall work; G.N.: study inception and design, manuscript editing, supervised overall work. All of the authors read and approved the final manuscript.

Funding: This research received no source of funding.

Acknowledgments: We thank Jess Haines and David W.L. Ma for providing feedback and comments that improved the manuscript.

Conflicts of Interest: The authors declare no conflicts of interest.

References

1. Canadian Dairy Commission. Available online: http://www.cdc-ccl.gc.ca/CDC/index-eng.php?id=3805 (accessed on 2 November 2018).
2. National Health and Medical Research Council. *Australian Dietary Guidelines*; National Health and Medical Research Council: Canberra, Australia, 2013.
3. Garriguet, D. Nutrition: Findings from the Canadian Community Health Survey. Overview of Canadians' Eating Habits. Available online: www.statcan.gc.ca/pub/82-620-m/82-620-m2006002-eng.pdf (accessed on 2 November 2018).
4. Nielsen, S.J.; Popkin, B.M. Changes in beverage intake between 1977 and 2001. *Am. J. Prev. Med.* **2004**, *27*, 205–210. [CrossRef] [PubMed]

5. Dror, D.K.; Allen, L.H. Dairy product intake in children and adolescents in developed countries: Trends, nutritional contribution, and a review of association with health outcomes. *Nutr. Rev.* **2014**, *72*, 68–81. [CrossRef]

6. Rizzoli, R. Dairy products, yogurts, and bone health. *Am. J. Clin. Nutr.* **2014**, *99*, 1256S–1262S. [CrossRef]

7. Tremblay, A.; Gilbert, J.A. Human obesity: Is insufficient calcium/dairy intake part of the problem? *J. Am. Coll. Nutr.* **2011**, *30*, 449S–453S. [CrossRef] [PubMed]

8. Wang, H.; Troy, L.M.; Rogers, G.T.; Fox, C.S.; McKeown, N.M.; Meigs, J.B.; Jacques, P.F. Longitudinal association between dairy consumption and changes of body weight and waist circumference: The Framingham Heart Study. *Int. J. Obes.* **2014**, *38*, 299–305. [CrossRef] [PubMed]

9. Nicklas, T.A.; Qu, H.; Hughes, S.O.; He, M.; Wagner, S.E.; Foushee, H.R.; Shewchuk, R.M. Self-perceived lactose intolerance results in lower intakes of calcium and dairy foods and is associated with hypertension and diabetes in adults. *Am. J. Clin. Nutr.* **2011**, *94*, 191–198. [CrossRef]

10. O'Connor, L.M.; Lentjes, M.A.; Luben, R.N.; Khaw, K.T.; Wareham, N.J.; Forouhi, N.G. Dietary dairy product intake and incident type 2 diabetes: A prospective study using dietary data from a 7-day food diary. *Diabetologia* **2014**, *57*, 909–917. [CrossRef] [PubMed]

11. Larsson, S.C.; Bergkvist, L.; Rutegård, J.; Giovannucci, E.; Wolk, A. Calcium and dairy food intakes are inversely associated with colorectal cancer risk in the cohort of Swedish men. *Am. J. Clin. Nutr.* **2006**, *83*, 667–673. [CrossRef] [PubMed]

12. Davis, K.; Christoffel, K.K. Obesity in preschool and school-age children: Treatment early and often may be best. *Arch. Pediatr. Adolesc. Med.* **1994**, *148*, 1257–1261. [CrossRef]

13. Skinner, J.D.; Carruth, B.R.; Bounds, W.; Ziegler, P.; Reidy, K. Do food-related experiences in the first 2 years of life predict dietary variety in school-aged children? *J. Nutr. Educ. Behav.* **2002**, *34*, 310–315. [CrossRef]

14. Marshall, T.A.; Eichenberger Gilmore, J.M.; Broffitt, B.; Stumbo, P.J.; Levy, S.M. Diet quality in young children is influenced by beverage consumption. *J. Am. Coll. Nutr.* **2005**, *24*, 65–75. [CrossRef] [PubMed]

15. Dubois, L.; Farmer, A.; Girard, M.; Peterson, K. Regular sugar-sweetened beverage consumption between meals increases risk of overweight among preschool-aged children. *J. Am. Diet. Assoc.* **2007**, *107*, 924–934. [CrossRef]

16. Yen, S.T.; Lin, B.H. Beverage consumption among US children and adolescents: Full-information and quasi maximum-likelihood estimation of a censored system. *Eur. Rev. Agric. Econ.* **2002**, *29*, 85–103. [CrossRef]

17. Hendrie, G.A.; Brindal, E.; Baird, D.; Gardner, C. Improving children's dairy food and calcium intake: Can intervention work? A systematic review of the literature. *Public Health Nutr.* **2012**, *16*, 365–376. [CrossRef] [PubMed]

18. Marquez, O.; Racey, M.; Preyde, M.; Hendrie, G.A.; Newton, G. Interventions to increase dairy consumption in adolescents: A systematic review. *Infant Child Adolesc. Nutr.* **2015**, *7*, 242–254. [CrossRef]

19. Cason, K.L. Evaluation of a preschool nutrition education program based on the theory of multiple intelligences. *J. Nutr. Educ.* **2001**, *33*, 161–164. [CrossRef]

20. Seward, K.; Wolfenden, L.; Finch, M.; Wiggers, J.; Wyse, R.; Jones, J.; Yoong, S.L. Improving the implementation of nutrition guidelines in childcare centres improves child dietary intake: Findings of a randomised trial of an implementation intervention. *Public Health Nutr.* **2018**, *21*, 607–617. [CrossRef]

21. Moher, D.; Liberati, A.; Tetzlaff, J.; Altman, D.G.; Altman, D.; Antes, G.; Tugwell, P. Preferred reporting items for systematic reviews and meta-analyses: The PRISMA statement. *PLoS Med.* **2009**, *6*. [CrossRef] [PubMed]

22. Akil, N. Evaluation of Effectiveness of Classroom-Based Nutrition Intervention on Changes in Eating Behavior in African American Parents/Caregivers and Their Children. Master's Thesis, Wayne State University, Detroit, MI, USA, 2013. Available online: https://digitalcommons.wayne.edu/oa_theses/224 (accessed on 25 June 2018).

23. Bender, M.S.; Nader, P.R.; Kennedy, C.; Gahagan, S. A culturally appropriate intervention to improve health behaviours in Hispanic mother-child dyads. *Child. Obes.* **2013**, *9*, 157–163. [CrossRef]

24. Harvey, S.P. The Results of a Home-Based Physical Activity and Nutrition Program of Preschool Children and Parent Perceptions of Barriers. Ph.D. Thesis, University of Kansas, Lawrence, KS, USA, 2008.

25. Kopetsky, A. A Healthy Snacking Intervention in Preschool-Aged Children. Master's Thesis, University of Delaware, Newark, DE, USA, 2017.

26. Korwanich, K.; Sheiham, A.; Srisuphan, W.; Srisilapanan, P. Promoting healthy eating in nursery schoolchildren: A quasi-experimental intervention study. *Health Educ. J.* **2008**, *67*, 16–30. [CrossRef]

27. Marquis, G.S.; Colecraft, E.K. Community interventions for dietary improvement in Ghana. *Food Nutr. Bull.* **2014**, *35*, S193–S197. [CrossRef] [PubMed]

28. Munday, K.; Wilson, M. Implementing a health and wellbeing programme for children in early childhood: A preliminary study. *Nutrients* **2017**, *9*, 1031. [CrossRef]

29. O'Sullivan, A.; Fitzpatrick, N.; Doyle, O. Effects of early intervention on dietary intake and its mediating role on cognitive functioning: A randomised controlled trial. *Public Health Nutr.* **2016**, *20*, 154–164. [CrossRef] [PubMed]

30. Roberts-Gray, C.; Briley, M.E.; Ranjit, N.; Byrd-Williams, C.E.; Sweitzer, S.J.; Sharma, S.V.; Palafox, M.R.; Hoelscher, D.M. Efficacy of the Lunch is in the Bag intervention to increase parents' packing of healthy bag lunches for young children: A cluster-randomized trial in early care and education centers. *Int. J. Behav. Nutr. Phys. Act.* **2016**, *13*, 1–19. [CrossRef] [PubMed]

31. Salehi, M.; Kimiagar, S.M.; Shahbazi, M.; Mehrabi, Y.; Kolahi, A.A. Assessing the impact of nutrition education on growth indices of Iranian nomadic children: An application of a modified beliefs, attitudes, subjective-norms and enabling-factors model. *Br. J. Nutr.* **2004**, *91*, 779–787. [CrossRef]

32. Schwartz, M.B.; O'Connell, M.; Henderson, K.E.; Middleton, A.E.; Scarmo, S. Testing variations on family-style feeding to increase whole fruit and vegetable consumption among preschoolers in child care. *Child. Obes.* **2015**, *11*, 499–505. [CrossRef]

33. Vereecken, C.; Huybrechts, I.; van Houte, H.; Martens, V.; Wittebroodt, I.; Maes, L. Results from a dietary intervention study in preschools "Beastly Healthy at School". *Int. J. Public Health* **2009**, *54*, 142–149. [CrossRef]

34. Racey, M.; O'Brien, C.; Douglas, S.; Marquez, O.; Hendrie, G.; Newton, G. Systematic Review of School-Based Interventions to Modify Dietary Behavior: Does Intervention Intensity Impact Effectiveness? *J. Sch. Health* **2016**, *86*, 452–463. [CrossRef] [PubMed]

35. Michie, S.; Ashford, S.; Sniehotta, F.F.; Dombrowski, S.U.; Bishop, A.; French, D.P. A refined taxonomy of behaviour change techniques to help people change their physical activity and healthy eating behaviours: The CALO-RE taxonomy. *Psychol. Health* **2011**, *26*, 1479–1498. [CrossRef]

36. Abraham, C.; Michie, S. A Taxonomy of Behavior Change Techniques Used in Interventions. *Health Psychol.* **2008**, *27*, 379–387. [CrossRef] [PubMed]

37. Albrecht, L.; Archibald, M.; Arseneau, D.; Scott, S.D. Development of a checklist to assess the quality of reporting of knowledge translation interventions using the Workgroup for Intervention Development and Evaluation Research (WIDER) recommendations. *Implement. Sci.* **2013**, *8*, 1–5. [CrossRef] [PubMed]

38. Scott, S.; Albrecht, L.; O'Leary, K.; Ball, G.; Hartling, L.; Hofmeyer, A.; Dryden, D. Systematic review of knowledge translation strategies in the allied health professions. *Implement. Sci.* **2012**, *7*, 70. [CrossRef] [PubMed]

39. Cochrane Handbook for Systematic Reviews of Interventions. Available online: http://handbook-5-1. cochrane.org/ (accessed on 15 January 2018).

40. What Is GRADE? Available online: http://clincialevidence.bmj.com/x/set/static/ebm/learn/665072.html (accessed on 15 January 2018).

41. Hawkins, R.P.; Kreuter, M.; Resnicow, K.; Fishbein, M.; Dijkstra, A. Understanding tailoring in communicating about health. *Health Educ. Res.* **2008**, *23*, 454–466. [CrossRef] [PubMed]

42. Grimm, G.C.; Harnack, L.; Story, M. Factors associated with soft drink consumption in school-aged children. *J. Am. Diet. Assoc.* **2004**, *104*, 1244–1249. [CrossRef]

43. Watterworth, J.; Mackay, J.M.; Buchholz, A.C.; Darlington, G.; Randall Simpson, J.; Ma, D.W.L.; Haines, J.; Guelph Family Health Study. Food parenting practices and their associations with child nutrition risk status: Comparing mothers and fathers. *Appl. Physiol. Nutr. Metab.* **2017**, *42*, 667–671. [CrossRef]

44. Birch, L.L.; Fisher, J.O. Development of eating behaviours among children and adolescents. *Pediatrics* **1998**, *101*, 539–549.

45. Faith, M.S.; Scanlon, K.S.; Birch, L.L.; Francis, L.A.; Sherry, B. Parent-child feeding strategies and their relationships to child eating and weight status. *Obes. Res.* **2004**, *12*, 1711–1722. [CrossRef]

46. Hanson, N.I.; Neumark-Sztainer, D.; Eisenberg, M.E.; Story, M.; Wall, M. Associations between parental report of the home food environment and adolescent intakes of fruits, vegetables and dairy foods. *Public Health Nutr.* **2005**, *8*, 77–85. [CrossRef] [PubMed]

47. Kratt, P.; Reynolds, K.; Shewchuk, R. The role of availability as a moderator of family fruit and vegetable consumption. *Health Educ. Behav.* **2000**, *27*, 471–482. [CrossRef] [PubMed]
48. Tunis, S.R.; Clarke, M.; Gorst, S.L.; Gargon, E.; Blazeby, J.M.; Altman, D.G.; Williamson, P.R. Improving the relevance and consistency of outcomes in comparative effectiveness research. *J. Comp. Eff. Res.* **2016**, *5*, 193–205. [CrossRef] [PubMed]

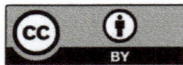

MDPI

St. Alban-Anlage 66

4052 Basel

Switzerland

Tel. +41 61 683 77 34

Fax +41 61 302 89 18

www.mdpi.com

Nutrients Editorial Office

E-mail: nutrients@mdpi.com

www.mdpi.com/journal/nutrients

www.ingramcontent.com/pod-product-compliance
Lightning Source LLC
Chambersburg PA
CBHW051710210326
41597CB00032B/5436